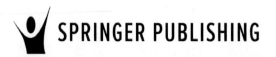 SPRINGER PUBLISHING

MW00997756

GET THE MOST FROM YOUR BOOK

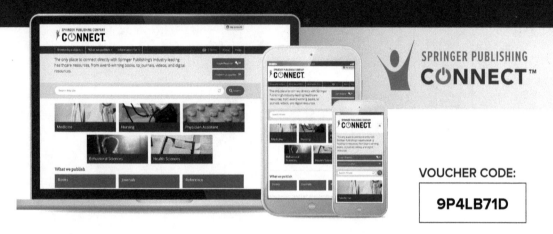

SPRINGER PUBLISHING
CONNECT™

VOUCHER CODE:

9P4LB71D

Online Access

Your print purchase of *Nurses Making Policy, Third Edition,* includes **online access via Springer Publishing Connect**™ to increase accessibility, portability, and searchability.

Insert the code at http://connect.springerpub.com/content/book/ 978-0-8261-6646-3 today!

Having trouble? Contact our customer service department at cs@springerpub.com

Instructor Resource Access for Adopters

Let us do some of the heavy lifting to create an engaging classroom experience with a variety of instructor resources included in most textbooks SUCH AS:

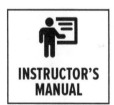

INSTRUCTOR'S MANUAL

POWERPOINTS

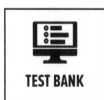

TEST BANK

Visit **https://connect.springerpub.com/** and look for the **"Show Supplementary"** button on your **book homepage** to see what is available to instructors! First time using Springer Publishing Connect?

Email **textbook@springerpub.com** to create an account and start unlocking valuable resources.

Nurses Making Policy

Rebecca M. Patton, DNP, RN, CNOR, FAAN, is the past, two-term president of the American Nurses Association (ANA; 2006–2010) and holds the inaugural Endowed Perioperative Nursing Chair, Lucy Jo Atkinson Perioperative Nursing Professor at Frances Payne Bolton School of Nursing, Case Western Reserve University. As a nurse, author, and lecturer, she has presented extensively throughout the world. Dr. Patton has testified before Congress and met with major policymakers—including Presidents Obama, Bush, and Clinton—when she lobbied on healthcare issues affecting nurses and the public. In response to concerns raised about the ethical treatment of prisoners, she was invited by President Bush to meet with the soldiers and nurses at the Guantanamo Detainee Camp in Cuba. Dr. Patton was selected twice by the U.S. State Department to serve on the U.S. delegation at the World Health Assembly in Geneva, Switzerland. Dr. Patton serves on the American Nurse Today (ANT) editorial board and has written chapters for books on medical–surgical nursing and for nursing journals. She has received numerous recognitions, including the American Nurses Association (ANA) Distinguished Membership Award and the Sigma Theta Tau International Founder Dorothy Garrigus Adams Award for Excellence in Fostering Professional Standards. She was named to the Modern Healthcare's "Top 100 Most Influential Persons in Healthcare" in 2009 and 2010. She is a fellow of the American Academy of Nursing.

Margarete L. Zalon, PhD, RN, ACNS-BC, FAAN, is a professor in the Department of Nursing and director of the Master of Science in Health Informatics program at the University of Scranton, Scranton, Pennsylvania, and a certified adult health clinical nurse specialist. She is an adjunct professor at the Marian K. Shaughnessy Leadership Academy at the Frances Payne Bolton School of Nursing, Case Western Reserve University. Dr. Zalon is the president of the Nursing Foundation of Pennsylvania. Dr. Zalon is a past board chair of the American Nurses Foundation and a former board member of the American Nurses Association. She also served as vice president, American Nurses Credentialing Center, and as president of the Pennsylvania State Nurses Association. Dr. Zalon is a fellow of the American Academy of Nursing and a member of its Acute and Critical Care Expert Panel. Her research focuses on vulnerable elders, and she has been funded by the National Institute of Nursing Research. She has authored articles in leading journals such as *Nursing Research, Applied Nursing Research*, the *Journal of Gerontological Nursing*, the *Journal of Nursing Scholarship*, the *Journal of Nursing Measurement*, the *Journal of Nursing Education*, and *Nurse Educator*. She has more than 100 professional publications and presentations at the local, state, national and international levels. Her contributions to the profession have been recognized with the Duke University School of Nursing Distinguished Alumna Award and the Pennsylvania State Nurses Association Distinguished Nurse Award.

Ruth Ludwick, PhD, RN-BC, APRN-CNS, FAAN, is professor emerita, Kent State University College of Nursing; adjunct graduate faculty at Northeast Ohio Medical University; and adjunct professor in the Marian K. Shaughnessy Nurse Leadership Academy at Case Western Reserve University. She is a research and policy consultant locally, nationally, and internationally. As a leader and an educator, Dr. Ludwick has transformed standards of nursing care of older people and the gerontological preparation of nurses. She is a fellow of the American Academy of Nursing and a member of its Aging Expert Panel. She has a sustained record of research and was recognized for this work by the Ohio Nurses Association with a Research in Nursing Excellence Award. Her numerous publications focus on challenging and significant gerontological nursing issues such as restraint reduction, health literacy, and advance care planning. Her funding includes grants from the Agency for Healthcare Research and Quality, the National Institute on Aging, the Institute of Museum and Library Services, and the National Palliative Care Research Center. She was a founding member on the editorial boards of the Online Journal of Issues in Nursing and the International Journal of Older People Nursing and continues in these editorial roles today. Her contributions to *OJIN: The Online Journal of Issues in Nursing* were instrumental in shaping dialogue about nursing issues beyond the United States and incorporating a regular column on ethics for the journal. She has authored more than 100 articles, book chapters, editorials, and compilations appearing in a variety of renowned journals, such as *Nursing Research, Advances in Nursing Science, The Gerontologist*, the *Journal of the American Geriatrics Society, Nursing Ethics*, and the *Journal of Pain and Symptom Management*. Dr. Ludwick was the first recipient of the Kent State University College of Nursing Distinguished Alumni Award. Some examples of her advocacy include serving on committees of the Ohio Nurses Association and the American Nurses Association, and on the board of the Ohio Health Literacy Partners (OHLP), a statewide collaborative dedicated to empowering Ohioans to make informed health choices through improved health literacy.

Nurses Making Policy

From Bedside to Boardroom

THIRD EDITION

Rebecca M. Patton, DNP, RN, CNOR, FAAN

Margarete L. Zalon, PhD, RN, ACNS-BC, FAAN

Ruth Ludwick, PhD, RN-BC, APRN-CNS, FAAN

Editors

Copublished With the American Nurses Association

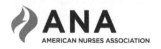

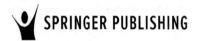

Springer Publishing Company, LLC
11 West 42nd Street, New York, NY 10036
www.springerpub.com
connect.springerpub.com/

Acquisitions Editor: Joseph Morita
Compositor: diacriTech

ISBN: 9780826166456
ebook ISBN: 9780826166463
DOI: 10.1891/9780826166463

SUPPLEMENTS:
Instructor Materials:

 Qualified instructors may request supplements by emailing
textbook@springerpub.com

Instructor's Manual: 978-0-8261-6647-0
Instructor PowerPoints: 978-0-8261-6648-7
Student PowerPoints: 978-0-8261-8856-4

22 23 24 / 5 4 3 2 1

Library of Congress Cataloging-in-Publication Data
Library of Congress Control Number: 2021921832

Contact sales@springerpub.com to receive discount rates on bulk purchases.

Publisher's Note: **New and used products purchased from third-party sellers are not guaranteed for
quality, authenticity, or access to any included digital components.**

Printed in the United States of America by Gasch Printing.

This book started with a dream to educate and inspire nurses. We dedicate this book to all nurses who dream and work to make it a reality.

Contents

Contributors

Michael Ackerman, PhD, RN, FCCM, FNAP, FAANP, FAAN   Director, Center for Healthcare Innovation and Leadership; Director Masters of Healthcare Innovation Program, Professor of Clinical Nursing, The Ohio State University College of Nursing, Columbus, Ohio

Kimberly D. Acquaviva, PhD, MSW, CSE   Betty Norman Norris Endowed Professor, The University of Virginia School of Nursing, Charlottesville, Virginia

Susan Apold, PhD, ANP-BC, AGNP, FAAN, FAANP   Dean and Professor of Nursing, College of Mount Saint Vincent, Riverdale, New York

Marianne Baernholdt, PhD, MPH, RN, FAAN   Associate Dean for Global Initiatives and Professor, Director PAHO/WHO Collaborating Center in Quality and Safety Education in Nursing and Midwifery, University of North Carolina School of Nursing, Chapel Hill, North Carolina

Taura L. Barr, PhD, RN, FAHA   Associate Professor of Clinical Practice, The Ohio State University College of Nursing, Entrepreneur in Residence, Co-Lead Center for Healthcare Innovation & Wellness, and Scientific Founder Valtari Bio Inc., CEO & Coach Deep Roots Healing LLC, Columbus, Ohio

Katherine Cardoni Brewer, PhD, RN   Assistant Professor, Towson University, Department of Nursing, Towson, Maryland

Ashley Leak Bryant PhD, RN-BC, OCN, FGSA, FAAN   Associate Professor, University of North Carolina School of Nursing, Anne Belcher Interprofessional Scholar in Nursing, Chapel Hill, North Carolina

Angela Clark, PhD, RN, CNE, FAAN   Interim Associate Dean, Executive Director of Undergraduate and Prelicensure Programs, University of Cincinnati College of Nursing, Cincinnati, Ohio

Sean P. Clarke, PhD, RN, FAAN   Executive Vice Dean and Professor, New York University Rory Meyers College of Nursing, New York, New York

Moriah Ellen, PhD, MBA   Associate Professor, Department of Health Policy and Management, Guilford Glazer Faculty of Business and Management, Faculty of Health Sciences and Chair, Israel Implementation Science and Policy Engagement Centre, Ben-Gurion University of the Negev, Be'er Sheva, Israel, and Assistant Professor, Institute of Health Policy Management and Evaluation, Dalla Lana School of Public Health, University of Toronto, Toronto, Canada

Greer Glazer, PhD, RN, CNP, FAAN Professor and Dean Emeritus, University of Cincinnati, College of Nursing, Cincinnati, Ohio

Linda K. Groah, MSN, RN, CNOR, NEA-BC, FAAN Chief Executive Officer/ Executive Director, Association of periOperative Registered Nurses, Denver, Colorado

Amy L. Hader, JD General Counsel and Director of Government Affairs, Association of periOperative Registered Nurses, Denver, Colorado

Debbie Dawson Hatmaker, PhD, RN, FAAN Enterprise Chief Program Officer, American Nurses Association, Silver Spring, Maryland

Lauren Inouye, MPP, RN Chief Program Officer, American Academy of Nursing, Washington, District of Columbia

Amy Jauch, DNP, RN, CNE Assistant Professor of Clinical Nursing, Director, Pre-Licensure Programs, The Ohio State University College of Nursing, Columbus, Ohio

Jessica Keim-Malpass, PhD, RN Associate Professor, University of Virginia School of Nursing, Charlottesville, Virginia

Colleen Leners, DNP, APRN, FAAN, FAANP Director of Policy, American Association of Colleges of Nursing, Washington, District of Columbia

Lori A. Loan, PhD, RN, FAAN Associate Professor and Executive DNP Pathway Director, University of Alabama at Birmingham School of Nursing, Birmingham, Alabama

Paul Logan, PhD, CRNP, ACNP-BC Assistant Research Professor, Ross and Carol Nese College of Nursing, The Pennsylvania State University, State College, Pennsylvania

Ruth Ludwick, PhD, RN-BC, APRN-CNS, FAAN Professor Emeritus, Kent State University College of Nursing, Kent, Ohio, Adjunct Graduate Faculty, Northeast Ohio Medical University, Rootstown, Ohio, Adjunct Professor, Frances Payne Bolton School of Nursing, Marian K. Shaughnessy Nurse Leadership Academy, Cleveland, Ohio

Bernadette Mazurek Melnyk, PhD, APRN-CNP, FAANP, FNAP, FAAN Vice President for Health Promotion, University Chief Wellness Officer, Dean of the College of Nursing and Helene Fuld Health Trust National Institute for Evidence-based Practice, Professor of Pediatrics and Psychiatry, College of Medicine; The Ohio State University, Columbus, Ohio

Patricia A. Patrician, PhD, RN, FAAN Professor and Rachel Z. Booth Endowed Chair in Nursing, University of Alabama at Birmingham School of Nursing, Birmingham, Alabama

Rebecca M. Patton, DNP, RN, CNOR, FAAN Lucy Jo Atkinson Scholar in Perioperative Nursing, Case Western Reserve University Frances Payne Bolton School of Nursing Cleveland, Ohio; Past President, American Nurses Association, Silver Spring, Maryland

Janice M. Phillips, PhD, RN, CENP, FAAN Director of Nursing Research and Health Equity, Rush University Medical Center, Chicago, Illinois

Tim Raderstorf, DNP, RN, FAAN Chief Innovation Officer and Assistant Professor of Clinical Nursing, The Ohio State University College of Nursing, Head of Academic Entrepreneurship, The Erdős Institute, Chief Operations Officer NursesEverywhere, Columbus, Ohio

Judith Shamian, PhD, RN, DSc (Hon), LLD (Hon), FAAN   President Emerita, International Council of Nurses, Toronto, Ontario, Canada

Eileen M. Sullivan-Marx, PhD, RN, FAAN   Dean and Erline Perkins McGriff Professor, New York University Rory Meyers College of Nursing, New York City, New York

Lisa Summers, DrPh, FACNM   President and Director, Healing Politics, Baltimore, Maryland

Karen Tomajan, MS, RN, NEA-BC   Independent Educator and Consultant, Hercules, California

Shanita D. Williams, PhD, MPH, APRN   Deputy Division Director, Data Division, Office of Strategic Business Operations, Bureau of Primary Health Care, Health Resources and Services Administration, U.S. Department of Health and Human Services, Rockville, Maryland

Margarete L. Zalon, PhD, RN, ACNS-BC, FAAN   Professor, Department of Nursing and Director, MS in Health Informatics Program, The University of Scranton, Scranton, Pennsylvania

Foreword

Now in its third edition, *Nurses Making Policy: From Bedside to Boardroom*, edited by Patton, Zalon, and Ludwick, gives nurses an all-access pass to a panoply of expert knowledge and advice. These experts and the contributing authors describe successes and failures, as well as challenges and solutions for transforming words and ideas into action for effective health policies in local, state, regional, national, and global arenas.

We have consistently called upon nurses to influence the health of the world, far beyond the caring and curative interventions we deploy in treating illness. That means changing social conditions that threaten the health of marginalized populations, committing to health equity, and advocating for a range of solutions that rest in the control of our elected officials, community leaders, and others who do not see through the lens of nursing or healthcare. Chapter 1 makes the case for continuing to address the pressing issues in healthcare where permanent solutions have been elusive. These challenges include access to care and assuring safe work environments. Then authors also draw attention to contemporary issues of social justice and the environment and well-being, each of which reflect national crises that affect not only nurses but also the very viability of our health systems throughout the world.

In this book nurse leaders are telling their stories. Chapter by chapter, examples illuminate the courage, skill, creativity, and tenacity of nurses to influence change, one at a time, or with the power of collective action—it's all here. The third edition continues the unique approach of "policy on the scene" to illustrate the experiences of champions, influencers, and nurses who amplified their passion for patients into passion for action. Among the many updates is introduction of the Patton-Zalon-Ludwick (PZL) Policy Assessment Framework to assess one's policy expertise. The model introduces interdependent dimensions of policy engagement stratified by scope and shaped by partnerships.

Advocacy may or may not come naturally beyond care delivery at the bedside, yet we are confronted by the question of, if not us, then who? Our professional nursing Code of Ethics compels us to embrace our duty of advocacy. That means every nurse, not just associations must advocate for patients and for quality healthcare for patients and communities, locally, nationally, and globally. The responsibility is ours as professional nurses.

In Chapter 11, focused on the nexus between innovation and policy, the authors remind us that the essence of our work invokes innovation to create change and policies that improve health and care delivery. For more than a decade, aggressive action has resulted in significant achievements to increase the level of education for nurses, the appointment to nurses on boards across a spectrum of interests, and more nurses serving in public office. By continuously building the confidence and competence of nurses we will increase the talent and expertise necessary to continue the accelerated pace of change. The instruments of that change are embedded in the pages of this text, not only for students, but also for any nurse who wants to engage in making change.

Nurses in every role and setting have the power to shape health policy and change healthcare. We not only can, we must. Perhaps it is time to move beyond the editors' declaration that "health policy competence is an essential fit for nursing" and declare health policy competence a "survival skill for the profession."

We have seen the grit of nurses throughout the pandemic, during which much of this book was written. Nurses have the answers for better health, better care, and better health policies. We encourage you to use the tools in the pages that follow to learn new skills, hone your messages and become an influencer.

Pamela F. Cipriano, PhD, RN, NEA-BC, FAAN
President, International Council of Nurses
Dean and Sadie Heath Cabaniss Professor of Nursing
University of Virginia School of Nursing
Charlottesville, Virginia
Past President, American Nurses Association

Joyce J. Fitzpatrick, PhD, MBA, RN, FAAN, FNAP
Director, Marian K. Shaughnessy Nurse Leadership Academy
Elizabeth Brooks Ford Professor of Nursing
Frances Payne Bolton School of Nursing
Distinguished University Professor
Case Western Reserve University
Cleveland, Ohio

Preface

Being a nurse can be challenging. It requires balancing multiple roles and professional responsibilities in fulfilling nursing's contract with society. We recognize and champion that all nurses have a significant advocacy role in promoting health and advancing the profession, whether in highly visible positions or working behind the scenes. Policies are essential opportunities for nurses to take ownership of advocacy.

This completely updated third edition provides a hands-on approach to help nurses across a variety of settings to develop health policy competencies for managing an ever-changing health and uncertain policy arena. Four major units provide a framework for our approach as the chapters of the book take the reader on a journey through all the steps of the policymaking process. Leadership, ethical, and social justice principles are unifying concepts integrated across chapters. Throughout each new or revised chapter, policy development is exemplified from the grand scale of global or national to the local level. We believe that policymaking at all these levels is essential. Often, however, the interplay between levels is not always recognized or acknowledged.

The key features of each chapter cover specific aspects of the policymaking process including learning objectives, an introduction, policy challenge and solutions, policies on the scene, key concepts, future implications, summary, learning activities, and e-resources. These features in each of the 15 chapters have been thoroughly revised. Each chapter introduces a key aspect of the policy-making process framing the important details for the reader. The *Policy Challenge* presents a particular dilemma or issue in policy with a *Policy Solution* illustrating the outcome at the end of the chapter. *Policies on the Scene* provide short vignettes about the policy journeys of nurse leaders and aspiring policy activists. *Implications for the Future* describe projected developments in nursing and healthcare that have the potential to influence policy. *Key Concepts* aid learning by taking readers through the steps of the policy process to enhance their policy skills. The *Learning Activities* are designed to enhance critical thinking. They include examining policy issues at all levels, and they can be carried out by individuals or as part of a group. *E-Resources* reflect key information from a variety of sources important for policy savvy nurses (e.g., key documents, government websites, videos, podcasts, etc.). These *E-Resources* were designed to be used for classroom teaching or independent learning.

NEW TO THIS EDITION

Updates include major revisions to the chapters. New authors and coauthors have joined our team providing a new perspective from experts on the frontlines of change and policy. Of the 15 chapters, eight chapters bring 16 new experts as contributors for this edition. Recognizing the value of innovation, a new chapter, "Transforming Policy With Innovation," has been added to illustrate the links among innovations and policies. Our expanding network of contributors illustrates the diverse opportunities that nurses have for influencing policy.

The new and revised *Policy Challenges, Solutions,* and *Policies on the Scene* portray the multiple arenas for nurses' advocacy, policy work, and the expansion of policy journeys to bring a real-world practical emphasis to policy development. Incorporated into this edition are the numerous reports issued to advance nursing, written to influence the direction of the nursing profession and its work including the *Future of Nursing 2020–2030: Charting a Path to Achieve Health Equity* report and the World Health Organization's *State of the World's Nursing-2020* report. Expanding on these reports, content related to diversity, equity, and inclusion; social justice; and the social determinants of health have been integrated throughout the book.

In this edition, the Patton–Zalon–Ludwick (PZL) Policy Assessment Framework is described. The framework illustrates three dimensions of policy competency development: policy engagement, policy partnership, and policy scope. This framework provides a visual guide for self-assessment of one's policy journey.

Appreciating the power of messaging, color has been incorporated into this edition for the ease of reading. New pictures, figures, and exhibits have been added to emphasize key events, documents, and resources that present information in a succinct and clear manner. PowerPoint presentations that include a student version and a version with talking and discussion points in the notes are available for instructors who email Springer Publishing Company at *textbook@springerpub. com.* An instructor's manual is also available to faculty that includes guidance for purposeful classroom discourse for each chapter.

Rebecca M. Patton
Margarete L. Zalon
Ruth Ludwick

Acknowledgments

The success of this book is a testament to the vision, commitment, and ideas of the diverse authors of the current and the previous editions about the essential value of policy in nursing. We are inspired by the numerous individuals who have worked hard to disseminate and advance policy. We appreciate the insights and questions of students we encounter in our policy work. We honor nurses around the world who in a multitude of roles provided or supported care for individuals during the COVID-19 pandemic. Their work made all the more visible the importance of good policy; it strengthened our commitment to advance policy and support nurses' development of policy expertise. *All 100% of the editors' royalties for the third edition, as in previous editions, will go toward funding the Washington Policy Fellowship at the American Nurses Foundation (www.nursingworld.org/foundation/programs/washington-policy-fellowship).*

We are extremely grateful for the collaboration among colleagues who made this book possible. We thank and acknowledge policy champions whether they are working late to write overdue policies, running for elected office, campaigning for candidates, speaking up about failed policies, or taking a myriad of actions to advance policy.

Without a doubt we owe endless thanks to the contributors—the esteemed authors of each chapter—and those who shared their real-life stories in the Policy Challenges and Policies on the Scene. We acknowledge the contributions of Ashley Badders, MSN, RN, CCRN, Hollie Gentry, MSN, WHNP-BC, CNE, and Holly Ma, MS, BSN, RN, NPD-BC, students in the Doctor of Nursing Practice (DNP) program at the Frances Payne Bolton School of Nursing, Case Western Reserve University, who provided background support. This third edition could not have been completed without the support of the people who contributed chapters to the first and second editions.

This edition, like previous editions, reflects the support of numerous family members and friends. Our families have provided us with ongoing support throughout our policy journey in actualizing the dream of this book.

In the Patton family, we thank mother Mary Ellen, a distinguished nurse leader; sister Betty Jane—also an RN—and brothers Bob and John.

In the Zalon family, we thank husband John.

In the Ludwick family, we thank husband John, son Tom, and Tom's wife Sara, and acknowledge the joy brought by grandchildren, Caleb and Carly.

As you read our acknowledgments, we encourage you to thank those who are supportive to you in your personal, work, and policy lives.

Contributors to the Previous Editions

SECOND EDITION CONTRIBUTORS

Susan Apold, PhD, ANP-BC, AGNP, FAAN, FAANP   Clinical Professor of Nursing, New York University Rory Meyers College of Nursing, New York City, New York

Pamela F. Cipriano, PhD, RN, NEA-BC, FAAN   President, American Nurses Association, Silver Spring, Maryland, Research Associate Professor, University of Virginia School of Nursing, Charlottesville, Virginia

Sean P. Clarke, PhD, RN, FAAN   Professor and Associate Dean, William F. Connell School of Nursing, Boston College, Boston, Massachusetts

Joanne Disch, PhD, RN, FAAN   Professor ad Honorem, University of Minnesota School of Nursing, Minneapolis, Minnesota

Linda K. Groah, MSN, RN, CNOR, NEA-BC, FAAN   Chief Executive Officer/Executive Director, Association of periOperative Registered Nurses (AORN), Denver, Colorado

Amy L. Hader, JD   General Counsel and Director of Government Affairs, Association of periOperative Registered Nurses (AORN), Denver, Colorado

Debbie Dawson Hatmaker, PhD, RN, FAAN   Enterprise Chief Program Officer, American Nurses Association, Silver Spring, Maryland

Lauren Inouye, MPP, RN   Vice President for Public Policy and Government Affairs, Council of Graduate Schools, Washington, District of Columbia

Ingrid Johnson, DNP, MPP, BSN   Senior Director of Operations and Policy, Colorado Center for Nursing Excellence, Denver, Colorado

Jessica Keim-Malpass, PhD, RN   Assistant Professor, University of Virginia School of Nursing, Charlottesville, Virginia

Colleen Leners, DNP, APRN, FAANP   Director of Policy, American Association of Colleges of Nursing, Washington, District of Columbia

Pamela B. Linzer, MSN, RN   Doctoral Candidate, William Connell School of Nursing, Boston College, Boston, Massachusetts, Employee Health and Infection Control Consultant, Winchester Hospital, Lahey Health System, Andover, Massachusetts

Ruth Ludwick, PhD, RN-BC, APRN-CNS, FAAN   Professor Emeritus, Kent State University College of Nursing, Kent, Ohio, Adjunct Graduate Faculty, Northeast Ohio Medical University, Rootstown, Ohio

Kathy Malloch, PhD, MBA, RN, FAAN President, KMLS, Glendale, Arizona, Professor of Practice, College of Nursing and Health Innovation, Arizona State University, Tempe, Arizona, Clinical Professor, College of Nursing, Ohio State University, Columbus, Ohio

Suzanne Miyamoto, PhD, RN, FAAN Chief Policy Officer, American Association of Colleges of Nursing, Washington, District of Columbia

Rebecca M. Patton, DNP, RN, CNOR, FAAN Lucy Jo Atkinson Scholar in Perioperative Nursing, Case Western Reserve University Frances Payne Bolton School of Nursing Cleveland, Ohio, Past President, American Nurses Association, Silver Spring, Maryland

Janice M. Phillips, PhD, RN, FAAN Director of Nursing Research and Health Equity, Rush University Medical Center, Chicago, Illinois

Tim Porter-O'Grady, DM, EdD, APRN, FAAN Senior Partner, Health Systems, Tim Porter-O'Grady Associates, Inc., Atlanta, Georgia

Audra N. Rankin, DNP, APRN, CPNP, CNE Instructor, Johns Hopkins University School of Nursing, Baltimore, Maryland

Judith Shamian, PhD, RN, DSc, LLD, FAAN President Emerita, International Council of Nurses, Toronto, Ontario, Canada

Michelle McHugh Slater, DNP, RN, CNOR Nurse Manager and Quality Fellow, Cleveland Veterans Administration Medical Center, Cleveland, Ohio

Eileen M. Sullivan-Marx, PhD, RN, FAAN Dean and Erline Perkins McGriff Professor, New York University Rory Meyers College of Nursing, New York City, New York

Karen Tomajan, MS, RN, NEA-BC Independent Consultant, Hercules, California

Kathleen M. White, PhD, RN, NEA-BC, FAAN Professor, Johns Hopkins University School of Nursing, Baltimore, Maryland

Shanita D. Williams, PhD, MPH, APRN Deputy Director, Northeast Health Services Division, Office of Northern Health Services, Bureau of Primary Health Care, Health Resources and Services Administration, U.S. Department of Health and Human Services, Rockville, Maryland

Margarete L. Zalon, PhD, RN, ACNS-BC, FAAN Professor, Department of Nursing, Director, Online MS in Health Informatics Program, University of Scranton, Scranton, Pennsylvania

FIRST EDITION CONTRIBUTORS

Sheila A. Abood, PhD, RN Adjunct Faculty, Grand Valley State University, Kirkhof College of Nursing, Grand Rapids, Michigan

Virginia Trotter Betts, MSN, JD, RN, FAAN President, Health Futures, Inc., Nashville, Tennessee

Josepha E. Burnley, DNP, RN, FNP-C Nurse Consultant/Project Officer, Nursing Practice and Workforce Development, Division of Nursing, Health Resources and Services Administration, U.S. Department of Health and Human Services, Rockville, Maryland

Pamela F. Cipriano, PhD, RN, NEA-BC, FAAN President, American Nurses Association, Silver Spring, Maryland, Research Associate Professor, University of Virginia School of Nursing, Charlottesville, Virginia

Sean P. Clarke, PhD, RN, FAAN Associate Dean for Undergraduate Programs, Professor, William F. Connell School of Nursing, Boston College, Boston, Massachusetts

Deborah Colton, MSW Senior Vice President for Strategic Communication, Massachusetts General Physicians Organization, Boston, Massachusetts

Joanne Disch, PhD, RN, FAAN Professor ad Honorem, University of Minnesota School of Nursing, Minneapolis, Minnesota

Marianne Ditomassi, MSN, MBA, RN Executive Director for Patient Care Services Operations and Magnet Recognition, Massachusetts General Hospital, Boston, Massachusetts

Jeanette Ives Erickson, DNP, RN, FAAN Senior Vice President for Patient Care and Chief Nurse, Massachusetts General Hospital, Boston, Massachusetts

Rose Iris Gonzalez, PhD, MPS, RN Independent Consultant, Past Director, Government Affairs, American Nurses Association, Silver Spring, Maryland

Linda K. Groah, MSN, RN, CNOR, NEA-BC, FAAN CEO/Executive Director, Association of periOperative Registered Nurses, Denver, Colorado

Amy L. Hader, JD Director, Legal and Government Affairs, Association of periOperative Registered Nurses, Denver, Colorado

Debbie Dawson Hatmaker, PhD, RN, FAAN Executive Director, American Nurses Association, Silver Spring, Maryland

Mathew Keller, BSN, JD, RN Regulatory and Policy Nursing Specialist Minnesota Nurses Association, St. Paul, Minnesota

Ruth Ludwick, PhD, RN-BC, CNS, FAAN Independent Consultant, Director of Nursing Research, Robinson Memorial Hospital, Ravenna, Ohio, Professor Emeritus, Kent State University, College of Nursing, Kent, Ohio

Kathy Malloch, PhD, MBA, RN, FAAN President, KMLS, LLC, Associate Professor of Practice, Arizona State University College of Nursing and Health Innovation, Phoenix, Arizona, Clinical Professor, The Ohio State University College of Nursing, Columbus, Ohio, Clinical Consultant, API Healthcare, Hartford, Wisconsin

Suzanne Miyamoto, PhD, RN Director of Government Affairs and Health Policy, American Association of Colleges of Nursing, Washington, District of Columbia

Rebecca M. Patton, MSN, RN, CNOR, FAAN Past President, American Nurses Association, Lucy Jo Atkinson Scholar in Perioperative Nursing, Frances Payne Bolton School of Nursing, Case Western Reserve University, Cleveland, Ohio

Janice M. Phillips, PhD, RN, FAAN Director of Government and Regulatory Affairs, CGFNS International, Inc., Philadelphia, Pennsylvania

Tim Porter-O'Grady, DM, EdD, ScD(h), APRN, FAAN, FACCWS Senior Partner, Tim Porter-O'Grady Associates, Inc., Associate Professor, Leadership Scholar, College of Nursing and Health Innovation, Arizona State University, Phoenix, Arizona, Clinical Professor, Leadership Scholar, The Ohio State

University College of Nursing, Columbus, Ohio, Adjunct Professor, Dean's Advisor, Emory University, Atlanta, Georgia

Eileen M. Sullivan-Marx, PhD, RN, FAAN Dean and Erline Perkins McGriff Professor, New York University College of Nursing, New York, New York

Karen Tomajan, MS, RN, NEA-BC Director, Professional Practice, John Muir Medical Center, Concord, California

Susan Tullai-McGuinness, PhD, MPA, RN Adjunct Associate Professor, Case Western Reserve University, Frances Payne Bolton School of Nursing, Cleveland, Ohio

Eileen Weber, DNP, RN, PHN, JD Clinical Assistant Professor, University of Minnesota School of Nursing, Minneapolis, Minnesota

Kathleen M. White, PhD, RN, NEA-BC, FAAN Director, Master's Entry Into Practice Program, Associate Professor, Johns Hopkins University School of Nursing, Baltimore, Maryland

Loretta Alexia Williams, BSN, RN Graduate Research Assistant and Instructor, Jonas Nursing Leadership Scholar (2012–2014), University of Tennessee Health Science Center College of Nursing, Memphis, Tennessee

Shanita D. Williams, PhD, MPH, APRN Branch Chief, Nursing Practice and Workforce Development, Division of Nursing, Health Resources and Services Administration, U.S. Department of Health and Human Services, Rockville, Maryland

Margarete L. Zalon, PhD, RN, ACNS-BC, FAAN Professor, Department of Nursing, University of Scranton, Scranton, Pennsylvania

Instructor Resources

Nurses Making Policy, Third Edition: From Bedside to Boardroom includes quality resources for the instructor and the student. Faculty who have adopted the text may gain access to these resources by emailing textbook@springerpub.com.

Instructor resources include:

- Instructor's Manual
- PowerPoint Presentations
  - Student Version
  - Instructor Version With Talking and Discussion Points in the Notes

UNIT |

Making the Case: Valuing Policy

CHAPTER 1

Marching to Lead in Policy

REBECCA M. PATTON, MARGARETE L. ZALON, AND RUTH LUDWICK

No system shall endure that does not march.
—Margretta Styles

OBJECTIVES

1. Critique nurses' elemental responsibilities to society for policy engagement.
2. Critically examine the perspectives that are foundational in formulating policies that affect health.
3. Differentiate between health policy and policies that affect health.
4. Appraise the potential of nursing's influence and impact on access to care, workplace and workforce needs, well-being, and the environment.
5. Analyze the leadership roles of nurses in influencing health policy at the local, state, and national levels.

Nurses have had a meaningful influence that has resulted in new or revised policy solutions for the last 100 years or more. Their influence and policy solutions have not always been recognized. Today that is changing. What the profession needs in 2021 and beyond are nurses equally competent in practice, advocacy, and policy. Policy is important to practice across all settings, interactions within healthcare organizations, and the health of communities and citizens around the globe.

Building on the work of Florence Nightingale, Margretta Styles, international nurse leader and architect of advanced practice credentialing, challenged us to do more than take a step forward. It is a call to action for working together to advance the healthcare and profession through policy. At no time in our recent history has nurses marching to advance the health of the communities we serve been more necessary. Nurses are "marching," advancing solutions in their workplace, communities, and the profession.

Nurses are aligned and identified with caring about issues, especially those that directly affect health. Nurses are known for their passion, commitment to patients, and understanding of the intricacies of providing care. These characteristics have galvanized nurses to march for policy solutions. Nurses are visible across the country championing causes such as climate change, racism, health inequities, and responses to the COVID-19 pandemic. However, in order to effectively advocate for others, it is also essential that nurses take care of themselves and take care of each other. The well-being of nurses is garnering more attention with the designation of 2020 and 2021 as the Year of Nurse and Midwife since it coincides with the worst pandemic in 100 years. The stressors of the last year have called attention to the issues surrounding mental health and have also cast light on the topic of nurse suicide, a topic that is difficult to discuss, stigmatized, and buried from view. The Policy Challenge addresses nurse suicide in the context of policy.

Did I miss the signs? What could have been done differently? What will happen to the family? What will the unit be like without my colleague? How did it happen? Such an excellent nurse. A sad and unnecessary loss. Everyone loved ... Why didn't we know what was going on? When someone close to us commits suicide, we all second-guess ourselves and wonder what we could have done to prevent it. Asking these questions and mourning the loss is a natural response. Nurses' poignant descriptions of the aftermath of a suicide illustrate the struggles faced in coping with the loss: *"Many weeks later, after ... many sad and mournful days in our unit, we were told Penny's death was ... intentional ... "* ... *"No one at work would ever suspect."* *"I transferred to another unit"* (Davidson et al., 2018, "Nurses as Whole People").

Suicide is the 10th-leading cause of death in the United States, touching the lives of family members, friends, and colleagues left behind. Tragically, the suicide rate among nurses is significantly higher than that of the general population. When comparing female nurses to women, nurses have almost double the suicides per 100,000 than women in the general population (Davis et al., 2021). Aside from the usual risk factors, for example, depression and substance use disorders, suicide in nurses is also associated with workplace and job performance issues. Suicide touches everyone personally and professionally.

With 4.3 million RNs in the United States comprising the largest professional group of healthcare providers, suicide among nurses cannot be ignored. Nurses are integral to our healthcare system, a fact that became more apparent to the public during the COVID-19 pandemic. Nursing is stressful, and the COVID-19 pandemic exacerbated that stress for many. The burden of responsibilities carried by nurses adds stressors knowing that crushing workloads inhibit them from providing the care deemed necessary. In addition, the second victim syndrome or guilt over an error adds stressors, which may be considered so traumatic that it requires emergency care (Denham, 2007). Complicating this problem further, nurses often face the same challenges in accessing quality mental health services as the public does. In addition, it is too soon to know the full result of the pandemic on nurses' well-being and resilience in handling new stressors, although early empirical reports indicated a heightened impact on the stress of healthcare professionals, including nurses (Hummel et al., 2021).

Complicating this issue is that tracking suicide is a complex endeavor. The Centers for Disease Control and Prevention (CDC) tracks suicide in the National Violent Data Reporting System (NVDRS), but data are not available from even half of all states (CDC, 2021). No national group tracks nurse suicide.

This Policy Challenge illustrates one of the many difficult issues that nurses face personally and professionally. Daily, nurses see how policy decisions, such as access to care, affect patients, their families, and themselves and how organizational staffing policies may harm patients and adversely affect nurses and their work environment. Suicide among nurses is one such poignant example.

Each nurse's job is to identify when policy solutions are needed. Many issues may not necessarily have an obvious policy solution, and others may have an obvious solution that is not always recognized or acted on. Nurses are uniquely qualified to lead the multifaceted work of policy and have the requisite duty to take on those responsibilities individually and collectively. The International Council of Nurses (ICN), the American Nurses Association (ANA), and other policy stakeholders, including the report *Future of Nursing 2020–2030: Charting a Path to Achieve Health Equity* (National Academies, 2021), call for nurses to actively contribute through engagement and leadership at all levels of health policy.

Policy and political involvement are not solely defined by one's position. Nurse managers, educators, researchers, and administrators are often viewed as having more obvious roles in setting direction for the successful articulation of federal and state regulations and implementation of institutional policies. Nurses live at the sharp edge of those policies and regulations and the politics surrounding them, an advantage that is vital to informing, shaping, monitoring, and evaluating policy. The COVID-19 pandemic clearly illustrates nurses' living at the sharp edge and the need to use their expertise.

ESSENTIAL POLICY AND POLITICAL SKILLS FOR NURSES

It is with great certainty that once policy skills are understood and practiced, nurses can successfully engage in advocacy through policymaking. These skills are essential to nurses in the trenches, performing direct care across all settings, and nurses in leadership, education, and research positions. Thus, policy work is the role of every nurse.

Policy refers to the actions taken by a government or organization to achieve a specific goal. Thus, there are public policies that are achieved through the implementation of laws, regulations, and standardized practices. Policies also include rules and standards set forth by organizations, as well as the budgetary processes, to support their actions and programs. There are many opportunities for nurses to use their expertise to provide formal and informal input in the public and private sectors.

Nurses, like many, see politics as a dirty word, that it is nurses' place to remain neutral. However, very little in healthcare, or any work environment is apolitical. Politics is a process and reflects an attitude. As a process, it refers to the activities of individuals in groups or organizations working together to achieve agreed-on goals. As an attitude, being "political" is shaped by one's life experiences, education, and environment. Not being involved in politics or policy is as much of a decision as being actively involved.

A famous journalist, Shapiro (2021, p. 317), aptly stated that "people often say, with pride, 'I'm not interested in politics.' They might as well say, 'I'm not interested in my standard of living, my health, my job, my rights, my future or any future.'" To take this further, for nurses to manage their work environment, advance the profession, and provide effective care for their patients, being politically active is the only option.

POLICY AS A FIT FOR NURSING

Health policy competence is an essential fit for nursing. Nursing skills such as problem-solving, communication, versatility, and resourcefulness equip the nurse in this arena. The everyday practical lens of nurses facilitates the identification and implementation of actions on issues requiring policy solutions. Nurses experienced in policy at the national, state, local, or organizational level know that they possess healthcare system knowledge, especially at the point of care, and essential skills that can be adapted for application to successful policymaking. Montalvo (2015), in her integrative review, indicates that nurses with political competencies are able to evaluate and react to organizational dynamics in order to achieve desired outcomes (e.g., patient care quality).

Many organizations (e.g., professional associations, think tanks, accrediting bodies) strongly recommend that all nursing education programs have health policy education incorporated in the curriculum and nurses' organizations across the world advocate policy action. Shared governance and other forms of collective action (e.g., alliances, unions) at their core are about nurses providing input for decision-making at the policy table developing policies for practice.

Nurses frequently voice that they have no control over policy. A frequent excuse heard is that there is no time in the fast-paced world of healthcare, with the numerous rules and regulations, to become policy experts. Nurses need to be at policy tables. Despite policy tables being everywhere, nurses are often underrepresented at those tables whether it be at the hospital board level or a committee. These tables are where decisions influencing nursing practice and patient care are made. When nurses are not at policy tables, others quickly fill the void, but they may not represent the needs of nurses regarding patient care or their work environments. Sometimes the policy tables may be uneven with nursing not being adequately represented. Being silent implies unspoken endorsement or agreement with policies, actions, governance, the actions proposed, or the status quo. It facilitates others making their voices heard in the void of our silence.

HARNESSING PASSION

Embracing passion, acknowledging personal circumstances, and tackling current events are often what draws nurses into policy, albeit sometimes with reluctance. Nurses are committed to their patients but sometimes hesitant to be involved in policy. When nursing is highlighted in the public's eye, the focus is on passion and caring. Passion is only one of the compelling reasons that nurses engage in policy. Karen Daley, past ANA president, had her passion for improving workplace safety through policy fueled after a devastating needlestick injury (see her story at www.youtube.com/watch?v=C3wNc9fcBds). Ernie Grant, ANA president until 2022, is an expert clinician who treated life-altering burn injuries, devoting his life to using a health-in-all-policies (HiAP) approach to educating people, especially children about fire safety, progressing to national and international leadership and persuading policymakers on issues related to water temperature safety, pyrotechnic safety, and fire-safe cigarettes. Margaret Flinter, PhD, APRN, FAAN, a family nurse practitioner and community health center executive, has a passion for getting involved and encouraging others to become involved through her weekly radio show, *Conversations on Health Care*. She engages top thought leaders on healthcare issues that also readily available to the public via podcasts (www.chradio.com).

There is no shortage of issues about patients and the nursing profession that fuel nurses' passions. The Royal College of Nursing (RCN, 2020) conducted a survey completed by almost 42,000 members that showed a large majority (88%) of nurses continue to be passionate about their role. But it is not passion alone that drives nurses' involvement in policy. Nurses share a unique intimacy with patients that brings critical understanding and potential solutions to many high-profile, complex healthcare issues, such as access, quality, cost, and value. This positions nurses with an exceptional lens to appreciate the convergence of policy and politics in healthcare. It is often the convergence of these that fuels the emerging realities in which action is needed.

These stories of passion also hold the key to nurse political activation, as they also provide rich stories that put faces to an issue and help outsiders, such as legislators or board members, understand the richness and the complexity of

EXHIBIT 1.1   INTERVIEW WITH THE HON. GALE ADCOCK, MSN, RN, FNP, FAAN, FAANP, NORTH CAROLINA GENERAL ASSEMBLY, HOUSE DISTRICT 41

What got you interested in running for office or engaging in policy work?	I grew weary of trying to persuade elected officials—who were powerful but no smarter than I—to make good decisions about legislation affecting my patients' health and healthcare and my day-to-day nursing practice. When it hit me that pushing for a better health policy was pointless without an equal push for improvement in the social determinants of health (education, employment, socioeconomic status), I decided to run.
Why do you stay at the state level and not run for national office?	State government is the best fit for my skill set, policy interests, and bipartisan philosophy. My focus continues to be evidence-based state policy that determines healthcare access (including full-practice authority), addresses health disparities, funds public education from preK through the community college/university system, and creates pathways to economic independence for all North Carolinians.
What gives you the most joy or satisfaction in this role?	Making policy problems "relatable" through the use of stories from my decades of varied nursing experience.

healthcare issues facing frontline nurses as they provide care to their constituents. The passion that often comes from personal experiences in professional caregiving or from within one's personal life may be a catalyst, but passion alone does not account for political activism. Many nurses indicate that their life experiences from education and family play a role in their political activism. Gale Adcock, a family nurse practitioner who is a member of the North Carolina Nurses Association (see Chapter 3) and has served in the state legislature since 2015, answers key questions about her legislative role in Exhibit 1.1.

POLICY APPROACHES

Nurses have a duty to address issues of concern through policy. The ANA Code of Ethics (2015) mandates nurses' moral obligations to address social justice through political advocacy. Advancing policies requires nurses to understand approaches to policy and be knowledgeable and strategic in politics. This may seem foreign to nurses if they assume political activism means being involved in campaigns or working with legislators. However, being active in policy can span a wide spectrum. The impact of policies can be considered at the macro or micro level. Three commonly utilized approaches are big "P" versus little "p," upstream versus downstream, and HiAP.

Policies carried out at the microlevel and processes associated with nurses' work environments are called little "p." These policies are not less important; the term is used to convey a difference in scope. Examples of little-p policies might include implementing a no-lift policy in a clinical agency or addressing bullying and violence in school settings. These policies could also evolve into national standards for practice, or they might be incorporated into legislation and regulation. Conversely, established policies at the macro level, or the big-P level will influence policies or practice standards at the local level. The big-P level policy very often implies holding office in a major organization or the government, working actively to pass state and federal laws related to safe patient care or some such similar activity. We refer to *policies* on this grand scale as policies with a big P. The differentiation with little-p and big-P helps recognize who has jurisdiction over the issues (see Chapter 6).

Nurses may be more familiar with advocacy within the context of the nurse–patient relationship because we have traditionally focused our efforts and energies on encouraging nurses to be advocates at the individual level or at the point of care. When addressing issues, nurses need to move beyond the point-of-care approach, which is considered essential but a downstream approach. Nurses need to consider an upstream approach. This approach addresses primary prevention, root causes of disease and disability, system change, and/or the social determinants of health (see Chapter 13). The familiar classic public health parable that highlights the differences between upstream and downstream is that of rescuers frantically working to pull people out of a river instead of going upstream to figure out why people are falling into the river and preventing that from happening in the first place. Not only is an upstream approach necessary, but the strategies to influence upstream decisions necessarily also involve collaborative or team efforts and/or political action. Upstream approaches are important in addressing social determinants of health.

Nurses need to have a broad perspective and use nontraditional approaches. Health is influenced by policies and practices that are implemented across the board. An example is a city regulation requiring sidewalks in all new housing developments. Without sidewalks, walking is limited. Opportunities to walk safely influences people's exercise habits and health. Addressing this and similar issues is known as an HiAP approach. A HiAP approach is important in addressing the social determinants of health such as housing, education, food security, and transportation (Williams et al., 2018). The *Future of Nursing 2020–2030 Report* (National Academies, 2021) emphasized the essential nature of nursing in addressing the social determinants of health and health equity. Recognizing the health impact of policies is important for nurses to be global citizens (see Chapter 14).

We argue that the profession and nurses need to be advocates at all levels, big-P and little-p, upstream and downstream, with attention to a HiAP approach, to achieve our healthcare and population health goals. These goals cannot be achieved without attention to healthcare disparities and inequities. The advocacy competencies nurses learn at the point of care can be readily transferred to these multiple policy arenas.

BEING POLITICAL

Being political is influencing policy and politics at local, state, and federal levels, much like nursing, and is an art and a science. It is a process that requires nurses to be savvy in multiple arenas. That all people are political is not always recognized or acknowledged. We try every day to influence others based on our beliefs, values, and knowledge. Nurses routinely exert influence no matter their role.

While everyday examples are easily identified, being politically active is still often misunderstood (Ellenbecker et al., 2017). Being political can be seen as less than desirable in a world where it is may be associated with disingenuous elected officials, and political campaigns are perceived as increasingly divisive and negative. Some will use this as an excuse not to vote. In the past, elections, except for 2020, the United States often trailed most developed countries in voter turnout (Desilver, 2020).

These negative views fuel a reluctance to get involved and may contribute to advocacy hesitancy or apathy. For example, a staff nurse may be uneasy about writing a letter to the editor in response to a negative article on breastfeeding because she did not want to be viewed as "too political." On further exploration, she said she did not want to seem "too radical." Notably, in the software program Microsoft Word, the word *radical* is listed as a synonym for *political*. Aside from being reluctant to take part in what is perceived as political, nurses may also believe that they do not have the competencies necessary for taking political action. This may be reinforced by faculty and other leaders who believe that nursing and nurses be apolitical, who themselves may not necessarily have political skills or appreciate their importance. Nurses, as a group, are good at work-arounds and soothing hot-tempered families, patients, and coworkers, but have trouble seeing that these nursing skills are transferable and necessary to success in being political.

The need and call for nurses' to be politically involved is only growing. We find nurse activists in all levels of government across the world, holding elected and appointed office. Examples at the federal level include RNs who have been elected to the 117th U.S. Congress. Eddie Bernice Johnson (D-TX), who is the "dean" of the Texas Congressional delegation, the first and longest serving nurse (since 1992) previously served as a state legislator (first woman and African American from the Dallas area to serve as a senator since Reconstruction), and was chief psychiatric nurse at the Dallas Veterans Administration Hospital. Lauren Underwood (D-IL), who worked for the Obama administration on the rollout of the Patient Protection and Affordable Care Act (ACA), was the youngest African American woman serving in Congress when she was first elected in 2018 at the age of 32. Legislation that she introduced in the 116th Congress covering insulin costs and veterans' care quality were passed into law. Cori Bush (D-MO) is the newest nurse; she is also an ordained pastor, a community activist, and the first African American woman from Missouri to serve in Congress. At the state level, Bethany Hall-Long, the lieutenant governor of Delaware, previously served as a representative and senator in the state legislature. Lourdes Aflague "Lou" Leon Guerrero is serving as governor of Guam and previously served as a senator in its legislature. Numerous nurses serve in elected positions in state houses across the country and local government as well as in appointed positions at local, state, and federal levels. Obviously, more nurses are needed at this grander scale, given that there are more than four million licensed RNs in the United States. Other professionals, such as physicians with approximately one million in their ranks have done proportionally a better job with four senators and 16 representatives serving in the 117th Congress.

Obviously, we need more nurses elected and appointed to public office, but nurse advocacy goes well beyond these positions, which are only some of many arenas in which nurses can do policy work. Some nurses may assume significant advocacy roles by holding appointed office or key positions at the local level. For example, a very common entrée into public life is election to a local school board. Other opportunities to influence policy that also require being political include holding elected or appointed office in professional associations both nursing and interdisciplinary and consumer groups and serving on boards of healthcare organizations or community agencies. Nurses may also become involved in organizations or groups focused on a single issue or advocating for change related to a single issue in their workplace or where they live.

In 2011, the Institute of Medicine (IOM, now the National Academy of Medicine [NAM]) made a clarion call for action for nurses in its first *Future of Nursing: Leading Change, Advancing Health* report to "have a voice in health policy decision making and be engaged in implementation efforts related to healthcare reform" (p. 8). This call to action is historic because it provides a plan for nursing advocacy in healthcare at the national level and is coupled with initiatives in each state that are designed to make it happen. Responding to the mandate, the Nurses on Boards Coalition (NOBC) was created in 2014 to get nurses appointed to boards and other policy tables for the purpose of advancing the health of communities and the country. The first *Future of Nursing* report recognized the unique perspective that nurses bring to boards at the local, state, and national levels. The NOBC provides resources to assist nurses in building leadership and policy skills and serves to connect nurses to organizational board opportunities. This initiative has brought much attention to the policy power of nurses. In early 2021, the NOBC achieved its original goal to have 10,000 nurses on boards.

Being apolitical is not acceptable, nor is it a reality. Florence Nightingale admonished, "I think one's feelings waste themselves in words, they ought all to be distilled into actions, which bring results" (Cook, 1913, p. 94). Not being political limits what we do for patients and our profession. Overshadowing the long-standing negative connotations of "politics" has traditionally resulted in nurses deliberately avoiding politics at the local, state, or federal levels. Making a difference at the local level may be much easier for nurses, in recognition of the long-standing admonition that all politics is local. We are at a unique juncture in the history of nursing because of the alignment of forces that encourage and enhance nurses' opportunities to be visible and political across multiple settings.

POLICY JOURNEY

The policy journey requires an understanding of factors that influence the development and implementation of policy. Ideally, nurses should be guided by the nursing profession's contract with society, its *Code of Ethics for Nurses* (ANA, 2015), practice standards (ANA, 2021), and their personal values and beliefs in their approaches to policy. However, nurses are often thrust into policy when the day-to-day demands of their work require a solution. Addressing patient needs, incidents, interprofessional dynamics, or just being assigned to develop or revise a policy often pushes nurses into the policymaking arena. Policy work is pervasive in nursing and all aspects of healthcare.

One's policy journey varies depending on the context of the situation. The processes associated with the policy journey are both formal and informal. Being prepared for policy is an ongoing process that has many facets. For example, it requires an examination of one's values and beliefs, a grounding in basic civics and organizational structures and procedures, harnessing scientific evidence, an understanding of the policy process and analysis, and ongoing assessments of one's own policy expertise. One's values and beliefs are addressed with the examination of the nurse's role in advocacy in Chapter 2, civics and organizational structures and procedures are addressed in Chapter 3, and harnessing scientific evidence is addressed in Chapter 5. The steps of policymaking are the same, but the journey for those involved in the process may vary depending on roles and the situation. Regardless of one's personal journey, policymaking involves readiness for policy, an understanding of the applicable policy processes and analysis, and an ongoing self-assessment of one's policy competencies.

INDIVIDUAL READINESS FOR POLICY

Starting points for policy trajectories vary and may include family, education, employment, and networking, which are often coupled with chance political involvement (Betts et al., 2015; Gebbie et al., 2000). These attributes are illustrated by the stories of the 19 nurses interviewed by Betts et al. (2015) in the first edition, and a different group of nurse leaders discussed in Chapter 11 of this edition. The stories of these individuals illustrate the commonalities of policy journeys, numerous avenues to policy roles, and the variety in pathways to success. The stories can provide an inspiration to take the first steps to a more active role in policy. In the words of Dorothy Cornelius, who was president of both the ANA and the ICN, *"every nurse can make a difference."*

Influencing policy requires that nurses be prepared. Preparation for policy is an ongoing process and comes in many forms. Historically, nurse leaders have increasingly called for strengthening educational standards that prepare students in policy. Despite the need for nurses to be involved in policy, most would agree that policy education and widespread policy involvement are still lacking. Sadly, some nurses have limited exposure to policy and, thus, find it difficult to appreciate the important role that nurses can and should play in policy. The specific, interrelated approaches for policy readiness addressed here include educational preparation, defining and appraising one's values, knowing the policy terrain, and networking within one's organization and beyond. Policy on the Scene 1.1 illustrates the interplay of being prepared for the advocacy role, aligning advocacy with one's values, and expanding one's horizons to advocate more broadly.

POLICY ON THE SCENE 1.1: HEARING THE VOICES OF NURSES

Joan O'Hanlon Curry, MS, RN, CPNP, CPON®
Administrative Director, Pediatric Clinical Services
University of Texas at MD Anderson Center, Children's Cancer Hospital,
Houston, TX

In 2018, I successfully ran for president-elect of the Association of Pediatric Hematology/Oncology Nurses (APHON). I had just completed two terms as secretary, and although I had attended all our board meetings, and worked with several of our committees, I felt that I was less than knowledgeable about our advocacy group and its work. Part of their initiative was to educate nurses on policies that impact our profession and our patients. To assist in achieving that goal, APHON awards two members with scholarships to attend the Nurse in Washington Internship (NIWI) annually. I felt this would be an invaluable experience for me and help inform me about the advocacy work our committee is engaged in as I prepared for my 2-year term as APHON president.

In March 2019, I attended the NIWI in person. The first day provided an informative orientation and general information about policy and advocacy. Although my subspecialty is pediatric hematology and oncology, I recognized, and NIWI reinforced, that the attendees represented all of nursing, and therefore, one focus was spreading the word about Title VIII funding and the nursing workforce. Grouped by state, we spent time reviewing what we wanted to say to our U.S. representatives and senators and tips for effective communication.

Because my own representative was not available, I joined a group that met with Congressman Dan Crenshaw's (R-TX) legislative aide, who told us that the representative's concerns were about the high price of end-stage renal disease, diabetes, hypertension, and cancer care. She asked what nurses could do to address these costs. We explained that prevention was key because it is difficult and costly to get these illnesses under control once they manifest. I made the point that prevention and good habits start in childhood and that there are not enough school nurses. We also talked about the lack of primary and preventative care in rural areas and underserved areas and that the evidence shows that nurse practitioners can safely and effectively provide that care, which can be enhanced with full-practice authority. We pointed out the importance of increasing the nurse workforce and tuition support.

We learned that Congressman Crenshaw spoke later that day on the floor regarding healthcare, emphasizing the points we made earlier with his aide about the need for preventative care. His had aide heard what we said, and it resonated. It was so inspiring and really taught me that we can make a difference in educating legislators about patients' needs and the full scope of what nurses can do.

This ignited a fire in me that had not been there before. It made me think about how I can give back to nurses as I progress in my career. How can we increase the number of nursing students? How can we change the face of healthcare with prevention and advanced practice registered nurses (APRNs) practicing in the community to make sure everyone has access to care? We need people to understand the importance of nursing research and how it affects patients.

My policy world has expanded. This year, in addition to attending the NIWI, I participated in the Alliance for Childhood Cancer Action Day. It was rewarding to advocate for the patients and families I work with daily. At the NIWI, I was able to emphasize even more the importance of Title VIII funding and the nursing workforce in the face of the pandemic. I was so inspired with advocacy that I applied and was selected to be an ambassador in training for the Friends of the National Institute of Nursing Research. This is another avenue to advocate for nursing, nursing science, and, in particular, pediatrics to start making lasting changes in our healthcare system. Part of being a nurse is advocating for our patients. This responsibility isn't just at the bedside or in the clinic. If we truly want to make a difference, we need to find the cause that speaks to each of us individually in order to make change whether it be on the local, regional, state, or national level. My advocacy journey is really in its infancy, and I am excited to see where it takes me.

EDUCATIONAL PREPARATION

Policy and the roles of nurses in policy have a critical place in nursing education in forming professional values and facilitating the lifelong engagement of nurses in policy. The American Association of Colleges of Nurses (AACN), National League for Nursing (NLN), and numerous specialty nurses associations call for nurses' involvement in policy. In turn, consistently actualizing these mandates in educational programs will bolster nurses' abilities to partner with other healthcare professionals in the redesign of the U.S. healthcare system as recommended in the *Future of Nursing* report (IOM, 2011). The latest *Future of Nursing 2020–2030* report (National Academies, 2021) emphasizes that strengthening social determinants of health (SDOHs) content is essential to preparing nurses to fully engage in policy related to social justice and health equity.

Nursing education programs can indeed provide a robust environment for the development of professional values related to policy through learning activities, exposure to a wide variety of perspectives, robust discussion in class and clinical settings, and a broad range of clinical practice experiences. At the baccalaureate level, formal education prepares nurses at the entry level to be generalists in health policy. In Chapter, 11 the Policy Challenge introduces the reader to Marcus Henderson and how his education helped launch his policy work. See nurse educator policy role in Chapter 15.

Developing expertise in policy is a lifelong process that is informed by practice, continuing education, and immersion in policy experiences. At all levels of policy engagement, relationships with peers, mentors, role models, and leaders inside and outside of healthcare are equally necessary. These all provide a foundation for the development of capital, which is further described in Chapter 7.

APPRAISING ONE'S VALUES

Defining and appraising one's values and one's positions are necessary for going beyond the acquisition of knowledge about policy. Personal values play a role in the choice of nursing as a career and in one's subsequent career path. Professional values and value clarification are foundational content in nursing education. When both professional and personal values align with the day-to-day nursing practice, values are often not given much consideration. In the real world of practice, however, one's personal and professional values are often challenged, resulting in ethical conflicts and moral distress.

The *Code of Ethics for Nurses* (ANA, 2015), *Nursing's Social Policy Statement* (ANA, 2010), and *Nursing: Scope and Standards of Practice* (ANA, 2021) provide nonnegotiable standards that succinctly outline the basic values and obligations of the nurse across all settings and roles. These documents that underpin all nursing share the value of advocacy for equity and social justice. However, sources of conflict arise when one's personal values, professional values, and the values embodied in the workplace, educational settings, organizations, and communities are not aligned. Value conflicts can be small and additive or overwhelming and contribute to moral distress, which is known to be a cause of nurse burnout. Chapters 2 and 13 illustrate in depth some of the structural components in place that support values such as equity and social justice as well as potential areas of conflict.

KNOWING THE POLICY TERRAIN

Knowing the terrain for policy involves having an understanding of the structure and processes for policy implementation in one's work environment, professional associations, and community organizations in the context of societal issues such as equity and climate change. Understanding of and subsequent essential engagement in the policy terrain is essential for professional development, as it leads to interpersonal effectiveness and the ability to navigate the work environment safely and effectively. This involvement, in turn, is vital to the health of organizations and facilitates the achievement of patient outcomes. One can begin to navigate a complex work environment by volunteering for projects and/or appointments to committees, with the eventual goal of assuming policy leadership roles.

Professional associations and community organizations provide nurses with a different and necessary perspective of the policy terrain. This engagement often provides information about policy issues ranging from local to regional to global. These groups also have an advocacy function that includes navigating policymaking arenas such as legislation and regulation.

Depending on the mission of the organization, advocacy may be focused on a single issue or be multifaceted. The latter is typical of ANA and state and specialty nurses associations that address broad issues impacting practice (e.g., staffing, safety and quality, full-practice authority). This is illustrated by the ongoing work to end violence against nurses done by ANA (www.nursingworld.org/practice-policy/work-environment/end-nurse-abuse) and the joint work done by the American Organization of Nurse Executives (now the American Organization for Nursing Leadership (AONL) and the Emergency Nurses Association (ENA) (2015) (www.aonl.org/system/files/media/file/2019/04/Mitigating-Violence-in-the-Workplace-Toolkit.pdf).

Professional associations inform nurses, the public, and policymakers about legislative and regulatory needs related to practice, such as workplace violence. Involvement in associations increases the likelihood that nurses are more informed about legislative and regulatory initiatives, processes, and opportunities. The number of states that have passed legislation to protect nurses and other healthcare workers from violence is increasing. Legislation may have different approaches in terms of coverage of healthcare workers, with some states covering nurses only in emergency department (ED) or mental health settings. The coverage for some workplace violence prevention programs has been limited, for example, having requirements in place only for public employers. Very often a critical mass of states passing legislation on an issue is required before interest in the legislation can be marshaled at the federal level. In the 117th Congress (2021–2022), legislation with bipartisan support was reintroduced in the House of Representatives to address the rising rates of workplace violence now exacerbated by the COVID-19 pandemic that faces healthcare and social service workers. The proposed legislation, which never advanced to the Senate in the previous Congress, has broad coverage of employees and calls for the establishment of an occupational safety and health standard to require healthcare employers to develop and implement a comprehensive workplace violence prevention plan. Professional associations like the ANA are great resources for knowing the terrain for policy initiatives and progress through environmental scanning and their ongoing tracking efforts.

Community organizations provide the opportunity to expand one's terrain through collaboration and marshaling a broader set of resources to accomplish policy goals. Very often working with community organizations allows one to expand from a focus on individual actions and facility policies to support health through involvement in community initiatives that can provide greater opportunity to improve population health. For example, at the personal level, nurses can be involved in the formulation of policies related to safe routes to schools (walking, busing, drop-offs) that include parents, school nurses, administrators, city council members, and community leaders to support the health and safety of children. Working from a community perspective may have a greater value because it involves understanding a health problem from a wider lens. See Chapter 6, Policy on the Scene 6.1 for a real-world example about school recess policies.

Professional associations and community organizations provide nurses with a broader lens. It is important to be as inclusive as possible to broaden the effectiveness of policies. In some states, legislation may include other healthcare workers. The nursing lens is valuable in developing policy (see Chapter 11). The intersectionality of nursing with health provides broad entrée for nurses to become involved in local issues in one's community as well as issues in the forefront on the national level and beyond. To move policy forward, nurses need to apply their lens while building an advocacy base beyond nursing that involves stakeholders: colleagues, other healthcare professionals, leaders from broad sectors in communities as well as consumers (see Chapter 4).

NETWORKING

Networking is an important part of policymaking at the bedside and boardroom. It involves exchanging information and ideas with professionals inside and outside of one's organization and community leaders as well. It involves expanding one's sphere of influence and bringing others along with you to help them expand their influence. Networking occurs with every encounter. Thus, each encounter with a professional colleague, staff member, administrator, stakeholder, or government official should be done in mind with the goal of achieving positive communication outcomes. See Policy on the Scene 1.2 and Figure 1.1 for examples of such an encounter. This will facilitate steady growth in one's ability to extend one's

---

POLICY ON THE SCENE 1.2: WHY AN ELEVATOR SPEECH IS KEY IN ADVOCACY

Meredith Foxx, MSN, MBA, NEA-BC, APRN
Executive Chief Nursing Officer, Cleveland Clinic Health System, Cleveland

As a member of the most trusted profession year after year, I have learned throughout my career the importance of advocacy at many levels. Nurses are advocates for their patients, the families of their patients, their profession, and, on a bigger scale, healthcare in their communities. As professionals who are the front lines impacting lives, it is key that nurses feel confident to advocate.

Nurses are experts and have a role in health policy. But first they must understand and be educated about health policy and politics and the best way to make a change. In my career, I have been fortunate to have opportunities to speak on behalf of patients, families, and the profession. To do this you have to expand your knowledge, know your audience, and develop confidence in your delivery.

As a nursing leader and an APRN, I made it my goal to have a down to earth, layperson "elevator speech" that I could convey to a neighbor while walking my dog, to a cashier in a grocery store, or to a legislator or their aide expressing the importance of APRNs in providing healthcare to all people. The questions I asked myself were, "What do people know and understand about APRNs, what is most important for their healthcare delivery, what matters most to them, and what do APRNs offer to improve their health?"

My elevator speech has evolved over time. The first time I realized I needed one was at a legislator's local town hall when I was asked for about APRNs. That made me think that I needed a real-life example of a rule, law, or bill that would touch them or their constituents personally and, therefore, be meaningful and easily explained. I used an example of who had the authority to order a diagnostic test (physician, APRN). I asked them to imagine that having taken off work, they had shown up for a test but found out the test could not be performed because an APRN ordered it. This was a real-life example in which resources, time, and full-practice authority were all demonstrated.

The first time I delivered my refined elevator speech was outside an elevator in Washington, D.C., when my senator came off the elevator. The senator asked where we were coming from and if we had anything we wanted to discuss. At first everyone was quiet. Then I "leaned in" and said I would like to share my thoughts with him on advanced practice nursing and providing healthcare to Ohioans. I confidently shared my speech that I had practiced over and over. I was succinct, clear, and was able to articulate my thoughts. The elevator speech works!

See Figure 1.1.

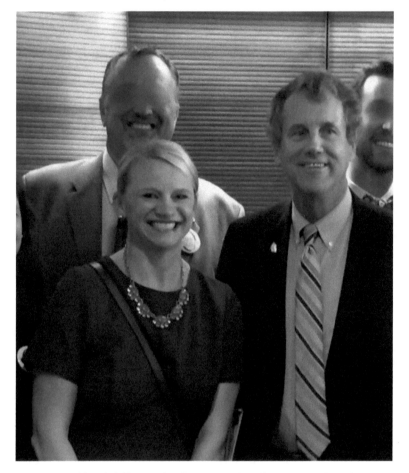

FIGURE 1.1 Meredith Foxx and colleagues give an elevator speech in the capital to Sen. Sherrod Brown (OH-D).

influence. Take the time to get to know the people you work with and to meet others in your organization. Volunteering for councils or committees will allow you to meet people from other units or other disciplines. The value in this process is that when you have a question or concern, one has a wider circle of contacts with whom to share ideas and ask questions. Furthermore, when a complex issue comes up, you have already established the relationship, and you do not have to negotiate that while getting a problem addressed.

Networking outside of one's organization provides opportunities for developing relationships with others who have similar professional interests whether one agrees with their positions. One can learn about different approaches to a problem or work together on solutions to reach a wider group. It provides yet another opportunity to not only learn about handling of issues outside of one's immediate sphere but also expand one's influence. Colleagues in one's networks can provide information to bolster one's policy positions as well as support the development of strategies to achieve policy goals. As one develops networks, one can call on one's network for assistance or referral to someone with expertise on the issue or policy. It is consistent with the expectations of the *Code of Ethics for Nurses* (ANA, 2015) that nurses collaborate with other health professionals and the public and work through professional organizations. Participation in professional associations is foundational to networking success.

Networking can take many forms; it is not limited to face-to-face contact. It utilizing a wide variety of modalities, often including technology. Successful strategies include participating in virtual events and implementing modifications in accordance with the environment. Networking is an opportunity to build trust through open and transparent communication. It provides an avenue for identifying people who may be interested in one's issues or supportive of one's positions and is a means of expanding one's social capital (see Chapter 7).

Learning about policy, understanding one's values, knowing the terrain, and networking all facilitate preparation for taking on a more substantive role in policy. Assessing areas for further development is essential for engaging in a policy journey.

POLICY PROCESS AND ANALYSIS

Understanding policymaking involves understanding the steps of the policy process, as well as the process for the analysis of potential policy options. This allows nurses to more clearly identify strategies to advance policies and the possible points of intervention for advocacy. A brief overview is presented here, with more details provided in Chapter 4.

PROCESS

Engaging in policy requires knowledge and comprehension of the policy process so that one's actions have a better chance of achieving the desired results. The basic phases of the policymaking process have much in common with the steps of the nursing process, and the comparison is helpful in beginning to demystify the policy process. Like the steps of the nursing process, policymaking is viewed as cyclical, involves continued feedback, and may take longer in certain phases, depending on the project being undertaken. Although this four-phase process is not fully comprehensive of all the steps in policymaking, the comparison provides a solid starting point for nurses reviewing and developing policy. Much like the work nurses do every day, it starts with the identification of a problem after assessment of a patient or a situation and then logically follows the problem-solving and decision-making steps used to solve everyday patient problems.

All nurses have the potential to identify, formulate, implement, and evaluate change based on their work setting, their community, and their passion. However, the number of steps and the details involved in policymaking vary. The most basic approach to policy identifies three policy-development phases: recognition and identification, formulation, and implementation. Because policymaking is an ongoing, evolutionary process, we have added a critical but often overlooked step, monitoring and evaluating, which is consistent with the fourth phase of the nursing process. Policymaking is easier to understand by breaking down the steps into pieces small enough to study, and seeing the pieces helps us understand the whole.

ANALYSIS

Integral to the policymaking process is policy analysis, which involves the detailed examination of various policy options in terms of their desired outcomes. Analyzing policy is a social and political activity because it can improve or hurt the well-being of large numbers of people and because the process involves professionals and interested stakeholders (Bardach & Patashnik, 2020). One approach often used to understand policy is to take an existing policy and/or problem and conduct an in-depth analysis to provide direction for the way forward. Policy analysis, similar to the nursing process, involves detailed steps and is an iterative process between defining the problem and developing the proposed policy. Bardach and Patashnik's (2020) eightfold path for policy analysis includes (a) defining the problem, (b) assembling some evidence, (c) constructing alternatives, (d) selecting criteria by which to evaluate the alternatives, (e) projecting the outcomes, (f) confronting trade-offs, (g) stopping to focus, narrow, and deepen the choices and deciding, and (h) communicating the policy. Developing skill in policy analysis is an important leadership competency in the complex world of healthcare whether it is done at the little-p or the big-P level. It involves understanding the broader picture. Policy analysis is an attempt to understand the desired and possible outcomes of policies, as well as their pitfalls or unintended consequences.

Improving policy is a task that numerous individuals, groups, organizations, legislative bodies, and governments seek as a goal to improve health. The recommendations of the IOM (2011) *Future of Nursing report:* are a call to action for nurses to take a leadership role in the healthcare systems of the future. To take on this leadership role, one must be well versed in the strategies and tools of policy, and the IOM recommendations, when achieved, will help provide the needed base structure for larger nurse involvement in policy from bedside to boardroom.

As the world, healthcare, and nursing have become progressively multifaceted, uncertain, changeable, and interconnected, the policymaking process has become more complex. Throughout the book, we discuss more detailed steps, tools, and techniques that are necessary for policymaking from bedside to boardroom.

POLICY AND ADVOCACY SELF-ASSESSMENT

Nurses may not realize the critical importance of honing their existing skills and developing new policy competencies to leverage nursing's potential power to influence healthcare and nursing practice locally and globally. Often they do not know where to start (Haebler & Fitting, 2018). Nurses, because of their education and experience, have the skill sets to be successful in policy. These include analytical skills, the ability to grasp the whole picture, communication, and organization, to name a few (Maryland & Gonzalez, 2012). For example, a psychiatric nurse or a nurse educator with experience in conducting groups may be able to transfer this skill to conducting a focus group to determine which message strategy for a proposed policy might resonate best with those traditionally opposed to a position.

Health policy competencies are multidimensional. Analyzing one's skills and competencies is an important foundational step in building policy skills, advocacy strategies, and the key considerations in providing a nursing lens in making policy (see Chapter 11). It is recognized that nurses may have different levels of policy competency. Completing an assessment will identify areas of strength, opportunities to leverage expertise, and areas for self-growth.

The ability to analyze problems, grasp the whole picture, communicate with persons holding diverse viewpoints, and organize are all skills that can be applied to the policy arena from the local community to the world stage. A useful method to assess one's political expertise or capital is the PZL (Patton–Zalon–Ludwick) Policy Assessment Framework©. The three faces of the model reflect its dimensions: policy engagement, partnership, and scope (see Figure 1.2). These facets are

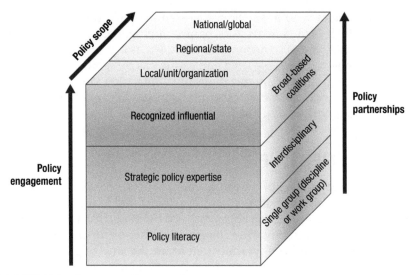

FIGURE 1.2 PZL Policy Assessment Framework.

interdependent and reflect complexities associated with the development of policy expertise. It can be used by nurses who feel they are new to the policy arena or more experienced in one or more dimensions.

POLICY ENGAGEMENT

The first dimension is policy engagement, which includes the progression from being policy literate to having strategic policy expertise and becoming a recognized policy influencer. This progression is universal, applying to everyone, not only nurses. Policy literacy is the beginning step. It includes civics (see Chapter 3), professional education, and clarification of one's values. Policy literacy is comprehending the context and processes by those who have decision-making authority. It includes having a basic knowledge of policy structures, processes, and outcomes within organizations and government. Furthermore, beginning competencies are demonstrated by engaging in basic activities that are reflective of that literacy, such as writing letters, meeting with officials, posting on social media, and/or taking part in other grassroots activities.

Strategic policy expertise refers to the use of one's leadership talents to advance specific policy goals. It is akin to an emotional quotient regarding one's ability to navigate the dynamic interaction of forces in policy development. It helps in positioning oneself and the group you are working with to develop, analyze, and provide insights. Strategic policy expertise involves knowing the terrain related to an issue or problem as well the processes involved in developing, changing, implementing, or evaluating policies.

Having this expertise enables nurses to be effective in using the tools of the policy process to achieve results. The need is great for nurses to have strategic policy expertise and for the voices of nurses to be heard to address the many issues involving practice and promote the health of the public. Having this expertise is essential if nurses are to fulfill the first *Future of Nursing* report's recommendation that nurses be "full partners, with physicians and other health professionals, in redesigning healthcare in the United States" (IOM, 2011, p. 7).

At the peak of policy engagement is becoming an influencer either regarding a specific issue, within an organization, or a more broadly recognized role in policy leadership. Nurses who have taken this step have the opportunity to influence care beyond their own patients. A recognized influential can be at any level, local, state, or national, and is someone who is known as a grasstop. These individuals are highly connected and respected and as such have significant sway with one or more people or groups or organizations or countries making decisions. Influence can come from any form of capital or combinations of capitals: intellectual, social, financial, or political, as described in Chapter 7.

POLICY PARTNERSHIPS

Moving to the second face of the framework are policy partnerships. Regardless of the setting, partnerships form an essential network and foundation for the achievement of common goals. Partnership work can be conducted within a single group (e.g., discipline or work group), an interdisciplinary team, or a broad-based coalition. The problem itself will typically determine the level of partnership needed.

Initially, nurses may be very comfortable within their single unit, or community group. They are familiar and comfortable with the values, beliefs, and responses of their colleagues at this level. Becoming involved in interdisciplinary groups provides the opportunity to gain new perspectives, diversity of opinions, and expand one's network, all of which can then be used to advance a policy agenda when faced with a problem that requires an interdisciplinary solution. Having experience outside of one's comfort zone will then enhance one's ability to bring together more diverse groups in coalitions to develop policy solutions for more complex problems. The diversity of problems and the range of their complexity can be addressed within a single group, or beyond (e.g., breastfeeding, firearm safety, school starting-time policies, recycling). For example, a policy focus may be limited to ensuring that schoolchildren have access to physical activities on days when the weather is bad. The next level may be an extension of the partnership beyond a single focus to an interdisciplinary level (e.g., working with other healthcare professionals) in addressing this concern across a school district or region. The transdisciplinary level includes working with broad coalitions (e.g., health professionals, community, consumer, and/or business groups) to initiate changes in schools across the country. Leadership in health policy, of necessity, is going to involve working with members of other disciplines and a diversity of stakeholders.

POLICY SCOPE

Policy scope refers to where one's policy activities are situated, whether it is a micro or macro level, whether it be within a self-contained clinical unit to an organizational or national policy. Specifically, we include whether policy activities are being conducted at little-p level or at the big-P level, upstream and downstream, and HiAP as described earlier. The scope needs to be considered because efforts to achieve policy goals may need to be implemented at multiple levels at the point of care, within an organization, through statewide regulation as with full practice authority, or on the national level with the Affordable Care Act (ACA). Policies related to a single issue such as full-practice authority can be formulated for the organizational, state, or national level to illustrate policy scope. At the organizational or little-p level, policies related to full-practice authority may be related to hospital privileges. At the state level, it may involve prescriptive authority or collaborative agreement requirements. At the federal level, it may involve differential reimbursement policies. Another example is workplace violence, clearly a local issue that can be addressed with organizational policies. It has also been addressed with legislation at the state level, which has considerable variation. Then, at the federal level, there are regulations promulgated by OSHA, as well as legislation, the Workplace Violence Prevention for Health Care and Social Workers Act that has been introduced in the 117th Congress.

In summary, it is recognized that these dimensions, policy engagement, policy partnerships, and policy scope are not isolated but that they overlap, often intersect, but are not linear. Nurses can be at different levels of policy competency for each dimension. Developing one's policy expertise involves being strategic about where one can broaden one's scope to increase policy influence. In completing such the assessment, it is important to consider how changes in the environment, the issue at hand, and specifically, the political environment influence the competencies that are needed.

ENDURING ISSUES IN NURSING: THE LONG VIEW

Key enduring issues in the forefront for nurses requiring a long view include access to care, workplace, and workforce needs, nurse well-being, and the environment. Each of these issues speaks to the advocacy for the profession and society. The importance of these issues are varyingly highlighted in the *Future of Nursing 2020–2020* report (National Academies, 2021), and the *Global Strategic Directions for Nursing and Midwifery* (2021–2025; World Health Organization [WHO], 2021). Access to care is embedded in each component of the Quadruple Aim of healthcare: improving the experience of care, improving population health, reducing costs, and improving the work life of healthcare providers (Bodenheimer & Sinsky, 2014).

ACCESS TO CARE

The term access to healthcare conjures up many images about the inadequacies of the delivery of healthcare system among the myriad of stakeholders. According to the Agency on Healthcare Research Quality (AHRQ, n.d.), access to healthcare means having "the timely use of personal health services to achieve the best health outcomes" (para. 1). Four areas considered by AHRQ regarding access to care include coverage, available services, timeliness of care, and adequacy of the workforce. Nurses can inform policies about access because of their experiences on the frontlines directly observing care, bureaucratic hurdles, and gaps.

Coverage is how people get entered into the healthcare system. Major stakeholders in influencing access to healthcare are insurance providers. Insurance coverage both private and public facilitates access to healthcare, but gaps remain, with the uninsured being less likely to receive timely services and having worse health outcomes. These problems vary from state to state and within states. For example, health outcomes in states that have not expanded Medicaid options are worse (Guth & Ammula, 2021). See this interactive link for state by state coverage: www.kff.org/medicaid/issue-brief/status-of-state-medicaid-expansion-decisions-interactive-map/.

Removing practice barriers to the full scope of one's education is a key strategy in increasing healthcare coverage. Over half of the states still have restrictions on APRN practice. Although barriers to practice are typically discussed in the context of APRNs (clinical nurse specialists, certified nurse midwives, certified

RN anesthetists, nurse practitioners). RNs providing direct care also face barriers related to their scope of practice. Removing barriers for both RNs and APRNs will increase coverage and the availability of services and decrease delays due to bureaucratic processes. The AARP is a strong supporter of ensuring that nurses are able to contribute to the full extent of their education, skills, and certification.

APRNs have had an integral role in the delivery of care in retail-based health clinics because they provide access points for more individuals to enter the health-care system (ANA, 2009). The urgent need to increase primary care capacity led to a high-level policy discussion, sponsored by the Josiah Macy Jr. Foundation (2016), regarding the role of RNs as team members in primary care. The ensuing report indicated that RNs need to be appropriately prepared and used to meet the primary care needs of the nation. Two of the key recommendations include strengthening primary care content and learning experiences in prelicensure RN and RN baccalaureate education, as well as redesigning primary care practice to use RNs' abilities. The appropriate use of RNs in primary care has been demonstrated to improve health outcomes, reduce cost, and improve patient satisfaction (Josiah Macy Jr. Foundation, 2016). RNs can be used to enhance transitional care, medication reconciliation, care coordination, chronic disease management, and patient education, to name a few primary care roles.

Services are defined as having a usual source of care for everyday healthcare needs, and for screening and preventive services. Creative ways to use nurses effectively in the provision of services include federally qualified health centers; home health, transitional care, care coordination, and case management; and school-based, nurse-managed, retail, and employer-based clinics. These creative models and subsequent policy changes can enhance access to services. For example, nursing has taken a leadership role in care coordination—one of the profession's traditional roles and a vital element in healthcare reform. Care coordination helps ensure that patients' needs and preferences regarding health services and information sharing are met over time and involve the deliberate organization of patient care activities to facilitate the appropriate healthcare service delivery.

Timeliness is the ability to provide care within an appropriate time frame after a need is identified. Alleviating provider shortages is critical to timely care. For example, the wait for a new appointment with a behavioral health provider may be 4 months or longer. If a person or family is experiencing a mental health crisis, the choice is often to wait or seek emergency department care. These shortages also burden primary care providers who have not been adequately prepared educationally for the influx of patients with behavioral health problems. Similarly, delays in other arenas, such as cancer care, have serious long-term consequences.

Workforce shortages are a chronic, recurring problems impacting access. The federal government classifies shortage areas by area, population, or facility with different designations (e.g., health professions shortage areas, medically underserved areas, medically underserved populations, exceptionally underserved populations; Health Resources and Services Administration [HRSA], n.d.). to plan for workforce needs. In 2021, there were 84 million Americans living in health professions shortage areas (HRSA, 2021). Not having enough nurses decreases the quality of care across all healthcare settings. Without adequate numbers of well-prepared nurses in the workforce, is it not possible to meet the needs for coverage, services, and timeliness of care.

Nurses have a critical role to play in access to care through the recognition of their value and the removal of barriers that restrict their contributions. Nurses have numerous opportunities to influence policy through individual advocacy, collectively through nurses organizations and special interest groups, collaboration with consumer groups and other stakeholders (e.g., Robert Wood Johnson Foundation, Josiah Macy Jr. Foundation). For example, the Robert Wood Johnson Foundation and AARP created the Future of Nursing: Campaign for Action with affiliates in all 50 states to strengthen nursing through collaboration with other providers, businesses, educators, and consumers, and so forth.

WORKPLACE AND WORKFORCE NEEDS

Workplace and workforce needs are intertwined. *Workplace* refers to the setting for the delivery of services and the related structural elements. *Workforce* refers to the body of individuals employed. These areas have long been recognized as critical for quality patient outcomes and safety and, therefore, comprise an important arena for policy monitoring, development, and implementation. Both have long been championed by the ANA, state nurses associations, and specialty nurses associations. These needs are supported by research evidence linking Magnet™ recognition with improvement in the quality of work environment and patient and nurse outcomes (Kutney-Lee et al., 2015). According to the Lucian Leape Institute of the National Patient Safety Foundation (NPSF, 2013), now part of the Institute for Healthcare Improvement (IHI), "if we expect the workforce to care for patients, we need to care for the workforce. Workplace safety is also inextricably linked to patient safety. Unless caregivers are given the protection, respect and support they need, they are more likely to make errors, fail to follow safe practice, and not work well in teams" (p. 1). The World Health Assembly endorsed the WHO's *Global Strategic Directions for Nursing and Midwifery* and adopted a resolution that calls upon countries to not only protect and safeguard the nurse workforce but also to invest in the workforce (WHO, 2021). What is notable is that this was the first time the World Health Assembly adopted a nursing strategy (Ford, 2021). This is even more important with the advent of the COVID-19 pandemic.

Ongoing challenges for nursing include the shortage of nurses, workforce needs, and the workplace environment. The overlapping workplace/workforce needs of the profession can be broadly categorized into professional development, safety, staffing, respect and civility, health, and conditions of employment. See Exhibit 1.2 for a listing of potential areas for nursing policy development. Although not meant to be exhaustive, these areas provide opportunities for nurses to make improvements in their work environment, as well as to advance issues of relevance to the profession. In examining the range of these work-related issues, it is clear that opportunities for policy involvement exist at the little-p level within organizations or at the big-P level through local, state, federal, and even international initiatives. It also important to include upstream approaches, such as Title VIII funding, as well as the downstream interventions implemented at individual work sites.

One of the reasons nurse leaders established the ANA in 1896 was to address deplorable working conditions. The complexities of nurses' workforce needs are illustrated by the changing landscape of the workday that cuts across issues related to patient safety, staffing, fatigue, mandatory overtime, and overtime compensation. In 1903, the first nurse practice act was passed in North Carolina. The ANA and state nurses associations have been at the forefront of addressing and improving the poor working conditions of nurses. One area of workforce that needs highlighted here is working hours.

EXHIBIT 1.2   NURSING WORKPLACE AND WORKFORCE NEEDS

Workplace safety	Musculoskeletal injuries Occupational exposures to communicable diseases Occupational exposures to hazardous substances Reproductive rights and hazards Resources for impaired nurses Safe needles, sharps, and devices Safe patient handling Slips, trips, and falls Violence Work release during a disaster
Staffing and support services	Adequacy of access to medications, supplies, and equipment Adequacy of support (e.g., pharmacy, housekeeping) Fatigue Healthy work hours and schedules Mandatory overtime Safe staffing levels
Employment conditions	Continuing education Credentialing and privileging Disabilities Diversity, equity, and inclusion Family medical leave Full practice authority for advanced practice nurses Mandatory vaccinations Overtime Paid time off Pay for performance Preemployment screening (smoking, weight) Reimbursement for advanced practice nurses Sick time Union representation Wage compression

In 1934, the ANA House of Delegates approved a resolution, for example, calling for an 8-hour workday for nurses (ANA, n.d.). Working hours remain an issue today. Many hospitals transitioned to 12-hour shifts in the late 1970s to provide an attractive incentive for nurse recruitment and retention. This scheduling flexibility was a boon for some facilities, allowing nurses to return to school and providing more days and weekends off, for example. Now, nearly 50 years later, research findings justify reexamination of long working hours. Disadvantages include adverse health effects for nurses and quality issues for patients (e.g., care continuity). The increasingly robust accumulation of evidence demonstrates the extent of these adverse effects (Griffiths et al., 2016; Rogers et al., 2004; Sagherian et al., 2017; Westley et al., 2020).

For many years, nurses associations, including the ANA, and unions indicated that nurses should determine whether they could safely work an additional shift or accept an overtime assignment. Policy initiatives restricting the use of mandatory overtime for nurses have not been addressed in all states. This policy debate will continue. However, some organizations are reframing the issue by taking a more holistic approach by examining fatigue, sleep deprivation, human performance factors, and role expectations, in addition to shift length. Some widely publicized errors and research that extended working hours can be detrimental to patient safety have led to more awareness of the potential negative consequences of not addressing mandatory overtime. Despite the evidence related to the negative outcomes of longer work shifts, developing policies to address the needs of nurses while maintaining patient safety is challenging. Staff nurses need and want fair scheduling of their work hours.

Policies developed to address working hours and a host of other work needs must be fair, conducted using a deliberative process, and reflect the interests of diverse stakeholder groups. These efforts are ongoing and cut across the spectrum of policy development in healthcare from policy with the little-p (e.g., how a nurse handles the response to a supervisor's request to work overtime or take on a heavier patient workload) to big-P policies addressed with legislative proposals.

WELL-BEING

Nurses have always been concerned with the well-being of others. The participation of more than 100,000 nurses since 1976 in the Nurses' Health Study (2016) is one obvious example of nurses being willing to take part in research for the betterment of healthcare. Unfortunately, nurses' own health has often not been the priority of many. According to Pam Cipriano, PhD, RN, NEA-BC, FAAN, ANA past president, "While nurses are committed to caring for others, they often struggle to care for themselves, due to long work hours, lack of sleep and lack of access to healthy food" (ANA, 2017a, para. 2). Without a healthy nurse workforce, it is difficult to promote the health of the nation. Key stakeholder organizations within nursing and beyond with a mission of improving health and safeguarding the well-being of nurses have launched initiatives to address this problem. These include the IHI's Joy in Work and the ANA's Healthy Nurse, Healthy Nation (Hume, 2018).

Organizations are recognizing the importance of well-being by joining forces in the provision of resources. The American Nurse's Foundation's (2020) Well-Being Initiative has partnered with the ANA, the American Association of Critical Care Nurses, the American Psychiatric Nurses Association, and the ENA. Not only are the organizations providing services and resources to nurses, but they are also joining forces to advance policy initiatives to prioritize the well-being of the workforce and making the work environment more hospitable to workers.

Healthcare organizations themselves, have made changes in the environment including policies that support well-being by creating a safe and productive workplace. These innovations have included healthy vending and menu choices, walking meetings, and fitness activities like yoga and mindfulness. Benefits have been redesigned to reward prevention and wellness. Exhibit 1.3 illustrates some of the more common areas for the development of initiatives to support nurse well-being.

Nurses' well-being is enhanced by professional development, respect and civility and health. Some of these issues faced by nurses may be named differently, but have persisted over time, for example, "incivility," "bullying," "lateral violence," "workplace violence," and "nurses eat their young," are all descriptors illustrating the breadth, depth and complexity of a recurring workplace issue related to how nurses are treated by their colleagues. These concerns have been addressed by nurses and organizations over time, yet they still continue.

Healthcare organizations are recognizing the value of investing in the health of their own community as a strategic business initiative. These programs are

EXHIBIT 1.3   INITIATIVES SUPPORTING NURSES' WELL-BEING

Professional development	Adequacy of the supply of nurses Distribution and use of nurses and advanced practice nurses Diversity, equity, and inclusion Education International recruitment Role, practicing to full scope of education and skills
Respect and civility	Blame-free environment, just culture Bullying Harassment, sexual harassment Physical and verbal abuse Respect for all team members
Health	Healthy nurse Work engagement Work–life balance

important to the well-being of the nurse workforce. However, nurses need to be at the policy tables when planning, implementing, and evaluating these initiatives. This is another arena in which the value of nurses needs to be recognized. Certain settings in healthcare have well-known workplace/workforce needs that require tailored interventions to improve the well-being of the nursing staff (e.g., violence in psychiatric and ED settings, bullying in operating rooms, physical injuries in long-term care, etc.). With the advent of COVID-19, in 2020, jobs in nursing homes have been identified as one of the deadliest (Lewis, 2021). All these may require programmatic improvements, but without policy, changes may not be long-lasting.

THE ENVIRONMENT

Nurses have long recognized the role of the environment in maintaining health. Florence Nightingale emphasized that the environment should promote health and in no way be harmful. Her views were that the provision of fresh air, light, a quiet environment, nutrition, warmth, clean water, sanitation, and cleanliness was essential to this vision. Nurses today are continuing these efforts for the environment at the patient level and in our communities and globally. The newest revision of the Nursing: Scope and Standards of Practice addresses an important update regarding the environment in standard 18 moving from practice that is environmentally safe and healthy to nurses having the obligation to "practice in a manner that advances environmental safety and health" (ANA, 2021). Advancing safety and health necessitates action via policy.

Environmental factors are central to the elimination of healthcare inequities around the world. Access to clean water is vital to preventing and treating life-threatening diarrhea, which kills yearly over a half million children younger than age 5 (World Health Organization, 2017). Cleaner air in the community where we live and work means that children are less likely to get asthma. Every day, we learn more about the relationship of certain diseases to the environment: asthma, allergies, emphysema, cancer, heart disease, and stress. In fact, it is difficult in the course of a day to come across a patient whose health is not impacted by the environment. These increasing numbers and everyday experiences with our patients are a call to action for policies that help make improvements to the environment and strengthen public health so that everyone can live to their fullest potential (see Chapters 13 and 14).

Nurses are ideal natural advocates for environmental health because of our professional commitment to social justice and our skills in working with our communities. Nurses are uniquely situated to understand environmental issues and can articulate them to the public to garner support and build coalitions for action that can improve environmental health at work, in schools, in hospitals, and in communities. Whether nurses care for workers experiencing lung diseases from mines, factories, or farms across the world or, more regionally, care for children with lead exposure from contaminated water, they have a vital role to play to prevent harm in the environmental policy arena.

Disasters, whether natural (e.g., climate-change-induced storms, fires) or human-caused (e.g., terrorist attacks, mass shootings, civil unrest), often have a high impact on those with the least reserves, the most vulnerable in society. The increase in the number of heat waves and storms has resulted in more death and devastation. The effects of climate change on health outcomes are far-reaching and include numerous arenas where nurses can work on policies and also mitigate their effects. See Figure 1.3 from the CDC. Socioeconomic and demographic inequities easily translate into increased healthcare disparities when disaster hits. In every year between 1994 and 2013, more than 200 million persons were harmed in some way by the almost 7,000 recorded disasters (United Nations Centre for Research on the Epidemiology of Disasters [CRED] and United Nations Office for Disaster Risk Reduction [UNDRR], 2015). Natural disasters have shown the need for, and provided the opportunity to address, environmental health issues. Nurses

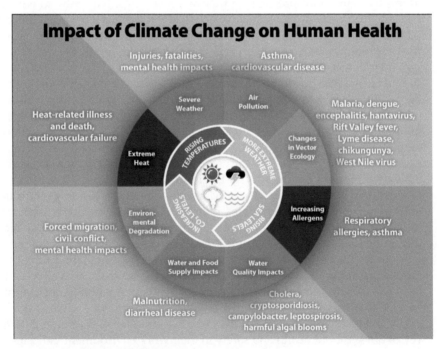

FIGURE 1.3 Climate effects on health.

Source: Centers for Disease Control and Prevention. (2021). *Impact of climate change on human health.* https://www.cdc.gov/climateandhealth/effects/

have responded individually and collectively when disasters have hit, often focusing their efforts broadly but also working to help the poor and often the elderly, who have fragile support systems and often bear the brunt of a disaster.

Nurses and their professional associations along with innumerable charitable and volunteer agencies have traditionally played an important role in disasters. The ANA (2017b) has actively pursued examining and advocating for legal and ethical roles of nurses in natural disasters and, as a result, issued a brief, *Who Will Be There? Ethics, the Law, and a Nurse's Duty to Respond in a Disaster.* The brief discusses some of the ethical and personal issues related to the duty of a nurse to respond to disasters and raises questions to consider before disaster strikes. Also contained in the brief are principles that need to be included when developing standards of care for all healthcare providers involved in disasters, as well as information on the ANA's involvement with other interprofessional groups. Leading the way internationally have been the ICN and the World Association for Disaster and Emergency Medicine, which conducted a review of the use of the ICN Framework for Disaster Nursing Competencies (Hutton et al., 2016).

The latest *Future of Nursing 2020–2030* (National Academies, 2021) report calls for strengthening nurses' competencies with regard to disaster preparedness and public health emergencies as a strategy for addressing the social determinants of health, equity, and population health in future decades. The CRED developed the Sendai Framework for Disaster Risk Reduction 2015–2030 to serve as a roadmap for to prevent new risk, reduce existing risk, and increase resilience (UNDRR, 2020–2021).

If we can consider the familiar phrase that all politics is local, we need not look very far for an opportunity to improve environmental health. Nurses themselves, as briefly addressed in the chapter so far, may be at risk for harm from environmental hazards in their own work settings and may contribute to environmental harms by using poor practices in their work settings. Not only do we have more research that demonstrates the link between the work environment of nurses and patient outcomes, but also we have the link between the work environment and the health of nurses. Nurses can and should be at the forefront of efforts to ensure that their working conditions are safe.

Nurses may be informed about the hazards associated with chemotherapeutic agents, but they may not even know about the nature of the hazards associated with chemicals such as cleaners, solvents, disinfectants, and pesticides despite ubiquitous safety data sheets. Hospitals and other healthcare organizations expose employees to a wide range of hazards: biological, chemical, ergonomical, physical, and psychological. A 2007 survey of more than 1,500 nurses across the United States (sponsored by the ANA, Environmental Working Group, Health Care Without Harm, and University of Maryland School of Nursing) indicates that a third of nurses had high exposures, defined as being exposed at least twice a week, to at least five chemicals and other hazardous substances for 10 or more years (Environmental Working Group, 2007). These data indicate the need for nurses to work to implement strategies at the little-p level by marshaling forces to replace hazardous materials and instituting engineering controls, as well as at the big-P level to institute necessary legislative and regulatory action to ensure that nurses and their coworkers have a healthy and safe environment to deliver quality care.

It is not just hazardous chemicals that are a concern for nurses. A 2011 ANA survey of nurses about health and safety in their work environment indicates nearly all nurses say that they have worked despite experiencing musculoskeletal pain. Nurses' top two health and safety concerns were (a) the acute or chronic effects of stress and overwork and disabling musculoskeletal injury, and (b) concerns about on-the-job assault, which have increased (ANA, 2011). In a Healthy Nurse® survey (2018), 14%

EXHIBIT 1.4   REPRESENTATIVE ORGANIZATIONS ADDRESSING
ENVIRONMENTAL ISSUES IN HEALTHCARE

Agency for Toxic Substances and Disease Registry, Environmental Health Nursing Initiative: www.atsdr.cdc.gov
Alliance of Nurses for Healthy Environments: www.envirn.org
American Nurses Association, Healthy Work Environment: www.nursingworld.org/practice-policy/work-environment/
Health Care Without Harm: www.noharm.org
National Environmental Health Foundation: www.neefusa.org
Practice Green Health: www.practicegreenhealth.org

of nurses report nodding off or falling asleep while driving in the last 30 days. In 2019's Healthy Nurse survey, 77% of nurses reported that workplace stress put them at a significant level of risk. The results of these surveys and the evidence drawn from the world indicate that there is much work to do and that each nurse needs to be involved in making environments at work and the community safer for all.

Consider the possibilities for one's level of involvement. Numerous organizations address environmental issues in healthcare (see Exhibit 1.4). Nurses can become part of these groups or access numerous resources available on their websites.

Nurses are also tackling broader issues of environmental concern. The Pennsylvania State Nurses Association (PSNA) submitted a proposal that was adopted by the ANA's House of Delegates calling for a national moratorium on new permits of unconventional oil and natural gas extraction (fracking) until human ecological safety could be ensured (McDermott-Levy et al., 2013). The PSNA's bold move gave a national voice to a problem experienced at the local level. It also illustrates the potential within the nursing community to address environmental health problems. Access to clean water for communities, as so vividly brought to the forefront by the Flint, Michigan, crisis is central to the national debate on this issue. Acting upon the issue of safe water supplies for communities, the Alliance of Nurses for Healthy Environments (2017) released a report in 2017 designed to provide nurses with the advocacy tools for strengthening the protections for clean water, which is critical for not only for good health but also safe nursing practice.

IMPLICATIONS FOR THE FUTURE

Nurses' engagement in policy roles must increase in the future. Healthcare has become increasingly complex, the population is aging, and the population is increasingly experiencing more health problems because of chronic diseases and the opioid epidemic. This confluence of trends means that the need for nursing services will increase. At 4.3 million strong, nurses will continue to be the largest healthcare professional group. The public will continue to depend on nurses and trust them for the delivery of high-quality healthcare. We have had dramatic increases in the overall educational preparation of the nursing workforce. This means that nurses are prepared to take on a more significant role in policy from the little-p to the big-P level. The public will come to expect nurses to take on a more active role in policy at the upstream level.

The death of a nurse colleague, let alone one that resulted from a suicide, is devastating and very often engenders feelings of helplessness. This is compounded with the mantra of thinking about suicide as being always preventable and the culture of silence surrounding suicide and mental health. Nurses have an integral role in examining and advocating for policies in the workplace that can provide nurses and other healthcare professionals with concrete guidance. Likewise, they can join with nurses associations and other advocacy groups in lobbying for the establishment of programs and resources. While downstream policies and services that address mental health/behavioral health issues are essential, upstream approaches are needed as well.

At the little-p level, most commonly those at the workplace, policies that support mental health and foster a "mental health–friendly culture," which is consistent with efforts to support diversity, equity, and inclusion are needed. Advocating for work environment policies supportive to mental health and well instituting educational policies is critical. Healthcare employers can proactively develop policies and protocols to screen and implement strategies to reduce nurse suicide. Understanding and reducing contributing risk factors will play a role in prevention and create a culture of wellness. Educating managers and nurses to recognize nurses at risk is essential. Employee wellness programs, including their mental health components, must be easily accessible and accepted as valid and helpful programs. Ensuring nurses have access to behavioral health services when involved with or exposed to traumatic events, such as sentinel events, should be incorporated into employee wellness programs. With mergers and acquisitions, the country's now very large healthcare systems have no excuse to not put mental health issues front and center in creating a healthy work environment.

At the big-P level, a multipronged policy approach is needed to address access to quality prevention and treatment services, mandatory reporting and data collection, and education. Access to services at the workplace and in health in general is needed. The Dr. Lorna Breen Health Provider Protection Act was introduced in both the 116th and 117th Congresses in the Senate and House of Representatives. This act, strongly endorsed by the ANA, is designed to decrease burnout among healthcare providers, provide grants for suicide prevention training, improve programs for behavioral health promotion for providers caring for patients with COVID-19, and require the CDC to develop related policy recommendations.

Mandatory reporting of nurses' deaths by suicide is necessary for data collection. One recommendation is for states to report occupational data to the NVDRS at the CDC. Suicide data can be evaluated by boards of nursing, which could then lead to further policy recommendations such as mandatory educational requirements. Analysis of statewide data collection can identify gaps that need to be addressed more fully in order to implement policies related to mental health services.

Education related to mental health services and specifically suicide prevention includes education and the provision of resources for all nurses, enhanced education for healthcare providers, including APRNs without specialized psychiatric background, and enhanced opportunities for growing the mental health workforce in nursing and beyond. Mandatory continuing education for nurses can increase awareness and early intervention. Many such programs have been established. These multiple opportunities to improve education and thus the provision of mental health resources require a variety of policy strategies at the local, state, and national level. Nurses can join with efforts at each of these levels through their workplace and then professional associations at the local, state, and national level.

The ANA has taken a leadership role in practice and advocacy for nurse suicide prevention and resilience as part of the ANA Enterprise Healthy Nurse Healthy Nation initiative (www.nursingworld.org/practice-policy/nurse-suicide-prevention/). ANA's website provides resources for nurses as well as identifies opportunities for nurses to become involved in additional resource and policy development. Nurses can get involved not only in ANA's initiatives but also those of other associations, such as the American Organization for Nursing Leadership, and the American Association of Nurse Anesthesiology, the latter being particularly hard hit by nurse suicides.

Nurses are positioned to take on more substantial policy roles. Nurses have opportunities to engage in policy work because they are intimately connected to patients who are experiencing life's most difficult and challenging moments as they struggle with healthcare transitions (e.g., acute illness, management of chronic illness, illness at birth, death, and transfer from one health state to another). These experiences enable nurses to identify policy problems and craft workable policy solutions.

Nurses are at different stages of policy engagement. They may not know how or when work, family, personal life, community, education, or other circumstances prompt taking on a more active policy role. However, because of nurses' unique perspectives, nurses need to be nimble to take advantage of opportunities to influence population health and/or advance the profession.

Work in policy is the opportunity to influence care beyond the immediate circumstance of direct care for one patient, several patients, or a larger number of patients in a practice. Nursing has a history of singular leaders who have made phenomenal strides to advance nursing and promote health. However, the increasingly interconnected, regulated, and global world of healthcare means that advancing health and promoting health will require the ability to work in interdisciplinary teams and have exquisite policy-making skills. Nurse educators in formal educational programs and practice settings have embraced the opportunity to prepare nursing students and nurses in interprofessional collaboration. This, coupled with having advanced education, being a member of professional groups, and having a network, are critical foundational steps for influencing policy. Gale Adcock, day in and day out, saw the needs of patients in her clinic and spent years advocating as a professional nurse. These experiences provided her with the perspectives and the passion to pursue policymaking in a legislative role.

People enter the nursing profession because they are passionate about caring for people and promoting their patients' health and well-being. Participation in policymaking can extend that passion upstream. The uncertainties presented in the current healthcare environment in the United States have ignited passions across the country, and it is anticipated that greater activism of nurses who are aligned with professional and consumer groups will be seen, and more nurses will pursue unique causes on their own. Professional associations and consumer groups need to be ready to marshal the forces of this increased activism to advance their agendas.

Being silent within an organization has repercussions for the safety and well-being of patients. Being silent within our society, organizations, associations, community, and government has repercussions for the advancement of the profession and the health of the population. Action is needed to protect the policymaking processes of democracy to protect the rights of the people served by nurses and the most vulnerable among them. Shaping policy not only is critical for improving healthcare and improving the practice environment for nurses but is an ethical responsibility of all nurses, not just a dedicated few. The challenge is to increase the commitment of all nurses, not only those working in tandem for broader issues but also those working on issues germane to a very specialized area of practice. Taking an active role in policy is every nurse's responsibility as a member of our profession.

KEY CONCEPTS

1. The policy process includes recognition and identification of problems, formulation of policies, their implementation, and then monitoring and evaluating the results.

2. Nurses, by being at the sharp end of care and having intimate knowledge of the healthcare system, are critical to the development, monitoring, and evaluation of policy related to safety and quality.

3. Nurses must have substantive roles in policy at all levels.

4. Nurses are well prepared for adapting their skills to the policy arena.

5. Passion about an issue often fuels policy activism.

6. Key documents and reports from the ANA, the ICN, WHO, and the NAM all describe the essential roles and responsibilities of nurses not only for improving health but addressing the social determinants of health.

7. Being political is an essential component of nursing practice.

8. The PZL Policy Assessment Framework is a useful tool for analyzing one's policy engagement, partnership, and scope in developing one's policy journey.

9. Enduring issues for nurses include efforts to address access to care, workplace and workforce needs, nurse well-being, and the environment.

10. Being silent is not an option as it is detrimental to the well-being of patients; action is necessary to protect vulnerable patients and the ability of nurses to provide care.

SUMMARY

Nurses are an essential part of healthcare delivery, and as such, they have an integral leadership role and responsibility in the development of health policy. Nurses have myriad opportunities to be involved in health policy on the continuum from providing direct care to the boardroom, with the formulation and implementation of policy at the top echelons of complex organizations at the state, national, and even international levels. Some forces influencing nursing practice and healthcare include access to care, workplace and workforce needs, well-being, and the environment. Nurses are increasingly being called on to be leaders regardless of their position. Being a nurse means being a leader, being a leader means being involved in policy. Policy work is every nurse's work. It involves multiple areas and alignment of multiple forces and stakeholders to achieve a common goal in advancing health. Addressing a policy in one arena very often leads to new issues and new policy directions. Nurses are well positioned to lead the way in policy, from the bedside to the boardroom.

END-OF-CHAPTER RESOURCES

LEARNING ACTIVITIES

1. Discuss your earliest experiences related to civics and policy with a problem that had a policy component.
2. Compare and contrast current policy activities of the ANA and one specialty nursing organization.
3. Identify one or two policy activities that you will accomplish while in school, and then determine what three to five goals related to policy you will accomplish within 3 years of graduation.
4. Describe your goals for your policy involvement in the next 3 to 5 years and the steps necessary to achieve them.
5. Develop an elevator speech to counteract misinformation about nurses' roles in policy.
6. On a daily basis for a week, read a paper and/or watch a news show and identify a political issue that is discussed. For every issue, discuss at least three reasons why the issue is important to nursing and/or healthcare and how a nursing lens is important to policy solutions.
7. At your workplace or clinical practicum site, identify three policy issues that are currently under discussion. What is the impetus for those policies? Describe your role, or potential role, and the impact that the policy will have on you.
8. Describe the status of policies to mitigate violence at your workplace, organization, and state.
9. Create a short advocacy video that can be used to present an issue to the public, stakeholders, or policy makers.
10. Select an issue that has inconsistent policies or inconsistent application of policies (e.g., mandatory vaccinations) for a debate.
11. Determine if a nurse is holding an elected office in your state, city, or local government or any position that changes the health of the community.
12. What is your specialty nurses group doing about suicide prevention?
13. Determine how long your state has submitted data to the NVDRS. Using WISQARS, determine your state's data for suicide compares to the reported suicide rates for nurses. https://www.cdc.gov/violenceprevention/datasources/nvdrs/index.html
14. Track recent legislation at the state and federal level to address violence against nurses, full practice authority, clean air or water quality, or another issue related to nursing practice or community health.

E-RESOURCES

- AARP. Advanced Practice Registered Nurse. APRN https://states.aarp.org/tag/advanced-practice-registered-nurse-aprn
- Agency for Healthcare Research and Quality. PSNet, Patient Safety Network https://psnet.ahrq.gov/
- American Academy of Nursing. Edge Runners http://www.aannet.org/initiatives/edge-runners
- American Association of Critical-Care Nurses. Well-Being Initiative https://www.aacn.org/nursing-excellence/well-being-initiative

■ American Association of Nurse Practitioners. COVID-19 state emergency response: Temporarily suspended and waived practice agreement requirements https://www.aanp.org/advocacy/state/covid-19-state-emergency-response-temporarily-suspended-and-waived-practice-agreement-requirements

■ American Association of Suicidology. Workplace Suicide Prevention https://suicidology.org/2019/10/10/workplace-guidelines/

■ American Nurses Association. Advocacy https://www.nursingworld.org/practice-policy/advocacy/

■ Centers for Disease Control and Prevention. National Violent Data Reporting System (NVDRS) https://www.cdc.gov/violenceprevention/datasources/nvdrs/index.html

■ Congress: https://www.congress.gov

■ Dr. Peggy Berry Talks Occupational Health https://podcasts.apple.com/us/podcast/nhe-season-3-13-dr-peggy-berry-talks-occupational-health/id1316089858?i=1000472009745

■ Future of Nursing Campaign for Action https://campaignforaction.org/wp-content/uploads/2020/11/APRN-Practice-two-pager-1-4-2021-FINAL.pdf

■ Introduction to Upstream https://www.youtube.com/watch?v=qarQXqKbmLg&feature=youtu.be

■ Nurses on Boards Coalition www.nursesonboardscoalition.org/

■ Office of Disease Prevention and Health Promotion. Social Determinants of Health https://health.gov/healthypeople/objectives-and-data/social-determinants-health

■ Suicide Prevention Resource Center https://www.sprc.org

■ University of Guelph. *Florence Nightingale and public health policy: Theory, activism and public health administration* http://www.uoguelph.ca/~cwfn/nursing/theory.htm

■ World Health Communication Associates. International Council of Nurses. *Promoting health: Advocacy guide for health professionals* https://www.whcaonline.org/uploads/publications/ICN-NEW-28.3.2010.pdf

REFERENCES

Agency for Healthcare Research and Quality. (n.d.). *Access to care*. https://www.ahrq.gov/topics/access-care.html

Alliance of Nurses for Healthy Environments. (2017). *Water and health. Opportunities for nursing action*. https://envirn.org/water-and-health/

American Nurses Association. (n.d.). *Historical review*. https://www.nursingworld.org/globalassets/docs/ana/ana-expandedhistoricalreview.pdf

American Nurses Association. (2009, December 11). Additional access to care: Supporting nurse practitioners in retail-based health clinics. https://www.nursingworld.org/practice-policy/nursing-excellence/official-position-statements/id/additional-access-to-care/

American Nurses Association. (2010). *Nursing's social policy statement. The essence of the profession* (3rd ed.). Author.

American Nurses Association. (2011). *2011 ANA health and safety survey*. Author https://www.nursingworld.org/practice-policy/work-environment/health-safety/health-safety-survey/

American Nurses Association. (2015). *Code of ethics for nurses with interpretive statements*. Author.

American Nurses Association. (2017a, February 2). ANA Enterprise announces Sage Products as sponsor of its Healthy Nurse, Healthy Nation™ grand challenge. https://www.nursingworld.org/news/news-releases/2017-news-releases/ana-enterprise-announces-sage-products-as-sponsor-of-its-healthy-nurse-healthy-nation-grand-challenge/

American Nurses Association. (2017b). *Who will be there? Ethics, the law, and a nurse's duty to respond in a disaster*. Author. https://www.nursingworld.org/~4ad845/globalassets/docs/ana/who-will-be-there_disaster-preparedness_2017.pdf

American Nurses Association. (2021). *Nursing: Scope and standards of practice* (4th ed.). Author.

American Nurses Foundation. (2020, May 19). *American Nurses Foundation launches national well-being initiative for nurses*. https://www.nursingworld.org/news/news-releases/2020/american-nurses-foundation-launches-national-well-being-initiative-for-nurses/

American Organization of Nurse Executives, & Emergency Nurses Association. (2015). *Toolkit for mitigating violence in the workplace*. https://www.aonl.org/system/files/media/file/2019/04/Mitigating-Violence-in-the-Workplace-Toolkit.pdf

Bardach, E., & Patashnik, M. (2020). *A practical guide for policy analysis: The eightfold path to more effective problem solving* (6th ed.). Sage.

Betts, V. T., Tullai-McGuiness, S., & Williams, L. A. (2015). Serving the public through policy and leadership. In R. Patton, M. Zalon, & R. Ludwick (Eds.), *Nurses making policy: From bedside to boardroom* (pp. 397–431). Springer Publishing Company; American Nurses Association.

Bodenheimer, T., & Sinsky, C. (2014). From triple to quadruple aim: Care of the patient requires care of the provider. *Annals of Family Medicine, 12*(6), 573–576. https://doi.org/10.1370/afm.1713

Centers for Disease Control and Prevention. (2021). *National Violent Death Reporting System*. https://www.cdc.gov/injury/wisqars/nvdrs.html

Centre for Research on the Epidemiology of Disasters, & United Nations Office for Disaster Risk Reduction. (2015). *The human cost of weather related disasters: 1995–2015*. Centre for Research on the Epidemiology of Disasters. https://www.unisdr.org/2015/docs/climatechange/COP21_WeatherDisastersReport_2015_FINAL.pdf

Cook, E. T. (1913). *The life of Florence Nightingale* (Vol. 1, 1820–1861). MacMillan. http://www.gutenberg.org/files/40057/40057-h/40057-h.htm

Davidson, J., Mendis, J., Stuck, A. R., DeMichele, G., & Zisook, S. (2018). *Nurse suicide: Breaking the silence. NAM Perspectives*. Discussion Paper, National Academy of Medicine. https://doi.org/10.31478/201801a

Davis, M. A., Cher, B., Friese, C. R., & Bynum, J. (2021). Association of US nurse and physician occupation with risk of suicide. *JAMA Psychiatry, 78*(6), 1–8. https://doi.org/10.1001/jamapsychiatry.2021.0154

Denham C. R. (2007). TRUST: The 5 rights of the second victim. *Journal of Patient Safety, 3*(2): 107–119. https://doi.org/10.1097/01.jps.0000236917.02321.f

Desilver, D. (2020, November 3). *In past elections, U. S. trailed most developed countries in voter turnout*. Pew Research Center. https://www.pewresearch.org/fact-tank/2020/11/03/in-past-elections-u-s-trailed-most-developed-countries-in-voter-turnout/

Dr. Lorna Breen Healthcare Provider Protection Act. S.610. 117th Cong. (2021–2022). https://www.congress.gov/bill/117th-congress/senate-bill/610?q=%7B%22search%22%3A%5B%22s+610%22%5D%7D&s=2&r=1

Ellenbecker, C. H., Fawcett, J., Jones, E. J., Mahoney, D., Rowlands, B., & Waddell, A. (2017). A staged approach to educating nurses in health policy. *Policy, Politics and Nursing Practice, 18*(1), 44–56. https://doi.org/10.1177/1527154417709254

Environmental Working Group. (2007). *Nurses' health. A survey on health and chemical exposures*. https://www.ewg.org/research/nurses-health/about-survey#.WxfhovVrzcs

Ford, M. (2021, June 1). World's governments urged to get behind new global nursing strategy. *Nursing Times*. https://www.nursingtimes.net/news/workforce/worlds-governments-urged-to-get-behind-new-global-nursing-strategy-01-06-2021/

Gebbie, K. M., Wakefield, M., & Kerfoot, K. (2000). Nursing and health policy. *Journal of Nursing Scholarship*, 32(3), 307–315. https://doi.org/10.1111/j.1547-5069.2000.00307.x

Griffiths, P., Ball, J., Murrells, T., Jones, S., & Rafferty, A. M. (2016). Registered nurse, healthcare support worker, medical staffing levels and mortality in English hospital trusts: A cross-sectional study. *BMJ Open*, 6(2), e008751. https://doi.org/10.1136/bmjopen-2015-008751

Guth, M., & Ammula, M. (2021, May 21). *Building on the evidence base: Studies on the effects of Medicaid expansion, February 2020 to March 2021*. https://www.kff.org/medicaid/report/building-on-the-evidence-base-studies-on-the-effects-of-medicaid-expansion-february-2020-to-march-2021/

Haebler, J., & Fitting, M. (2018). Advocacy at the bedside and beyond. *The American Nurse Today*, 13(1), 39. https://www.myamericannurse.com/

Healthy Nurse Healthy Nation. (2018). *Year one highlights 2017-2018*. https://www.healthynursehealthynation.org/globalassets/all-images-view-with-media/about/hnhn17-18highlights.pdf

Healthy Nurse Healthy Nation. (2019). *Year three highlights 2019-2020*. https://www.healthynursehealthynation.org/globalassets/all-images-view-with-media/about/2020-hnhn_sup-8.pdf

Health Resources and Services Administration. (2021, July 1). Bureau of health workforce. Designated health professional shortage areas statistics. Third quarter of fiscal year 2021 Designated HRSA annual summary. https://data.hrsa.gov

Hume, L. (2018). An investment in staff well-being. *Nursing Management*, 49(12), 9–11. https://doi.org/10.1097/01.NUMA.0000547833.17955.8a

Hummel, S., Oetjen, N., Du, J., Posenato, E., Resende de Almeida, R. M., Losada, R., Ribeiro, O., Frisardi, V., Hopper, L., Rashid, A., Nasser, H., König, A., Rudofsky, G., Weidt, S., Zafar, A., Gronewold, N., Mayer, G., & Schultz, J. H. (2021). Mental health among medical professionals during the COVID-19 pandemic in eight European countries: Cross-sectional survey study. *Journal of Medical Internet Research*, 23(1), e24983. https://doi.org/10.2196/24983

Hutton, A., Veenema, T. G., & Gebbie, K. (2016). Review of the International Council of Nurses (ICN) framework of disaster nursing competencies. *Prehospital and Disaster Medicine*, 31(6), 680–683. https://doi.org/10.1017/S1049023X1600100X

Institute of Medicine. (2011). *The future of nursing: Leading change, advancing health*. The National Academies Press. https://doi.org/10.17226/12956

Kutney-Lee, A., Stimpfel, A. W., Sloane, D. M., Cimiotti, J. P., Quinn, L. W., & Aiken, L. H. (2015). Changes inpatient and nurse outcomes associated Magnet Hospital Recognition. *Medical Care*, 53(6), 550–557. https://doi:10.1097/MLR.0000000000000355

Lewis, T. (2021, February 18). Nursing home workers had one of the deadliest jobs of 2020. *Scientific American*. https://www.scientificamerican.com/article/nursing-home-workers-had-one-of-the-deadliest-jobs-of-2020/

Josiah Macy Jr. Foundation. (2016). *Registered nurses: Partners in transforming primary care. Recommendations from the Macy Foundation Conference on preparing registered nurses for enhanced roles in primary care*. http://macyfoundation.org/docs/macy_pubs/201609_Nursing_Conference_Exectuive_Summary_Final.pdf

Maryland, M., & Gonzalez, R. (2012). Patient advocacy in the community and legislative arena. *OJIN: The Online Journal of Issues in Nursing*, 17(1), 2. https://doi.org/10.3912/OJIN.Vol17No01Man02

McDermott-Levy, R., Kaktins, N., & Sattler, B. (2013). Fracking, the environment, and health. *American Journal of Nursing*, 113(6), 45–51. https://doi.org/10.1097/01.NAJ.0000431272.83277.f4

Montalvo, W. (2015). Political skill and its relevance to nursing: An integrative review. *The Journal of Nursing Administration*, 45(7–8), 377–383. https://doi.org/10.1097/NNA.0000000000000218

National Academies of Sciences, Engineering, and Medicine. (2021). *The future of nursing 2020–2030: Charting a path to achieve health equity*. National Academies Press.

National Patient Safety Foundation (NPSF). (2013). *Through the eyes of the workforce: Creating joy, meaning and safety health care*. http://www.ihi.org/resources/Pages/Publications/Through-the-Eyes-of-the-Workforce-Creating-Joy-Meaning-and-Safer-Health-Care.aspx

Nurses' Health Study. (2016). About NHS. https://nurseshealthstudy.org/about-nhs

Rogers, A. E., Hwang, W. T., Scott, L. D., Aiken, L. H., & Dinges, D. F. (2004). The working hours of hospital staff nurses and patient safety. *Health Affairs, 23*(4), 202–212. https://doi.org/10.1377/hlthaff.23.4.202

Royal College of Nursing. (2020, August 21). *Survey responses reveal members' experiences of working during the pandemic*. https://www.rcn.org.uk/news-and-events/news/uk-passionate-but-pushed-to-the-limit-covid-19-200820

Sagherian, K., Clinton, M. E., Abu-Saad Huijer, H., & Geiger-Brown, J. (2017). Fatigue, work schedules, and perceived performance in bedside care nurses. *Workplace Health and Safety, 65*(7), 304–312. https://doi.org/10.1177/2165079916665398

Shapiro, F. R. (Ed.). (2021). *The new Yale book of quotations*. Yale University Press.

United Nations Office for Disaster Risk Reduction. (2020–2021). *What is the Sendai framework for disaster risk reduction?* https://www.undrr.org/implementing-sendai-framework/what-send-ai-framework

Westley, J. A., Peterson, J., Fort, D., Burton, J., & List, R. (2020). Impact of nurse's worked hours on medication administration near-miss error alerts. *Chronobiology International, 37*(9–10), 1373–1376. https://doi.org/10.1080/07420528.2020.1811295

Williams, S. D., Phillips, J. M., & Koyama, K., (2018). Nurse advocacy: Adopting a health in all policies approach. *OJIN: The Online Journal of Issues in Nursing, 23*(3), 1. https://doi.org/10.3912/OJIN.Vol23No03Man01

World Health Organization. (2017, May). *Diarrheal disease*. Fact sheet No. 330. http://www.who.int/mediacentre/factsheets/fs330/en/index.html

World Health Organization. (2021). *Health workforce: Global strategic directions for nursing and midwifery*. Report by the Director-General. Seventy-Fourth World Assembly Provisional Agenda Item 15. https://apps.who.int/gb/ebwha/pdf_files/WHA74/A74_13-en.pdf

CHAPTER 2

Advocating for Nursing and for Health

KAREN TOMAJAN AND DEBBIE DAWSON HATMAKER

Never doubt that a small group of thoughtful, committed citizens can change the world; indeed, it's the only thing that ever has.
—Margaret Mead

OBJECTIVES

1. Investigate advocacy as a means to improve the safety and quality of healthcare delivery.
2. Demonstrate the competencies needed to be an advocate in different healthcare settings.
3. Describe the relationship of social justice and ethics to the work of advocacy.
4. Discuss the public's view of nursing in healthcare advocacy.
5. Identify barriers that can impact the success or failure of advocacy.
6. Select key resources to support advocacy initiatives.

In this time of unprecedented uncertainty about the future of the healthcare system lies opportunities for nurses and the nursing profession. A greater voice in healthcare policy, expanded employment opportunities, and an enhanced image for nurses and the profession are a few of the potential outcomes. Despite the opportunities afforded by being the largest healthcare group, the diversity of the scope of the nursing profession, and the unique relationship nurses share with the public, the full potential for influence is yet to be realized (Institute of Medicine, 2011; Jurns, 2019; Tomajan, 2012). After a decade of unresolved debate, the future of healthcare remains unclear. Current economic strife, political divisiveness, and social unrest compound system ineffectiveness and highlights health disparities and inequities. As the nation emerges from this difficult time, nurses must be strategically positioned to seize opportunities and leverage the forces of change in partnership with others in the evolution of healthcare.

The evolution of modern nursing began in the late 1800s as Florence Nightingale published her views about how nurses should be educated and patient care should be provided (Hegge, 2011). Although Nightingale did not directly use the word *advocacy* in her writings, her works were consistently about advocating for change (Selanders & Crane, 2012). Her own words speak to the importance she placed on action and change: "I think one's feelings waste themselves in words; they ought all to be distilled into actions and into actions which bring results" (Cook, 1913, p. 94).

Since the inception of the profession, nurses have been actively involved in advocacy and activism on behalf of patients, families, communities, and patient populations and have worked tirelessly to address healthcare and social justice issues that impact health. The concept of advocacy is part of professional nursing. Advocacy involves a complex interaction among nurses, patients, professional colleagues, and the public at large (Selanders & Crane, 2012). To be an effective

Linda Minnich RN, BSN, Nurse Clinician, is a staff nurse on the postoperative recovery unit in a community hospital. She attended a pain management conference and was inspired to bring what she had learned back to improve care for patients in her work setting. She was aware of the impact of postoperative pain, and the detrimental effects of sustained opioid use. Linda was a member the shared governance council that provided a forum for collaboration with nurses from other hospital units and found universal interest in new practice innovations to improve patient experiences of pain and discomfort.

Linda had some ideas which included focusing on orthopedic surgery patients, a high-volume population for her hospital. She was ready to advocate for patients but didn't quite know how to begin. She sought assistance from her hospital's director of professional practice to help her determine how she could best apply what she had learned.

She was looking for answers to questions such as:

- What is the most effective way to advocate for culture change in various nursing units?
- What is the organization's philosophy about advocating for culture change?
- Which competencies are needed to be an advocate?
- What resources are available within the work setting to facilitate new procedures?
- What advocacy organizations will be helpful in promoting these changes?
- What standards, guidelines, or best practices are available to provide evidence-based support to the advocacy process?

nursing professional, a nurse must understand and embrace the role of advocate—advocating for health and for the nursing profession.

This chapter provides an overview of the concept of advocacy, the nurse's advocacy roles, and expectations of society and the profession regarding advocacy. The American Nurses Association's (ANA, 2015) *Code of Ethics for Nurses* is used as a framework to describe the application of advocacy. In addition, competencies for advocacy, resources for becoming an advocate, and advocacy arenas are identified. Advocacy exemplars are used to illustrate the various possible outcomes of nurses' advocacy efforts. See the Policy Challenge, which describes how a nurse was inspired to improve the care of patients experiencing pain after attending a pain management conference. She worked within the organization to introduce new pain management modalities, train the staff, and influence hospital policy development.

ADVOCACY DEFINITIONS

Advocacy is defined as "the act or process of pleading, supporting, or recommending a cause or course of action. Advocacy may be for persons (whether an individual, group, population or society) or for an issue such as potable water or global health" (ANA, 2015, p. 41). Advocacy can take many forms and may require working through formal decision-making bodies to achieve positive results. This could include working through committees, an administrative chain of command, state commission, regulatory body, or state/federal legislative entity.

The term *advocacy* was first included in the profession's codes by the International Council of Nurses (ICN) in 1973 (Vaartio & Leino-Kilpi, 2005). Nursing education documents prior to the mid-1970s did not reference advocacy as a clear expectation in nursing. In fact, early nursing education historically emphasized conformity, obedience, and subservience (Selanders & Crane, 2012). Since that time, advocacy has increasingly been associated with the role of the professional nurse. This evolution of nursing practice from loyalty to advocacy has put forward a metaphor of the nurse as an advocate of patients' rights, which has been readily embraced by nurses. In recent years, there has been an ever-increasing mandate for the profession's further evolution to encompass a broader social justice advocacy model while retaining individual commitment to patient–nurse advocacy. This has been a challenging transition that continues to evolve today (Florell, 2020; Paquin, 2011). As U.S. healthcare moves to a more socially just system, it is important that nurses leverage their sizable political clout to help drive this change. As the largest and most trusted professional group, nurses are expected to actively lead with a social justice mindset. This requires the ability to push "nursing advocacy to move beyond the bedside and outside the walls of the institutions in which most nurses work" (Paquin, 2011, p. 67).

In a review of empirical literature from 1990 to 2003, Vaartio and Leino-Kilpi (2005) identified three themes related to patient advocacy: advocacy motivated by the patient's right to information and self-determination, advocacy stemming from the patient's right to personal safety, and advocacy as a philosophical principle in nursing. Bu and Jezewski (2007) discuss three core attributes of nursing advocacy: safeguarding patient autonomy, acting on behalf of patients who are not able to act for themselves, and championing social justice.

In recent years, increased focus on patient safety and continuity of care has helped spotlight the vital role nurses play in every setting to ensure patients receive safe, effective care and their rights are protected. Nurses have played a key role in the evolution of healthcare, with the recognition that there is a more expansive role for the profession that could and should be realized.

While nurses readily accept the requirement of the professional nurses' advocacy role as it applies to their patients; advocacy activities that extend to broader groups or for global issues are less consistently evident. Two of the ANA's core documents, the *Code of Ethics for Nurses with Interpretive Statements* (ANA, 2015) and *Nursing: Scope and Standards of Practice* (ANA, 2021), delineate the professional nurse's responsibility to advocate at multiple levels: nurse–patient, nurse–nurse, nurse–self, nurse–others, nurse–profession, nurse–society, and nursing–society (Bazdak & Turner, 2015).

The ANA's (2021) *Nursing: Scope and Standards of Practice* clearly identifies "advocacy" within the scope of nursing practice, suggesting that it is fundamental to practice, and identifies four levels of advocacy:

- **Individual:** The nurse educates healthcare consumers to consider actions, interventions, or choices related to their own personal beliefs, attitudes, and knowledge to achieve desired outcomes.

- **Interpersonal:** The nurse empowers healthcare consumers by providing emotional support, assistance in attaining resources, and necessary health through interactions with families and significant others in social support networks.

- **Organization and community:** The nurse supports the cultural and social transformation of organizations, communities, or populations and helps inform environmental and societal conditions related to health, wellness, and care of the healthcare consumer.

- **Policy:** The nurse promotes the inclusion of the healthcare consumer's voices into policy, legislation, and regulation about such issues as access, cost reductions, and protection of the healthcare consumer and the environment.

The ANA's (2015) *Code of Ethics for Nurses with Interpretive Statements* (2015) identifies multiple advocacy expectations for the professional nurse. These expectations include a commitment to patients, families, communities, and populations served. Nurses also have an obligation to advocate for the profession through teaching, mentoring, peer review, involvement in professional associations, community service, and knowledge development and dissemination. These activities and skills are foundational to the advocacy role of the professional nurse.

Advocacy is based on a foundation of ethical principles that include autonomy, beneficence, nonmaleficence, fidelity, and justice. It is essential that advocates act in the interest of those they represent in the advocacy process and align their actions with these principles (ANA, 2015; Butts & Rich, 2016):

- **Autonomy:** Autonomy is respect for another's right to self-determine a course of action and support for independent decision-making. Nurses should protect the autonomy of those for whom they are acting, which includes involvement in decision-making.

- **Beneficence:** Beneficence is acting to help others and to protect them from harm. The desire to "do good" and help others is a core principle of advocacy.

- **Nonmaleficence:** Nonmaleficence is the avoidance of harm or hurt. This principle is sometimes described as "do no harm" and is likewise an important role of the advocate.

- **Fidelity:** Keeping one's promises and being truthful and loyal to those represented are unequivocal expectations of the advocate. Disclosing personal interests and being cognizant of one's own goals prevent conflict of interest when advocating on behalf of others.

- **Justice:** Justice is a "moral concept of fairness and equality . . . [and includes] treating people equally, without prejudice and equitable distribution of benefits and burdens" (Butts & Rich 2016, p. 46.).

CODE OF ETHICS FOR NURSES

Advocacy carries with it a significant ethical dimension; therefore, principles of ethics can help to evaluate a nurse's effectiveness as an advocate. A code of ethics is fundamental for any profession. It provides ethical and legal guidance to the members of the profession, as well as a social contract with the population served. ANA published its original *Code of Ethics* (www.nursingworld.org/codeofethics) in 1950. Through seven revisions, the code "retains nursing's historical and ethical values, obligations, ideals and commitments" (Fowler, 2015, p. ix). Several significant changes have occurred since the Code's original publication: (a) the conceptualization of "patient" has expanded from that of an individual receiving treatment to include the family, community, and population; (b) a provision that recognizes the nurse's responsibilities for self-care; and (c) emphasis on social justice, health as a universal right, and a responsibility to advocate for global health issues such as poverty, violence, and oppression (Fowler, 2015). Each of the nine code provisions includes an aspect of advocacy.

PROVISION 1

The nurse practices with compassion and respect for the inherent dignity, worth, and unique attributes of every person (ANA, 2015, p. 1).

Respect for inherent dignity, worth, unique attributes, and human rights are fundamental to nursing practice. Nurses establish relationships based on trust and free from bias or prejudice. Factors such as culture, values, religious or spiritual beliefs, lifestyle, social support system, sexual orientation or gender expression, and primary language must be considered when planning care. Nurses provide the same level of care regardless of diagnosis, ethnicity, or economic status. Therefore, the nurse is ethically bound to care and advocate for all. The nurse supports the patient's autonomy and self-determination, including informed consent, by providing accurate, complete, and understandable information that supports the patient's decision-making process. This obligation of respect for others extends to all individuals with whom the nurse interacts and defines the nurses' responsibility to create an ethical environment and culture of civility.

PROVISION 1 EXEMPLAR: Right to Self-Determination

Richard James is 87 years old and a resident in an assisted living center. He is single; however, he has a very close family with seven nieces and nephews in the area. Six months ago, while living in his own home, he experienced a small stroke that left him with memory and balance deficits. Since admission to assisted living, his condition has improved. He has decided that he is going to go back to his own home. His oldest niece, Lydia Grant, is his healthcare proxy and executor of his estate. Mr. James's entire family is very concerned about his safety at home. Lydia talks with the director of nursing, Sylvia Sanchez, seeking her opinion about Mr. James's ability to manage his home situation, particularly related to safety. Nurse Sanchez points out that Mr. James has steadily improved over the months he has been in the facility and reminds his niece that the decision to return home is ultimately Mr. James's. Nurse Sanchez sets up a care conference with the facility physician, social worker, Lydia, and Mr. James. Based on the discussions, Mr. James will have home health assistance and a part-time housekeeper to assist him several days per week with cooking, shopping, and transportation for errands and medical appointments. Nurse Sanchez works with Lydia to coordinate his move out of the facility. In addition, Nurse Sanchez reassures Mr. James that he can return to the facility if his condition changes.

PROVISION 2

The nurse's primary commitment is to the patient, whether an individual, family, group, community, or population (ANA, 2015, p. 5).

Ethical dilemmas arise as the nurse attempts to balance a commitment to the patient, the family, and the community; however, this provision is clear that the nurse's primary obligation is to the patient. "Nurses address such conflicts in ways that ensure patient safety, guard the patient's best interests, and preserve the professional integrity of the nurse" (ANA, 2015, p. 5). Interpretation of this provision speaks to distributive justice when resources are limited, collaboration when caring for a patient in the complexity of the healthcare environment, and professional boundaries within the nurse–patient relationship. Therefore, advocacy has its limits and limitations that must be observed.

PROVISION 2 EXEMPLAR: Commitment to the Patient

Karen Anderson, RN, works in the role of patient relations liaison. She receives a telephone call from Rachel Carr, who had been cared for earlier that day in the ED for back pain. Ms. Carr was quite upset, saying that during the visit the physician had been rude, called her a "drug seeker," and did not offer any pain-relief treatment or medication. Ms. Carr explained that she has a chronic back injury had just moved to the area and reinjured her back while unpacking boxes. Although she has a future appointment with a local physician, she has not yet been seen, and the physician's staff referred her to the ED. Nurse Anderson meets with the ED nurse manager and medical director and arranges for Ms. Carr to be reevaluated later that day.

PROVISION 3

The nurse promotes, advocates for, and protects the rights, health, and safety of the patient (ANA, 2015, p. 9).

Provision 3 addresses the patient's right to privacy and confidentiality, safeguarding research participants, and addressing incompetent practice (whether it involves impairment or lack of knowledge or skill). "The nurse has a duty to maintain confidentiality of all patient information, both personal and clinical in the work setting and off duty in all venues including social media or other means of communication" (ANA, 2015, p. 9). The nurse must always weigh the patient's right to privacy with protecting the patient from harm. Provision 3 outlines the nurse's role in promoting a culture of safety, which includes responsibilities for reporting errors and near misses and for addressing the problem of incompetent practice. Whether the incompetence is due to impairment or a lack of knowledge, the nurse must report the issue to the appropriate person in the organization. If not acted on, the nurse must then take the next step in the organizational hierarchy or even consider reporting to an outside accrediting or regulatory body. Such advocacy skills as maintaining standards of care, advocating for impaired colleagues, or whistle-blowing may come into play with this provision.

PROVISION 3 EXEMPLAR: Addressing Impaired Practice

John Smith, RN, has just completed his first year of practice on the telemetry unit. His nurse preceptor, Linda Nelson, has been a great support during his orientation, and he is feeling very confident as he enters his second year. Linda has recently separated from her husband of 20 years and has not seemed herself lately. John notices that she is arriving late for work, looks strained, and is disorganized. Linda has verbally blown up while interacting with several coworkers in the past week. He noticed alcohol on her breath the past 2 days that she has come to work, and he is really concerned about Linda and her patients. When John identifies that Linda almost administered an incorrect medication—a "near-miss" error—he realizes he must take his concerns to their nurse manager. Ethically, he is bound to address his colleague's impaired practice and ensure the safety of patients.

PROVISION 4

The nurse has authority, accountability, and responsibility for nursing practice; makes decisions; and takes action consistent with the obligation to promote health and provide optimal care (ANA, 2015, p. 15).

Accountability for actions is the cornerstone of a profession due to the implied social contract with the public. Nursing has been identified repeatedly as the most honest and ethical profession because its practitioners take the issue of accountability seriously. This accountability includes self-assessing competency, seeking educational resources when less than competent to perform care, and delegating appropriately to other healthcare providers. This provision highlights the need for nurses' acceptance of accountability and self-assessment to be effective advocates.

PROVISION 4 EXEMPLAR: Accountability for Nursing Judgment and Action

Stacy Samuels, RN, a faculty member, who teaches pediatric nursing in a baccalaureate nursing program, works per diem in the summer on the pediatric or mother-baby units of a community hospital. One Saturday, she reports to the pediatric unit only to learn she has been assigned to float to the sixth-floor adult oncology unit due to low pediatric census. Nurse Samuels has never been oriented to any of the adult units and has not taken care of adult oncology patients since she graduated from nursing school 10 years ago. She does not feel safe in providing nursing care to oncology patients. She calls the house supervisor; however, the call has not yet been returned. She reports to the sixth-floor nurses' station and tells the charge nurse that she will agree only to take patient vital signs and do patient personal care. When the supervisor makes rounds, Stacy intends to inform her that she cannot ethically take accountability for complete care of these patients since she does not have the knowledge, competence, and experience to engage safely in their care.

PROVISION 5

The nurse owes the same duties to self as to others, including the responsibility to promote health and safety, preserve wholeness of character and integrity, maintain competence, and continue personal and professional growth (ANA, 2015, p. 19).

Provision 5 addresses moral self-respect, professional growth, and the maintenance of competence, wholeness of character, or integration of personal and professional values. Self-advocacy is inherent in this provision. Nurses should model health promotion and maintenance, including rest, diet, exercise, healthy relationships, and work/life balance. Nurses may face threats to integrity when confronted with verbal threats or abuse from patients, families, or coworkers. Preservation of nurses' integrity under this provision would also allow for the concept of "conscientious objection" when a treatment, intervention, or activity is morally objectionable to the nurse. Although nurses cannot abandon their patients, they must make it known to the administration when situations place them in moral dilemmas that they find objectionable (Lachman, 2015).

PROVISION 5 EXEMPLAR: Wholeness of Character

Patsy Williams is a 56-year-old patient diagnosed with stage IV metastatic breast cancer and is on an aggressive chemotherapeutic regimen. She is experiencing extreme nausea and anorexia unresolved by medications. Her goals are to spend quality time with her family and friends and to continue to teach third grade as long as possible. Leah Donnelley, RN, is an oncology nurse in the freestanding outpatient oncology center caring for Patsy. Patsy asks Nurse Donnelley's opinion of medical marijuana to alleviate

POLICY ON THE SCENE 2.1: ARIZONA NURSES ADVOCATING FOR HEALTH AND SAFETY

Dedicated staff nurses Jasmine Bhatti, Jade Juriansz, Laruen Leander, and Brittiany Schilling demonstrated public health advocacy when they learned that a rally was planned at the Arizona State Capitol for individuals protesting the governor's stay-at-home orders and other COVID-19 pandemic mitigation measures. They joined others at the Capitol and stood in defense of public health and the safety of colleagues doing everything possible to save lives. Photos of the nurses went viral and became a flashpoint in the national debate (Ruelas, 2020).

After the media attention subsided, the nurses used their notoriety to help raise money for underserved communities hit hardest by COVID-19. In May, they helped launch the Navajo and Hopi Community Relief Fund via the online platform GoFundMe. The effort raised over $287,000 for the Navajo and Hopi people. These donations helped support critical COVID relief efforts, purchasing food, water, personal protective equipment (PPE), medical supplies, and other relief for families and healthcare workers in these communities (Navajo-Hopi Observer, 2020). As a result of her work, Lauren Leander received a John F. Kennedy Profile in Courage Award in November 2020 (John F. Kennedy Presidential Library, 2021).

her nausea symptoms. Patsy has explored this option on the internet and brings her informed questions to Nurse Donnelley. Patsy asks for help in exploring this modality. Although medical marijuana is approved for use in this state, Nurse Donnelley personally opposes the use of marijuana under any circumstances. However, Nurse Donnelley is an experienced RN and knows that while she could voice her opinion, ethically she should assist Ms. Williams in clarifying her own values in reaching an informed decision, thus avoiding unintentionally persuading her one way or another. Nurse Donnelley agrees to investigate the latest evidence on the effectiveness of cannabis for chemotherapy-induced nausea. She also calls a team conference with Ms. Williams, her oncologist, and the center's dietitian and pharmacist to formulate a comprehensive plan to address Ms. Williams's nausea and to help her determine if and how she might best make use of this modality.

PROVISION 6

The nurse, through individual and collective effort, establishes, maintains, and improves the ethical environment of the work setting and conditions of employment that are conducive to safe, quality healthcare (ANA, 2015, p. 23).

Provision 6 extends the nurse's obligation to advocate for an ethical work environment that supports the values central to nursing. The reciprocal relationship between the nurse and the work environment is inherent in this provision. The work environment can either obstruct or support nursing values and ethical obligations. This provision sets forward an expectation of moral activism; the nurse should work to change the environment if it is obstructive. The goal is for nurses to work with the administration to create an environment that supports safety and quality patient care (Lachman, 2015; Lachman et al., 2015). Advocacy on a large scale is possible when nurses join with their professional associations and participate in collective action such as workforce advocacy, collective bargaining or legislative days (see Figure 2.1). When this is not possible and an organization refuses to support patient rights or puts nurses in a position that violates professional standards of practice, nurses may have little choice but to leave the organization.

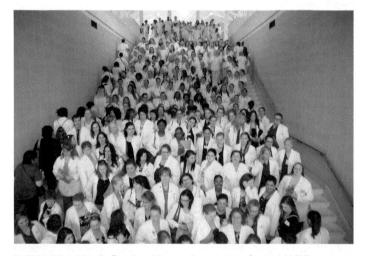

FIGURE 2.1 North Carolina Nurses Association Capitol Hill Day

Source: Reproduced with permission from the North Carolina Nurses Association.

PROVISION 6 EXEMPLAR: Improving the Healthcare Environment

Patricia Brown is a staff nurse in a critical care unit. She is very committed to her colleagues and believes that maintaining a healthy work environment is the responsibility of every nurse. She overhears Angela Nelson, one of her colleagues, speaking condescendingly to a new nurse who has asked a question regarding the unit routine. After the conversation concludes, Patricia pulls Angela aside and relates what she heard between the two nurses. She shares her feelings that Angela was too harsh with the new nurse and relays her concern that this is an example of incivility. She informs Angela that harsh communication with new staff is detrimental to the development of a positive unit environment and relays her belief that every staff member should feel comfortable asking questions of any colleague without fear of reprisal. Patricia discusses the situation with her manager who supports her actions and offers to intervene if there are further issues.

PROVISION 7

The nurse, in all roles and settings, advances the profession through research and scholarly inquiry, professional standards development, and the generation of both nursing and health policy (ANA, 2015, p. 27).

Advancement of and advocacy for the nursing profession is the focus of this provision. Many activities are representative of this obligation: mentorship, service on organizational shared governance committees, leadership in professional associations, and civic activity at the local, state, national, or international levels. Nurses contribute through knowledge development, research and scholarly inquiry, development and enactment of professional standards, and participation in nursing and health policy development. Nurses advocate through role-specific responsibilities that include the nurse educator's responsibility for nursing education standards, the nurse researcher's support of clinical practice by providing practice-based evidence, and nurse administrators' advocacy in creating environments that support the ethical integrity of staff.

PROVISION 7 EXEMPLAR: Advancing the Profession

State nurses associations routinely review new bills being presented in state legislatures to determine the impact on the health of citizens as well as the impact on the profession. A bill has been forwarded to the state legislature that allows clerical staff in public schools to administer medications to students. The association's legislative committee believes that passing this bill could compromise the safety of school children and that a better alternative would be to increase funding to hire more school nurses across the state. They partner with school nurses and involve their specialty organization, the National School Nurses Association, to jointly lobby against this bill in the legislature, citing the potential risks to children.

PROVISION 8

The nurse collaborates with other health professionals and the public to protect human rights, promote health diplomacy, and reduce health disparities (ANA, 2015, p. 31).

Provision 8 addresses advocacy for health concerns in the larger world, calling on nurses to advance health and human rights and to reduce disparities. This provision identifies health as a universal right, which includes access to healthcare, basic sanitation, potable water, food security, immunizations, injury prevention, and health promotion. Nurses are called to collaborate with others to bring attention to human rights violations such as poverty, abuse, rape, hate crimes, genocide, human trafficking, and exploitation and to address the needs of special populations such as the homeless, mentally ill, and elderly. This provision also addresses situations in which nurses are required to practice under extreme conditions, such as during disasters, epidemics, and fields of battle.

PROVISION 8 EXEMPLAR: Raising Awareness of Health Disparities

Ernest Grant, PhD, RN, FAAN, was elected president of the American Nurses Association from 2018 to 2022. His area of practice is burn nursing, and he is well known nationally and internationally as an educator on burn care and prevention. Dr. Grant is the first male president of the ANA, and is also the first African American male to serve as the president of the North Carolina Nurses Association. In 2020, Dr. Grant participated in a COVID-19 Phase III vaccine trial at the University of North Carolina. Because the virus was disproportionately affecting communities of color, he felt compelled to participate in the trials, to assure there was enough evidence to determine the vaccine's efficacy in these populations. He also felt he could serve as an influencer to encourage people of color to take the vaccine if they knew individuals who look like them participated safely in the trial. Dr. Grant served as a role model to encourage nurses and other health providers to get vaccinated when the national program launched.

PROVISION 9

The profession of nursing, collectively through its professional organizations, must articulate nursing values, maintain the integrity of the profession, and integrate the principles of social justice into nursing and health policy (ANA, 2015, p. 35).

Who advocates for the nursing profession? The focus of Provision 9 is on the profession through its associations rather than the individual nurse. It calls for nurses associations and organizations to act collectively with one voice, in

POLICY ON THE SCENE 2.2: USE OF TRUSTED INFLUENCERS IN ADVOCACY INITIATIVES

At the outset of the COVID-19 pandemic, morbidity and mortality statistics indicated significant disproportionate levels of severe complications and death among members of the Black, Latinx, and Native American populations. Surveys also indicated that these same populations held deep-seated distrust of the healthcare system, based on legitimate historical experiences, particularly as it related to vaccines and other "experimental" therapies. In planning for the COVID-19 vaccine distribution, one key concern was that these patient populations would not accept the vaccine. Plans for distribution of the newly developed COVID-19 vaccines were targeted for early administration to members of these communities to stop transmission of this deadly pathogen. However, this presented an ethical dilemma. Given the requirements for storing and distributing the vaccine vials, it was essential to act rapidly to increase the trust and willingness of these groups to be vaccinated. With the help of the Ad Council, a not-for-profit foundation with expertise in formulating population-specific ads, a vaccination communication plan was developed and implemented in a matter of days. One key strategy was to involve "trusted influencers" from within these communities in the planning process. Trusted influencers included religious leaders—pastors, priests, medicine men, and shamans—as well as physicians, nurses, athletes, pop stars, and political leaders in a tailored communication strategy designed with the input of each target group. This resulted in a higher level of vaccination than would otherwise have been expected. The ANA was one of 18 partner organizations that contributed to videos highlighting the importance of COVID-19 vaccination. ANA President Ernest J. Grant, PhD, RN, FAAN contributed the following statement in association with this initiative:

> I am grateful for the courage and dedication of those on the frontlines of the pandemic. I was proud to participate in a COVID-19 vaccine clinical trial as a way to demonstrate my confidence in the safety and efficacy of the development process and in this Ad Council initiative to reach nurses and physicians with timely and important information. I encourage nurses to be informed and to get vaccinated as soon as possible, to protect themselves and as a role model for others, so that we can achieve widespread vaccination and return to normal activities.

solidarity across all specialties, roles, and practice settings to articulate nursing values, maintain the integrity of the profession, and integrate the principles of social justice to reduce health disparities. The integrity of the profession is based on the covenant between nursing and society through a code of ethics, standards of nursing practice, and educational requirements for practice, knowledge development, and continuing evaluation of professional nursing actions. A specific focus on social ethics reflects nursing's historical interest in how health and illness affect society.

PROVISION 9 EXEMPLAR: Articulating Nursing Values and Maintaining Professional Integrity

Following the devastating hurricanes in Louisiana, Mississippi, Florida, and Texas in 2006, the ANA acted, along with other professional associations and regulatory agencies, to define the responsibilities of nurses and other healthcare professionals in disaster situations. The ANA worked with state and national agencies and disaster-relief organizations such as the American Red Cross to define the role of the RN in a disaster, establish structures to coordinate disaster response through the Medical Reserve Corps, and define potential legal protections for nurses acting in good faith in catastrophic situations (ANA, 2017). These actions are examples of the association's advocacy for nursing as a profession, which impacts all nurses, not just ANA members.

This laid the groundwork to facilitate the responses of nurses in subsequent disasters. The ANA's collaboration among state nurses associations, nursing specialty organizations, allied health groups, governmental and public service organizations provided a useful network that was activated to efficiently and effectively advocate for healthcare professionals during recent disasters, particularly the COVID-19 pandemic.

CLINICAL PRACTICE AND MORAL DISTRESS: THE REALITY OF PRACTICE ADVOCACY

Nurses in clinical practice encounter ethical issues that can lead to moral distress—negative feelings that result when one knows the ethically correct action to take but feels powerless to take that action (ANA, 2015; ANA Professional Issues Panel, n.d.; Rushton, 2017, Rushton et al, 2017). For nurses to be effective advocates, they must understand and accept their ethical responsibilities to the patient, family, community, and profession. However, when nurses are unable to advocate due to practice barriers, fear, or lack of skills—moral distress ensues. Moral distress results in psychological distress and feelings of anxiety, irritability, frustration, anger, fatigue, or depression. When left unchecked, moral distress undermines safety and quality of care, disrupts interprofessional relationships, contributes to burnout, stress disorders, and results in turnover and the loss of nurses from the profession (Rushton, 2017). Causes of moral distress include conflict between the nurse's responsibility to the patient and duty to the employer; a lack of colleague support; perceived a lack of power; fear of reprisal from colleagues, physician, or supervisor; inadequate resources to meet patient needs; and a lack of education or skills. When surveyed, nurses have identified ethical priorities that include the following (Pavlish et al., 2011):

- **Patients' Quality of Life:** an obligation to treat distressing symptoms, pain, or suffering.

- **Promoting Patient Autonomy:** the notion that patient preferences should prevail over family wishes or healthcare team values.

- **Substandard Healthcare:** situations in which the healthcare team either did not adhere to standards of care, were severely conflicted over treatment options, or had inadequate resources to provide the usual standard of care.

Many healthcare agencies have processes and policies that establish the chain of command to address ethical concerns, which may include an ethics committee tasked with addressing ethical dilemmas. Nurses increasingly have a voice in advocating for their patients within these organizations. However, these processes are often inadequate.

New approaches to assist nurses and other healthcare professionals to cope with the impact of moral distress and to promote the development of moral resilience are being implemented. Moral resilience is the ability to recover from or healthfully adapt to the challenges of stress, adversity, or trauma and to be "buoyant" in the event of adverse circumstances. Interventions for cultivating moral resilience include mindful meditation, cognitive reappraisal, biofeedback, and organizational support such as ethics rounds, debriefings, and consultations. Educational strategies include training on ethical principles and decision-making, conflict resolution, change management, mindfulness, spiritual well-being, and self-care (ANA, n.d.; Rushton, 2017; Rushton et al., 2017).

SOCIAL JUSTICE

Social justice is defined as the belief in equality for all people, including the distribution of the advantages and disadvantages among the individuals in a society (Butts & Rich, 2016). A strong commitment to social justice requires professional nurses to advocate for the health of all persons. Advocacy activities are an expected outcome for a health profession that promotes the concept of social justice. Social justice advocacy is an inherent expectation of all nurses as expressed in the professional codes that guide nursing practice (ANA, 2015; Paquin, 2011).

Nursing has long maintained a strong commitment to advocacy for vulnerable populations and has embraced social justice as a core value since the inception of the profession. Early nursing leaders were strong advocates for the healthcare needs of the vulnerable and disadvantaged. In recent years, the profession has been called on to reinvigorate its commitment to social justice advocacy and to build on nursing's distinguished history of leadership on social issues (Florell, 2020; Matwick & Woodgate, 2016; Valderama-Wallace, 2017).

EQUITY

An important role of the advocate is to promote equity and eliminate or mitigate the effects of health disparity at both the individual and system levels. One of the features of healthcare reform has been to address disparities and promote equity within the healthcare system. Health equity "means that everyone has a fair and just opportunity to be as healthy as possible. This requires removing obstacles to health such as poverty, discrimination and their consequences including powerlessness and lack of access to good jobs with fair pay; quality education and housing; safe environments; and healthcare" (Braveman et al., 2017, p. 2). Health disparity is defined as the differences in health outcomes attributed to inequities in healthcare delivery (Butts & Rich, 2016). Disparities contribute to infant mortality, disability, decreased life expectancy, and higher incidence of preventable hospitalizations (Braveman et al., 2017; see Chapter 13).

As a profession, nurses have led the way among healthcare professionals in their work to promote a healthcare system that is accessible to all and to address issues of disparity and inequality. In the advocacy role, nurses have worked to address the equity needs of individual patients and patient populations and to advance health policy at the healthcare system level.

DISCRIMINATION AND RACISM

Contributors to health inequity and social injustice are discrimination and racism. *Discrimination* exists when a person is treated unfavorably or unjustly according to a particular characteristic such as race, age, gender, or religion (ANA, 2018). Racism is a complex term that includes prejudice, bias, and discrimination directed toward an individual or group based on membership in a particular racial or ethnic group, typically one that is a minority or marginalized. Racism also exists across systems, institutions, and societies resulting in practices that disadvantage minority populations (Annie E. Casey Foundation, 2020).

"Racism is a public health crisis that impacts the mental, spiritual and physical health of all individuals. *The Code of Ethics for Nurses* obligates nurses to be allies and advocates and speak up against racism, discrimination and injustice" (ANA, 2020, para. 2). In the weeks and months following the 2020 deaths of George Floyd and Breonna Taylor, citizens including nurses and other healthcare professionals took to the streets to protest, calling for law enforcement reform and changes in public policy to end racism. In June 2020, the ANA's Membership Assembly adopted the "Resolution on Racial Justice for Communities of Color," which reaffirmed previous positions on discrimination and condemned law enforcement cruelty and abject racism. The resolution also sought to advance institutional and legislative policies that promote diversity, equity, inclusion, and social justice for all. The ANA (2020) established a collaborative among nursing organizations to further develop education and advocacy actions to end systematic racism at the state and national levels.

PUBLIC EXPECTATION FOR ADVOCACY

You are traveling in a foreign country where you do not know the culture or language. How will you get your needs met? You may use nonverbal cues like gestures or pictures, but you are not certain you will be understood. What if you had an advocate, someone who knows the language, culture, and belief system? The U.S. healthcare system is foreign and challenging for many patients. There are technical terms, abbreviations, jargon, and euphemisms that complicate communication. Hospitals have hierarchies, policies, standards, routines, and rituals that are mysterious to patients, families, visitors, and students (Bosek & Savage, 2007).

The public has come to expect nurses to serve in the role of advocate, assisting them to migrate through the "foreignness" of the healthcare system. Although no single profession "owns" the role of advocate, nursing has traditionally seen this role as integral to good nursing care. The American public also sees the nurse in the role of advocate in that they have rated RNs as the most honest and ethical profession for the past 19 years, according to Gallup's annual survey (Saad, 2020). Nurses are increasingly recognized as leaders in transforming the healthcare system to meet the burgeoning demand for services, with a focus on improving quality and managing costs. In a 2019 survey conducted by the *New York Times*, Commonwealth Fund, and Harvard T. H. Chan School of Public Health, respondents rated nurses' recommendations for healthcare system redesign as the most trusted, over that of doctors, hospitals, or the government (Rappleye, 2019).

Although the public has come to know nurses' advocacy activities through their patient care experiences, they do not always see nurses in key leadership roles. A 2010 Gallup poll of 1,500 health opinion leaders indicated they wanted nurses to have more influence in a variety of areas: reducing medical errors, increasing quality of care, and promoting wellness. They also believed that nurses should have more influence in policy development (Khoury et al., 2011). However, in contrast, an American Hospital Association survey of 1,000 U.S. hospitals found that nurses accounted for only 6% of hospital board members. This contrasts with the number of physicians (20%) and other clinicians (about 5%) on boards (Van Dyke et al., 2011). In 2014, the Robert Wood Johnson Foundation and the Center to Champion Nursing in America formed the Nurses on Boards Coalition (NOBC). A goal for adding 10,000 nurses to boards of directors by 2020 was established, resulting in a threefold increase in the number of board appointments in a 4-year time frame. Nurses bring a unique perspective to boards, panels, and commissions in their understanding of health needs across the care continuum and the issues of front-line healthcare providers. They also bring critical thinking, active listening, communication, and change management skills (Harper & Benson, 2019). The NOBC announced at the end of 2020 the goal had been achieved with more than 10,035 nurses appointed to a variety of decision-making boards.

COMPETENCIES NEEDED TO BE AN ADVOCATE

Two of ANA's foundational documents, the *Code of Ethics for Nurses with Interpretive Statements* (2015) and *Nursing: Scope and Standards of Practice* (2021), address the professional nurse's responsibilities for advocacy. The documents cover the required competencies and activities of professional nurses, through the care of patients, teaching, mentoring, peer review, involvement in professional associations, community service, and knowledge development and dissemination. The skills of problem-solving, communication, influence, collaboration, and resource identification are also useful to support a cause on behalf of a patient, a family, a community, a population, the profession, or one-self (Tomajan, 2012).

Problem-Solving

Since advocacy is directed at problems in need of a solution, the problem-solving process is a necessary skill for the effective nurse advocate. The steps in problem-solving and strategies to achieve each are illustrated in Figure 2.2.

This problem-solving process should feel very familiar to nurses, as it parallels the steps in the nursing process. Figure 2.2 provides guideposts for planning and implementing advocacy efforts. Getting Help (under "Analyze the problem") is important and should occur early in the advocacy process. Novice advocates are advised to seek advice from trusted colleagues, supervisors, or mentors who know the organization and the decision-making process. Their perspective of the current state and appropriate timing will be invaluable to the development of a successful action plan.

Communication

Communication is key to an effective advocacy strategy. Verbal, written, and electronic forms of communication are used when advocates pull individuals together to work collectively on a problem. It is important that all messages are based on

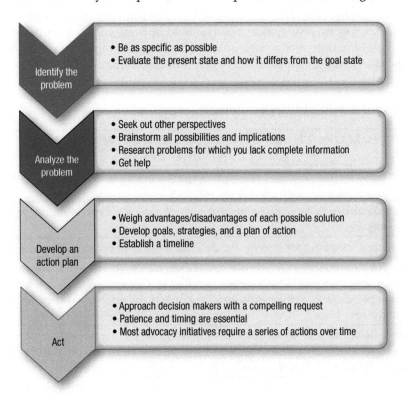

FIGURE 2.2 **Problem-solving process.**

fact and that messaging across time is consistent. Although advocates are often "armed" with facts and figures when they attempt to influence decisions-makers, it is equally important to tell the story of the impact of the problem, particularly as it affects people. Giving specific examples of patient care situations or how individuals within the community are affected by an issue (without violating privacy) can demonstrate how the problem and suggested solution(s) have a real-world impact.

Influence

To be effective, the nurse advocate must be able to influence others. Influencing an individual or group's thoughts, beliefs, or actions is essential and built on competence, credibility, and trustworthiness (Tomajan, 2012). Advocates use influence to effect change in a number of ways. Access to decision-makers may be gained through strategies such as telephone calls, town hall meetings, face-to-face interactions, letter-writing campaigns, legislative testimony, financial contributions, or joining organizations with missions that align with the advocacy initiative.

Using an influential leader or spokesperson can bring attention to an issue. Celebrities, such as Michael J. Fox for Parkinson's disease research and Marlo Thomas for cancer in children, are regularly tapped to bring their influence on important issues. An influencer may also be a leader or influential member of a target group asked to promote an issue or solution. An influencer may be able to reach groups whose trust level with the advocate is low. To influence most effectively, the advocate must build a compelling case for change by using facts, figures, and examples. Equally important, the advocate must be able to influence others with a strong delivery. Developing an "elevator speech" is a valuable tool for the advocacy toolkit (see Table 2.1; see also Chapter 10). Written materials distributed in association with an elevator speech should be brief, succinct, and align with the verbal presentation. A one-page bulleted document is highly recommended, with the request being made stated clearly. Contact information for follow-up should be included.

TABLE 2.1: Key Elements of a Good Elevator Speech

FOLLOW THESE GUIDELINES WHEN PREPARING AN ELEVATOR SPEECH:
▪ **Keep It Short:** After hearing a few sentences, your audience should know what you do and what you want. Limit your pitch to 60 seconds.
▪ **Have a "Grabber":** An opening line that grabs the person's attention and piques interest in hearing more.
▪ **Show Your Passion:** Your energy and dedication will help sell your proposal.
▪ **Make a Request:** At the end of your speech, mention what you need. Do you want that person's business card? Do you want to schedule a meeting? Ask for a referral? Getting the person to take the next step is crucial. It is the reason you came up with your speech in the first place.
▪ **Practice:** Rehearse your elevator speech so that when the opportunity to use it comes up, you can do it well. Always be prepared to give your pitch so you can use it in a chance encounter. Memorize it. Revise as needed to keep it fresh and updated.

Source: Reprinted with permission. Copyright ©2021, HealthCom Media. All rights reserved.

Adapted from Pagana, K. D. (2013). Ride to the top with a good elevator speech. *American Nurse Today, 8*(3), 14–16. https://www.americannursetoday.com/ride-to-the-top-with-a-good-elevator-speech

Collaboration

In the complex world of healthcare, few changes are made in isolation. In fact, advocacy should be considered a team sport. Collaboration and partnership are necessary to effect major change. Collaboration is a process of working with others for a common purpose. Collaborative ventures involve the development of common goals, strategies, and activities that will achieve those goals (Tomajan, 2012). Successful collaboration can be a time-intensive process requiring ongoing communication with those involved, validating information, and reporting on progress toward the goal. The ANA, in collaboration with the Association of Nurse Executives (AONE now known as the American Organization for Nursing Leadership [AONL]), developed Principles for Collaborative Relationships to guide nurses in communicating with supervisors, and leaders within and outside the workplace (ANA/AONE, n.d.).

When collaborations are developed, it is helpful to consider all possible stakeholders to strengthen the advocacy efforts. Nurses may partner with other nurses or nursing organizations when the issue is directly related to professional nursing practice, but collaboration with other healthcare providers or even community-based groups can strengthen the advocacy efforts and message. An example of a coalition designed to address issues for advanced practice nurses and other healthcare providers is the Coalition for Patients' Rights (CPR). This coalition consists of 14 healthcare organizations working to offset the efforts of the American Medical Association's Scope of Practice Partnership (SOPP) initiative that was developed to limit patients' choices of healthcare practitioners. The CPR is predicated on the principle of patients having the right to choose their type of provider and having access to the right type of care at the right time (www.patientsrightscoalition.org).

Resource Identification

Another important skill for the nurse advocate is the ability to identify valuable resources. Although this competency is necessary for any problem-solving process, searching for health information is an essential skill when it comes to advocacy (White et al., 2010). Searching the internet for resources is commonplace; however, with the explosion of web-based information, much of it lacking credibility validation, the task can be daunting. Steps to a successful health policy internet search are illustrated in Figure 2.3.

Credible resources on the internet that the nurse advocate should use include peer-reviewed and professional databases (e.g., PubMed, the Cumulative Index to Nursing and Allied Health Literature), professional associations (e.g., ANA, the American Association of Critical-Care Nurses [AACN]), health policy organizations (e.g., the Robert Wood Johnson Foundation [RWJF], the Kaiser Family Foundation), and governmental entities (e.g., the Centers for Medicare & Medicaid Services [CMS], the Centers for Disease Control and Prevention). The

Formulate a clear, concise issue statement that describes and quantifies the problem

Identify the target audience for the advocacy efforts

Identify key words and phrases to search for information using an internet search engine

FIGURE 2.3 **Steps for successful health policy searches on the internet.**

following criteria are suggested for evaluating websites for use in advocacy activities (Binghamton University, 2020; White et al., 2010):

- **Accuracy and Expertise:** The qualifications, affiliations, and reputations of the authors are vital for reliability and credibility. Attention to details, especially in relation to scholarly references, is a hallmark of quality.

- **Content and Focus:** The website should be examined for a complete, balanced, and unbiased presentation of information. Reputable websites often include a mission statement, are clear about their perspective and intended audience, and include contact information.

- **Currency:** The information should be recent unless it is of historical nature. Broken uniform resource locator (URL) links and websites without recent update information indicate a poorly maintained website and raise questions about credibility.

- **Organization and Ease of Use:** Navigation should be user-friendly. The information may have limited use if the web pages, documents, and portable document format (PDF) files do not load easily and quickly. Member-based organizations often place valuable information behind a "For Members Only" section.

Extra care to ensure information accuracy is essential. Given the environment of fake news, alternate facts, and the myriad of misinformation available on the internet, it is incumbent on the nurse advocate to validate the accuracy and currency of information. *Misinformation* is false or inaccurate information that may be the result of mistakes or misunderstanding, whereas *disinformation* is false information intended to mislead or even cause harm (Binghamton University, 2020). Nurses should be members of their professional associations and other groups that support their advocacy work to get the most current and complete information (see Chapter 10).

ARENAS FOR ADVOCACY

Nurses have numerous opportunities for advocacy. The one that most often comes to mind is the workplace; however, advocacy also occurs in the community, state, national, and global arenas.

Workplace

Nurses most frequently use their advocacy skills in the workplace—whether it is a hospital, public health clinic, long-term care facility, or primary care office. Advocacy works best in environments that encourage its activity, where leaders are supportive, and where tools are available to make change happen.

The work environment of nurses has been studied extensively, with strong links to patient and nurse outcomes. Factors that define the work environment include workload, staffing, managerial support at the unit and organizational level, work team dynamics, and interprofessional relationships. The work environment impacts patient outcomes, including the patient experience, the incidence of infections, falls, pressure injuries, and mortality. Nurse-focused outcomes that are the result of work environment factors include job satisfaction, turnover, exhaustion and burnout, and perceptions of quality of care (Lake et al., 2019; Press Ganey, 2015).

The AACN (2016) developed the *AACN Standards for Establishing and Sustaining Healthy Work Environments* that address not only the physical environment but also fewer tangible barriers to staff and patient safety. The AACN highlights the ingredients for success as skilled communication, true collaboration, effective decision-making, appropriate staffing, meaningful recognition, and authentic leadership. These standards are guidelines that the nurse as advocate can use to support a healthy work environment. Mounting evidence is making the connection between positive work environments and patient and nurse outcomes (Lake et al., 2019; Press Ganey, 2015).

In 2017, the ANA launched the Healthy Nurse Healthy Nation (HNHN) initiative to address health issues of nurses. On all measures other than smoking, nurses are less healthy than the general population. The HNHN's vision is to "improve the nation's health one nurse at a time." The initiative involves partnership with multiple organizations to improve nurses' health in five domains—physical activity, nutrition, rest, quality of life, and safety; and provides online resources to support nurses' self-care goals. In 2020, strategies were added to address financial health. In 2020, more than 183,000 nurses were participating in opportunities for self-advocacy and role modeling for patients (HNHN, 2020).

Along with its partners and through its organizational relationships, ANA is a leader in promoting improved work environments. It protects, defends, and educates nurses about their rights as employees by addressing occupational hazards such as needle stick safety, back injuries, and workplace violence. The ANA and specialty organizations have developed a number of position statements and resources to support advocacy in the workplace. These resources are available at www.nursingworld.org/practice-policy/nursing-excellence/official-position-statements/.

Community

When nurses are advocating in their community for increased access to care or other healthcare resources, the respect they have from the public strengthens their ability to persuade others to create the needed changes regarding patient care and services. The cost of healthcare continues to create barriers for patients. Patients and families often share with the nurse the difficulties they are experiencing in obtaining needed care due to the costs of treatments and medications. Nurses find themselves advocating at the individual and community levels on access issues and funding to address the patients' ability to receive appropriate healthcare services. Nurses have been engaged in identifying community resources for patients and establishing resources when they are inadequate. Because of the high expense of prescription drugs, many patients forego treatment when they do not have the funds to obtain needed medication. Nurses may be aware of community resources for drug discounts or even pharmaceutical companies' resources to obtain needed treatment. Nurses have established community-based clinics for those who do not have adequate access to healthcare. These nurse-managed health centers under the direction of APRNs provide primary, secondary, and tertiary prevention services to the uninsured and underinsured populations; there are more than 200 such centers across the country (Holt et al., 2014; Valdez, 2017).

State

Although nurses may feel comfortable taking on the advocate role within their workplace or community, they may hesitate to take it to the next level and use their advocacy skills at the state level. They may not feel confident about their presentation skills or believe that others know more about the issue than they do (Jurns, 2019). However, they quickly find that their passion and healthcare knowledge will take them far in state advocacy. The ANA represents the interest of over 4.3 million RNs across the United States through its constituent and state nurses associations and its specialty nursing and affiliate organizations. With the implementation of the Patient Protection and Affordable Care Act, more commonly known as the ACA, and the ongoing state-level scope of practice issues that are barriers to APRNs, there is much to be done at the state level. One important provision of the ACA that highlights the need for effective state and national partnerships was the establishment of state insurance exchanges. These exchanges—online marketplaces where individuals can purchase health plans—have been established at the state level. The ANA works with the CMS to use language that includes APRNs to ensure that patients have improved access to care. With the continuing debate about healthcare reform, this collaboration is even more important to ensure that these gains continue within the structures of any new or revised legislation passed by Congress. Most barriers to APRN practice are at the state level as the result of state laws and regulations, including each

POLICY ON THE SCENE 2.3: REMOVING SCOPE OF PRACTICE BARRIERS

In September 2017, Elizabeth Ellis, DNP, RN, APRN, FNP-BC, FAANP, CRHCP, opened the B.I.S. Community Clinic in rural Bedias, Texas. The B.I.S. Clinic is a CMS-designated Rural Health Clinic that serves Bedias, Iola, Singleton, and surrounding communities. One of the many challenges that Elizabeth encountered was the inconvenience and strain of having to drive 2 hours to meet face-to-face monthly with her collaborative physician as a requirement of her nurse practitioner prescriptive authority agreement (PAA). This requirement took her away from the only healthcare facility in northern Grimes County.

Just 2 months prior to the opening of B.I.S Community Clinic, the Texas legislature passed Senate Bill 1625 with an amendment allowing physicians assistants to meet virtually with their supervising physicians in place of a face-to-face meeting. Unfortunately, APRNs were not included in this bill. Frustrated with the disparity, as well as the significant time and travel demands the outdated mandate imposed on her and her delegating physician, Elizabeth worked with members of the APRN Alliance to get the legislation changed. The APRN Alliance is a partnership of Texas APRN organizations that represent certified nurse-midwives, nurse anesthetists, clinical nurse specialists, nurse practitioners, and the Texas Nurses Association (TNA). The APRN Alliance met as an informal collaborative to improve the APRN practice environment in Texas. The alliance coordinates the efforts and communication between the organizations to sure consistent messaging.

Leading the APRN Alliance on this issue were TNA staff members who utilized their relationship with Representative Tom Oliverson to argue that this was not the best use of the APRN's or physician's time, especially when they have telemedicine capability. Representative Oliverson agreed and introduced House Bill 278. On February 27, 2019, Elizabeth testified on behalf of the bill. The proposed legislation passed unanimously through both the House (141–0) and Senate (31–0) and was signed into law on May 16, 2019. This example demonstrates the value of coalitions, unity, and speaking with one voice, which requires good communication and maximizing the talent and resources of each member.

State nurses associations and state-based coalitions have been vital to moving advocacy and lobbying activities and educating nurses to take on the additional responsibilities that are required at this level. State lobby days are one of the many activities held to educate nurses about important practice issues and ways they can make a difference when speaking to legislators, mayors, city council members, community activists, or the public at large.

state's respective nurse practice act. It is vital for nurses to advocate within their state for removing practice barriers such as requirements for physician supervision and prescriptive authority restrictions.

National

Moving advocacy to the national level typically takes nurses from their familiar practice settings to the unfamiliar world of policy and politics, a world in which many nurses do not feel prepared to effectively maneuver. Successful policy advocacy requires one to have the power, will, time, and energy, along with the political skills needed to "play the game" in the legislative arena. This move into national advocacy is challenging and time-consuming but offers the nurse a unique opportunity to make a difference in patient care and the satisfaction of playing a role in improving the healthcare system.

Many nurses who are active in the national arena honed their skills first through experiences with policy and legislative events sponsored by their state nurses association. Policy fellowships and workshops can also provide the needed opportunities to learn more about healthcare issues and the legislative process (see the Section "E-Resources"). There are multiple ways to get actively involved: Write a letter or email, make a call to your representative in Congress, attend a state or national Lobby Day event, educate your colleagues on national aspects of health policy such as healthcare reform, or even run for elective office. There are currently several nurses serving in the U.S. House of Representatives.

Many complex health policy issues require collaboration and sustained efforts to effect and maintain change. Organized nursing groups, the assistance of professional lobbyists, and sustained activity for months or even years are required when issues are as complex as healthcare reform or changing models of care delivery. Nurses who participate in their state and national nurses associations have access to important resources and can strategize collaboratively to bring nursing's perspective to legislative or regulatory decision-makers. Professional nursing organizations, such as the ANA, monitor public policy as their core work and educate their members about the impact of policy issues. This is illustrated by the ANA's collaborative work conducted over many years in support of healthcare reform.

Global

Advocacy on the global stage seems quite daunting. The ICN leads the profession in these efforts, representing the interests of nearly 28 million nurses worldwide. ICN seeks to align and integrate nursing actions around global health priorities and to influence the World Health Organization (WHO) and other decision-making bodies to shape health policy at the global level. The ICN publishes and disseminates position statements and educates nurses and the public at large about key health issues. The ICN advocates for policies that contribute to social justice, global health, sustainable development, and just treatment of nurses and healthcare professionals.

The ICN and other international health agencies have worked for many years to ban nuclear weapons. In 2021, an updated position statement was published by the International Committee of the Red Cross, ICN, International Federation of Medical Student Associations, International Physicians for the Prevention of Nuclear War, World Federation of Public Health Associations and World Medical Association that defines the threat and supports international efforts to ban nuclear weapons (ICN, 2021). In 2016, the ICN took its Leadership for Change™ (LFC) program to China to develop stronger nursing leaders at the national level. The LFC program is now established in more than 40 countries and focuses on the development of nursing knowledge and leadership skills. As a federation of more than 130 national nurses associations, the ICN works to effect global change (ICN, 2016) (see Chapter 14).

In 2018, the WHO created a new position, chief nursing Officer, and appointed Elizabeth Iro, a public health nurse and midwife from the Cook Islands (McSpendon, 2018). Ms. Iro has the opportunity to give voice to nearly 28 million nurses from around the world. In 2020, the WHO and the ICN published the *State of the World's Nursing: Investing in Education, Jobs and Leadership*, outlining the challenges and opportunities related to the global nursing workforce. The WHO, in collaboration with the ICN, designated 2020–2021 as Year of the Nurse and Midwife to commemorate the 200th anniversary of Florence Nightingale's birth and provide a platform to bring attention to the many contributions of nurses worldwide.

Increasingly, social and healthcare issues are global as opposed to simply national or regional. Global health issues transcend national boundaries and involve complex interagency and interprofessional cooperation for planning, prevention, and response. Solutions that respect health equity among nations often involve governments, nonprofits, and many times corporations and foundations. Examples of global issues include emerging infectious diseases including pandemics, human trafficking, maternal–newborn mortality, climate change, food insecurity, and hunger. These issues are influenced by the worldwide maldistribution of healthcare professionals (Edmonson et al., 2017).

Nurses across the globe are focused on the concept of advocacy as they provide care to their patients. Scandinavian nurse researchers examined how advocacy is defined by patients and nurses (Vaartio et al., 2006). Turkish nurses studied how ICU nurses make decisions about the distribution of scarce beds to their patients (Ersoy & Akpinar, 2010), and Iranian nurses developed their own patients' bill of rights and code of ethics while studying the extent of involvement in patient advocacy among their country's nurses (Negarandeh & Dehghan Nayeri, 2012; Salehi et al., 2010). The newly revised ICN Code of Ethics for Nurses (ICN, 2021, p. 7) indicates that nurses "advocate for equity and social justice in resource allocation, access to healthcare and other social and economic services."

WHEN ADVOCACY FAILS/WHEN ADVOCACY SUCCEEDS

One needs only to review the case example of U.S. healthcare reform to understand the arduous and complex nature of advocacy. From President Theodore Roosevelt's efforts toward national health insurance in the early 20th century to the creation of Medicare and Medicaid under President Johnson in 1965 and finally to the 2010 passage of the ACA under President Obama, the advocacy efforts of more than 100 years have brought us many improved programs but with many challenges left unresolved.

If advocacy is such an important aspect of nursing care, why do efforts sometimes fail? What are the barriers that prevent nurses from being effective advocates on behalf of their patients, themselves, or their profession? In a concept analysis of barriers to nursing advocacy, Hanks (2007) identified the most common barriers as conflict of interest between the nurse's responsibility to the patient and the nurse's duty to the employer, a lack of support, lack of power, time constraints, threats of punishment, the nurse's lack of education, and the historical barrier of being in a feminine profession with a tradition of subservience to the medical profession.

Institutional barriers to advocacy are challenging and often difficult to address. Nurses must know the legal scope of practice in their state and in their healthcare facility. Knowing the statutes and regulations assists nurses in being more effective advocates. If more assistance is needed with the state nurse practice act or practice guidelines, nurses should contact their state nurses associations; however, it is important for nurses to understand that membership organizations can best support only those dues-paying members who contribute to their profession.

Clear, effective communication is central to overcoming advocacy barriers. The nurse's ideas and suggestions are more effective when spoken clearly and without overt emotion such as anger and frustration. Even body language makes a difference. Using a loud voice, leaning into another person's space, pointing fingers, or crossing arms conveys hostility and prevents the nurse's message from being received. Patient-centered language is the best approach when seeking to be an effective advocate. Written documentation may also prove important if the situation escalates or there are negative patient outcomes.

The nurse must understand and use the employer's chain of command. There are important organizational policies for reporting concerns and issues that arise. The employer may have an administrative structure that includes committees supporting advocacy efforts (e.g., ethics, shared governance, staffing).

Education has a major role to play in teaching effective advocacy. Faculty must teach the issues related to nursing advocacy, as well as role model what it means to be an advocate—at the individual patient level and the political/policy level. The practicing nurse should seek a preceptor, mentor, or sponsor who demonstrates strong advocacy skills to assist in navigating difficult clinical issues and organizational processes. The following advocacy exemplars illustrate the range of issues, the forms an advocacy effort might take, and the different outcomes for the advocacy efforts.

Advocacy Exemplar: Understaffing

Labor and delivery nurse Mary Washington was tired, frustrated, and worried—her unit had been dealing with high census and low staffing for many months. The staff nurses were concerned for a while and had met with the unit manager to voice their concerns. Mary had even presented her professional organization's staffing guidelines to nursing leadership in an effort to make the case for improved staffing. However, it seemed that cost constraints were not allowing new staff to be hired, and Mary knew it was just a matter of time before understaffing would cause a problem. Some signs of fetal distress might be missed, and then a negative outcome would throw light on the consequences of the unit's staffing patterns. She was just a few years out of her undergraduate program, so Mary consulted with one of her maternal–child health faculty members, who gave her suggestions for advocacy efforts. She also consulted with her state nurses association to see if there were any regulations or other guidelines that might apply. She took all the suggestions to her unit manager and division director to advocate for safe patient care and protection of her own practice. Ultimately, Mary realized that she was being labeled a "troublemaker," so after discussing the situation with her colleagues, she determined she had no recourse but to resign and take a position at a different hospital in the city with safer staffing levels.

Advocacy Exemplar: Removing Scope of Practice Barriers

The value of APRNs is increasingly recognized by policymakers and consumers. As nursing practice is regulated by state boards of nursing, the United States continues to have a jumble of different regulations across state boundaries. However, a shift to full practice authority for APRNs is taking hold across the country as a result of nurses associations' advocacy and consumers' demand for better access to primary care providers. States are continuing to pass legislation to allow full practice authority for nurse practitioners (see Chapter 1).

Advocacy Exemplar: The Whistle-Blowing Nurses From Winkler County, Texas
In 2009, two nurses, Anne Mitchell and Vickilyn Galle, anonymously reported Dr. Rolando Arafiles Jr. to the Texas Medical Board for unsafe care. Dr. Arafiles urged the county sheriff and county attorney to uncover who made the report and then struck back at the nurses who were charged with misuse of official information, a third-degree felony, and fired from their jobs. After their case was nationally publicized by the TNA and the ANA, Dr. Arafiles's attempts to retaliate against the two whistle-blower nurses were uncovered. Subsequently, Dr. Arafiles was charged with misuse of official information and retaliation, also a third-degree felony. He was sentenced to 60 days in jail and fined $5,000. Three others involved in the case received jail sentences and lost their jobs as a result of the roles they played: Sheriff Robert Roberts Jr., Attorney Scott Tidwell, and Hospital Administrator Stan Wiley. Nurses Mitchell and Galle were completely exonerated and received a civil suit settlement of $375,000.

ADVOCACY ORGANIZATIONS

Nurses advocate to support patient autonomy and rights; however, they are less effective when challenging problems such as inadequate staffing or patient access to care unless they collectively respond to such systemic issues. Within direct-care clinical situations, individual nurses are staunch patient advocates, yet this focus of patient advocacy overlooks systemic problems that can cause harm to all patients (Florell, 2020). Although patient advocacy is most often framed in terms of an obligation to individual patients, it must include social and political advocacy and activism to address the full spectrum of patient care issues. Collective activism for nurses is best accomplished through professional associations. For professional nurses associations to effectively advocate for their professionals, they must rely on their members to report instances of inadequate and substandard care, as well as participate in the process of raising awareness.

Professional nurses organizations in the United States began two decades after formal education programs were established. The first training school for nurses in the United States opened in 1873, and by 1893, nursing school administrators worked to form the American Society of Superintendents of Training Schools for Nurses (later becoming the National League for Nursing) to network, share best practices, and maintain a universal standard for training nurses (Matthews, 2012). When graduate nurses were seeking consistent standards in education and competency, they formed the Nurses Associated Alumnae of the United States and Canada (later renamed the ANA) in 1896 to elevate the standards of nursing education, establish a code of ethics, and promote the interests of nursing. Three documents developed by the ANA form the foundation of nursing as a profession and establish the role of advocacy for the professional nurse: the *Code of Ethics for Nurses with Interpretive Statements* (2015), *Nursing: Scope and Standards of Practice* (2021), and the *Nursing's Social Policy Statement: The Essence of the Profession* (2010).

The director made arrangements for Linda to join the hospital's interprofessional pain committee, and she become involved in the implementation of nerve block therapy for joint replacement patients. Linda worked collaboratively with nurses from the inpatient orthopedic unit and physical therapists to assure staff knew how to safely care for the patient with a nerve block. She worked with the nursing education department to plan and implement training and developed a reference guide for staff who work infrequently with this modality. Standards of practice for pain management and other evidence-based resources were used to develop the training processes and support new policy development. Patient ratings for pain control during hospitalization improved for 10 consecutive quarters. Once this project was completed, the Pain Committee set its sights on several new projects—the use of ketamine and lidocaine infusions for patients with acute and chronic pain and the use of aromatherapy. These projects were much easier to plan and implement based on the process that was developed by Linda and the Pain Committee. Over the course of several following years, committee members presented their findings at regional and national conferences and were published in several professional journals.

Depending on the classification, there are approximately 100 national nurses associations in the United States. Most are specialty-focused, demonstrating the maturation, increased demands, and specialization that have occurred in nursing over the past 120 years. These organizations focus on missions that include legislative and broad-scale advocacy, education, professional development, and support for the professional nurse and patients' rights. These organizations with differing strategic plans have identified the value of working collaboratively on a large number of issues. Formal structures such as the Nursing Organizations Alliance (www.nursing-alliance.org) and the ANA's Organizational Affiliates (www.nursingworld.org/FunctionalMenuCategories/AboutANA/WhoWeAre/AffiliatedOrganizations), as well as informal coalitions and groups, come together to address a specific problem or issue. See the Policy Solution for how nurses can address issues in their practice.

IMPLICATIONS FOR THE FUTURE

Advocacy at its best is about transformation. Wolf (2012) uses complexity science to demonstrate how events, patterns, and system structures can be helpful in transforming an organization. Successful nurse advocates can look beyond the events of today, see patterns and trends that are occurring, and map the direction needed for tomorrow. Future orientation causes the nurse advocate to ask: What type of care will patients look for in the future? What patterns need to change to improve the care given today? What outcomes require focus now? How might our patient population be different in future years, and what must we do to prepare for that? What structures would support that difference? What policies need to change? "The changes that are needed for patients will drive the changes that are needed for professional practice and become the source of advocacy" (Wolf, 2012, p. 309). The importance of transformational leaders to drive toward this future view of advocacy is vital.

As nursing leaders explore the facts and observe how patterns fit together, they develop goals and objectives that will move the organization forward. They must use their influence to build collaboration and confidence, seeking staff input on how changes impact patient care, nurse satisfaction, and patient outcomes. When advocacy works best, all in the organization feel valued and engaged. Transformation in healthcare occurs only when advocacy is embraced by healthcare professionals and seen as an inherent part of their practice.

KEY CONCEPTS

1. The concept of advocacy is an integral part of professional nursing.
2. Nurses readily accept the requirement of the professional nurse's advocacy role as it applies to their patients; however, opportunities to advocate on behalf of colleagues, the profession, or even oneself are often missed.
3. The *ANA Code of Ethics for Nurses with Interpretive Statements* defines expectations for the professional nurse's engagement in advocacy.
4. A strong commitment to social justice requires professional nurses to advocate for health for all persons.
5. The American public sees the nurse in the role of advocate in that they have rated RNs as the most honest and ethical profession and have called for nurses to be more involved in healthcare decision-making.
6. Nurse advocates need to have the competencies of problem-solving, communication, influence, collaboration, and resource identification.
7. Advocacy works best in environments that encourage its activity, where leaders are supportive, and tools are available to make it happen.
8. Moving advocacy to the state, national, and global levels typically takes nurses from their familiar practice settings to the unfamiliar world of policy and politics, a world in which many nurses do not feel prepared to effectively maneuver.
9. Common barriers to advocacy include conflict of interest between the nurse's responsibility to the patient and duty to the employer, a lack of support, a lack of power, time constraints, threats of punishment or retaliation, or the nurse's lack of education.
10. Stress is a common workplace issue that can have serious effects. This experience can be minimized through self-advocacy measures that include mindfulness, education, a healthy lifestyle, and organizational support.

SUMMARY

As a profession, nurses "stand on the shoulders of giants" as it relates to the contributions of historical nurse leaders—championing social justice and access to care. Their contributions are still felt today. Healthcare is undergoing dramatic changes and the role of the professional nurse is evolving. In this time of evolution, nurses are in the rooms where decisions are being made. The importance of nursing advocacy and activism cannot be overstated. More than 20 million uninsured in the United States gained access to healthcare under the provisions of the ACA and until the ACA reaches its full capability, the future of care for millions of Americans remains in question. Every nurse can take active measures to foster their own voice, and collectively join together to amplify the voice of nursing to transform healthcare. Every nurse in every setting has the opportunity and responsibility to make a positive difference in the lives of patients and the quality of nursing care. Advocacy is the key.

END-OF-CHAPTER RESOURCES

LEARNING ACTIVITIES

1. Describe two specific actions you could use to advocate for a culture of safety.
2. Describe one example of how you could infuse the *Code of Ethics for Nurses* into your daily practice.
3. Evaluate the resources available in your state to support nurses who have been reported to the Board of Nursing for impaired practice.
4. Explore the programs available to assist with advocacy efforts in your workplace or state. Identify three individuals you could consult to assist you with workplace concerns.
5. Identify a current issue that you have experienced or read about, and identify advocacy and/or activist strategies to promote solutions to address the issue.
6. Explore the lives and accomplishments of a historical nursing leader. What are their enduring contributions to society? Examples of nursing leaders include, but are not limited to, Dorothea Dix, Jane Delano, Lillian Wald, Mary Breckinridge, Clara Barton, Florence Nightingale, and Margaret Sanger.

E-RESOURCES

- Advocacy Project http://advocacynet.org
- Agency for Healthcare Research and Quality http://www.ahrq.gov
- American Association of Nurse Practitioners State Practice Environment Map https://www.aanp.org/advocacy/state/state-practice-environment
- American Nurses Association http://www.nursingworld.org
- American Nurses Association Advocacy Toolkit, Governmental Affairs https://ana.aristotle.com/SitePages/toolkit.aspx
- American Nurses Association. *Code of Ethics for Nurses* http://www.nursingworld.org/codeofethics
- American Nurses Association Policy & Advocacy http://www.nursingworld.org/MainMenuCategories/Policy-Advocacy
- American Public Health Association. Advocacy & Policy https://www.apha.org/~/media/files/pdf/advocacy/power_of_advocacy.ashx
- Centers for Medicare & Medicaid Services http://www.cms.gov
- Child Health Advocacy Institute https://childrensnational.org/advocacy-and-outreach/child-health-advocacy-institute
- Commonwealth Fund http://www.commonwealthfund.org
- Department of Health and Human Services http://www.hhs.gov
- Healthy Nurse Healthy Nation https://www.healthynursehealthynation.org/
- House of Representatives http://www.house.gov
- Institute for Healthcare Improvement http://www.ihi.org
- Institute of Safe Medication Practice https://www.ismp.org
- International Council of Nurses http://www.icn.ch

- National Academy of Medicine http://www.nam.edu

- National Conference of State Legislatures http://www.ncsl.org

- Nurse-Family Partnership NFP Nurse Advocacy Toolkit https://www.nursefamilypartnership.org/public-policy-and-advocacy/advocacy-toolkit-for-nurses/

- Occupational Safety and Health Administration https://www.osha.gov

- Robert Wood Johnson Foundation Health Policy Fellows Program https://www.healthpolicyfellows.org/

- Senate http://www.senate.gov

- Trust for America's Health https://www.tfah.org/

REFERENCES

American Association of Critical-Care Nurses. (2016). *AACN standards for establishing and sustaining healthy work environments* (2nd ed.). https://www.aacn.org/~/media/aacn-website/nursing-excellence/standards/hwestandards.pdf

American Nurses Association. (2010). *Nursing's social policy statement: The essence of the profession* (2nd ed.). Author.

American Nurses Association. (2015). *Code of ethics for nurses with interpretive statements.* https://www.nursingworld.org/practice-policy/nursing-excellence/ethics/code-of-ethics-for-nurses/

American Nurses Association. (2017). *Who will be there? Ethics, the law and nurse's duty to respond in a disaster* (ANA Issue Brief). https://www.nursingworld.org/~4ad845/globalassets/docs/ana/who-will-be-there_disaster-preparedness_2017.pdf

American Nurses Association. (2020). *ANA's Membership Assembly adopts resolution on racial injustice for communities of color.* https://www.nursingworld.org/news/news-releases/2020/ana-calls-for-racial-justice-for-communities-of-color/

American Nurses Association. (2021). *Nursing: Scope and standards of practice* (4th ed.). Author.

American Nurses Association & American Association of Nurse Executives. (n.d.). *Principles for collaborative relationships between clinical nurses and nurse managers.* https://www.nursingworld.org/~4af4f2/globalassets/docs/ana/ethics/principles-of-collaborative-relationships.pdf

American Nurses Association Professional Issues Panel. (n.d.). *A call to action: Exploring moral resilience toward a culture of ethical practice.* https://www.nursingworld.org/~4907b6/globalassets/docs/ana/ana-call-to-action--exploring-moral-resilience-final.pdf

American Nurses Association. (2018). The nurses' role in addressing discrimination. Protecting and promoting inclusion, strategies in practice settings, policy and advocacy. https://www.nursingworld.org/practice-policy/nursing-excellence/official-position-statements/

Annie E. Casey Foundation. (2020). *Equity vs. equality and other racial justice definitions.* https://www.aecf.org/blog/racial-justice-definitions/?gclid=EAIaIQobChMInZGO9ZeT7gIVIQh9Ch-1Q8QPgEAAYASAAEgI-yPD_BwE

Bazdak, L., & Turner, M. (2015). 2015 Code of Ethics for Nurses with interpretive statements: Summary of revisions to the 2001 code. *American Nurse Today, 10*(3), 18. https://www.myamericannurse.com/

Binghamton University. (2020). *Smart sharing in the age of mis and dis-information.* Center for Civic Engagement. https://libraryguides.binghamton.edu/c.php?g=1042510&p=7718852

Bosek, M. S. D., & Savage, T. A. (2007). *The ethical component of nursing education: Integrating ethics into clinical experiences.* Lippincott Williams & Wilkins.

Braveman, P., Arkin, E., Orleans, T., Proctor, D., & Plough, A. (2017). *What is health equity? And what difference does it make?* http://www.rwjf.org/content/dam/farm/reports/issue_briefs/2017/rwjf437393

Bu, X., & Jezewski, M. A. (2007). Developing a mid-range theory of patient advocacy through concept analysis. *Journal of Advanced Nursing, 57*(1), 101–110. https://doi.org/10.1111/j.1365-2648.2006.04096.x

Butts, J. B., & Rich, K. L. (2016). *Nursing ethics: Across the curriculum and into practice* (4th ed.). Jones & Bartlett.

Cook, E. T. (1913). *The life of Florence Nightingale: Vol. 1, 1820–1861.* Macmillan. http://www.gutenberg.org/files/40057/40057-h/40057-h.htm

Edmonson, C., McCarthy, C., Trent-Adams, S., McCain, C., & Marshall, J. (2017, January 31). Emerging global health issues. *OJIN: The Online Journal of Issues in Nursing, 22*(1), 2. https://doi.org/10.3912/OJIN.Vol22No01Man02

Ersoy, N., & Akpinar, A. (2010). Turkish nurses' decision-making in the distribution of intensive care beds. *Nursing Ethics, 17*(1), 87–98. https://doi.org/10.1177/0969733009349992

Florell, M. C. (2020). Concept analysis of nursing activism. *Nursing Forum, 56*(1), 136–140. https://doi.org/10.1111/nuf.12502

Fowler, M. D. M. (Ed.). (2015). *Guide to the code of ethics with interpretive statements: Development, interpretation and application* (2nd ed.). American Nurses Association.

Hanks, R. G. (2007). Barriers to nursing advocacy: A concept analysis. *Nursing Forum, 42*(4), 171–177. https://10.1111/j.1744-6198.2007.00084.x

Harper, K. J., & Benson, L. S. (2019). The importance and impact of nurses serving on boards. *Nursing Economic$, 37*(4), 209–212.

Healthy Nurse Healthy Nation. (2020). *Healthy Nurse Healthy Nation.* https://www.healthy-nursehealthynation.org/

Hegge, M. J. (2011). The lingering presence of the Nightingale legacy. *Nursing Science Quarterly, 24*(2), 152–162. https://doi.org/10.1177/0894318411399453

Holt, J., Zabler, B., & Baisch, M. (2014). Evidence-based characteristics of nurse-managed health centers for quality and outcomes. *Nursing Outlook, 62*(6), 428–439. https://doi.org/10.1016/j.outlook.2014.06.005

Institute of Medicine. (2011). *The future of nursing: Leading change, advancing health.* National Academies Press. https://doi.org/10.17226/12956

International Council of Nurses. (2021). The ICN Code of Ethics for Nurses. https://www.icn.ch/system/files/2021-10/ICN_Code-of-Ethics_EN_Web_0.pdf

International Council of Nurses. (2021). International health care humanitarian organizations welcome the entry into force of the treaty on the prohibition of nuclear weapons. https://www.icn.ch/sites/default/files/inline-files/FINAL-English-Global-Health-Statement.docx_.pdf

John F. Kennedy Presidential Library. (2021). Celebrating COVID Courage. Lauren Leander, Intensive Care Nurse, Arizona. https://www.jfklibrary.org/events-and-awards/profile-in-cour-age-award/award-recipients/covid-courage/lauren-leander

Jurns, C. (2019). Policy advocacy motivators and barriers: Research results and applica-tions. *OJIN: The Online Journal of Issues in Nursing, 24*(3). https://doi.org/10.3912/OJIN.Col24No033PPT63

Khoury, C. M., Blizzard, R., Wright Moore, L., & Hassmiller, S. (2011). Nursing leadership from bedside to boardroom: A Gallup national survey of opinion leaders. *Journal of Nursing Administration, 41*(7–8), 299–305. https://doi.org/10.1097/NNA.0b013e3182250a0d

Lachman, V. D. (2015). Conscientious objection in nursing: Definition and criteria for acceptance. *Medsurg Nursing, 23*(3), 196–198.

Lachman, V. D., Swanson, E. O., & Winland-Brown, J. (2015). The new "code of ethics for nurses with interpretive statements" (2015): Practical clinical application, Part II. *Medsurg Nursing*, 24(5), 363–366, 368. http://www.medsurgnursing.net

Lake, E. T., Sanders, J., Duan, R. Riman, K. A., Schoenauer, K. M., & Chen, Y. (2019). A meta-analysis of the associations between the nurse work environment in hospitals and 4 sets of outcomes. *Medical Care*, 57(5), 353–361. https://doi.org/10.1097/MLR.0000000000001109

Matthews, J. H. (2012). Role of professional organizations in advocating for the nursing profession. *OJIN: The Online Journal of Issues in Nursing*, 17(1), 3. https://doi.org/10.3912/OJIN.Vol17No01Man03

Matwick, A. L., & Woodgate, R. L. (2016). Social justice: A concept analysis. *Public Health Nursing*, 34(2), 176–184. https://doi.org/10.1111/phn.12288

McSpendon, C. (2018). World Health Organization's Chief Nursing Officer. *American Journal of Nursing*, 118(9), 69–70. https://doi.org/10.1097/01.NAJ.0000544986.95312.c6

Navajo-Hopi Observer. (2020, November 18). Arizona nurses stand in solidarity with Navajo and Hopi neighbors in pandemic. https://www.nhonews.com/news/2020/sep/01/arizona-nurses-stand-solidarity-navajo-and-hopi-ne/?fbclid=IwAR1C48X-DQYTBLc7wdNoMi-2Am4e1WCz5_DcMpU9HalkqUTTHnqaGwSZBcf4

Negarandeh, R., & Dehghan Nayeri, N. (2012). Patient advocacy practice among Iranian nurses. *Indian Medical Ethics*, 9(3), 190–195. https://doi.org/10.20529/ijme.2012.063

Pagana, K. D. (2013). Ride to the top with a good elevator speech. *American Nurse Today*, 8(3), 14–16. https://www.myamericannurse.com/

Paquin, S. O. (2011). Social justice advocacy in nursing: What is it? How do we get there? *Creative Nursing*, 17(2), 63–67. https://doi.org/10.1891/1078-4535.17.2.63

Pavlish, C., Brown-Saltzman, K., Hersh, M., Shirk, M., & Rounkle, A. (2011). Nursing priorities, actions and regret for ethical situations in clinical practice. *Journal of Nursing Scholarship*, 43(4), 385–395. https://doi.org/10.1111/j.1547-5069.2011.01422.x

Press Ganey. (2015). *Nursing special report: The influence of nurse work environment on patient, payment and nurse outcomes in acute care settings*. http://www.pressganey.com/about/news/nursing-special-report-the-influence-of-nurse-work-environment-on-patient-payment-and-nurse-outcomes

Rappleye, E. (2019, October 30). Nurses are most trusted to improve the US healthcare system. *Becker's Hospital Review*. https://www.beckershospitalreview.com/hospital-management-administration/nurses-are-most-trusted-to-improve-the-us-healthcare-system.html

Ruelas, R. (2020, April 24). 'That's the one there: A photo of a protesting nurse in Phoenix goes viral.' Arizona Republic. https://www.azcentral.com/story/news/politics/arizona/2020/04/24/how-photo-protesting-nurse-phoenix-went-viral/3023111001/

Rushton, C. (2017). Cultivating moral resilience: Shifting the narrative from powerlessness to possibility. *American Journal of Nursing*, 117(2 Suppl. 1), S11–S15. https://doi.org/10.1097/01.NAJ.0000512205.93596.00

Rushton, C., Schoonover, K., & Kennedy, M. (2017). Executive summary: Transforming moral distress into moral resilience in nursing. *American Journal of Nursing*, 117(2), 52–56 https://doi.org/10.1097/01.NAJ.0000512298.18641.31

Saad, L. (2020, December 22). U.S. Ethics Ratings rise for medical workers and teachers. https://news.gallup.com/poll/328136/ethics-ratings-rise-medical-workers-teachers.aspx?version=print

Salehi, T., Dehghan Nayeri, N., & Negarandeh, R. (2010). Ethics: Patients' rights and the code of nursing ethics in Iran. *OJIN: The Online Journal of Issues in Nursing*, 15(3). https://doi.org/10.3912/OJIN.Vol15No03EthCol01

Selanders, L., & Crane, P. (2012). The voice of Florence Nightingale on advocacy. *OJIN: The Online Journal of Issues in Nursing*, 17(1), 1. https://doi.org/10.3912/OJIN.Vol17No01Man01

Tomajan, K. (2012). Advocating for nurses and nursing. *OJIN: The Online Journal of Issues in Nursing*, 17(1), 4. https://doi.org/10.3912/OJIN.Vol17No01Man04

Vaartio, H., & Leino-Kilpi, H. (2005). Nursing advocacy—A review of the empirical research 1990–2003. *International Journal of Nursing Studies*, 42(6), 282–292. https://doi.org/10.1016/j.ijnurstu.2004.10.005

Vaartio, H., Leino-Kilpi, H., Salanterä, S., & Suominen, T. (2006). Nursing advocacy: How is it defined by patients and nurses, what does it involve and how is it experienced? *Scandinavian Journal of Caring Sciences*, 20(3), 282–292. https://doi.org/10.1111/j.1471-6712.2006.00406.x

Valderama-Wallace, C. P. (2017). Critical discourse analysis of social justice in nursing's foundational documents. *Public Health Nursing*, 35(1), 1–7. https://doi.org/10.1111/phn.12327

Valdez, B. (2017, January). The effect of regulation on innovation in healthcare delivery. *Social Innovations Journal*. https://socialinnovationsjournal.org/75-disruptive-innovations/2271-the-effect-of-regulation-on-innovation-in-healthcare-delivery

Van Dyke, K., Combes, J., & Joshi, M. (2011). *AHA health care governance survey report*. Center for Healthcare Governance. American Hospital Association.

White, P., Olsan, T. H., Bianchi, C., Glessner, T., & Mapstone, P. (2010). Legislative: Searching for health policy information on the Internet: An essential advocacy skill. *OJIN: The Online Journal of Issues in Nursing*, 15(2). https://doi.org/10.3912/OJIN.Vol15No02LegCol01

Wolf, G. (2012). Transformational leadership: The art of advocacy and influence. *Journal of Nursing Administration*, 42(6), 309–310. https://doi.org/10.1097/NNA.0b013e3182573989

CHAPTER 3

Navigating the Political System

EILEEN M. SULLIVAN-MARX AND SUSAN APOLD

All politics is local.
—*Tip O'Neill, Jr., 55th Speaker of the U.S. House of Representatives*

OBJECTIVES

1. Compare and contrast functions among the executive, legislative, and judicial government branches in the creation and implementation of policy.
2. Critique policy solutions obtained through regulatory and legislative processes.
3. Differentiate among local, state, and federal jurisdictions.
4. Analyze strategies to create or influence policy during all phases of the policy cycle.

In the United States, more than 200 years ago, the Founding Fathers envisioned a government in which democratic principles would rule the nation. Fundamental to a democratic system is the participation of all citizens in the creation and evolution of that government. The U.S. system was created to specifically address the needs of its people to ensure that the voices of the people would be heard and that no one entity had the power to overrule the voice of the people. This system, while over 200 years old, is relatively new in the history of governance, but it has persisted in this nation, and it appears that this "Great Experiment" is here to stay. It can survive only if its basic premise is upheld and carefully nurtured: The people must participate and diligently protect our democracy. All citizens of our nation have the opportunity and responsibility to participate in and nurture our democracy. As the largest healthcare workforce in the country, with more than 4 million practicing nurses have unprecedented power to exert influence on almost any aspect of life in the United States but most particularly their area of expertise: the healthcare needs of our nation and the profession itself. The National Council of State Boards of Nursing (NCSBN, 2021) reports that as of, December 2021 there are 4,311,704 RNs in the United States. This translates to approximately one RN for each 1,000 people. Gallup polls consistently rank nursing as number one for ethics and honesty (Saad, 2020). Paradoxically, although society holds nursing in high esteem, only 14% of American opinion leaders from the public and private sector, academia, and trade organizations believed nurses were likely to exert a great deal of influence on healthcare in comparison to 75% and 56%, respectively, for government and insurance executives (Khoury et al., 2011).

Nurses have exerted exceptional influence on individual patients, families, and communities; however, they have not historically harnessed the power of their numbers, knowledge, or economic force into a cohesive unit with the potential for a powerful collective voice in healthcare. Nursing has reacted and responded to a number of healthcare policies; however, nurses' reactions remain peripheral to policymaking. Nurses have the potential political power to make momentous

71

contributions to the national healthcare system. Although a cadre of individual nurses has exhibited exceptional records of accomplishments in policymaking as a unified profession, nurses have historically experienced tension between their perceived role as caretakers and their role as political activists.

Politics is often perceived as dirty and dishonest, and nurses often do not embrace the reality that in their role as patient advocates, political engagement with its solutions and challenges, is an essential responsibility in keeping nursing's social contract with society (Des Jardin, 2001). Nurses need to look no further than their own professional documents to discover their imperative to engage in the policy process. Nursing arises out of society's need for the promotion of health and care of the sick; it is society that entrusts nursing with autonomy and responsibility for addressing these needs. The American Nurses Association (ANA, 2010) defines *nursing* as "the protection, promotion, and optimization of health and abilities, prevention of illness and injury, alleviation of suffering through the diagnosis and treatment of human response, and advocacy in the care of individuals, families, communities, and populations" (p. 3). The *Nursing's Social Policy Statement* (ANA, 2010), which describes the social contract between society and the nursing profession, requires that the profession advocate for public health; organization, delivery, and financing of healthcare; expansion of healthcare resources and health policy; and planning of health policy and regulation (see Chapter 2).

To embrace the full responsibility for the privilege of serving as a professional RN, individual nurses must participate in politics and the policymaking-making process. Realizing the Triple Aim, improved patient healthcare experiences, decreased healthcare cost, high-quality healthcare, and now the Quadruple Aim, with the addition of care of the provider, cannot be achieved without the voice of nursing at every table where healthcare is discussed—hospitals, colleges, universities, professional nursing organizations, government agencies, and board rooms of every company in this nation (Berwick et al., 2008; Bodenheimer & Sinsky, 2014).

Nurses can be engaged with a full cycle of policy activities through a continuum of engagement, from local municipalities to international venues from participation in workplace committees to election to public office. Nurses are well recognized as a potent political force when they coalesce through organized campaigns to write letters, speak through nursing leadership, and represent themselves as a significant voting bloc. Despite these abilities and strides, nurses remain relatively invisible in the policy process. Few nurses run for elected office, hold a political appointment, work as a staff member for a legislator, or work on a candidate or issue campaign. They are more commonly employed in staff positions within government administrative agencies, where they are responsible for implementing administrative policies and clarifying and informing their respective employing agency regarding health and nursing issues. However, these positions are not widely known in nursing.

This chapter discusses opportunities for nurses to engage in the policy process not as widely known or as visible. These include actively participating in professional association memberships, contributing to political action committees (PACs), writing letters, sitting on local community boards (e.g., parent–teacher associations), registering to vote and voting, engaging in the development of proposed legislation, testifying, writing comments on federal or state regulatory rulemaking, working on campaigns, and vetting local politicians for endorsement by organizations. Before the details of these activities are examined, the key features of governmental processes are discussed because understanding these processes is vital to accepting policy opportunities. Much of the focus of this chapter is on the processes at the federal level, recognizing that there are similarities but diversity in the structures and processes at the state and local levels. Equally important is appreciating the long view of policy; creation and implementation can take years, with many different stakeholders.

Many nurses who have become involved in policy didn't necessarily plan their involvement. Often, an issue impacting their practice or their community inspired them to take action. This policy challenge illustrates how a direct care nurse can influence policy and make a difference. Engagement in policy doesn't always follow a direct path and is different for everyone.

Often, numerous stakeholders, years of work, and various political and policy strategies are needed for effective long-term defensible solutions. An example of an issue specific to nursing policy is the evolution and status of the Doctor of Nursing Practice (DNP) degree. The dramatic changes in healthcare and prominent reports cited the need for a better and differently educated workforce using a seamless and efficient strategy for nursing education. These reports included the *Recreating Health Professional Practice for a New Century* (O'Neil & the Pew Health Professions Commissions, 1998), *Crossing the Quality Chasm* (Institute of Medicine [IOM], 2001), *Health Professions Education* (Greiner & Knebel, 2003), and *The Future of Nursing: Leading change, advancing health* (IOM, 2011). Specifically, the identified need was for the development of advanced competencies for increasingly complex clinical, faculty, and leadership roles, along with the need for enhanced knowledge to improve nursing practice and patient outcomes.

| POLICY CHALLENGE | A Different Path to Nursing: Building Influence and Creating Change |

Hollie Gentry, MSN, WHNP-BC, CNE
Lecturer, Rutgers School of Nursing, New Brunswick, NJ

I like to say that I've taken the long way to nursing. After high school, I completed an undergraduate degree in English at The Ohio State University. I always thought I would become a teacher or perhaps go to law school. One of my roommates worked as a page at the Ohio Senate, and she asked me if I would want to work there, too. I thought, "Hey, that sounds like an interesting job—maybe I'll meet some important people or get to do some exciting things." During my last 3 years at Ohio State, I ran errands for senators, took phone messages from constituents, and attended committee meetings and full Senate sessions. I even became the personal office page for one state senator, assisting with constituent correspondence, preparing recommendations for recognition of achievements, and helping set up for committee hearings. I was able to see how the political process works from an insider's perspective—how a bill is initiated, who is involved with writing the legislation, and how much work actually goes into getting a bill to become a law. I also came to understand how important it is to build and maintain relationships with key partners. I really enjoyed this work and thought about continuing as a legislative aide after graduation. However, when I finished my degree, I got married and move out of state, leaving behind my Ohio Statehouse connections and friendships.

Eventually, I moved back to Ohio and decided that nursing was the next step for me, but I always remained interested in policy and politics. When I first became a women's health nurse, I realized there was a lot I did not know about infant and maternal mortality. I learned that Cuyahoga County, Ohio, and Cleveland in particular, had one of the worst infant mortality rates in the United States. I also discovered that Black babies were two to three times more likely to die in their first year of life than their White or Hispanic counterparts. Additionally, the statistics on maternal mortality and morbidity, especially for black women, were startling to me as I watched the U.S. maternal mortality rate continue to increase, even when a majority of these deaths are preventable. My eyes were opened to these issues and I just could not look away.

How was I going to contribute to the solution? What did I bring to the table?

The first nursing doctoral program was established in 1924 at Teachers College at Columbia University. It was a program designed for nurses interested in the science of nursing education and conferred an EdD. In 1934, the first PhD program was offered to nurses at New York University and concentrated on advanced knowledge in nursing and nursing science (Apold, 2008). Within the profession, conversations emerged regarding the need for a clinical doctorate, a terminal degree for nurses that focused on the implementation of nursing research, development of quality science in nursing, and the further development of clinical expertise. Attempts were made to provide such a degree, with DNS and DNSc programs emerging to fill that need; however, these programs soon closely resembled traditional PhD programs. A nursing doctorate (ND) program was introduced in 1979 as an innovative clinical entry-level program at Case Western Reserve University Frances Payne Bolton School of Nursing in Cleveland, Ohio (Patzek, 2010). This was designed as the first clinically focused doctoral program in nursing in the nation. With the increasing need for and growth of nursing research, PhD and DNSc programs continued the focus on developing researchers to create the evidence base for nursing. However, the changing perspectives on nursing education called for visionary leadership to guide future policy discussion and decisions, create parity with other health professions, and address advanced clinical education for nurses. Stakeholders were convened and made a recommendation to the American Association of Colleges of Nursing (AACN) that a clinical doctorate, the DNP, be established and standardized as the terminal clinical degree for nurses. The DNP has emerged as the terminal graduate clinical degree for advanced nursing practice preparation (e.g., clinical nurse specialist, nurse practitioner [NP], certified nurse-midwife, certified registered nurse anesthetist, and other nursing leaders). The National Organization of Nurse Practitioner Faculties (NONPF) now recommends that the DNP be considered entry-level preparation for NPs. In addition, the American Association of Nurse Anesthesiology recommended that all nurse anesthesia programs move to a practice-oriented doctoral degree so that all graduates will have a doctorate when entering practice as certified registered nurse anesthetists (CRNAs) by 2025.

UNDERSTANDING THE SYSTEM

To navigate the system, nurses need to understand it. Often, nurses and the U.S. public, in general, avoid policy and politics because the system of government appears complex and confusing. The following section provides a brief overview of the system and structure of government in the United States. (For a more comprehensive understanding of the U.S. government, see www.congress.org.)

The U.S. Constitution is the legal basis for all government and governmental activity. It consists of a (a) preamble containing perhaps, the most famous words in our nation, "We the People"; (b) seven original articles defining the branches of government, providing for interaction between state and federal government and providing for the process of amendment and ratification; and (c) amendments (27), the first 10 of which compose the Bill of Rights. The Constitution is based on "Six Big Ideas" (Exhibit 3.1) that underscore the values of the Founding Fathers and the American people.

As laid out in the Constitution, each branch of government has specific powers to ensure that no one branch gains too much control or has too much power (see Exhibit 3.2). The Constitution provides for a federalist system whereby governance is shared between federal and state entities. It is essential for nurses to understand which branches of government are responsible for which laws, policies, and

EXHIBIT 3.1 "SIX BIG IDEAS" IN THE U.S. CONSTITUTION

CONCEPT	APPLICATION
Limited government	The restriction of the power that government has over its people
Republicanism	A government that requires the active involvement of its people
Checks and balances	The division of power such that the power to govern does not rest completely in any one branch
Federalism	Shared government between the federal and state governments
Separation of powers	Established branches of government, each with its own responsibilities
Popular sovereignty	Government ruling at the consent of its people through elected officials

EXHIBIT 3.2 BRANCHES OF THE U.S. GOVERNMENT

BRANCHES	LEGISLATIVE (MAKES LAWS)	EXECUTIVE (ENFORCES LAWS)	JUDICIAL (EVALUATES LAWS)

Composition	Congress
	■ U.S. Senate
	  ● 50 members
	  ● Elected every 6 years
	  ● U.S. House of Representatives
	  ● 435 members
	  ● Elected every 2 years
		■ President
		■ Vice president
		■ Cabinet secretaries of federal agencies
		■ Executive Office of the White House
			■ Supreme Court
			■ Appellate courts
			■ District courts

Powers and duties	■ Both Houses create new or amend existing laws
	■ Both Houses must agree on a bill before it can become a law
	■ Congress can override a Presidential veto
	■ U.S. Senate
	■ Confirms presidential appointments
	  ● Ratifies treaties
	  ● U.S. House of Representatives
	■ Initiates revenue bills
	■ Approves budget
	■ Impeaches federal officials
	■ Elects the president in the event of an electoral college tie
		■ Executes and enforces laws created by Congress
		■ Executes and enforces treaties
		■ Commands the armed forces
		■ Determines military deployments
		■ Signs legislation or vetoes bills
		■ Appoints more than 1,000 positions in federal agencies and judiciary, including Supreme Court
		■ Issues executive orders
			■ Interprets the Constitution
			■ Protects individual constitutional rights
			■ Determines constitutionality of laws
			■ Determines constitutionality of executive actions
			■ Resolves legal disputes
			■ Provides the check over the power of executive and legislative branches

regulations; for example, professional licensing and insurance laws and regulations are under the jurisdiction of the states, and civil rights and immigration laws fall under federal jurisdiction. This distinction is important when speaking with policymakers to ensure that the right issues get to the policymaker or legislator that has jurisdiction over them. The U.S. government was designed to allow for a thoughtful, contemplative, and lengthy decision-making process. It takes years, sometimes decades, for legislation to be enacted.

The doctrine of "states' rights" is secured by the U.S. Constitution. Each state, therefore, has a constitution and a formal government structure that is like the federal governmental structure. All states have an executive branch (led by the governor), a legislative branch (usually a bicameral legislature consisting of a state senate and state house of representatives or state assembly), and a judicial branch. State constitutions cannot conflict with the U.S. Constitution; when a conflict arises, the federal constitution prevails. The formal legislative process is depicted in Figure 3.1. The informal legislative process is the stuff of politics.

Policy not only happens in formal political and governmental arenas. As former Speaker of the House Tip O'Neill famously stated, "all politics is local." All systems are political! Local governments are often the place where issues close to the people are identified as problems requiring political action and policy solutions. Professional associations are also the source of many contributions to formal policymaking. Most organizations have structures similar to governmental structures. These include constitutions (bylaws), governing bodies with elected and appointed positions (presidents, executive directors, and boards of directors or trustees), and committees who conduct business and make recommendations (see Chapter 11). Navigating any political system requires a thorough understanding of its bylaws (constitution), structure, governance, mission, vision, and processes. As nurses become increasingly involved in all systems political, navigating those systems requires careful consideration of political and structural processes.

LEGISLATIVE PROCESS

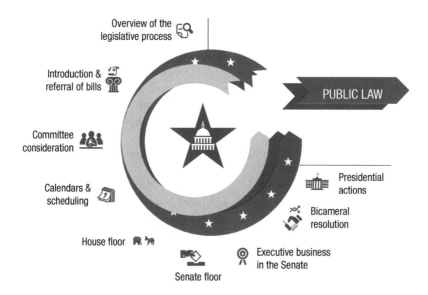

FIGURE 3.1 **The legislative process.**

Source: From Congress.gov. (n.d.). *The legislative process.* https://www.congress.gov/content/legprocess/legislative-process-poster.jpg

THE LEGISLATIVE PROCESS

The first step in the legislative process at the local, state, or federal level is the introduction and referral of bills. What happens before a bill is referred is as important to understand as the legislative process itself. Once a bill becomes a law (statute), the opportunity for influence does not end. Nurses have an enormous role in the development of a regulation. After a bill is passed and signed into law, it is sent to the agency responsible for proposing rules and regulations so that it can implement the law. This phase at the federal or state level is a great opportunity to influence policy. Each rule in the regulation has the potential to be an effective, powerful policy. At the federal level, the executive branch is responsible for developing final regulations. Prior to the publication of proposed rules, however, interested parties can recommend language and meet with agency staff responsible for rulemaking to express points of view. Even if nurses did not fully support a newly formed law, they can use their influence to address specific issues or mitigate action in proposed regulation that may be detrimental to nursing's position.

It is not easy to get legislation passed. This is by design. Before laws are passed, careful assessment of the values underpinning them must be made, stakeholders engaged, intended and unintended consequences evaluated, and economic, legal, social, and political costs determined. Like many policy issues, legislative solutions usually occur over time and with representation from many stakeholders representing a variety of special interest groups. While considered complex, the legislative process is a series of well-documented steps in which a bill can become a law. The process is essentially the same for both state and federal legislation. However, it is very common that a bill, once introduced, never becomes law. Since the 109th Congress, fewer than 5% of bills introduced became law, with the 116th Congress passing only 95 of the 3,160 bills introduced in 2019 (Ballotpedia, n.d.).

Nurses can influence the development and implementation of policy and legislation at every step of the process. Specific examples of active participation in the legislative process are listed in Exhibit 3.3. Policymaking takes place in many forums. Frequently, as one considers policy solutions, legislation is often seen as the most obvious one. However, multiple options exist for nurses to exert influence and activities in other venues both legislative and nonlegislative. Nurses are included in many panels and provide input into expert clinical decision-making. Nurses are employed in, and serve as consultants to, many powerful organizations that inform healthcare policy, including the Centers for Medicare and Medicaid Services (CMS) and the National Council on Quality Assurance (NCQA). Strategies for influencing policymaking are most often planned after a policy agenda is formulated. Where to take the issue, how to get it there, and how to make sure it moves forward are all points discussed when planning the implementation of a policy agenda. By virtue of nurses' education, clinical expertise, and advocacy roles, they are well situated to engage in a variety of strategies to influence at every level where policy needs discussion.

Laws may be written in such a way that they are funded for a limited time and then must come back to a legislative body for reenactment or funding. Anticipating reenactment legislation and expressing opinions early on why a particular program or piece of legislation remains important or how it can be updated and renewed for the current healthcare environment is very important.

An important example of necessary vigilance occurs in states with sunset clauses in their legislation and regulations for governmental agencies and boards. These sunset clauses need monitoring because they require periodic legislative action to reauthorize or extend the law. Agencies, such as boards of

EXHIBIT 3.3 LEGISLATIVE STEPS IN WHICH NURSES HAVE INFLUENCE

- Electing legislators whose positions are aligned with the nursing profession's views and values
- Drafting legislative language
- Participating in committee hearings
- Testifying at local, state, or federal committee hearings
- Informing congressional offices before voting on legislation
- Informing the White House before the president signs or vetoes passed legislation
- Providing comments to agency-proposed regulations to implement legislation
- Alerting and informing stakeholders about common legislative issues
- Attending legislative forums such as town halls

nursing (BONs) in some states, are susceptible to these regulations and may possibly change or be eliminated if action is not taken. Some states have witnessed their BON come precipitously close to dissolution and elimination. Without renewed legislation, these BONs would not exist or therefore have no authority to regulate nursing. The unintended consequence is that anyone would be allowed to practice nursing, that newly graduated nurses or nurses moving to the state would not be able to obtain licensure and/or employment, and that no one would investigate nurse practice violations. Typically, it is nurses (through state nurses associations) who monitor these activities to ensure that any sunset legislation is managed through review and reauthorization to protect the practice of nursing within their states. Most laws and BONs do not have sunset clauses and therefore remain in force indefinitely. However, it is the responsibility of nurses to be aware of such legislation and to make sure that such processes go smoothly. Another example is the funding for nursing education, which needs annual reauthorization.

STRATEGIES FOR INFLUENCING POLICYMAKING

Living in a nation where people are free to use their voice, whether in support or opposition to government, is a cherished freedom, one that was hard won and requires constant vigilance. Showing up is the first step. When presented with an opportunity to represent nursing and patients, always say yes. These affirmative replies will offer nurses experiences to develop advocacy skills or a career focus in policy. Conversation is a valuable tool in the arsenal of the policy-savvy nurse. Use informal conversations to learn about people, their organizations, and policy positions, as well as to identify possible opportunities for policy engagement. These will present themselves, sometimes when you least expect it, like when a position is open, or a new initiative is being planned. Whether influencing legislators or serving on committees, boards, or expert panels, there are some standard strategies for influencing policymaking (see Figure 3.2). Professional engagement requires only two ingredients: interest and showing up.

Engaging With Professional Associations

All RNs in the United States have an opportunity and an obligation to join a professional nurses association. Professional associations collectively speak for the profession and patients. Membership allows for nurse representation at every table when healthcare and health policy are discussed. Nurses' professional

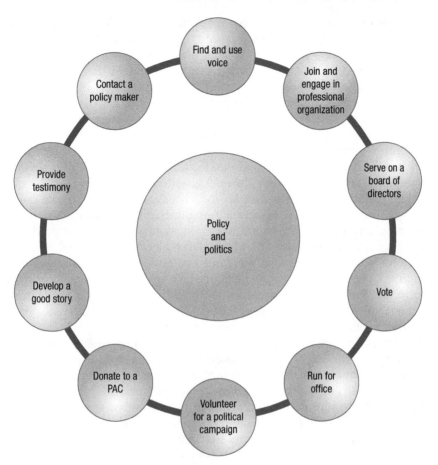

FIGURE 3.2 Strategies for influencing policy and politics.

associations promote nursing's position on issues of importance in the political arena. Associations with larger memberships (and, therefore, resources) can hire staff and lobbyists from PACs to back candidates who support nursing's agenda and engage in the political process. Professional associations have played strong roles in identifying nursing and healthcare issues needing scrutiny; lobbying for legislation, regulation, or policy change; monitoring the progress of pending legislation; moving legislation through committees and onto the House and Senate floors; crafting rulemaking language and options after laws are passed; overseeing the implementation of newly passed legislation; and monitoring the impact of legislation for intended and unintended consequences.

Healthcare delivery and finance are important issues, and the public needs to hear a nursing voice and perspective. Professional nurses associations have played a major role in healthcare reform conversations, which are partisan, passionate, personal, and political. National nurses associations have taken the position that access to high-quality healthcare should be guaranteed. During the specified implementation timeline (2010–2018) of the Affordable Care Act (ACA), a focused nursing community remained engaged to achieve the intent of the legislation. At times, monitoring the *Federal Register* (www.gpo.gov/fdsys) resulted in a call to action for the profession to react or suggest draft language for regulation and implementation of the ACA's hundreds of provisions. For example, because agencies determine who can be eligible healthcare providers in new, patient-centered team-based models of care, such as "medical homes" and "accountable care orga-nizations," draft language was submitted urging that APRNs be specifically iden-tified as primary care providers. At other times, the judicial processes are essential to upholding the legislation's interpretation and intent. For example, the ANA joined five other healthcare groups representing millions of healthcare profes-sionals in filing an amicus brief with the U.S. Supreme Court in support of the ACA minimum coverage provision, or "individual mandate" (ANA, 2012; see the Opportunities to Influence Judicial Actions section in this chapter and Chapter 6). As frontline witnesses to those who are uninsured and defer needed care, nurses have a unique perspective to share and guide the Supreme Court regarding the consequences of changes to healthcare legislation.

More expansive opportunities for individual nurses to influence policy often emerge from professional association engagement. A powerful mechanism for informing and influencing legislators is providing testimony at public hearings and congressional committees. Public hearings not only are held on a variety of topics for legislation but also are routinely held by congressional committees, appointed commissions, and federal or state agencies seeking information (see Figure 3.2). Professional associations work with their members to identify oppor-tunities to provide testimony, select articulate members to provide testimony, and prepare the remarks to be made during hearings.

Hearings, as a part of a formal process, provide a distinct opportunity for providing detailed reports and answering questions at all levels of government. Hearings are often a major step toward enactment of legislation and symbolize its importance. Legislative committees use this method to assemble informa-tion and solicit opinions from officials of the executive branch, other members of Congress, representatives of interest groups, experts, and concerned citizens. Hearings include written testimony that can be submitted alone or with an oral presentation and questioning by members of Congress. Presenters usually repre-sent organizations such as the ANA or state nurses associations, but individuals can provide both written and oral testimony. See www.rnaction.org for selective testimony presented by the ANA or www.loc.gov/law/find/hearings.php for the Law Library of Congress, which has a collaborative collection of the library's com-plete collection of printed hearings.

Processes for hearings are typically well established with common expec-tations. Exhibit 3.4 lists commonsense approaches to hearing preparation and presentation. The committee chairperson or host of the hearing selects the num-ber and timing of oral presenters. Nurses can participate in several important ways in the testimonial process by providing (a) contextual information on the topic, (b) examples that emphasize the critical nature of the topic, or (c) oral testimony and answering questions. Individual nurse clinicians and researchers who present as members of their organization and who have a close working knowledge of the topic are often able to bring a sense of proportion and reality to the discussion. Exhibit 3.5 lists some of the congressional committees that often play a role in issues that impact nursing and healthcare and that often conduct hearings.

Because nurses are trusted by the public and represent many potential voters, they are valued participants during hearings. Having multiple presentations by representatives from numerous nurses associations supporting an issue creates a powerful presence. It is critical that the presentations are accurate and reflect con-sistency in voice as appropriate. Working and coordinating with nurses associa-tions in which you hold membership is a benefit. The association can help support

EXHIBIT 3.4   APPROACHES TO HEARING PREPARATION AND PRESENTATION

- Follow specific hearing guidelines.
- Talk ahead of time with the staff member assigned to the hearing chairperson.
- Dress well—professional business attire.
- Come early, be on time, and be prepared to spend the entire day.
- Rehearse your spoken testimony before the hearing.
- Keep it under time limits.
- Address legislators politely and answer questions if asked. Say "thank you" for the opportunity to speak.
- Be courteous and respectful of the legislators, regardless of their opinion, as well as respectful and courteous to all who testify.
- "Pass" when called to speak if you are uncomfortable or answer simply, "Representative/Senator, I will have to look into your question and get back to you."
- Realize that elected and/or appointed officials come in and out of the room during the hearing.

EXHIBIT 3.5   SELECTED ISSUES IMPORTANT TO NURSING AND THE RELATED FEDERAL AGENCY

ISSUE	RELATED FEDERAL AGENCY
Lead poisoning	Environmental Protection Agency
Food safety Healthy eating	Department of Agriculture
Affordable housing	Federal Housing Finance Agency
Disabilities Aging Home care	Department of Health and Human Services
Brain injuries Posttraumatic stress disorders Family health	Department of Defense Department of Veterans Affairs

individuals participating in hearings by providing collaboration and background information that can further enhance talking points. This additional help and the presence of a representative of the association at the hearing to supplement responses can help build confidence and reassure the presenters.

Numerous federal and state agencies appreciate the working relationship with nurses associations when there is an alignment of interests with the agencies' core missions. Examples of issues that nurses can address by working with specific agencies are illustrated in Exhibit 3.5.

Nurses in practice, research, and education can provide data and context for these agencies when developing hearing testimony or public statements. Exhibit 3.6 lists selected congressional committees and governmental agencies that play a role in issues impacting nursing and healthcare. It is also important to consider the work of Congressional Nursing Caucuses, with bipartisan membership, one in the House of Representatives and in the Senate. The role of the caucuses is to educate members of Congress about legislative issues important to nurses, and the impact nurses have on healthcare in America. The House Nursing Caucus

EXHIBIT 3.6 CONGRESSIONAL COMMITTEES FOR NURSING AND HEALTHCARE ISSUES

SENATE	HOUSE OF REPRESENTATIVES
Appropriations Committee Controls the federal purse strings and determines federal funding for all government functions, from defense to biomedical research	**Appropriations Committee** Controls the federal purse strings and determines federal funding for all government functions, from defense to biomedical research
Labor, Health and Human Services, Education, and Related Agencies Appropriations Subcommittee Determines federal funding for federal agencies, including the HHS, NIH, CDC, and HRSA, which administers the nursing workforce development programs	**Labor, Health and Human Services, Education, and Related Agencies Appropriations Subcommittee** Determines federal funding for federal agencies, including the HHS, NIH, CDC, and HRSA, which administers the nursing workforce development programs
Health, Education, Labor, and Pensions Has jurisdiction over all non-Medicare and non-Medicaid healthcare policy issues	**Energy and Commerce Committee and Its Health Subcommittee** Has policy jurisdiction over the Medicaid program, Part B of the Medicare program, and all non-Medicare and non-Medicaid healthcare issues
Finance Committee and Its Healthcare Subcommittee Has policy jurisdiction over Medicare and Medicaid	**Ways and Means Committee and Its Health Subcommittee** Has policy jurisdiction over the Medicare program (shares jurisdiction over certain parts of Medicare with the House Energy and Commerce Committee)
Committee on Veterans Affairs Provides oversight of U.S. veterans' issues	**Veterans Affairs Committee** Has oversight responsibility and monitors and evaluates the operations of the VA
Special Committee on Aging Serves as a focal point for discussion and debate on matters relating to older Americans and reviews Medicare's performance, pension coverage, and employment opportunities for older Americans	

CDC, Centers for Disease Control and Prevention; HHS, Health and Human Services; HRSA, Health Resources and Services Administration; NIH, National Institutes of Health; VA, Veterans Administration.

was founded in 2003 under the auspices of Rep. Lois Capps (D-CA), an RN, and Rep. Ed Whitefield (R-KY) after the Nurse Reinvestment Act was signed into law. The Senate launched its Nursing Caucus under the auspices of Sen. Jeff Merkley (D-OR), Mike Johanns (R-NE), and Barbara Mikulski (D-MD) 7 years later in 2010. The nursing caucuses have been instrumental in peer-to-peer outreach to support nursing issues. An example is facilitating efforts to secure funding for Title VIII legislation to support nursing education. Therefore, check the official government website of one's senators and representative to determine their membership in the caucus. If one's representatives are a member of the caucus, thank them for their involvement. If they are not members, encourage them to join.

Writing proposed legislation for federal statutes occurs in congressional committees. Thus, committees have enormous power, for it is here where issues are discussed, debated, and negotiated. Legislation must move through and out of committee before legislation can get to the floor of the House or Senate for a vote. Constituents do play an important role in moving legislation through committees because they have the power to influence their legislators by contacting them through a variety of means and encouraging them to move or hold legislation.

Attending public hearings as a speaker or as an observer, as well as attending in numbers at all levels (local, state, federal) can be strategic. Moreover, being at hearings provides an excellent opportunity to network with staff and other interested stakeholders. Exchanging contact information, discussing an issue, or commenting on presentations can lead to future opportunities. Building relationships is an invaluable task in policymaking. Sharing an interest or assisting someone in policymaking duties will be greatly appreciated and could lead to future contacts and opportunities related to other issues. Federal hearing schedules are published in advance and can be viewed in the *Federal Register*. Tracking hearing schedules requires regular review of the *Federal Register* (www.federalregister.gov), committees' and agencies' websites, or local publications for schedule announcements. Typically, state governments also have established mechanisms to review hearing schedules and can be acquired by contacting your state legislator for assistance. State nurses associations often publish state hearing schedules and identify nurse experts to deliver comments. Some associations have created databases of experts to provide critical presentations.

It is not enough to just belong. Nurses must support and engage with their professional associations economically by paying dues and serving on committees and philosophically by contributing to white papers, accepting invitations for the delivery of public testimony, attending public hearings, contributing to PACs, and responding to requests for action.

Reaching Out to Policymakers and Legislators

Whether through Lobby Days sponsored by professional nurses associations, letter writing, or meeting individually with representatives in the community, one of the most powerful ways to influence policy and navigate the political system is to get to know the legislator and staff responsible for representing the district that you live and vote in and to communicate with them regularly. Nurses initially may find meeting with their legislators an intimidating task, but legislators need to hear from their constituents. They need to understand the position of their constituents and are profoundly interested and invested in maintaining their legislative positions. Nurses who get to know legislators are powerful influencers of the political system. Generally, congressional visits are handled by staff who welcome information about issues of importance to their legislator. Staff and legislators alike are generally gracious and welcome the opportunity to speak to constituents. Exhibit 3.7 provides an overview of when nurses should make visits. One should investigate the legislator's views on an issue prior to the visit. When visiting a legislator to ask for support, never leave without clarifying where the legislator stands on an issue. Always leave materials (e.g., a policy brief, fact sheet) for the staff to review (see Chapter 10). Exchange business cards and offer to be available to answer questions.

EXHIBIT 3.7 TIPS AND CONSIDERATIONS FOR CONTACTING LEGISLATORS

- Introducing yourself as a constituent and as an RN
- Speaking on behalf of your professional association
- Offering your assistance as an expert on healthcare
- Presenting your positions on important legislative and policy issues
- Determining interest and potential support or opposition for an issue
- Requesting sponsorship or cosponsorship of a bill
- Seeking information on a legislator's position on a bill
- Asking that a bill move from a committee to a floor vote/after a vote to the executive branch for signature
- Thanking legislators for their support and work on behalf of issues important to a policy agenda

Reaching Out to Policymakers and Legislators

When visiting a legislator, it is useful to have a compelling story that illustrates why the legislator should put resources into the issue, a story that will convince the legislator of the legitimacy of nursing's position. Well-planned, well-articulated stories about how an issue affects a constituent are the keys to making a legislator understand. Stories, far more than statistics, grab a legislator's attention (see Policy on the Scene 3.1).

Visits are not the only way to communicate with a legislator; letter writing is powerful. With the widespread and mainstream use of electronic communication, it is no longer necessary to produce a physical letter; indeed, for a variety of reasons, letters sent to legislators through the mail may never be opened. However, communication in the form of an email, and the use of an association's legislative communication tools can send powerful messages. Letters in support of or in opposition to legislation are categorized as such and counted so that legislators can get a sense of their constituents' positions. Professional associations often request that members send letters; these requests are also accompanied by sample letters or data to assist nurses with preparing letters. Letters must be professional, addressing the legislator by the correct title; focused; and polite and respectful. For example, legislation requiring RNs to obtain a baccalaureate degree in nursing within 10 years of initial licensure was passed in New York's Assembly and Senate. While the bill awaited the governor's signature, colleges, universities, and professional associations across the state encouraged nurses to write letters of support to the governor to demonstrate nursing's commitment to this legislation. Nurses' support for this legislation was communicated to Governor Andrew Cuomo, who signed the bill into law in 2017. New York State is the first state in the nation to have such legislation. Nurses exerting influence on their legislators made the difference.

Exerting policy influence can be accomplished not only by working with legislators but also by working with other key stakeholders. It is essential that nurses network and seek mentors in a variety of settings. Professional associations are an excellent place to start this work. Many opportunities to engage in this process happen because nurses show up and become involved. The ANA's Healthy Nurse Healthy Nation™ (HNHN) initiative provides opportunities to not only promote the health of nurses but also examine opportunities for the development of related state and federal policies, regulations, and/or legislation (See Policy on the Scene 3.2).

POLICY ON THE SCENE 3.1: LOSE THE JARGON AND ALIGN THE MESSAGE

The Honorable Gale Adcock, MSN, RN, FNP FAAN, FAANP
North Carolina General Assembly, House District 41

I am an NP, former corporate chief health officer, and legislator in my fourth term serving my community. I know from my personal experiences that APRNs play significant roles in the improvement of healthcare outcomes; and more importantly, evidence supports this. However, we often fail to follow basic communication ground rules when our audience is a legislator. I see NP colleagues making communication blunders that I have been guilty of myself in the past: using technical jargon, getting emotional, offering obscure facts, and relying on a ream of research studies to make our case. I often hear NPs bitterly complain after legislative visits, "All the data and logic are behind us! Why do they not get it?" Sometimes, they do not get it because we use the same message, the same words, and the same context for every legislator regardless of who they are, what they do for a living, and what experience they have had with our issues—and with us. I know effective NPs do not take this approach with patients. We understand in our clinical work that each patient is different and that we must change our style of talking to better match their style of listening and learning.

Nurses' messages become most effective when they can be related to what legislators already care about. We can learn to make our point—and make our message memorable—by using background knowledge plus the language and key concepts already familiar to them. Here is one example straight from my experience in the North Carolina House of Representatives. I use this knowledge, key concepts, and language to tell this story and make my points about full practice authority:

■ North Carolina spends a lot on public education—only healthcare expenditures top education expenditures.

■ Most of the state's NP programs are part of the UNC system, which is heavily subsidized by state funds.

■ Every legislator touts their support of education in their campaign and in their voting record.

■ North Carolina spends a lot on transportation, especially interstate highways. We have been referred to as "the good roads" state for decades.

■ North Carolina's current legislative majority prides themselves on cutting government spending, lowering taxes, and giving taxpayers a good return on their investment (i.e., taxes).

If the state of North Carolina spent $100 million to build a six-lane highway, would it make sense to you to have a state law that limits drivers to the use of only three lanes? Of course not. Subsidizing the education of hundreds of nurse practitioners who graduate from the UNC system and who are then restricted—by state law—from using every bit of their taxpayer-subsidized education to benefit North Carolina's citizens is just like building that six-lane highway and wasting money on the three lanes that no one can use.

Notice not one statistic or study is mentioned. There is not a hint of emotion. Instead, it is a story that resonates with the intended audience because their language and their values are paramount. It is a pithy and memorable story. And believe me, they get it.

NP, nurse practitioner; UNC, University of North Carolina.

POLICY ON THE SCENE 3.2: GRAND CHALLENGE FOR GRAND BENEFITS

Peter Stoffan, MPA, BSN, RN, CCRN, NEA-BC, CPXP
Regional Director, Human Experience
Hackensack Meridian Health, Hackensack, NJ

Nurses are prone to poor health due to work and environmental factors, including, but not limited to, stress, high demand, and working hours (National Academies, 2021). Due to the stresses put on the healthcare workforce during the SARS-CoV-2 global pandemic, now more than ever, there is a need to address self-care among nurses (Adam & Walls, 2020). The National Academy of Medicine's (formerly known as the Institute of Medicine) latest Future of Nursing Report supports there must be an improved focus to reverse the global phenomena surrounding the poor health of nurses (National Academies of Sciences, Engineering, and Medicine, 2021). Nurses must take care of themselves prior to acting as role models for patients, families, team members, and community members. What support structures exist to empower the nurse to effectively prioritize self-health?

The phrase so often heard on airplanes—"please place your own oxygen mask on before helping others"—can be directed toward nurses in all roles. *The Future of Nursing: Charting a Path to Achieve Health Equity* report (National Academies, 2021) argues that the improved health of the nursing workforce requires both the individual will to engage in self-care behaviors and the support of organizational and systemic stakeholders. Self-care promoting agendas tailored to the specific needs of nurses may represent a fundamentally significant and potentially cost-effective means for building a sustainable and healthy nursing workforce.

One such self-care promoting agenda was created by the ANA realizing that the nursing workforce is paradoxically one of the unhealthiest groups of workers. Identifying the need for positive change, the ANA (2021) created "HNHN," stating "if all four million registered nurses increased their personal wellness and then their families, co-workers and patients followed suit, what a healthier nation we could live in!" (ANA, para. 1). The ANA hopes to create a snowball effect of healthier people nationwide through their large-scale health promotion and supportive digital engagement platform. The HNHN "Grand Challenge" aims to foster connections with nurses and institutions to improve health in five areas: physical activity, nutrition, rest, quality of life, and safety (ANA, 2021).

Organizations, including, but not limited to, nursing schools, employers of nurses, and healthcare institutions have joined and adopted ANA's HNHN campaign. Some of the large organizations that have been recognized by HNHN as champions include large healthcare systems such as University of Texas Southwestern Medical Center in Texas and Ochsner in Louisiana, specialty nurses associations, such as the American Psychiatric Nurses Association, the Emergency Nurses Association, and state nurses associations, such as the Kentucky Nurses Association and the Georgia Nurses Association (HNHN, 2021). See additional champions at www.engage.healthynursehealthynation.org/blogs/24.

The HNHN campaign has helped raise awareness of the need to support nurses in all areas of their health. By partnering with HNHN, positive outcomes may be expedited to benefit nurses and all healthcare workers and consumers. Institutions and individuals can engage in HNHN, but what could assist in driving the message home for those who don't subscribe to health promotion? Some institutions already provide incentives for those who engage in healthy lifestyle modifications (e.g., tobacco cessation, health and wellness program participation, health screenings, etc.), so why shouldn't participation in ANA's HNHN be an additional component? Companies want to reduce spending through individual insurance usage while supporting the health of the individual and, therefore engage in external health-promoting policies, agendas, and platforms may be an underutilized cost-neutral opportunity.

ANA, American Nurses Association; HNHN, Healthy Nurse Healthy Nation.

Additional Strategies for Influencing Policy

Exerting influence requires a variety of approaches that yield a cumulative effect to achieve policy goals. These include, for example, capitalizing on opportunities presented by current events, seeking key positions, volunteering, and providing financial support.

Seizing the Moment With the Nursing Voice

No one has a nursing perspective on healthcare except nurses (see Chapter 9). Nurses view healthcare through an authentically holistic framework, with a unique understanding of health and illness as it is lived and experienced by individuals, families, and communities every single day. Our values are clear to us as professionals and to a society that consistently views us as trustworthy and ethical. The nursing perspective on health, illness, people, and systems is essential to an improved healthcare system. Nursing historically has not been known for "speaking truth to power."[1] However, it is no longer acceptable (it never has been acceptable) for nurses to remain silent or disengaged. Nurses must use every forum, political, social, educational, employment, and organizational, to speak about the issues and concerns of our profession and ourselves. Our voices, our knowledge, and our experiences are valued. The development of a nursing voice is essential when articulating issues of concern to legislators and policymakers. Using this voice can be risky; it requires a measure of courage.

On July 26, 2017, RN Alex Wubbels was discussing a blood-draw procedure with a police officer at the University Hospital in Salt Lake City. The officer, a member of the police department's blood-draw team, had been sent to the hospital to draw blood for an alcohol level from the unconscious accident victim. Nurse Wubbels refused to allow the officer to draw blood, explaining hospital policy under which he could draw blood: patient consent, a warrant to obtain the blood, or an arrest of the victim. She explained: "I'm just a nurse trying to protect a patient." Nurse Wubbels was arrested for obstruction of justice. She was released 20 minutes later. Nurse Wubbels's responsibilities were clear, the hospital policies were clear, and the law was clear. She used her voice to advocate for her patient. She released a video of the incident that sparked national outrage. Ms. Wubbels's actions created a national conversation forcing an examination of policies and procedures. Often, as noted by Wubbels's lawyer, these types of incidents do not have this corroboration. Nurses' associations have seized the moment to draw attention to the violence that nurses and healthcare workers experience on the job. This is illustrated by the then ANA president Pam Cipriano's statement to a national news reporter: "Nurses should not be subject to any kind of violence . . . we feel

---

[1]*Speaking truth to power* refers to taking a stand and mobilizing societal action. It was a phrase popularized by Quakers in the 1950s with the publication of their book with the same name. The phrase is also attributed to Bayard Rustin, a civil rights leader.

so strongly, particularly in this situation, where another type of worker who the public needs to trust acted in an unconscionable way" (Almendrala, 2017, para. 2).

Being an advocate is not easy. Nurse Wubbels states she waited to release the video until September because she needed to deal with it personally. She soon realized that it needed to be released to change policy. It exemplifies the importance of seizing the moment and strategically using a nursing voice.

Registering, Voting, and Communicating With Elected Officials

A vote is a unit of political power. A vote is the ultimate expression of support or opposition to a formalized set of values. In the United States, careers have been built, wars have been fought, and lives have been lost over the acquisition and exercise of this right. Even in the 21st century, our nation continues to engage in strategies and enact laws and regulations to ensure that every citizen has the unencumbered right to vote. Exercising the right to vote is one of the most influential actions a nurse—or any citizen—can perform. With rights come responsibilities. Registering to vote and then voting is a fundamental civic duty. Nurses can encourage their friends, families, and colleagues to vote. When nurses point out to legislators at the local, state, and federal levels that they are voting members of their constituency, legislators pay attention. Nurses have earned the respect of many and are in positions to influence others with their thoughtful comments and the power of their vote.

Registering and voting help create credibility and influence beyond the poll booth. The central goal of all legislators is to obtain and then keep their office. When speaking or writing to a legislator, be sure to communicate that you are an RN and a voting constituent and state your role in nursing. Most important, your vote influences all branches of government. Votes elect legislators at the local, state, and federal levels who make the laws, and votes elect executives—the president, governor, and mayor, who make appointments to the executive branch, the implementer of laws and regulations, and to the judiciary, the evaluator of laws. Nurses must vote.

Volunteering to Work on a Campaign

Nurses are welcome additions to political campaigns. Candidates need volunteers to make their campaigns effective. Campaign volunteerism can be as all-encompassing as full-time work or as brief as participating in telephone polls, posting signs, or getting out the vote. Volunteering provides firsthand experience about the political system. Nurse volunteers provide candidates, their staff, and others with valuable knowledge about nursing and healthcare. Working on political campaigns and educating candidates about issues can be invaluable in the long run. If elected, the candidate, now legislator, will remember your support during the campaign but more important, will be potentially influenced about issues discussed. Other activities related to navigating campaigns can be found in Chapter 7.

Seeking Board Positions

The report *The Future of Nursing* (IOM, 2011), was a game changer for the profession. Key messages of the report require that the profession look both out of the window to external forces that regulate the profession and in the mirror to identify the changes that nursing itself must make to stand as equal partners in the healthcare system and with credible voices in the healthcare policy conversations. A major initiative that addresses developing nursing leadership and expanding nursing's influence beyond the profession itself is the Nurses on Boards Coalition (NOBC, 2021). Organized in 2014 and composed of national nursing and other organizations, the NOBC addresses one of the most challenging recommendations of *The Future of Nursing* report that nurses serve in critical decision-making roles on boards to improve health and patient care. The NOBC goal to have 10,000 nurses serving on corporate and health-related boards, panels, and commissions by 2020 was achieved. Disch and Kingston (2021) recommend that the new goal for the next 5 years should be that there is one nurse on every board of a "hospital, health system and agency affecting the health of the public." The coalition provides support to nurses seeking board positions. This support provides nurses with opportunities to influence healthcare beyond the profession and beyond healthcare venues by improving health and building healthier communities. However, the road to nurses' representation on major hospital and healthcare system boards has not been easy. A number of misconceptions and obstacles remain (see Exhibit 3.8).

Running for Office

The ultimate influence on a system comes from within that system. Only three nurses have seats in the U.S. House of Representatives in the 117th Congress, Cori Bush (D-MO), Edie Bernice Johnson (D-TX), and Lauren Underwood (D-IL). No nurses are serving in the U.S. Senate. Lourdes Aflague Leon Guerrero serves as the governor of Guam, and Bethany Hall-Long serves as the lieutenant governor of Delaware. Nurses do serve in their state legislatures. However, more nurses need to seek public office. Gale Adcock, FNP, as noted earlier, has a long history of holding political office. More than 20 years ago, she was on a mission: to influence healthcare in her state through politics. She carefully planned her political career, engaged her community, and, ultimately, sought and won office in local government (council member in Cary, North Carolina) and in state office as assemblywoman for the 41st North Carolina District. She is the only NP to have

EXHIBIT 3.8 MISCONCEPTIONS AND OBSTACLES VERSUS THE REALITY OF NURSES SERVING ON BOARDS

MISCONCEPTIONS AND OBSTACLES	REALITY
Too nurse-centric	Decisions based on what is best for patient/community
Considered functional doers	Possess a wide range of skills including communication, process improvement, complex problem-solving
Not decision-makers traditionally	Strategist, uses the nursing process to reach decisions
Face pressure to put the profession ahead of the hospital	Holistic view of issues
Misogyny	Continues to be a subtle underlying issue
Socio-politico-economic differences	Educated to care/see all individuals regardless of race/background
Don't have deep pockets	Trade-off; can volunteer their time
Networks are limited	Successful relationship-based engagement

ever served in her state. Rep. Adcock has introduced, sponsored, and cosponsored legislation running the gamut of the interests and needs of her constituency. Her very presence in the Assembly elevates nursing and gives voice to the possibilities that nurses offer the communities in which they live and work (See Policy on the Scene 3.1).

Contributing to a PAC

PACs are groups that form around issues to support candidates who can represent those interests and influence legislation supportive of them (see Chapter 7). PACs provide financial support to candidates on both sides of the aisle who support issues important to nurses and patients. Campaigns are expensive. Advertisements, debates, and other strategies to reach out to a constituency cost money. When nurses contribute to a PAC, they are demonstrating their influence by providing financial support to candidates who support nursing.

OPPORTUNITIES TO INFLUENCE THE EXECUTIVE BRANCH OF GOVERNMENT

The executive branches of federal and state governments are responsible for implementing laws and, consequently, oversee the agencies that are responsible for programs and services supported by legislation. One of the ways to influence policy at the executive branch level is through professional associations. It is part of their organizational mandate to forge strong relationships with staff and agencies in the executive branch of government. Professional associations have the connections and resources to influence appointments, regulatory processes, and important decisions impacting nursing and healthcare. In turn, the professional associations will reach back to engage members in grassroots support. Vast opportunities exist for nurses to influence the implementation of services and programs. All agencies need to hear from those with real information, expertise, research evidence, and stories about how it affects patients or their local communities.

Executive Orders

Under the power granted in the U.S. Constitution, the president can issue executive orders to officials and federal agencies. Executive orders are instructions to government agencies and departments. Executive orders have the full authority under the law and may be made pursuant to certain congressional actions that explicitly delegate discretionary power to the agency and the president. Executive orders can significantly influence internal government operations and the focus of federal agencies, but they cannot reverse congressional legislation, and their scope is not as wide-ranging as legislation; in essence, as an option, the president can issue executive orders that create policy where and when legislation fails or does not exist.

Executive orders have been issued by every president since George Washington. Some presidents have been accused of abusing executive orders and using them to make laws without congressional approval or alter existing laws from their original mandates. Like legislation and regulations, executive orders are subject to judicial review and may be struck down if deemed by the courts to be unsupported by statute or the Constitution. President Franklin D. Roosevelt had more than 3,500 executive orders, whereas recent presidents had fewer than 400 each. The entire listing can be viewed online at the nonprofit, nonpartisan American Presidency Project by searching the document category "executive orders" (www.presidency. ucsb.edu).

Federal Agency Appointment Selection

In any given presidential term, several thousand individuals are appointed. The *United States Government Policy and Supporting Positions* (Committee on Oversight and Government Reform, 2020) document, known as the Plum Book, lists more than 9,000 federal civil service support and leadership positions in the federal government that may be subject to noncompetitive appointment. Such positions include justices in federal courts, the presidential cabinet, members of boards, heads of agencies and their immediate subordinates, policy executives and advisors, and aides who report to these officials. As described in Chapter 11, the ANA and other nurses associations can make recommendations for appointments to key policy positions in governmental agencies. As evident with recent presidents, nurses' efforts were successful in lobbying for appointments. President Clinton appointed nurses to key senior leadership positions. Beverly Malone, PhD, RN, FAAN, was appointed to serve as a deputy assistant secretary for health in the U.S. Department of Health and Human Services (DHHS), whereas Virginia Trotter Betts, MSN, JD, RN, FAAN, was appointed a member of President Clinton's HealthCare Reform Task Force and senior advisor on Nursing and Policy to the secretary and assistant secretary of the DHHS. President Obama appointed Mary Wakefield, PhD, RN, FAAN, as administrator of the Health Resources and Services Administration (HRSA); Marilyn Tavenner, MHA, RN, as administrator of the CMS; and Linda S. Schwartz, PhD, RN, FAAN, as assistant secretary of Veterans Affairs for Policy and Planning. Nurses have served in the Surgeon General role. Rear Admiral Sylvia Trent Adams, PhD, RN, FAAN, was appointed as Surgeon General by President Trump, and Rear Admiral Susan Orsega, MSN, FNP-BC, FAANP, FAAN, was appointed as acting Surgeon General. Mary Wakefield served on the Biden transition team, which facilitated the appointment of key individuals in his new administration. At the state level, Karen Murphy, PhD, RN, for example, was Pennsylvania's secretary of health. These individuals and other nurses who have been selected in presidential or gubernatorial appointment processes are in ideal positions to influence health policy.

OPPORTUNITIES TO INFLUENCE JUDICIAL ACTIONS

The third governmental branch is the judicial system; it is less well known and less involved in the nursing profession's policy efforts. Historically, the ANA has participated in U.S. Supreme Court proceedings with cases of broad implications and interest to the profession. Typically, these cases have dealt with nurses' rights, workplace issues, and human rights issues involving individual patient rights and access to healthcare.

At the federal judicial level, the Supreme Court is well known for its powers, which include interpreting the Constitution and reviewing laws. Unlike the criminal court system, the Supreme Court usually does not hold trials but, rather, interprets the meaning of a law, decides whether a law is relevant to a set of facts, determines how a law should be applied, and most important, determines whether a law or regulation is permitted under the Constitution or is unconstitutional. The

Supreme Court may hear an appeal from lower courts on any question of law, provided that it has jurisdiction. Once a decision is made, the lower courts are obligated to follow the precedent set by the Supreme Court when rendering decisions.

The justices on the Supreme Court are appointed by the president of the United States and confirmed by the U.S. Senate. Justices in lower courts can be appointed or elected depending on the jurisdiction and purpose of the court. Unlike the legislative and executive branches, one's ability to influence judicial decisions is greatly limited. The only opportunity to influence judicial decisions is prior to justices being elected or appointed. Many times, these elections or appointments do not receive the scrutiny that they deserve. Supporting and electing candidates running for judicial positions or judicial nominees is an acceptable mechanism to have potential justices that represent and align with your values and views. Lobbying justices or members of juries is considered inappropriate and would not be tolerated outside legal proceedings.

It is critical that information advantageous to the situation be presented in testimony or legal briefs from the involved parties, as well as from *amici curiae*, or "friends of the court." Amici curiae are most often advocacy groups, such as professional associations and unions, that file a brief known as an *amicus brief* to advocate for or against an interpretation of a law or regulation. Amicus briefs can introduce concerns or support about the broader implications and effects in the court rulings. Whether to admit the information is at the discretion of the court.

In prominent cases, amicus briefs are generally provided by organizations with available content expertise, legal, and financial resources to produce strong documents that present convincing information and argument to support their position.

Over the years, the ANA has filed several amicus briefs either as a single association or with others on common causes. For example, the ANA, American Association of Nurse Anesthetists, American Association of Nurse Practitioners, American College of Nurse-Midwives, National Association of Clinical Nurse Specialists, and Citizen Advocacy Center filed an amicus brief in support of the Federal Trade Commission's (FTC) rulings regarding restraint of trade and unfair competition (ANA, 2015). This brief was in support of nondentists' provision of teeth-whitening services. The case is important because regulations related to other providers may set precedence for nursing practice. The Supreme Court ruling on the FTC action in this case provides guidance on what constitutes a controlling number of decision-makers who are active market participants for the occupation regulated by a board. The rulings were supportive of healthcare professionals' ability to practice to the full extent of their professional education and training. The nature of the decision, in this instance, requires that nurses closely monitor state regulatory board actions.

Although the judicial branch plays a significant role in making policy through the interpretation of laws and rules, they do not make the laws, nor do they have the power to enforce laws and rules. It is essential that legislation and rules that are clear, appropriate, constitutional, and respectful of rights be written up front to avoid long, lengthy legal challenges. An example is the situation in California, *American Nurses Association v. Torlakson* (2013), which is further described, along with other legal strategies, in Chapter 6. This controversial ruling allows unlicensed personnel to administer insulin in the school system. Years later, the policy matter has not resolved. Various stakeholders with a complexity of interests remain engaged together for better solutions.

IMPLICATIONS FOR THE FUTURE

Nurses cannot afford to be reticent about engagement in the political and policy making processes. Discussions and debates will continue to take place in our

A Different Path to Nursing: Building Influence and Creating Change

Hollie Gentry, MSN, RNC-MNN, CNE

Wanting to improve maternal–child healthcare beyond my own practice, I was inspired to find ways to build on my experiences in the Ohio Senate. Communication, advocacy, and education were always some of my most valuable nursing skills. I became involved in efforts to decrease infant and maternal mortality through education and group prenatal visits. Working with Moms First, a city of Cleveland home visiting program for pregnant and new moms, I became an Infant Mortality Ambassador, providing education and support at community events. I helped my colleagues understand the importance of implementing best practices and policies focused on improving maternal–child outcomes as an active member of Fairview Hospital's Baby-Friendly Designation Committee. Baby-Friendly is a WHO/UNICEF joint initiative aiming to increase breastfeeding rates worldwide by setting standards of excellence in providing breastfeeding education and support. Because I understood the amount of time and effort that went into planning, funding, and executing these programs, I was persistent and dedicated to making them successful. I continued educating myself, getting immersed in the data and statistics, attending maternal–child health conferences, and connecting with maternal health experts on Twitter. I tried to find new ways to make a difference, including sharing ideas and resources with nursing students.

Most recently, I increased my commitment to AWHONN by participating in its Advocacy Day on Capitol Hill. I took the leap and applied for membership on AWHONN's Public Policy Committee, a national group with seven members. I was excited to receive this national appointment by AWHONN's board, which provides me with the opportunity to impact policy for the population I care so much about. As a public policy committee member, I understand the importance of connecting with key legislators, building rapport with them and their staff, following up with them as needed, and making sure that I don't waste their time. Having a solid background in how legislation is enacted has proved beneficial as we also determine the bills on which we are going to focus our advocacy and how we might persuade legislators to support our positions. These activities have given me the opportunity to combine my passion for moms and babies with my political expertise to create change through policy influence at any level. As I continue to expand my involvement, I recognize that a nurse influencer's power lies in their ability to connect with others, build relationships, and convert knowledge into action. For me, what started out as a way to make money during college turned into the foundation of my future policy work. What will be your path to your policy journey?

AWHONN, The Association of Women's Health, Obstetric, and Neonatal Nurses; UNICEF, United Nations Children's Fund; WHO, World Health Organization.

nation regarding the best way to implement healthcare that is high quality, affordable, and accessible to every citizen in our nation. Every decision made on Capitol Hill and in state legislatures throughout the nation touches the lives of nurses and our patients. As the single largest healthcare provider group in the world, it is nurses that must not only sit at the table when all healthcare conversations are held but also lead the discussion. This cannot happen if nurses continue to profess to be apolitical or disinterested in politics. Nurses must be proactive to introduce new legislation or be at the table during the process of writing and revising regulations (See ANA link for information about rulemaking: https://www.nursingworld.org/practice-policy/advocacy/federal/agencies-regulations/). Although nurses typically provide testimony on current issues pertinent to nursing practice, few nurses provide testimony reflecting the challenges faced by nurses in daily practice or on the larger issues related to healthcare policy. To be an influential voice in policy, more nurses must take on greater involvement in the political system.

Nurses have multiple opportunities for involvement in policy and political action as debates about issues affecting health and healthcare come to the forefront of the public's attention in the legislative and regulatory arena. The profession must embrace these opportunities to focus on issues such as eliminating healthcare disparities, fostering a culture of health, providing care to the swelling ranks of veterans and the aging population, ensuring that children live lives as healthy or healthier than their parents, and pursuing the improvement of health through technology. Such opportunities are all central to the values of the profession of nursing. Legislative polarization at the national level, of necessity, drives legislative initiatives at the state level. This will create additional opportunities for savvy nurses to develop close relationships with their legislators to advance specific initiatives. Increasingly, consumer groups may take a judicial approach to advance policy, and these approaches may have an impact on health or how nursing is practiced. Consequently, nurses will need to partner with consumer groups and be aware of specific claims to provide their expertise in support or opposition to a particular issue.

KEY CONCEPTS

1. There are numerous mandates and opportunities for nurses to be involved across a variety of policy strategies.
2. Passing legislation, implementing it, and evaluating policy provide an array of rich opportunities for nurses to speak out and take action.
3. Rulemaking is a critical step after legislation has been passed and is an opportunity to influence legislation implementation.
4. All types of legislation should be monitored; any reauthorization requirements should not be overlooked.
5. Nurses' associations play a significant role in promoting the voice of the nursing profession at tables when healthcare decisions are made. Professional association membership is crucial to the advancement of initiatives important to nurses and patients.
6. Although not often recognized, action through judicial processes has been used by nurses associations.
7. The appointment and election of judges are crucial because the normal lobbying activities in the judicial processes would be considered inappropriate.
8. Executive orders and appointments can be effective mechanisms to create policies when legislation is not an option or likely to occur.
9. Including nurses as board members is vital to successful board governance.

SUMMARY

The range of contributions and impact that nurses can have in policy areas is limitless. Nurses have unique perspectives on the healthcare of individuals, families, and communities that are characterized by advocacy, trust, action, accountability, and authenticity. To fully actualize the voice of nurses, engagement with stakeholders and policy activity requires individual and organized action. Broadening policy action for nurses beyond letter writing includes key strategies such as testimony at public hearings, legislative engagement with staff writing language for bills, and public comment on proposed technical rules following enactment of laws. These actions will amplify the nursing voice as an advocate for all.

END-OF-CHAPTER RESOURCES

LEARNING ACTIVITIES

1. Identify your local government leaders (e.g., mayor, councils, boards) and your legislative representatives at the state and federal governments. For three of these representatives, identify at least one position they have taken on a healthcare issue.

2. Identify one nursing issue that has been adjudicated in the state and federal court system. Discuss highlights of the decision and how it has impacted nursing. Are there ongoing efforts to appeal these decisions or refine legislation?

3. Locate testimony provided at the federal, state, or local level on an issue that is important to nurses or health in general. Critique the testimony. Identify what should be included to influence the opinions of the group holding the hearing.

4. Locate proposed rules and regulations pertaining to a nursing or health issue. Identify the appropriate mechanism for providing comments. Critique the proposed rules and regulations for their support of nursing and/or for the way that an important health-care issue is addressed.

5. Plan strategies to successfully gain support for a policy proposal at a mock city council meeting.

6. Prepare a 3-minute testimony that will be presented at a BON hearing regarding proposed nursing regulations that require an NCLEX® type of examination every 5 years for license renewal.

7. Develop a strategy for influencing an issue in a town hall or school board meeting.

8. Identify all departments and administrators in your state government holding responsibility and authority over matters of importance to the nursing profession.

9. Select one strategy identified in this chapter to influence politics and policy at the local level. Identify how you can use that strategy within the next week to influence an issue important to nurses and patients.

10. Identify executive orders that impacted healthcare in the past 50 years and what was, or could have been, nursing responses.

11. Using the Healthy Nurse Healthy Nation (HNHN) framework, identify a workplace policy that can be implemented with state or federal policy, regulation, or legislation.

E-RESOURCES

- American Nurses Association http://www.nursingworld.org
- American Nurses Association. Congressional Testimony http://www.rnaction.org/site/PageNavigator/nstat_congressional_testimony
- American Presidency Project www.americanpresidency.org
- U.S. Congress https://congress.gov
- Congressional Management Foundation http://www.congressfoundation.org
- The U.S. Constitution https://www.whitehouse.gov/1600/constitution
- Diffen: Federal vs. State Law https://www.diffen.com/difference/Federal_Law_vs_State_Law
- *Federal Register* https://www.federalregister.gov
- U.S. Government Accountability Office (GAO) http://www.gao.gov

- Government Agencies and Elected Officials https://www.usa.gov
- Government Publishing Office (GPO) https://www.gpo.gov
- A Guide to the Rulemaking Process http://www.federalregister.gov/uploads/2011/01/the_rulemaking_process.pdf
- Health Resources and Services Administration http://www.hrsa.gov
- U.S. House of Representatives http://www.house.gov
- How Our Laws Are Made How Our Laws Are Made—Learn About the Legislative Process https://www.congress.gov/resources/display/content/How+Our+Laws+Are+Made+-+Learn+About+the+Legislative+Process
- Judges as Policy-Makers http://www.youtube.com/watch?v=qhsO4L5LezU
- The Legislative Process: Overview https://www.congress.gov/legislative-process
- U.S. Library of Congress https://loc.gov
- National Conference of State Legislatures http://www.ncsl.org
- National Council of State Boards of Nursing: Contact Information https://www.ncsbn.org/contactbon.htm
- U.S. Senate http://www.senate.gov
- Tracking the United States Congress https://www.govtrack.us
- U.S. Congress and Health Policy Tutorial http://kff.org/interactive/the-u-s-congress-and-health-policy-tutorial
- United States Government Policy and Supporting Positions (Plum Book). https://www.govinfo.gov/content/pkg/GPO-PLUMBOOK-2020/pdf/GPO-PLUMBOOK-2020.pdf
- White House http://www.whitehouse.gov

REFERENCES

Adam, J., & Walls, R. (2020). Supporting the health care workforce during the COVID-19 global epidemic. *JAMA*, 323(15), 1439–1440. https://doi.org/10.1001/jama.2020.3972

Almendrala, A. (2017, September 1). Nurses endure a shocking amount of violence on the job: Usually, though, it's not at the hands of police officers. *Huffington Post*. https://www.huffingtonpost.com/entry/nurses-violence-police_us_59a9c2f9e4b0dfaafcf07093

American Nurses Association. (2010). *Nursing's social policy statement: The essence of the profession* (2nd ed.).

American Nurses Association. (2012, February). ANA to Supreme Court: 'Individual Mandate' needed to make health care work. *The American Nurse*, 44(1), 14. https://www.myamericannurse.com/

American Nurses Association. (2015). *Issue brief. North Carolina State Board of Dental Examiners v. FTC: Next steps for state action and for nurses.* https://www.nursingworld.org/~4af030/globalassets/docs/ana/ethics/issue-brief-nc-db-v-ftc-2015-6-17--2.pdf

American Nurses Association. (2021). *What is the Healthy Nurse, Healthy Nation Grand Challenge?* https://www.healthynursehealthynation.org/

American Nurses Association v. Tom Torlakson. (2013). S184583 Ct. App C061150 Sacramento County Super. Ct. No. 07AS04631. http://www.cde.ca.gov/ls/he/hn/documents/anavtorlakson2013.pdf

Apold, S. (2008). The doctor of nursing practice: Looking back, moving forward. *Journal for Nurse Practitioners*, 4(2), 101–107. https://doi.org/10.1016/j.nurpra.2007.12.003

Ballotpedia. (n.d.). *Key votes: 116th congress, 2019–2020.* https://ballotpedia.org/Key_Votes:_116th_Congress,_2019-2020

Berwick, D. M., Nolan, T. W., & Whittington, J. (2008). The Triple Aim: Care, health, and cost. *Health Affairs*, 27(3), 759–769. https://doi.org/10.1377/hlthaff.27.3.759

Bodenheimer, T., & Sinsky, C. (2014). From Triple to Quadruple Aim: Care of the patient requires care of the provider. *Annals of Family of Medicine*, 12(6), 573–576. https://doi.org/10.1370/afm.1713

Committee on Oversight and Government Reform. (2020). *United States government policy and supporting positions (Plum Book).* https://www.govinfo.gov/content/pkg/GPO-PLUMBOOK-2020/pdf/GPO-PLUMBOOK-2020.pdf

Congress.gov. (n.d.). *The legislative process.* https://www.congress.gov/content/legprocess/legislative-process-poster.jpg

Des Jardin, K. (2001). Political involvement in nursing—Politics, ethics, and strategic action. *AORN Journal*, 74(5), 614–618, 621–622, 628–630. https://doi.org/10.1016/s0001-2092(06)61760-2

Disch, J., & Kingston, M. B. (2021). Using activism to get nurses on boards. *Nursing Administration Quarterly*, 45(3), 208–218. https://doi.org/10.1097/NAQ.0000000000000474

Greiner, A. C., & Knebel, E. (Eds.). (2003). *Health professions education: A bridge to quality.* National Academies Press.

Healthy Nurse Healthy Nation (HNHN). (2021). *Blog home. Champion spotlight.* https://engage.healthynursehealthynation.org/blogs/24

Institute of Medicine. (2001). *Crossing the quality chasm: A new health system for the 21st century.* National Academies Press. https://doi.org/10.17226/12956

Institute of Medicine. (2011). *The future of nursing: Leading change, advancing health.* The National Academies Press.

Khoury, C. M., Blizzard, R., Wright Moore, L., & Hassmiller, S. (2011). Nursing leadership from bedside to boardroom: A Gallup national survey of opinion leaders. *Journal of Nursing Administration*, 41(7–8), 299–305. https://doi.org10.1097/NNA.0b013e3182250a0d

National Academies of Sciences, Engineering, and Medicine. (2021). *The future of nursing 2020–2030: Charting a path to achieve health equity.* The National Academies Press. https://doi.org/10.17226/25982.

National Council of State Boards of Nursing. (2021). *Active RN licenses: A profile of nursing licensure in the U.S.* https://www.ncsbn.org/6161.htm

Nurses on Boards Coalition. (2021). *About: Our story.* https://nursesonboardscoalition.org/about

O'Neil, E. H., & the Pew Health Professions Commissions. (1998). *Recreating health professional practice for a new century.* University of California San Francisco, Center for the Health Professions. https://healthforce.ucsf.edu/publications/recreating-health-professional-practice-new-century

Patzek, M. J. (2010). Understanding the DNP degree. *American Nurse Today*, 5(5), 49–50. myamericannurse.com

Saad, L. (2020, December 2020). *U.S. ethics ratings rise for medical workers and teachers.* Gallup. News. Politics. https://news.gallup.com/poll/328136/ethics-ratings-rise-medical-workers-teachers.aspx

UNIT II

Analyzing Policy

CHAPTER 4

Identifying a Problem and Analyzing a Policy Issue

LISA SUMMERS AND KATHERINE CARDONI BREWER

> *If they don't give you a seat at the table, bring a folding chair.*
> —Shirley Chisholm

OBJECTIVES

1. Explain the criticality of problem identification in the policy process.
2. Explain the different aspects needed for defining a policy problem.
3. Explain the importance of understanding the context of policy problems.
4. Explain the process of identifying diverse stakeholders in defining policy problems and formulating policy solutions.
5. Identify tools for conducting policy analysis.

Problems abound in today's healthcare system. We, as nurses, observe and experience problems every day in our practice settings and communities. The problems we see most often relate to the patients under our care. Let's say there is high turnover where you work, and staffing is often thin. The problem might seem limited to staffing issues but is likely more complex than just that one issue. For example, turnover on the unit might be a problem for staffing, but it can also contribute to decreased quality of care, decreased patient and nurse satisfaction, higher costs associated with recruiting and training new staff, and lower workplace morale.

The problems we face might be more widespread than we realize, and the possible solutions might be more common than we realize. Turnover, for example, might seem limited to a particular work unit, but it might also be an issue faced by entire hospitals, systems, geographical areas, perhaps even the entire nation. Solutions to turnover, shortages, and other workforce issues have an impact on the workforce in other countries as well.

Although problems can seem immense, policy is a critical aspect of solving them. Policy in this chapter is referred to as the written rules of engagement in healthcare at institutional and governmental levels. Institutional policy refers to the policies and procedures that dictate or guide healthcare practices and procedures within an organization, such as procedural policies or human resources regulations. Institutions can refer to healthcare organizations, professional associations, or groups. Governmental policy refers to those ordinances issued by the government in the regulation of healthcare services, such as legislation, executive orders, regulations, and rules. Nurses have a critical role in shaping these policies, whether it be during actual drafting of them, evaluating them in light of nursing practice and patient outcomes, and advocating for changes to reflect the needs of nurses and patients. Some refer to policy at the institution level as the little-p policy, whereas the policy at the government level is the big-P policy. This designation is not to imply that institutional policies are not as important in relation to practice as governmental policy but rather to discern how governmental policy has a wider reach and often entails multiple disciplines and stakeholders in its development (see Policy Challenge).

POLICY CHALLENGE | **Words Matter**

Words are interpreted through the prism of each person's understanding, which often can be unique. Similarly, words and language used when advocating and then writing policy can have multiple meanings and subsequent consequences.

Addiction is an example of how the same problem is viewed differently depending on your role, as a patient, family member, or role in the criminal justice or healthcare system, and so forth. Addiction was long viewed as a moral failing and an inability of an individual to control their own behavior. In the 1980s, the Reagan administration began the "War on Drugs" as a way to militaristically address the issue of addiction by framing those addicted to the drug and the groups selling it as the enemy. Although criminalization and politicizing drugs were not new, the words used to describe the issue were. Another issue became the increasing use of crack cocaine, a highly addictive and cheaply processed drug, in many poor communities of color in inner cities. The war then escalated the criminalization and penalization of those who were using and addicted to this drug. Although the "crack" epidemic diminished over the 1990s, other drug epidemics emerged, despite the billions spent on the "war."

In the early 2000s, addiction to prescription pain medications, particularly among rural White communities began to emerge, and by the early 2010s, the opioid epidemic was taking an immense toll throughout the United States. However, this time, instead of criminalization and punishment, there was a greater call for treatment instead of penalties. The epidemic was dubbed a national public health emergency, and billions of dollars were allocated for treatment and prevention programs as opposed to the billions spent on law enforcement during the crack epidemic. In this case, the problem was the same—addiction—but the words used to describe it were entirely different based on the population (and, to a bold degree, the racial demographics of the population) who was being affected by the problem. The words *war* and *crackhead* largely used in the 1990s were replaced with *public health crisis* and *person suffering from addiction* in the 2010s. As nurses and members of society, we are challenged to pay attention to words as they can influence and alter lives and the direction of policy.

This chapter is organized around three steps in identifying and analyzing a policy problem or issue. First, we discuss the need for clear *identification* of a problem, including specificity in defining it, quantifying the problem and its impact with data, and determining the cost. Next, we discuss the importance of understanding the *context* of a policy problem, as the intrinsic and extrinsic factors related to the problem can sometimes be confounders to policy solutions. Finally, we discuss the importance of identifying and engaging *stakeholders* in both the policy problem identification and the development of an advocacy strategy, including the consideration of political stakeholders. The last section of the chapter provides several *policy analysis tools* for use in both big-P and little-p policy problems.

It should be noted that although this chapter outlines these steps individually, policy analysis is rarely a linear process. For example, although stakeholders are identified as a distinct section in this chapter, stakeholders are integral to every step of policy analysis and identification. In addition, political influence is integrated into many aspects of policy work, regardless of whether the issue involves elected officials. Like the nursing process in providing patient care, the process of policy work is iterative and cyclical. Like the nursing process, the assessment of the issue—the problem identification and definition—are the very foundation of policy analysis. Although this process can be iterative, the fundamental importance of understanding the problem and all its facets cannot be underestimated.

IDENTIFYING A PROBLEM

Problem identification is a basic and often complex stage of the policymaking process. It involves determining if an issue is a condition or a problem, clarifying a distinct problem, and using data to quantify problems. Clarifying these aspects will help determine which, if any, policy changes are requisites to address the identified problem or if an existing policy needs to be changed or eliminated.

Conditions Becoming Problems

Kingdon (2011), often cited for his work in policy, identifies three streams that come together for capitalizing on a window of opportunity: (a) problem definition, (b) availability of realistic policy solutions, and (c) political motivation to create the movement necessary for action. In addressing problem definition, Kingdon (2011) points out that

> "there is a difference between a condition and a problem. We put up with all manner of conditions every day: bad weather, unavoidable and untreatable illness, pestilence, poverty, fanaticism. Conditions become defined as problems when we come to believe that we should do something about them" (p. 109).

What influences that belief? What values drive us to believe we should do something?

Values play a role in our individual and societal view of when conditions become problems. The healthcare debate in the United States has been defined, to some degree, as a debate over whether basic healthcare is a right that should be accorded each member of our society or it is a commodity that must be purchased. Comparing our healthcare to that found in other countries has been an important aspect of that debate: Should we emulate the sort of national health insurance found in other countries, or reject it as socialism?

A clear example of problem definition is found in "never events." These events are defined as "errors in medical care that are clearly identifiable, preventable, and serious in their consequences for patients, and that *indicate a real problem* [emphasis added] in the safety and credibility of a healthcare facility" (Centers for Medicare and Medicaid Services [CMS], 2006, "Background"). The increased awareness and attention to medical errors over the past decades are an example of how a "condition" (like medical errors) became a problem that became a focus of policy and legislation.

In some cases, problems vault into national attention as a result of a significant, large-scale event that has wide-reaching ramifications. Kingdon (2011) describes these as "focusing events" such as a "disaster that comes along to call attention to a problem" (Kingdon, 2011, p. 94). The global COVID-19 pandemic provides a dramatic example of a focusing event. The pandemic once again highlighted the need to better support our public health system and to provide healthcare workers a safe working environment. The pandemic has also tragically laid bare the inequities in the system as communities of color have disproportionately experienced illness and death. These issues have long been identified as problems in healthcare but had not been thrust into the national spotlight until the pandemic (Betancourt, 2020).

Clarifying a Distinct Problem

It can be helpful to approach a complex field like healthcare by thinking about problems broadly, with categories like cost, quality, and access. But when it comes to *defining* a problem, "lack of access to care" is not specific enough to be a helpful starting place. One approach to narrowing such a broad problem is to look to the literature to see, for instance, the documented obstacles to accessing care, such as transportation, provider shortages, or a lack of culturally competent care. It is also useful to frame the problem in a way that helps illuminate possible policy solutions. The Centers for Disease Control and Prevention (CDC, 2015a), in its Policy Analytic Framework, uses this example: "Providing safe places for people to be physically active in their communities" (which has clear policy solutions) instead of "increasing physical activity" (where the policy options are not as clear)" ("Step 1: Identify the Problem or Issue").

One of the most common problems facing students addressing clinical or policy problems, particularly for doctoral nursing students, is the tendency to try to solve all the world's problems or, metaphorically speaking, to "boil the ocean." Each step in narrowing the problem, to achieve a degree of specificity, seems to be leaving out so much of the problem. Most problems are multifactorial, and given the interrelation, it is difficult to omit any one aspect. However, to successfully address a problem, it generally needs to be specific and limited.

Using Data to Quantify Problems

Data, what Kingdon (2011) calls "indicators," play a role in identifying problems. The fact that we choose to count something—in surveillance or monitoring systems—reveals our attitude about that thing being a condition worth our attention (or not). And we set limits on what is acceptable: How many people is it affecting? How severe is the problem? What is the financial impact? What gets counted counts!

Nurses recognize the collection of data is the critical first step of the nursing process. It is not different in policy analysis—the collection and analysis of data to quantify a problem is the first step in identifying it. Just like patient care, in which nurses cannot formulate a plan of care and comfort for a patient without understanding what is wrong with the patient, a robust assessment of a problem must be conducted to develop a viable policy solution. Think of it as trying to fight a forest fire with a garden hose—when the problem is not clearly quantified and defined, the solution will more than likely fail.

A first step in identifying and defining a problem is determining how much of the problem exists and how many people are affected. Part of the latter is identifying the populations affected, including population-level disparities that can be identified. Take the forest fire example: It is not just enough to know that there is a "forest fire"; we also must know how many acres are currently burning, the temperature of the flames, how many people are in harm's way, how much property is at risk, and if particular populations that are most vulnerable than others. This specificity is important because we likely will not get the right kind of support (e.g., financial, logistic, or resource support) if we do not first determine how much and what kind of support we need.

One essential element of quantifying problems is to determine appropriate data. There is an adage in policy work: "In God we trust; all others bring data." Health policy is no exception! Nurses are evidence-based practitioners, and just like nursing practice changes based on the best quality evidence, policy is likewise based on evidence.

However, evidence is not always enough to impact change; one must bring the best available evidence and appropriately decipher that evidence. Similar to grading evidence to make a practice change, as discussed at length in Chapter 5, nurses must grade evidence to influence policy change. To do so, nurses use their basic understanding of research and statistics. Understanding this information will greatly enhance the ability to define problems and to advocate for policy solutions. See **Policy on the Scene 4.1**.

POLICY ON THE SCENE 4.1: WHEN POLICY MEANS DATA DEVELOPMENT

Sarah DeSilvey, DNP, FNP-C
Director of Clinical Informatics, The Gravity Project

An oft-overlooked area of health policy is the domain of health data and data standards, and their ability to support existing policies across the whole health system. This discussion of data in relation to health programs and policies relies on Alderwick and Gottlieb's (2019) social determinant, social risk factor, social need lexicon. As a clinical informaticist, medical/social care integration expert, primary care provider, and clinical representative for Vermont's value-based accountable care organization (ACO), I was well aware that the lack of terminology to define the social determinants of health limited our capacity to offer quality care. With inadequate terminology, it's very difficult to document social risks critical for health outcomes during a patient encounter. We cannot distinctly represent a social risk in prospective payments, nor can we efficiently develop social risk quality measures. Furthermore, our hands are tied in being able to quantify our outcomes in line with the Triple Aim of healthcare.

These problems needed solutions. I had been working with my colleagues at the University of California San Francisco (UCSF) Social Interventions Research & Evaluation Network (SIREN) for some time to map the current state of data for social risks. The next step was to develop a consensus process to assess and fill those social risk data gaps. With the support of the Robert Wood Johnson Foundation and the U.S. Department of Health and Human Services (USDHHS), and the partnership of UCSF SIREN with EMI Advisors for program management, we jump-started a project to solve some of these issues: the Gravity Project.

The Gravity Project, started in the spring of 2019, is a national project to develop consensus-driven data standards for the social determinants of health. The project gathers diverse stakeholders from the government, academic, clinic, and community ecosystem to develop the terminology needed for social risk domains, such as food insecurity, housing instability and homelessness, and financial strain. This terminology is then built into open technical standards that are able to be shared between systems, settings, vendors, and payors in a process called interoperability.

Once the terminology and standards are in hand, we begin to solve some of the policy problems related to coding. In less than 2 years, the Gravity Project submitted ICD-10-CM (US version) code suggestions that align with health risks to enable social risk–informed prospective payments and social risk stratification within value-based payment programs. It has collaborated to build social risk quality measures with the National Center for Quality Assurance. It has partnered to begin a national taxonomy of social programs to aid in clinical care and research. Data and data standards enable specific policies for health information technology. The Gravity Project is working with the USDHHS Office of the National Coordinator on a pathway for building social risk data competency into policy-mandated health record standards. The Agency of Community Living wrote the Gravity Project standards into a community data exchange grant program. Finally, the CMS partners in assessing current barriers, addressing them through innovation and pilots, and disseminating standards across the country.

Although the Gravity Project focuses on increasing shared terminology and coding of certain health issues, the project also exemplifies the work to quantify social determinants of health as a means of expressing problems and engaging stakeholders in developing solutions. Social determinants of health, such as poverty, food insecurity, and education, can sometimes be overlooked in clinically focused health areas, demonstrating that problem identification requires broad thinking and analysis of the root cause of issues. This innovative project represents how data and data systems can be used to give visibility to problems but can also be used as policy solutions.

Finding data to define the problem is sometimes the hardest part of problem definition. Sometimes a problem appears to be anecdotal (i.e., an "N = 1" problem) or may only affect a very small number of people. Data are needed to support the notion that these are valid problems. For example, when nurses are overheard talking at break about how many of one's colleagues in other units are declining getting an influenza vaccine. This raises a concern that vulnerable patients might be exposed to nurses who are ill with preventable influenza. At this point, this is an anecdotal problem because it's only something being "talked" about. To fully quantify this problem, data would be needed to determine how many nurses are, in fact, declining annual flu vaccinations at the hospital. Think about who might collect that data and how it might be reported, perhaps occupational health tracks vaccination rates among nurses. Think about if the issue is publicly reported or is part of a licensure/accreditation requirement for the hospital. Publicly reported metrics, such as influenza vaccination of hospital healthcare providers, will have data collected at the hospital level and would be readily available because it is required to be public.

Nurses addressing problems at the state or federal policy levels, such as advocating for equitable access to vaccines and protective gear for nurses across healthcare facilities, use data largely collected at the state or national level. For example, the CDC publishes annual reports of healthcare worker influenza immunization rates after conducting national surveys. These reports not only are helpful in determining the extent to which nurses are being immunized but also describe the data in detail for development and analysis of policy (CDC, National Center for Immunization and Respiratory Diseases, 2019).

Although not an all-inclusive list, the following section describes some common sources for health data. At the national level, there is a trove of public data collected by a variety of government agencies. This includes the CDC, the CMS, the Healthcare Services and Resources Administration (HRSA), and the Agency for Healthcare Research and Quality (AHRQ). Which agency collects and reports data depends on the problem: public health, access to care, quality metrics, underserved communities (another important reason to properly identify the problem). For example, the CDC collects data in a variety of scientific ways and publishes numerous datasets and reports for public use on the National Center for Health Statistics website (www.data.cdc.gov/). Data sets often used to determine the extent of health problems include the National Health and Nutrition Examination Survey (NHANES), and the Behavioral and Risk Factor Surveillance Survey (BRFSS).

State and local health departments also collect and report data at the geographic level, and these sources are useful when quantifying problems that are smaller in geographic scale. Organizations representing state and local health departments, such as the Association of State and Territorial Health Directors and the National Association of County and City Health Officials, also publish reports and issue briefs describing problems within communities.

Data may also be available at the individual hospital/healthcare facility level. These data require a little more time, effort, and rationale to collect because these are private data belonging to the facility itself. Data reported to the National Database of Nurse Quality Indicators (NDNQI) might be one source of hospital-level data for determining problems within nursing practice. NDNQI is a powerful data source for determining the extent of problems, such as nurse satisfaction, retention, infection rates, or falls. Data within the NDNQI require permission to obtain; thus, it is important to assure the rationale for the data is concrete and transparent. Hospitals' customer satisfaction data are also a source of valuable information for determining the extent of problems and may be available within the hospital.

In situations in which data are not already collected, it is important to conduct a data collection process, much like a nursing assessment, that is thorough and transparent. For example, if a nurse wanted to quantify the problem of patient violence toward healthcare workers on a hospital unit, the nurse might need to collect these data manually. Options include running queries in an electronic health record or surveying nurses about the number of incidents they have witnessed or documented.

It is vitally important, whether manually collecting data or querying existing systems, to be sure permission has been obtained to collect and store the data. Some data collection will require institutional review board approval if the data involve identifiable patient or nurse information or if it will be published as part of a report or study. Institutional-level permission might be needed. Be sure to determine your facility's policy for data collection and storage if your problem definition will involve data not publicly available.

Like the nursing process, data collection (i.e., the problem "assessment") is only the first step. Defining a problem using data requires adequate analysis of that data. A basic understanding of descriptive statistics, including frequencies and percentages, rates (incidence and prevalence), and means/averages—goes a long way when describing the data to other stakeholders.

The Financial and Human Costs of Problems

The quantification of policy problems must also include cost. At the policy and political levels, cost is a major driver of intention to focus on problems and cost often is a factor in driving a policy problem to the top (or bottom) of an agenda. The financial burdens of problems may be wholly visible or entirely invisible. Determining cost to those hurt by the problem directly and indirectly is an important part of analysis.

Cost data is often estimated to allow for an accounting of the direct and indirect cost. For example, the CDC estimates costs of injuries and preventable deaths using actual and estimated cost data and publishes this information on the WIS™: Web-based Injury Statistics Query and Reporting System website (CDC, 2020a). According to the WIS, the CDC estimates the cost of suicide in the United States to be $70 billion annually, accounting for medical and burial costs, lost productivity, and costs related to the physical and mental health of dependents and loved ones of the victim (CDC, 2020b). Cost estimates need not be expressed exclusively in terms of dollars spent on care or burial.

Another metric for quantifying the cost of a problem is a quality-adjusted life-year (QALY) lost estimate. These estimates help quantify the cost of morbidity and mortality of a health issue by estimating the value of productivity and weighting certain factors in calculating and overall cost (Dooling et al., 2018). QALY has been integrated into several policymaking deliberative procedures at the CDC, including considering QALY as part of the immunization policy recommendations made by the Advisory Committee on Immunization Practices. The U.S. Public Health Services Taskforce has also cited QALY in some of its recommendation statements. QALY is not without controversy, however, as some describe it as too robotic and easily biased (Neumann & Cohen, 2018).

Identifying the Outcomes of a Problem: Who Is Affected?

Another critical part of policy analysis is determining who is interested and engaged in defining and solving the problem. This can make a big difference in how large scale and visible the policy solution becomes. Although more thoroughly explored in the section of this chapter that discusses stakeholders, part of a problem definition is articulating who within nursing, healthcare, and the community has a stake in the problem.

Defining a problem also involves determining who is being affected negatively by the problem. This can also make a difference in who the stakeholders will need to be to analyze and determine policy issues, as described later in this chapter. Here again, data sources are valuable in determining which populations are affected by the problem. Data reports that break down health issues at demographic levels, such as race/ethnicity, age, identified gender, and/or sexual orientation, to help determine which populations are most affected.

Rate comparisons are instrumental in discussing problems affecting vulnerable populations. For example, in 2017, among all women ages 25 to 34 years, pregnancy, childbirth, and postpartum complications were the sixth-leading cause of death, accounting for 512 deaths and a mortality rate of 2.3 deaths per 100,000 women. However, when this statistic is analyzed for race, among Black women ages 25 to 34 years, the rate increased to 4.9 per 100,000, even though the overall number of 161 deaths was seemingly lower than the overall number. Among White women ages 25 to 34 years, the rate was 1.9 per 100,000. In this example, when put in perspective for population, Black women ages 25 to 34 had twice the rate of death for pregnancy, childbirth, and postpartum complications than White women (Heron, 2019).

The problem of disparities in maternal–infant mortality is not a new one but provides an example of what seems to be a "window of opportunity" opening. The American College of Nurse-Midwives (ACNM) has been working, with regulators, policymakers, and maternal and child health stakeholders to raise awareness of this problem and provide commonsense solutions for decades. One of the key elements to achieving equity and improving disparities is to increase racial and ethnic diversity in the maternal health workforce. The USDHHS (2020) released *Healthy Women, Healthy Pregnancies, Healthy Futures: Action Plan to Improve Maternal Health in America*, with the goal of making the United States one of the safest countries in the world for people to give birth. Following the release, the U.S. Surgeon General issued a complementary call to action to improve maternal health.

The National Partnership for Women and Families (2020) released *Improving Our Maternity Care Now: Four Care Models Decisionmakers Must Implement for*

Healthier Moms and Babies recommending concrete resolutions that can be implemented to address disparities and improve the culture of health for Black, Indigenous, and people of color. Both the USDHHS and National Partnership reports include several of the same recommendations, including better integration of midwives and midwifery-led care models to address structural inequities. The reports highlight the workforce as a problem and call for increasing capacity and diversity within the midwifery workforce. It also provides support for scaling up birth centers, promoting diverse maternity care teams in all settings, and centering culturally congruent maternity care as a way to improve maternal and child health outcomes. None of these ideas is new, but they are rising in the policy agenda.

Data to determine who is hurt by a problem can be somewhat harder to obtain than quantitative data because it is not a typical data collection strategy for public agencies or institutions. However, identifying qualitative data in the literature can be a valuable source of determining the extent to which individuals, communities, or populations are affected by a problem. Qualitative data differ from quantitative data because they represent spoken words and expression of emotion, representing people's lived experiences or their descriptions of their experiences with a life event or situation. Qualitative data provide another, richer perspective; provide context for information; and tell a story beyond numbers and statistics.

Credible journalistic sources, such as mainstream newspapers and televised interviews, are other sources for qualitative data. Although not considered as "gold standard" scientific evidence because it is not necessarily scientifically collected, professional journalists are trained to interview subjects for their stories similarly to how qualitative researchers are trained. These interviews and stories can be powerful and compelling descriptions of the extent to which problems are hurting people. However, just as a nurse should grade evidence from the literature for its quality, news stories should be graded for the publication or website in which the story appears. Not all news outlets hold their reporters and writers to journalistic standards of professionalism, so nurses should scrutinize the publication before citing news stories as part of the evidence base for a problem. Determining the validity of sources is an essential skill (See Chapter 10).

Storytelling is an important tool in advocacy, helping to humanize a problem and get it on the agenda (Fitzpatrick, 2020; Morrise & Stevens, 2013). Also known as narrative inquiry, storytelling is a way to allow people to share the details of their experience as a way of provoking an emotional response among those listening, particularly if the story is relatable and compelling (Kahn & Lynn, 2014). Many advocacy organizations train advocates and patients in the art of storytelling, establish story banks, and invite people impacted by problems to testify, visit legislators, and use their stories as part of an advocacy agenda. An example is illustrated in Policy on the Scene 4.2.

Engaging Others to Take Action

A critical part of defining a policy problem is determining who would care about the issue, especially considering some of the deeper social issues that might be framing how the problem is viewed. In these instances, the populations that are affected and the words used to describe the problem can be very powerful in determining how the problem is perceived. Words and language used when advocating and then writing policy can have multiple meanings and subsequent consequences.

POLICY ON THE SCENE 4.2: PROBLEM IDENTIFICATION DURING COVID-19: ARMED WITH STORIES ABOUT PERSONAL PROTECTIVE EQUIPMENT

Kendra McMillan, MPH, RN
Katie Boston-Leary, PhD MBA MHA, RN, NEA-BC
Cheryl Peterson, MSN, RN
American Nurses Association

The COVID-19 pandemic laid bare many challenges to the U.S. healthcare system's ability to respond to a significant infectious disease event. One significant challenge that quickly became apparent was access to a sufficient supply of PPE directly impacting the ability of nurses to respond, as well as their personal safety. Contributing to this challenge was a failure to plan at all policy levels—institutional, local/regional, state, and national—and a failure to pivot to use policy vehicles, like the Defense Production Act (DPA), to quickly address the PPE gap.

The media quickly began to report on the state of PPE for healthcare workers. Through a series of nurse surveys, the American Nurses Association (ANA) sought to quantify the problem. Findings from the ANA's (2020a) initial COVID-19 survey revealed that 74% were extremely concerned about PPE and 58% were extremely concerned about personal safety. The ANA's follow-up survey in May highlighted continued shortages with 45% reporting PPE shortages with critical shortages identified in long-term care and community health facilities. Seventy-five percent reported they were encouraged or required to reuse PPE with 36% reusing N95 respirators for 5 or more days, and 59% reported feeling unsafe with reuse practices (ANA, 2020b). Six months into the pandemic, stories of nurses experiencing severe PPE shortages continued. The ANA's follow-up PPE survey conducted from July 24 to August 14 revealed that one in three nurses reported they were "out" or "short" of N95 masks, 68% were required to reuse N95s, 58% reused N95s for 5 or more days, 62% felt unsafe reusing N95s, and 55% felt unsafe using decontaminated masks (ANA, 2020c).

Armed with data and stories of clinical nurses about the impact of ongoing PPE shortages, the ANA launched a grassroots advocacy campaign leveraging social media to issue a call to action for Congress to increase PPE that generated a response from more than 107,000 nurse advocates and 330,000 messages to Congress. The ANA engaged with national media outlets through television, radio, and print to raise awareness of the impact of COVID-19 on nurses, patients, and families. The ANA maintained communication with the Trump administration, House of Representatives, and Senate staff on legislative priorities for COVID-19 relief and urged the administration to invoke the DPA to increase the domestic production of PPE, medical supplies, and equipment. Despite numerous organizations, including the ANA, imploring the administration to use the DPA, which gives the president power over funding, production, and the distribution of critical supplies during crises, only three companies were funded by the DPA to produce N-95 masks (Contrera, 2020).

In Senate Finance Committee testimony, ANA President Ernest Grant used the ANA's data and nurses' stories to highlight the dire need for action and to call on Congress and the administration to

- report the state of the Strategic National Stockpile with respect to PPE, vaccines, medicines, and other supplies;
- require healthcare facilities to report monthly to the government supply to support early identification of shortages. Manufacturers of these items would also be required to report on production;

- engage in national planning to support purchasing of PPE to avoid competition across states and healthcare systems; and

- incentivize and prioritize the manufacturing of PPE, medications, and other supplies in the United States, which will have the side benefit of supporting the U.S. economic recovery (ANA, 2020d).

One day following the World Health Organization's declaration of the pandemic, a recommendation was issued in the United States to rely on crisis and contingency strategies to preserve PPE inventory. The world will face another pandemic, and better policy and planning can ensure that we have a very different and more positive outcome.

Timing and Duration of Problems

The timing and duration of a problem are other pieces in defining it. Sometimes a problem is entirely new, as with technology or other innovations that are new to healthcare. Some problems may present as crises, whether small or large, forecasted, or unexpected. Other problems may seem new but could be exacerbations of existing problems. The timing of the problem is also a consideration in the "Window of Opportunity" (Kingdon, 2011).

Some problems are largely reactive, such as a problem presented as a crisis or an emerging large-scale issue. Examples of these types of problems include major accidents, mass casualty events, or public health epidemics. These types of problems, even if they were discussed or predicted, such as a natural disaster, pandemic, or nursing shortage, still present as issues requiring immediate attention. These types of problems are a bit like sugar rushes in that they get large attention, publicity, and subsequent action but only in the short term. Sometimes the problems persist despite attention in the media diminishing. Reactive problems on a localized, or little-p level, might include sentinel events at the hospital, a short-term staffing crunch, or a labor strike.

There are also problems that persist despite ever becoming major issues that garner much publicity. These are what we might call "slow boil problems," in which there are still people being affected and costs being accrued but no major massive action or movement to addressing them. On the big-P level, these issues would include things such as access to care and insurance coverage, where insurance inequalities and lack of physical or economic access to care persist. Others might include scope of practice issues and nurse staffing for advanced practice registered nurses (APRNs). These are problems addressed and written about for years and remain almost perennially as items of discussion in health policy. Little-p problems might include nurse staffing decisions at the hospital level, hand hygiene compliance, and nurse satisfaction. Despite the longevity, these are still important problems to address. Patience and persistence are required to document and address these problems and to be ready to leverage the opening of the "Window of Opportunity" to move these slow-boil issues to the theoretical front burner.

UNDERSTANDING THE CONTEXT OF THE PROBLEM

It is important from the outset to consider the larger context of the problem as a part of problem identification and policy analysis. A useful tool is the Advocacy Strategy Framework (Coffman & Beer, 2015; Figure 4.1). This framework is a simple one-page tool combined with questions that can help advocates consider the change that is desired and the audiences that need to be engaged. It is sometimes

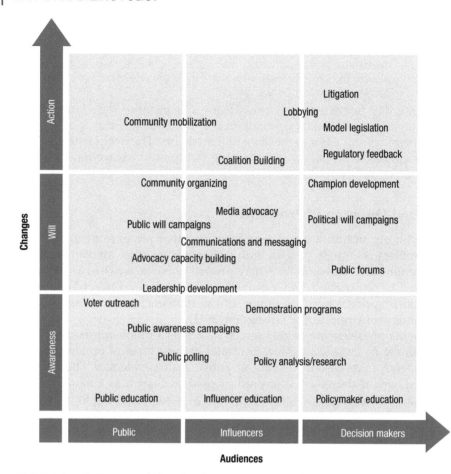

FIGURE 4.1 Coffman and Beer's advocacy strategy framework.

Source: Reproduced with permission from Coffman, J., & Beer, T. (2015, March). *The advocacy strategy framework.* Center for Evaluation Innovation. https://www.evaluationinnovation.org/wp-content/uploads/2015/03/Adocacy-Strategy-Framework.pdf

helpful to think about a problem in terms of the various strategies positioned within the framework. Is this a problem that needs public education? Could community organizing play a role? Would model legislation help address this problem?

With patient and community education a core component of nursing, the public awareness and education aspect of the framework (in the lower left) is likely an area nurses understand well. It is an area comfortable for nurses to engage, and nurses tend to be effective and well-received messengers (Saad, 2020). There is evidence, however that the profession has room for growth when it comes to engaging with and becoming decision-makers, particularly elected officials.

Despite an agreement that nurses have a professional and ethical responsibility to be politically involved (ANA, 2015; see Chapter 2) and a history that includes leaders who have engaged with decision-makers, nurses often avoid political engagement. Much has been written about the need to increase the political participation of nurses, particularly to better integrate political education in the nursing curriculum (Vandenhouten et al., 2011; Woodward et al., 2016). A host of activities, from attending advocacy training and contacting elected officials to working with other stakeholders and offering testimony can allow students to apply theoretical concepts, enriches their learning experience, and encourages political engagement.

An examination of political factors is critically important in the analysis of policy problems. For example, who holds elected office? What are the priorities of the political parties in power? Where are we in the election cycle, and how might this analysis evolve? When it comes to elected office and being decision-makers who can take action, nurses are sorely underrepresented. For example, the 117th Congress includes only three RNs (ANA, n.d.) and 17 physicians (American Medical Association, 2021). For more on political analysis, see the Tools for Analysis section of this chapter.

The face of electoral politics is changing. However, with a rise in the number of female and nontraditional candidates in recent years. In the words of one of the newly elected nurses, "I am the first nurse going to Congress from Missouri, in the middle of a pandemic. Nurses across the country have risked their lives to save others. Working class people need representatives who look like them and who have experienced their struggles. I am that champion" (Bush, 2020).

IDENTIFYING THE STAKEHOLDERS

Identifying stakeholders is critical to success in the policy process. In fact, stakeholder engagement and education are at the center of the CDC's (2015b) graphic depiction of the policy process (Figure 4.2).

In answering the question, *Who should you involve in your policy analysis,* the CDC offers three groups:

1. **People Who Can Provide and/or Interpret Information About the Policy:** Such as subject matter experts, economists, and community partners. Kingdon (2011) refers to these as "outside government," groups such as interest groups, academics, media, elections-related, public opinion. Professional associations are the north star for information about issues regarding policy.

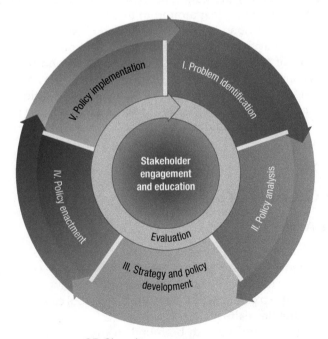

FIGURE 4.2 **CDC's policy process.**

Source: Centers for Disease Control and Prevention. (2015b, May 29). *CDC policy process.* https://www.cdc.gov/policy/polaris/policyprocess/index.html

2. **People Affected by the Policy:** Community members whose jobs or lives might be affected. There has been a growing trend toward including this group, exemplified by the Patient-Centered Outcomes Research Institute, established by the Patient Protection and Affordable Care Act (ACA). The ACA also requires tax-exempt hospitals to carry out a community health needs assessment, developed with community stakeholders, every 3 years.

3. **People Who Administer Resources Related to the Policy:** Public officials and administrators who understand the potential economic, budgetary, and legal implications. Kingdon (2011) refers to these as "inside government" groups: the administration, civil servants, Capitol Hill. As noted earlier, nurses are sorely underrepresented in this group.

The Advocacy Strategy Framework refers to "audiences," which are individuals and groups that are targeted as part of the strategy. Audiences also represent the important actors in the policy process, including policy influencers and stakeholders, such as other advocacy organizations and leaders in the business community.

One of the advantages of using the Coffman and Beer (2015) framework is that it allows for the mapping of multiple strategies carried out by multiple stakeholders. One of the six questions advocates are asked to answer is, "Who else is working on this and how?" Such an understanding helps avoid duplication of effort and allows each stakeholder to bring their strengths and expertise to the effort. One example of this is the way that APRNs have worked to address the scope of practice barriers along with physical therapists, psychologists, and a host of other healthcare professionals (Coalition for Patients' Rights, n.d.).

The process of identifying and refining policy problems is driven by what Kingdon (2011) calls "policy communities," made up of researchers, academics, interest group analysts, policy staff, and other specialists in a given policy area. His research showed the health community to be tightly knit, with a common language and ways of thinking (not to minimize sharp divides on strategy). He describes the way ideas float around in these communities as being like the way molecules floated around in "the primeval soup" before life came into being.

Which ideas survive and float to the top of this policy primeval soup depends on a number of factors such as technical feasibility and the perceived ability to withstand constraints that might be imposed. Values play a role as well and often are debated in the larger political arena. Nurses have a unique perspective on the importance of problems and the best ideas to address those problems and cannot shy away from or be intimidated by the policy process. It is critical that nurses be in this soup.

TOOLS FOR ANALYSIS

Root-Cause Analysis

Root-cause analysis (RCA) is a structured method of analyzing adverse events that came from industry and has been adapted to healthcare (AHRQ, n.d.). Given the widespread use of RCA in healthcare institutions today, many nurses will be able to think of a little-p example in their setting. This tool can be useful, however, with widespread public health problems as well.

An example of an RCA can be found in the case of lead poisoning in Flint, Michigan (Sologic, n.d.). In 2015, reports of increased numbers of children with elevated lead levels led clinicians to start mapping cases and determining clusters. Case clusters seemed centered on low-income neighborhoods of Flint, and a high percentage of the cases were among Black children. Investigations and case interviews led to the finding that the public water supply in the homes was contaminated. However, investigators could not explain why lead-contaminated water suddenly became an issue after decades of use of the same water infrastructure. Public health investigations helped uncover the root cause of the problem—changing the source of public drinking water from Lake Michigan to the Flint River. The water supply change had been made in an effort to save money and was largely driven by policymakers at the state level as a means of cutting expenses amid state budget deficits after the great recession of 2008. When the water supply was changed, the river water had not been adequately treated, and sediment in the water, which was different than the sediment in the lake water, began eroding the pipes that supplied water to homes, causing lead to leach out of the pipes and into the water supply.

The Flint water crisis exemplifies how RCA requires a deeper dive past the surface of a problem. Without the critical thinking and determination to determine the true root of the problem, the issue and the policy decisions that led to the problem might never have been uncovered. The RCA also spurred a national discussion on the social determinants of health, vulnerable populations, and the health implications of policy.

Environmental Scan

Part of the preparatory work essential in identifying a problem with a policy solution is conducting an environmental scan of external and internal factors related to a particular problem/issue. An environmental scan is a systematic way of examining an issue within the context of current events and situations. Environmental scans are commonplace in all planning across settings, from business to education to healthcare. The setting and purpose help define the environmental scan carried out. Environmental scans can be used for a variety of reasons: for an assessment of clinical issues, the adoption of clinical guidelines, or the climate for legislative or regulatory policies.

Healthcare policies do not exist in isolation, so taking the necessary time to conduct and analyze an environmental scan can pay off by identifying both positive and negative factors that may impact the problem. The scan should also consider the following: the stakeholders involved and the resources available, which of these factors will or will not influence the successful outcome, which factors can be influenced, and which factors are outside your scope of influence. The results of the scan and analysis of those results should help identify important trends and events in the larger external environment, which provide a basis for developing strategies to move the issue toward the policy agenda.

Environmental scanning is typically conducted through a group process. The stakeholder group proposing a legislative solution to an identified problem may form a small task force or an ad hoc committee to carry out the environmental scan or, depending on available resources, may hire an outside consultant to do this important work. There are no hard-and-fast rules for conducting an environmental scan, and it is only one component of an external analysis. The environmental scan can be informal and mainly observational and can consist of identifying and gathering existing information, or it can take on a more formal aspect in which new data are collected through surveys or other research methods. Information may be gathered through reviewing relevant publications; media resources; internet sites;

statements or opinions by social critics, experts, and activists; and other existing data.

Although determining what is important to scan or examine is usually specific to the problem being addressed, there are some common methods and considerations to help organize the environmental scan. It usually starts with an internal scan to identify and leverage the strengths within one's own interest group or organization. If any weaknesses are identified, the group can adapt and neutralize them as the issue moves through the legislative process. This internal scan, discussed in more detail later in this section, is often examined using a strengths, weaknesses, opportunities, and threats (SWOT) analysis.

PESTLE Analysis

One type of analysis that can be used for assessment focuses on the environment from the perspective of politics, economics, and sociocultural changes, or a PES analysis. The PES analysis is a robust examination of the factors that are influencing the policy environment and will likely make or break a policy proposal's success. It is key to consider each factor equally but to then consider the most influential factors on the policy proposal. These factors are likely impacting the conceptual understanding of a policy issue or proposal. The following provides examples of things to be considered in conducting a PES analysis—or, in some circumstances, when technological, legal, and environmental factors also need to be examined, a PESTLE analysis—for a policy issue:

- **Political Factors:** In the political environment, consider the current individuals who hold elected office and their political parties, priorities, governing philosophies, and agendas. It is also important to consider the interest groups aligned or allied with elected officials. In addition to elected officials, consider the appointees to various government positions and their backgrounds. Consider the level of the policy issue; that is, is the issue at the legislative, regulatory, or executive order level? Consider the current political climate, for example, election year, level of partisanship, level of cooperation among elected officials. One must also assess the underlying political will to address or take on a policy issue. This is typically dependent on many of the factors addressed earlier, such as priorities of elected officials and interest group activity.

- **Economic Factors:** Consider the general state of the economy by looking at key metrics such as markets indices, housing markets, unemployment, and consumer confidence. Health economics is likely a focus point of economic analysis because many nursing-oriented policy issues will involve these factors: reimbursement policies, actuarial forecasts, insurance coverage and capitation, and overall healthcare spending. Economic impact of a policy issue may include both monetary and nonmonetary costs of the policy proposals. Nonmonetary economic issues include things such as employment, community stability, and quality of life. Of particular focus in health policy is the healthcare workforce. Consider the workforce issues and employment standing in healthcare, such as nurse work environment, retention, employment stability, and wages.

- **Sociocultural Factors:** Consider the societal environment regarding various communities, particularly cultural groups based on race, class, economic status, employment, immigration status, gender identity, and sexual orientation. Consider the prevailing attitude toward societal issues and civic engagement. Consider the well-being metrics and quality-of-life indicators in various communities. Consider demographic trends and changes and the attitudes toward these changes. Consider the ethical implications of a policy issue or concern. Although there are clear designations between religion and state legal matters in the United States, a holistic analysis of the sociocultural environment should consider the religious aspects of a community; religious influence or cultural norms may have ramifications for policy and may influence attitudes of community members.

- **Technological Factors:** Consider the technological component to the issues. Consider how technology such as social media is influencing communities. Consider how technology innovations can be advantages or detractors to nursing practice and the workforce.
- **Legal Factors:** Consider the legal environment regarding litigation, legal boundaries, and liability.
- **Environmental Factors:** Consider the environmental (natural and man-made) factors influencing the policy issue. These would include the effects of the policy on the natural environment, such as climate, air, water, soil, forests, and wildlife. The built environment is also of consideration, such as how the built environment is impacting health and the policy considerations that influence the aesthetic and health factors of where people live, work, and recreate.

Understanding these dimensions in the environment is essential to anticipating opportunities, as well as constraints, and helps individuals and groups design more effective policies. Table 4.1 provides some preliminary questions to consider when exploring the political environment in greater depth before executing a strategic plan to advance an issue. These questions are often thought to relate to public policy, but in reality, they have applicability to all policy. The political aspects of the environment quite often get the most attention when examining an issue in depth.

After data collection for each of the selected environmental sectors, some analysis is necessary to assess the external opportunities and threats. Information gathered should be shared with the larger working group. Activities in some identified sectors may need to be tracked over time to monitor changes in the environment and to clarify information.

TABLE 4.1: POLITICAL CONSIDERATIONS FOR SCANNING THE ENVIRONMENT

Determine Leadership	<ul><li>Assess who has the ability or desire to lead the policy change</li><li>Recognize what individual or group has the capacity, expertise, reputation, and established relationships</li><li>Determine if this is an interprofessional issue</li></ul>
Consider Relationships/ Reputation	<ul><li>Anticipate how stakeholders will be impacted</li><li>Determine stakeholders' engagement with each other</li><li>Determine stakeholders' level of support of and/or opposition to the issue</li></ul>
Identify Possible Stakeholders	<ul><li>Assess what organizations or groups have a vested interest in the issue</li><li>Identify who will be impacted whether status quo is maintained or a change is implemented</li><li>Determine who supports, does not support, or is noncommittal</li></ul>
Examine Relationships	<ul><li>Assess whether a relationship exists between the groups and identified stakeholders</li><li>Evaluate if the group leading the policy forward is viewed as credible and speaking for all involved</li><li>Review groups with strong policy influence who may support or oppose the policy</li><li>Determine if any group participates in a coalition that could be built on</li></ul>

Strengths–Weaknesses–Opportunities–Threats

SWOT analysis is a widely used tool for assessing the viability of a project. It is a logical means of strategically examining an issue to better identify a pathway to success. The SWOT analysis is different from the PES analysis in that it can identify the strategic viability of a policy proposal. Table 4.2 provides factors that may

TABLE 4.2: ESSENTIAL ELEMENTS OF A SWOT ANALYSIS

INTERNAL	
Strengths	*Weaknesses*
■ Personal stories of patients, nurses, and/or health-care workers regarding the consequences of not dealing with the problem ■ Prominent individuals willing to speak out publicly and push the issue to the forefront ■ Data available describing the extent and pervasiveness of the problem or its consequences ■ Data about costs of the problem to individuals, healthcare organizations, or government ■ Qualifications and name recognition of key individuals who are experts on the problem ■ Resources of stakeholder organizations with experience in developing issue campaigns	■ Lack of media attention and lack of communication outlets and resources to share these stories of life-altering consequences ■ Competing agendas for stakeholder and policymaker involvement; too many issues to address. What is the priority issue? ■ Lack of sufficient association resources (staff, financial) to address the issue ■ Strong need to build an economic case on the issue to make a compelling message for those not familiar with the issue

EXTERNAL	
Opportunities	*Threats*
■ Nurses, nurses associations, unions, healthcare organizations, and consumer groups supportive of advancing a policy solution ■ Collaboration among important stakeholders ■ Increased calls for action because of the impact of the problem ■ New technologies and data analytics to address the problem ■ New communication strategies and social media platforms to get the word out about the problem ■ Multifaceted support from the public and private sectors, including professional associations representing different disciplines, healthcare organizations, industries, government, and consumer groups ■ Willingness of an organization to take the lead in addressing the issue ■ Endorsement of stakeholders for an organization to take the lead on an issue ■ Financial commitments from stakeholder groups	■ Costs of policy options ■ Opposition claiming that the burden of costs is prohibitive ■ Opposing organizations and the strength of their lobbying power ■ Compelling arguments put forth by opposing organizations ■ Lack of transparency about the extent of the problem ■ Lack of data or data being held and/or controlled by opposition groups ■ Reluctance to collect and disclose information related to the problem ■ Inconsistency in proposed solutions offered by stakeholder groups

be included when conducting a SWOT analysis for a specific issue. Using both SWOT and PES analyses is thought to reflect a more encompassing approach.

An SWOT analysis clearly outlines strengths and weaknesses that could impact the ability to advance an issue, even if the problems occur on the local or facility level. Nurse leaders at a local government health department used a SWOT analysis to determine the prevalence of problems within the tuberculosis case management nursing program. The SWOT analysis was instrumental in helping to determine the problems by engaging the public health nurses directly in the process. Once the SWOT analysis was used to determine the problems, solutions, including policy solutions at the department and state government levels, could be identified. Engaging the staff in the process secured buy-in for the outcomes and helped assure the nursing perspective and voice were included in the process. SWOT analyses at the national level, such as those conducted by the ANA, likewise assure that the problems affecting nurses are the focus of its work.

Scenario Analysis

Scenario analysis is a modeling tool to calculate future events (e.g., cost, frequencies) built using probabilities. Frequently used in cost analyses to determine probable monetary and quality-of-life costs related to disease, injury, or conditions. One example of its use is a study in which the probable costs per case and total costs of healthcare related to the incidence of COVID-19 were calculated (Bartsch et al., 2020). The study authors used several event trees of disease progression after infection with SARS COV-2, spanning asymptomatic disease to hospitalization for advanced respiratory distress syndrome. The model assumes an attack rate with assigned probabilities for each event in the tree based on current epidemiological data.

IMPLICATIONS FOR THE FUTURE

The sheer amount, breadth, and depth of problems in health and healthcare can seem overwhelming. Like sailing the ocean, it can feel like the more a problem is examined and analyzed, the deeper and wider the problem becomes. Nurses have an important vantage point in identifying and defining problems because of their training and competency in exploring the complexity of health from a holistic level. Policy problems require that same level of holistic assessment and analysis. Problems are unlikely to get any less complicated, particularly as problem identification in nursing and healthcare expands beyond traditional clinical medicine and health interventions. As highlighted in the *Future of Nursing: Charting a Path to Achieve Equity* report (National Academies, 2021) issues such as social determinants of health, health disparities, social justice in healthcare, and nurse well-being demand attention, analysis, and policy intervention. To address these problems, nurses will need to be equipped to collect and analyze data from a variety of sources and to translate this evidence into sound policy solutions. These issues have careened into the national spotlight during the COVID-19 pandemic, where health disparities, inequality in access to health services, national policy, leadership, and long-simmering racial inequalities became strikingly and tragically evident. The COVID-19 pandemic

POLICY SOLUTION | Words Matter

Nurses advocating a policy solution need to clearly define the issue with appropriate words as a first step in problem identification. Defining the issue begins by appreciating which words are universally understood and which can be emotionally or politically charged. In the Policy Challenge, the use of stigmatizing language can influence the public's and healthcare providers' perceptions of people negatively with a substance use disorder (SUD).

When addressing or referencing an individual with SUD, it is important to use person-first language that maintains the integrity of individuals as a whole human being. It is important to remove language that equates people to their condition or has negative connotations. Compare the difference when a person is described as a crackhead versus having a SUD.

While strides have been made to use words that are more appropriate when discussing SUDs, the need for vigilance continues for clinical problems and beyond. The appropriate use of terminology applies to each of us as nurses and as a profession. Words matter for our patients by our use of respectful language that is person-centered and does not have a pejorative connotation. Words matter for professionals to convey position, authority, and respect. Consider how are you referenced by title, how you are introduced, and what you call yourself. Compare these examples regarding role: *RN* versus *nurse*, *APRN* versus *mid-level provider*; *full practice authority* versus *independent practice*. While these might seem to be only a matter of words, there are real policy implications of terminology.

In Pennsylvania, for example, the official identification badge for an organization indicates that only titles as identified in its licensure laws may be used on a badge. This entitles physicians (MDs and DOs) to use "doctor" but prohibits persons with earned doctorates that are not part of the licensing structure from using their credentials on their official badge. Another policy consideration is state-by-state title protection for RNs, a long-term policy goal for the ANA and state associations.

Thus, words matter for policy in terms of the desired goal, need for collaboration, professional roles, and the achievement of healthcare outcomes. Examine how words influence, cause delays, or confusion or strengthen an approach to policy. When drafting and implementing policies, how issues are described and framed are crucial. Misunderstood policies can be dysfunctional or have unintended consequences. As a profession, our language and words are vital to our policymaking role and advocacy. Make your words count.

has increased the attention given to the mental, physical, and emotional toll on nurses and the responsibility of systems to provide for these needs. Nurses can be major stakeholders if we unite on common goals. Joining professional nurses associations builds diversity and strength in numbers to participate in advocacy activities, as well as shape favorable political circumstances. To address these issues, nurses need to also continue to cultivate allies to support and champion issues. As informed citizens, nurses engaged in full participation of the electoral process can better position themselves in boardrooms, political offices, and administrative leadership positions at the local, state, and federal level. Being an informed, data-driven professional positions nurses for leadership in presenting problems, engaging stakeholders, and increasing effective, sustained policy solutions.

KEY CONCEPTS

1. Words matter.
2. Problems are issues for which there is a concerted effort to solve them.
3. Societal values can be a significant factor causing a condition to become a problem.
4. Clarifying a distinct problem is essential to crafting solutions.
5. Quantification of problems involves using data to determine how much of a problem exists and how many people are affected.
6. Collecting, analyzing, and reporting data are crucial parts of problem identification and quantification.
7. Data can exist at many levels (national, state, local), and nurses should have a basic understanding of statistics to be effective in quantifying problems.
8. Cost is another critical part of problem quantification.
9. Defining problems also involves determining who is being harmed.
10. Qualitative data and storytelling are compelling methods of determining the emotional toll of problems.
11. The "window of opportunity" sometimes involves determining the right timing for identifying problems.
12. The context of the problem is a key part of analyzing problems and policy solutions.
13. Political activity is an important context of problem identification and one that nurses should embrace.
14. Stakeholder identification is crucial to assuring problems get the attention and resources needed for policy solutions.
15. Stakeholders include those within the government, external partners, and those affected by a policy.
16. Policy communities are ways in which nurses can engage with partners and stakeholders to be a part of a robust policy community.
17. Tools for policy analysis can assist nurses in engaging with stakeholders to identify problems and advocate for solutions.

SUMMARY

Learning how to identify, frame, and analyze problems; developing possible solutions; building stakeholder support; and evaluating the existing political circumstances are essential components in policymaking. Examining the environment through a scan, PESTLE analysis, or scenario analysis and taking stock of the internal and external environment with SWOT provide valuable information about the feasibility of a policy direction. Moving through these often nonlinear steps is preparatory for the recognition of the confluence of factors that create a favorable window of opportunity. Policy analysis using a well-defined process serves as an objective but critical step in determining the best course of action. Involving key stakeholders at key junctures in the process increases the chances for success when making a decision to move forward with a policy option. The policy process is iterative and will of necessity involve revisiting the analysis steps as the healthcare environment evolves. Several key examples demonstrated the challenges encountered when one advances a vision through policy.

END-OF-CHAPTER RESOURCES

LEARNING ACTIVITIES

1. Determine whether there are any regulations regarding the use of titles related to your position in your state.

2. Identify why each of these phrases might be divisive and how you would reframe them: "safe staffing," "gun control," "women's right to choose."

3. Identify a healthcare issue that, in your opinion, is a problem that calls for a policy solution. Explain how you would begin to gather data about the issue and develop a plan to address the problem. Discuss the tools that will help you in gathering the data.

4. Discuss some of the factors that indicate a problem that you identify has a window of opportunity opening. Use an example from a policy at work, school, or the community where you live to illustrate when a window of opportunity might open.

5. The Robert Wood Johnson Foundation, the Heritage Foundation, the Urban Institute, the Kaiser Family Foundation, and the Commonwealth Fund are all examples of research/policy organizations. Investigate the websites of at least three research/policy organizations to identify their organizational healthcare priorities.

6. Identify a current health story in the news that has potential policy implications. List the political institutions that are germane to the discussion about this health news issue. Brainstorm some possible policies that address this issue and then identify one policy from the list where a nursing voice can have the greatest impact.

7. Select one of the following e-resources to share with a work or school colleague or someone you supervise. Prepare a short summary of its purpose and applicability for policy tailored to the audience. Report back the audience's response.

8. Link to C-SPAN at www.c-span.org and select a topic that has implications for nursing. Discuss the problem identified and what contributions nursing can make to the definition of the problem.

9. Investigate the use of an advisory council where you work or go to school. Summarize its purpose, when it was developed, and current problems and solutions for which the group is being asked to provide advice or investigate.

E-RESOURCES

- Agency for Healthcare Research and Quality (AHRQ): Building Relationships Between Clinical Practices and the Community to Improve Care, Literature Review, and Environmental Scan http://innovations.ahrq.gov/linkages/report2.aspx

- Agency for Healthcare Research and Quality. Data Resources https://www.ahrq.gov/data/resources/index.html

- American Nurses Association. Advocacy: https://www.nursingworld.org/practice-policy/advocacy/

- Centers for Disease Control and Prevention. Data & Statistics https://www.cdc.gov/datastatistics/

- Centers for Medicare and Medicaid Services. Hospital Compare https://www.cms.gov/Medicare/Quality-Initiatives-Patient-Assessment-Instruments/HospitalQualityInits/HospitalCompare

- Gravity Project https://thegravityproject.net/

- Health Resources and Human Services Administration data.hrsa.gov

- National Resource Center for Participant-Directed Services (2013). *An Environmental Scan of Self-Direction in Behavioral Health: Summary of Major Findings* http://www.bc.edu/content/dam/files/schools/gssw_sites/ nrcpds/BH%20Scan/Summary_Scan%20of%20SD%20in%20BH_May2013. pdf

- National Black Justice Coalition. Words Matter Gender Justice Toolkit https://www.arcusfoundation.org/wp-content/uploads/2019/09/NBJC-Words-Matter-Gender-Bias-Toolkit-2019-vFINAL.pdf

- National Institute on Drug Abuse https://www.drugabuse.gov/ nidamed-medical-health-professionals/health-professions-education/ words-matter-terms-to-use-avoid-when-talking-about-addiction

REFERENCES

Agency for Healthcare Research and Quality. (n.d.). *Root cause analysis*. https://psnet.ahrq.gov/ primer/root-cause-analysis

Alderwick, H., & Gottlieb, L. M. (2019). Meanings and misunderstandings: A social determinants of health lexicon for health care systems. *The Milbank Quarterly, 97*(2), 407–419. https:// doi.org/10.1111/1468-0009.12390

American Medical Association. (2021). *Patients action network: Physicians of the 117th Congress*. https://patientsactionnetwork.com/physicians-117th-Congress

American Nurses Association. (n.d.). *Nurses serving in Congress*. https://www.nursingworld. org/practice-policy/advocacy/federal/nurses-serving-in-congress/

American Nurses Association. (2015). *Code of ethics for nurses with interpretive statements*. https://www.nursingworld.org/practice-policy/nursing-excellence/ethics/code-of-ethics-for-nurses/

American Nurses Association. (2020a). *COVID-19 survey*. https://www.nursingworld.org/ practice-policy/work-environment/health-safety/disaster-preparedness/coronavirus/ what-you-need-to-know/year-one-covid-19-impact-assessment-survey/

American Nurses Association. (2020b). *ANA personal protective equipment survey—May 2020*. https://www.nursingworld.org/~49cd40/globalassets/covid19/ppe-infograph-ic-june-5-2020.pdf

American Nurses Association. (2020c). *ANA personal protective equipment survey—July/August 2020*. https://www.nursingworld.org/~4a558d/globalassets/covid19/ana-ppe-survey-one-pager---final.pdf

American Nurses Association. (2020d). *Testimony from ANA president Ernest Grant to the senate finance committee regarding personal protective equipment*. https://www.nursingworld.org/ practice-policy/work-environment/health-safety/disaster-preparedness/coronavirus/ covid-19-interview-with-debbie-hatmaker-on-cnn/senfin-grant/

Bartsch, S. M., Ferguson, M. C., McKinnell, J. A., O'Shea, K. J., Wedlock, P. T., Siegmund, S. S., & Lee, B. Y. (2020). The potential health care costs and resource use associated with COVID-19 in the United States. *Health Affairs, 39*(6), 927–935. https://doi.org/10.1377/hlthaff.2020.00426

Betancourt, J. R. (2020, October 22). Communities of color devastated by COVID-19: Shifting the narrative. *Harvard Health Blog*. https://www.health.harvard.edu/blog/communities-of-col-or-devastated-by-covid-19-shifting-the-narrative-2020102221201

Bush, C. (2020, November 3). *I am the first nurse going to Congress from Missouri—In the middle of a pandemic*. [Tweet]. Twitter.com. https://twitter.com/CoriBush/status/132384139549751296 8?s=20

Centers for Disease Control and Prevention. (2015a, May 29). *CDC's policy analytical framework*. https://www.cdc.gov/policy/analysis/process/analysis.html

Centers for Disease Control and Prevention. (2015b, May 29). *CDC policy process*. https://www.cdc.gov/policy/polaris/policyprocess/policy_analysis.html

Centers for Disease Control and Prevention. (2020a). *Injury prevention and control*. WISQUARS. https://www.cdc.gov/injury/wisqars/

Centers for Disease Control and Prevention. (2020b). *Preventing suicide*. https://www.cdc.gov/violenceprevention/suicide/fastfact.html

Centers for Disease Control and Prevention, National Center for Immunization and Respiratory Diseases. (2019). *Influenza vaccination coverage among health care personnel—United States, 2018–19*. https://www.cdc.gov/flu/fluvaxview/hcp-coverage_1819estimates.htm

Centers for Medicare and Medicaid Services. (2006). *Fact sheet: Eliminating serious, preventable and costly medical errors—Never events*. https://www.cms.gov/newsroom/fact-sheets/eliminating-serious-preventable-and-costly-medical-errors-never-events

Coalition for Patients' Rights. (n.d.). *Coalition for patients' rights*. https://patientsrightscoalition.org/

Coffman, J. & Beer, T. (2015). *The advocacy strategy framework*. https://www.evaluationinnovation.org/wp-content/uploads/2015/03/Adocacy-Strategy-Framework.pdf

Contrera, J. (2020, September 21). N95 masks save lives. So why are they still hard to get this far into a pandemic? *The Washington Post*. https://www.washingtonpost.com/graphics/2020/local/news/n-95-shortage-covid/

Dooling, K. L., Guo, A., Patel, M., Lee, G. M., Moore, K., Belongia, E. A., & Harpaz, R. (2018). Recommendations of the Advisory Committee on Immunization Practices for use of herpes zoster vaccines. *MMWR. Morbidity and Mortality Weekly Report*, *67*(3), 103–108. https://doi.org/10.15585/mmwr.mm6703a5

Fitzpatrick, J. J. (2020, April 27). *Narrative nursing with Dr. Joyce Fitzpatrick, Frances Payne Bolton School of Nursing*. https://www.youtube.com/watch?v=DJqTVqBXKBY

Heron, M. (2019, June 24). *Deaths: Leading causes for 2017* (National Vital Statistics Reports, Vol. 68, No. 6). https://www.cdc.gov/nchs/data/nvsr/nvsr68/nvsr68_06-508.pdf

Kahn, R. & Lynn, J. (2014, July 14). *Storytelling: A tool for health advocacy*. The Colorado Trust. https://www.coloradotrust.org/wp-content/uploads/2016/08/PHC_IssueBrief_070214_FINAL.pdf

Kingdon, J. W. (2011). *Agendas, alternatives, and public policies* (2nd ed.). Longman.

Morrise, L., & Stevens, K. J. (2013). Training patient and family storytellers and patient and family faculty. *The Permanente Journal*, *17*(3), e142–e145. https://doi.org/10.7812/TPP/12-059

National Academies of Sciences, Engineering, and Medicine. (2021). *The future of nursing 2020–2030: Charting a path to achieve health equity*. National Academies Press.

National Partnership for Women and Families. (2020). *Improving our maternity care now: Four care models decisionmakers must implement for healthier moms and babies*. https://www.nationalpartnership.org/our-work/resources/health-care/maternity/improving-our-maternity-care-now.pdf

Neumann, P. J., & Cohen, J. T. (2018). QALYs in 2018—Advantages and concerns. *JAMA*, *319*(24), 2473. https://doi.org/10.1001/jama.2018.6072

Saad, L. (2020, December 22). U. S. ethics ratings rise for medical workers and teachers. *Gallup News*. https://news.gallup.com/poll/328136/ethics-ratings-rise-medical-workers-teachers.aspx

Sologic. (n.d.). *Flint water crisis*. https://www.sologic.com/en-us/resources/example-problems/flint-water-crisis

U.S. Department of Health and Human Services. (2020). *Healthy women, healthy pregnancies, healthy futures: Action plan to improve maternal health in America*. https://aspe.hhs.gov/system/files/aspe-files/264076/healthy-women-healthy-pregnancies-healthy-future-action-plan_0.pdf

Vandenhouten, C. L., Malakar, C. L., Kubsch, S., Block, D. E., & Gallagher-Lepak, S. (2011). Political participation of registered nurses. *Policy, Politics, and Nursing Practice*, 12(3), 159–167. https://doi.org/10.1177/1527154411425189

Woodward, B., Smart, D., & Benavides-Vaello, S. (2016). Modifiable factors that support political participation by nurses. *Journal of Professional Nursing*, 32(1), 54–61. https://doi.org/10.1016/j.profnurs.2015.06.005

CHAPTER 5

Harnessing Evidence in the Policy Process

LORI A. LOAN AND PATRICIA A. PATRICIAN

The acquisition of knowledge is the mission of research, the transmission of knowledge is the mission of teaching and the application of knowledge is the mission of public service.
—James A. Perkins

OBJECTIVES

1. Describe issues and resources that impact the translation of evidence into policy.
2. Analyze the types of evidence that have the potential to influence health policy.
3. Compare and contrast how evidence can be used at both the local level and beyond to influence policy.
4. Advocate for the implementation of policy initiatives based on evidence at different levels of policymaking.

The power of harnessing evidence for public policy can be easily traced in nursing from the data collected and analyzed by Florence Nightingale during the Crimean War and her advocacy efforts in the years that followed. Harnessing evidence, in this chapter, implies finding evidence and coupling it at the right times and places in the policymaking process. As illustrated in the lifelong work of Nightingale, the role of finding and using evidence to make policy change does not always follow a steady course in nursing or in healthcare generally.

Shortly after Florence Nightingale began her work, President Abraham Lincoln established the National Academy of Sciences (NAS) in 1863 to gather scientific information. It was not until 1930 that the Ransdell Act formalized the establishment of the National Institute of Health as a single agency whose research focus was biological and medical issues. In 1948, the singular National Institute of Health was renamed to the plural name, the National Institutes of Health (NIH) that we recognize today (Harden, 1998). In 1986, the National Center for Nursing Research (NCNR) was created, and then, in 1993, the National Institute of Nursing Research (NINR) was transitioned to institute status, 130 years after the NAS was established.

The institutionalization of research has not ensured a clear path for using scientific evidence for policymaking. There is currently much discussion on policies that were developed and are still operational; this discussion did not look at, or in some cases, seemed to ignore, convincing evidence contrary to those policies. Phrases heard at the big-P level, such as "when policy trumps science," and at the little-p level, such as "putting sacred cows to pasture," are testimony in common vernacular that attest to the disputes about the use of evidence in policymaking. The spectrum of policymaking has a myriad of examples in which evidence can be put to better use.

At the big-P level, policymakers often need help making sense of evidence and its practical relevance to policy. A great source of synthesized evidence for current policy topics is found in *Health Affairs' Health Policy Briefs*. These provide a synopsis of issues and relevant research related to healthcare improvement in the United States that concern policymakers, healthcare professionals, the public, and journalists. Originally (from 2009 to 2016), the policy briefs were produced by *Health Affairs* through a grant from the Robert Wood Johnson Foundation (RWJF) and included topics such as Patient Engagement, Implementing the Medicare Access and CHIP Reauthorization Act (MACRA), and the Two Midnight Rule. In 2017, *Health Affairs* began producing the briefs in collaboration with a variety of other partners.

A recent example is a *Health Affairs* brief authored by Julianne Holt-Lunstad (2020) focused on the culture of health, specifically social isolation and its impact on health. Professional associations, organizations, and other groups also use research to develop their policy briefs, testimony, and other dissemination venues (see Chapter 10). For example, the American Academy of Nursing's policy briefs developed by its expert panels often appear in its journal *Nursing Outlook*, as is illustrated by a brief on nurses' critical role to enhance health literacy (Loan et al., 2018).

Work at the little-p level may not be as easy to see or synthesize because this work does not often make it to the published literature. Further complicating the dissemination of little-p work is that so much work remains to be done to achieve the goal set by the Institute of Medicine (IOM, 2009; now the National Academy of Medicine) that 90% of clinical choices be based on evidence. However, as of 2017, only 18% of clinical recommendations are evidence-based (Ebell et al., 2017). Specific to nursing, Melnyk et al. (2016) found in a survey that more than 50% of the chief and executive nurse officers stated that the practice of evidence-based care was "low." There are, however, growing numbers of examples of how evidence is garnered and shared at the little-p level that can be seen on websites, in books, and in best practice stories from Magnet-designated organizations, such as those available at Johns Hopkins Medicine (https://www.hopkinsmedicine.org/evidence-based-practice/ebp_exemplars.html).

In this chapter, the Policy Challenge illustrates an example of a practice policy that was changed first at the little p-level followed by advocacy and policy change at the big-P level, both levels using evidence to make the practice policy change. Policy problems, even when it seems obvious that there would be universal support for a solution, are not always "simple." They often require multiple steps for implementation and success to improve outcomes. As discussed in the Policy Challenge, controversy often surrounds harnessing the evidence.

From ICU to State Capital: Policy Change Starting at the Bedside

Policymakers need data and this can come from a variety of sources. Often it starts with individual observations that ignite someone's passion and then extends to data collection within individual facilities, to statewide data and then to larger data repositories that may be nationally or globally based. Staff from North Children's Hospital Just for Kids Pediatric Critical Care Center in Louisville, Kentucky, noticed an increase in the number of children being treated for nonaccidental abusive head trauma. Although the trend was noticed in the ICU, these healthcare providers knew that significant change would occur only if they focused their efforts on educating the public on prevention strategies and warning signs of nonaccidental trauma. Justine O'Flynn, an RN on the unit, contacted the hospital's Public Relations and Child Advocacy departments, indicating that she wanted to write a letter to the editor to every newspaper in the state of Kentucky. The passion on the unit to educate others on preventing child abuse snowballed and resulted in an awareness campaign that greatly influenced the following actions:

- Developing a multidisciplinary child abuse task force focused on research on pediatric abusive head trauma
- Purchasing additional child abuse screening equipment within the hospital
- Establishing a Department of Pediatric Forensic Medicine at the University of Louisville
- Developing a "train the trainer" program, *Preventing Shaken Baby Syndrome*, in partnership with Prevent Child Abuse Kentucky
- Creating an educational video on child abuse-prevention strategies to play to families on all birthing units in the hospital system (KSPAN, n.d.)

This little-p project that started at the bedside took root with these efforts. Like many projects that have roots at the direct care level, it was time to be taken further.

See Policy Solution.

CONTROVERSY

Although much work remains to be done to fully use evidence, there is no doubt that its use to inform practice in healthcare has changed the healthcare environment. Increasingly, clinicians at all levels and points of care are held accountable to ensure that healthcare practices are based on the best available evidence. Those examining policy often question why the same attention has not been paid to using health services research to develop policies, with many articles written over the past 20 years on this question. The titles or phrases in some of those articles indicate the conundrum we face: "The Paradox of Health Services Research: If It Is Not Used, Why Do We Produce So Much of It?" (Lavis et al., 2002), "Translation of Research to Practice: Why We Can't Just Do It?" (Green & Seifert, 2005), and, more recently, "Bridging the Gap between Research and Policy and Practice" (McKee, 2019). These articles and many others suggest a gap, or even a chasm, exists between what we as a society *know* and what we *do*. Cairney and Oliver (2017) challenge researchers to consider that closing the gap requires a long view and recognition that evidence-based policymaking goes beyond a robust evidence base; it is often value and belief-driven. McKee (2019) recommends researchers partner with end users to keep their research relevant and policymakers having research translated for their use.

The notion of whether evidence-based policy is achievable has been questioned, and some have gone as far as declaring it a myth (Hammersley, 2013). There are numerous influences on policy, and evidence is not always the most definitive determinant of public health policy (Leuz, 2018). Grinspun et al. (2018) suggest a two-pronged strategy for advancing health policy: the evidence and the advocacy; to effect change in healthcare, nurses must be able to distill evidence to support a cause and have collective skills to create the "political will for change" (p. 470).

The term *evidence-informed policy* has gained considerable attention, with the recognition that research provides only one form of evidence. The World Health Organization (WHO) Europe explains that other essential forms of evidence include political and social climate, budgetary concerns, and timing of other priorities (WHO Europe, n.d). WHO formed an Evidence-Informed Policy Network (EVIPNet) in 2005 to promote the use of health research evidence for better decision-making and health policymaking, primarily focusing on low- and middle-income countries. The EVIPNet is a platform that fosters the translation of research results and other forms of knowledge into policy (WHO, n.d.). It is characterized by the systematic and transparent access to, and appraisal of, evidence as an input into the policymaking process. One may assume a linear process to policymaking, that is, that once a policy problem is identified, the evidence is obtained, and policies are implemented. Often, policymaking is not linear at all (see Chapter 1). The complexity of the policymaking process will be debated for years to come regarding the implementation, evaluation, and sustainability of the Patient Protection and Affordable Care Act (ACA).

CHALLENGES IN MOVING EVIDENCE INTO POLICY

The important role that research, in particular, plays in improving healthcare and the development of healthcare policies has been recognized for some time. Researchers and policymakers are "travelers in parallel universes" (Brownson et al., 2006, p. 164). Why are researchers and policymakers thought to be traveling in parallel universes? What are the issues?

Policymakers, whether at the big-P or little-p level, and researchers often have conflicting roles and needs. As early as 1979, Caplan sought to explain the issue by suggesting that there are cultural differences between researchers and policymakers, noting that these groups have different views of the world. Gaps exist between the two in values, language, reward systems, and professional affiliations. Researchers are mainly concerned with pure science and esoteric issues, whereas policymakers are more interested in immediate relevance and have an action orientation. Ellen et al. (2018) confirmed these differences in that policymakers perceived health services research findings were not immediately implementable. In contrast, researchers felt the lack of a coordinated effort between the two groups. These producers and users of research evidence varied greatly in their perceptions about the knowledge transfer exchange process.

McKee (2019) suggests that the research policy/practice gap must be closed from both directions. He recommends knowledge producers discuss researchable problems with end users to keep their research relevant and that users of knowledge have mechanisms in place to translate research for them.

This brings the issue of where the responsibility lies in ensuring the use of, or translating, new research into policy and practice to the forefront. The difficulty in identifying or assigning responsibility can be explained with technology transfer theory. This postulates that there is a unidirectional responsibility. There is either a science push or knowledge-driven model in which the information flows from researchers to policymakers, resulting in specific policy decisions, or a demand-pull or problem-solving model whereby information is commissioned from researchers by policymakers with the intent of addressing a well-defined policy problem.

Researchers have tried to determine (a) what barriers make the gap so hard to bridge and (b) the most effective strategies that help close the gap. Published systematic reviews provide strong evidence of numerous barriers in translating research into policy. Significant hindrances and facilitators in the use of evidence in developing health policy reported by most stakeholders include a lack of locally useful and concrete evidence, evidence on costs, and a lack of shared understanding. Factors influencing health policy development were users' characteristics and the role of media (van de Goor et al., 2017). Work examining the most effective strategies for translating evidence into policy is ongoing. One strategy that holds promise is the knowledge transfer and exchange approach, which is an iterative process of synthesis, dissemination, and application of evidence (Canadian Institute for Health Information, 2012; Ellen et al., 2018).

Public health laws are often perceived to be a strategy for infusing research into policy. "Model" public health laws consist of statutory language recommended by at least one organization for government adoption. Hartsfield et al. (2007) identified 107 model public health laws, but only in 6.5% of cases did the sponsors provide details demonstrating that the model law was based on scientific information (e.g., research-based guidelines). More recent model public health laws include food policy laws for obesity prevention (Hawkes et al., 2015) and public health initiatives to reduce opioid overdose (Alexandridis et al., 2017). Despite these efforts, public health laws are perceived to be a missed opportunity, in part because there is no systematic method for categorizing them and examining their effectiveness in achieving the desired change (Attaran et al., 2012).

A challenge faced by researchers and those charged with ensuring that their organizations are using the best evidence is how quickly can research be used and how is it decided that the evidence is sufficient. Several initiatives have been developed to address the underuse of evidence in practice and policymaking within the United States. The NIH created the National Center for Advancing Translational Sciences (www.ncats.nih.gov); it provides Clinical and Translational Science Awards (CTSAs) to address the complexity of conducting patient-oriented research and applies biomedical research to patient care delivery. The ACA established the Patient-Centered Outcomes Research Institute (PCORI, n.d.) to fund comparative effectiveness research that helps people make decisions about their healthcare. Studies funded by PCORI require that patients and other consumers are actively involved in the research process, empowering the end user's voice. Selected research entities supporting the use of evidence in practice and/or translational research are described in Exhibit 5.1.

EXHIBIT 5.1 SELECTED U.S. HEALTH RESEARCH ENTITIES

AGENCY AND YEAR ESTABLISHED	DESCRIPTION
AHRQ (1999)	U.S. Department of Health and Human Services agency that oversees health services research. It is complementary to the research mission of the National Institutes of Health. Originally known and established as the Agency for Health Care Policy and Research, it was reauthorized as AHRQ in 1999.
NAM, formerly IOM (1970)	Last of four federally authorized independent, nonprofit institutions called the National Academies established to provide expert, unbiased scientific information for health decisions. The other agencies include the National Academy of Sciences, the National Academy of Engineering, and the National Research Council.

(continued)

EXHIBIT 5.1   SELECTED U.S. HEALTH RESEARCH ENTITIES (CONTINUED)

NIH (1948)	U.S. Department of Health and Human Services agency that oversees 27 institutes and centers that conduct research to improve health and lengthen life, including length, and to decrease both illness and disability. Link to mission and goals: nih.gov/about/mission.htm
NINR (1993)	Originally established as a center in 1986, the mission of this institute is specifically research that increases the health of individuals, families, communities, and populations across the life span.
NCATS (2011)	One of six NIH centers. Its aims stress novel approaches and outcomes, and the use of evidence and technology to advance, establish, and publicize improvements in translational science. Its work is meant to complement the research of other NIH institutes and centers.
PCORI (2010)	Established as an independent nonprofit, nongovernmental organization to conduct research to help patients and their healthcare providers make decisions based on the best available evidence about prevention, treatment, and care options that is derived from research guided by patients, caregivers, and the broader healthcare community.

AHRQ, Agency for Healthcare Research and Quality; IOM, Institute of Medicine; NAM, National Academy of Medicine; NCATS, National Center for Advancing Translational Sciences; NIH, National Institutes of Health; NINR, National Institute of Nursing Research; PCORI, Patient-Centered Outcomes Research Institute.

Professional groups and patient advocacy groups are also working on translating evidence into practice. AcademyHealth (www.academyhealth.org), the professional organization representing health services researchers, created the Dissemination and Implementation Institute, with its sole purpose being helping researchers disseminate findings to policymakers. A private-sector initiative is illustrated with the Research-to-Policy Collaboration (RPC) that uses a cost-effective model combining strategic legislative needs assessments and a rapid-response researcher network to facilitate the translation of research into criminal justice prevention into practice by (a) engaging scientists with legislators, (b) connecting legislative offices with prevention researchers, and (c) eliciting requests from legislators for evidence to support prevention efforts (Crowley et al., 2018). This model has the potential to be replicated with other scientist groups. Advocacy organizations, often started and managed by patients and their families, frequently have scientific advisory boards and encourage members to become advisors to research studies through patient-powered registries and patient-powered research networks (Nowell et al., 2018; Workman, 2013). Although each of these initiatives has a different focus, they illustrate the value of evidence, dissemination to the public and policymakers, and efforts to move research evidence into practice and policy.

TERMINOLOGY

Another key piece in the puzzle to understanding the harnessing of evidence for policymaking is the variation in the use of terminology. Different terms, such as *research utilization* and *evidence-based practice* (EBP), have been used to explain the complex process of moving evidence to both practice and policy, with perhaps more attention given to practice. *Translational research* is a term initially designed for use in the medical world. The term emerged in response to concern over the long lag between scientific discoveries and changes in treatments, practices, and health policies that incorporate the new discoveries.

Titler (2018) defines translational research as "a dynamic continuum from basic research through the application of research findings in practice, communities, and public health settings to improve health and health outcomes." This continuum of translational research is also known as T0 (basic science), T1 (translation to humans, Phase I clinical trials), T2 (translation to patients, Phases 2 and 3 clinical trials), T3 (translation to practice, or effectiveness research), and T4 (translation to communities and populations; University of Wisconsin-Madison Institute for Clinical and Translational Research, n.d., www.ictr.wisc.edu/what-are-the-t0-to-t4-research-classifications/).

Further complicating the use of terminology is the confusion existing about the meaning of EBP, research, quality improvement (QI), and the interplay among them. Many practitioners misuse these three terms. Many nurses may have had little formal education in these processes. Nurses who have had such education may not have adequate opportunity to practice each of these separate but overlapping processes (Carter et al., 2017).

Evidence-Based Practice

The EBP approach is credited in medicine to Archie Cochrane in the early 1970s, so the term *evidence-based medicine* is often heard. The more generic term *EBP* is useful because it is not discipline-specific. EBP is "a problem-solving approach to the delivery of healthcare that integrates the best evidence from studies and patient care data with clinician expertise and patient preferences and values" (Melnyk et al., 2010, p. 51).

To ensure a practice based on evidence, healthcare providers are encouraged to use a framework or model to approach the search, critique, and translation of evidence for implementation into practice policy. Many nursing models of EBP are available for guiding practice. The Johns Hopkins Nursing Evidence-Based Practice (JHNEBP) model is defined as

> a powerful problem-solving approach to clinical decision-making, and is accompanied by user-friendly tools to guide individual or group use. It is designed specifically to meet the needs of the practicing nurse and uses a three-step process called PET: practice question, evidence, and translation. (Johns Hopkins Medicine, n.d., para. 1)

Three critical goals in using an EBP are the following: (a) to ensure that the highest quality of care is provided to achieve the best outcomes for patients, (b) to support rational decision-making (including structural changes) that reduce inappropriate variation in care, and (c) to create a culture of critical thinking and ongoing learning that grows a practice environment where the evidence supports clinical and administrative decisions (Newhouse et al., 2005). The highest quality is often assumed to be the biggest and latest finding but that might not necessarily be the case. Furthermore, it is just as essential to eliminate practices that are no longer valid as it is to institute new practices based on evidence.

An EBP inquiry is performed for many reasons, but most often, it is because nurses are questioning their practices and are concerned about practice outcomes. Some typical reasons why an EBP inquiry is performed include the following: improvement is needed for a high-risk, high-cost, and/or high-volume patient problem; adverse outcomes are being reported; variations in care are noticeable;

policy reviews are being completed; and/or healthcare team members are aware of new evidence or that their practice is different from the professional or community standard.

The EBP inquiry process, although designed for practice, can be used as an approach to policymaking at both the big-P and little-p levels. Some of the key steps in the EBP movement (searching, critiquing, appraising, synthesizing evidence) may be helpful to policymakers who are faced with how to find, evaluate, use, or discard scientific information in areas foreign to their background, such as healthcare. This problem is aptly called a "research glut and information famine" (Colby et al., 2008). Critical synthesis of evidence in relation to the scientific literature and making it relevant to policymakers are important steps in bridging the gap between the explosion of knowledge and the lack of information (Andermann et al., 2016). Nurses who are well acquainted with EBP could use its steps to provide policymakers with usable data to guide policy questions and subsequent policy development. Numerous professional associations provide their members with resources on EBP. See Policy on the Scene 5.1.

Research

Research is conducted to discover and generate new knowledge and evidence. The need to conduct research can result from an EBP inquiry when the search has found poor-quality evidence, conflicting evidence, or no evidence to support a

POLICY ON THE SCENE 5.1: A FRAMEWORK FOR EVIDENCE-BASED PRACTICE

Lisa Spruce, DNP, RN, CNS-CP, CNOR, ACNS, ACNP, FAAN
Director of Evidence-Based Perioperative Practice, Association of periOperative Registered Nurses, Denver, CO

Evidence-based practice is essential to promoting high-quality healthcare and safety because it provides a foundation for policies ensuring that decisions are made based on the evidence rather than on an individual provider's opinion. As one of the largest specialty nurses associations, the Association of periOperative Registered Nurses (AORN) has developed a model for the evaluation of research evidence that it uses to develop guidance for perioperative nurses, including its members. Smaller specialty nurses associations often may not have the capacity to evaluate practices germane to their clinical focus. The model set forth by AORN can be used by teams collaborating in the development of evidence-based practices and standards.

Clinical practice guidelines consist of recommendations developed from evidence and the evaluation of benefits and harms of various approaches to care. The AORN publishes national guidelines. These guidelines are based on a comprehensive, systematic review of research and nonresearch evidence; the individual references are appraised and scored, and the recommendations are rated according to the strength and quality of the evidence supporting the recommendation (AORN, 2021). Guidelines such as these provide a foundation for implementing evidence-based recommendations into state and national policy decisions.

AORN has created a framework for evidence-based practice that is used to appraise research studies and nonresearch projects and documents to develop a practice recommendation. These appraisal tools help evidence reviewers and authors who work on the AORN guidelines determine the type and the quality of study used and the strength of the findings. The AORN research appraisal tools can be used to appraise research evidence, including systematic reviews, randomized controlled trials (RCTs), quasi-experimental, nonexperimental, and qualitative studies. The AORN nonresearch appraisal tools can be used to appraise nonresearch evidence, which includes clinical practice guidelines, position or consensus statements, literature reviews, case reports, expert opinion articles, and quality improvement projects or organizational experiences (Spruce et al., 2016).

After the evidence is individually appraised, the collective evidence supporting each intervention within a specific recommendation is rated using the AORN Evidence Rating Model. Factors considered when applying this model to the collective body of evidence are the quality of research, the number of similar studies on a given topic, and the consistency of results supporting a recommendation. The recommendations in each guideline are given a strength rating that helps guideline readers or policymakers quickly understand the collective level of evidence used to support the practice recommendation.

Perioperative nurses and others can use these tools to evaluate research and nonresearch evidence from many disciplines. The tools should be used by nurses interested in learning more about evidence-based practice. Perioperative nurses and policymakers can be confident in the AORN evidence review process and in knowing that the evidence supporting the AORN Guidelines for Perioperative Practice is the highest quality available and that the guidelines provide reliable guidance to inform perioperative practice. The AORN appraisal tools and model are available at www.aorn.org.

practice or policy change. *Research* is a systematic investigation, including research development, testing, and evaluation, designed to develop new knowledge or contribute to generalizable knowledge (Office for Human Research Protections [OHRP], 2018).

Researchers must complete formal training to meet OHRP standards for the protection of human subjects and have their research protocols reviewed and approved by their organization's institutional review board (IRB). It is important that when embarking on a project that the team seeks clarification regarding whether the project is considered research, QI, or an evidence-based project and that the appropriate approvals are obtained. Oversight from these external bodies is designed to ensure that standards are met, individual rights are protected, and results are valid and can be used and disseminated.

The interplay between research and policy is an ongoing process. Researchers should seek to provide evidence for policy development. Research may also be used to examine existing policy effectiveness. Policy analysis is carried out to determine how well a policy has realized its intended outcomes, and whether it has resulted in any unintended outcomes (see Chapter 13). Policy analysis is often carried out by staff or commissioned by government agencies, organizations, or associations. Policy analysis is a systematic and formal approach that includes using specific criteria to examine and evaluate a policy problem. It involves developing policy alternatives or options, assessing the potential outcomes of each, and selecting a preferred alternative from among the proposed choices. The policy analysis process includes specific steps quite familiar to nurses: Define the problem, establish evaluation criteria, identify policy choices among alternative solutions, formulate the chosen policy, implement the policy solution, and evaluate the policy. Policy analysis tends to be issue-specific. An interprofessional approach, with nurses contributing to the process, is often effective.

Projects carried out that arise from everyday clinical questions often require the examination of evidence to determine the best direction for policy formulation. Nurses returning to school for advanced degrees can use their new skills in leading teams investigating these little-p issues. These little-p initiatives are often carried out based on the immediacy of a clinical problem.

At the big-P level, researchers can use their expertise and the results of their work to move policy forward. Collaborating with colleagues within and across disciplines can propel policy initiatives to a larger arena achieving a wider impact. An example of the big-P level of policy impact is illustrated in Policy on the Scene 5.2.

POLICY ON THE SCENE 5.2: MOVING YOUR RESEARCH INTO A POLICY FRAMEWORK: HEALTHCARE SERVICES FOR TRANSGENDER INDIVIDUALS

Carol Sedlak, PhD, RN, ONC, FAAN
Professor Emeritus, Kent State University, Kent, OH

Often an opportunity for research comes knocking at your door when least expected. This was an unplanned journey in a new area for this researcher who seized the opportunity to study transgender individuals, a marginalized population, which led to the development of a position statement for the American Academy of Nursing (AAN). As a nurse researcher, I was one of the first to explore osteoporosis prevention in women and men long before it became a public health concern, but a colleague discussed with me her research on transgender individuals' access to healthcare, a seemingly, unrelated topic. As we brainstormed and searched the literature, we realized our mutual individual research interest was transgender individuals' bone health and the effect of using cross-sex hormones. There were no nursing studies on this topic.

I immersed myself in the literature. I planned meetings with leaders in the transgender community and learned about the life of transgender individuals, their challenges, frustrations, and healthcare needs. These interactions informed my needs assessment, helped me gain the trust of key stakeholders, and establish myself as a credible and knowledgeable healthcare professional who wanted to help. I joined the research team of my colleague, Dr. Cyndi Roller, which was exploring how transgender individuals engage in healthcare. This was an invigorating opportunity leading to a publication on how transgender individuals navigate the healthcare system (Roller et al., 2015). Next, we developed a grant proposal addressing transgender individuals and osteoporosis prevention funded by the AAN and Sigma Theta Tau International. The research was a success ,and the results were published (Sedlak et al., 2017).

From my previous work as a researcher, I understood the relationship among research, policy development, change, and practice implementation. Acting on the responsibilities in the ANA Code of Ethics, I felt compelled to promote a greater awareness of the healthcare needs of transgender individuals and I joined the LGBTQ Health Expert Panel of the AAN's Panel. The purpose of the AAN Expert Panels is to promote knowledge development, collaboration, and shape health policy and practice for addressing the health needs of populations, including diverse populations. This can be in a variety of formats such as policy proposals, policy briefs, and position statements.

One of the AAN panel's goals focused on transgender individuals' healthcare. This was an opportunity to establish policy on the healthcare needs on healthcare services for transgender individuals, a marginalized population. A position statement was developed and approved by the AAN board, and published (Sedlak et al., 2016).

When opportunity knocks, don't be afraid to open the door. You may not know exactly where the research journey may take you, but you should always be considering where policy fits. Take a risk, and as you move forward, use your expertise and accomplishments to advance policy.

Quality Improvement

QI is a data-driven, formal approach to the analysis of performance and the systematic efforts to improve it (Devers, 2011). Analyzing performance requires techniques to better understand a problem, such as process mapping and measuring variation in a process or processes over time. Improving performance requires gathering existing evidence to support interventions, such as published studies or established guidelines; engaging the users in selecting interventions; trialing these interventions in iterative steps, sometimes called small tests of change; measuring the change longitudinally; and sustaining the effective interventions. Because QI is inherently focused on improvement by applying research and other evidence, patient care is expected to benefit. Context is very important in QI work and requires understanding the local setting and organizational culture. The QI work intends to describe and share lessons learned rather than creating new, generalizable knowledge.

One final comment should be made here concerning IRB oversight of QI. Because QI involves using existing effective interventions and its sole purpose is to improve clinical care, it should not require IRB review; however, IRBs at different facilities may view protocols and the application of regulations differently. Therefore, it is best to address issues of human subjects' protection early in the planning process, well in advance of any data collection procedures. This is particularly important when collaborating across several institutions. Clinicians undertaking QI projects should be familiar with OHRP standards and their own organization's policies.

Improvement and Implementation Science

Improvement science is an emerging field of study focused on the methods, theories, and approaches that facilitate or hinder efforts to improve quality and the scientific study of these approaches (Health Foundation, 2011). The science of improvement includes system thinking, understanding variation, the psychology of change, and the theory of knowledge that is applied to improve the performance of processes, organizations, and communities (Deming, 2000). The application of this science requires the integration of a set of improvement methods and tools with expert subject knowledge to develop, test, implement, and spread changes.

Implementation science, which can be thought of as a component of improvement science, is the "scientific study of methods to promote the systematic uptake of research findings and other evidence based practices into routine practice, and hence, to improve the quality and effectiveness of health services" (Eccles & Mittman, 2006, "Abstract"). A major difference between improvement/implementation science and clinical research is the active engagement with the context within which the intervention is implemented rather than controlling or tolerating it, as with clinical investigations (Bauer & Kirchner, 2020).

EVERY NURSE'S ROLE IN TRANSLATING EVIDENCE INTO POLICY

Translating evidence into policy (and practice) involves communicating new evidence to decision policymakers in an understandable and useful way. Once again, differing terms are often encountered in describing the process of translation. The term *knowledge transfer* is defined as a systematic approach for capturing, collecting, and sharing tacit knowledge for it to become explicit knowledge so that individuals and/or organizations can access and utilize essential information, which previously was known intrinsically to only one person or a small group of people (Graham et al., 2006). Another term, *diffusion*, refers to a broad process whereby knowledge or evidence is communicated throughout an organization or a larger system. Finally, the term *dissemination*, which is used frequently in the translation literature, refers to communicating knowledge or evidence in journals, at conferences, or through some other medium. The discussion of the nurses' role in translation refers to multiple avenues of communication.

The translation of evidence into healthcare practice and policy faces multiple challenges. Those challenges are found throughout the healthcare system, with individual providers or teams of providers at the organizational level and both public and private organizations at the local, state, and national levels, such as professional organizations and governmental agencies. See Exhibit 5.2 for a summary of key steps to enhance the use of evidence for policy.

It is important for all healthcare professionals to use evidence to make informed decisions about practice and policy, and yet we know this does not happen consistently (Guerden et al., 2014; Lockwood et al., 2014; Yost et al., 2014). In many organizations (e.g., health departments, clinics, hospitals, educational programs), internal data and benchmarks are used only when data may be available at a regional, state, or national level. Using internal data may, however, result in false reassurance about the effectiveness of a program. Internal data from a project, although useful, may not necessarily be subject to the rigor of external peer review.

EXHIBIT 5.2 KEY STEPS TO ENHANCING THE USE OF EVIDENCE IN THE FORMULATION AND IMPLEMENTATION OF POLICIES

1. Familiarize yourself with the evidence related to practice issues.
2. Understand the difference between research, EBP, and quality improvement.
3. Build relationships with policymakers at all levels (organizational, local, state, and national).
4. Raise questions about the evidence used in policies.
5. Lead the development of a research, EBP, or quality improvement project.
6. Develop an action plan for the dissemination of evidence.
7. Disseminate evidence in a variety of outlets pertinent to the policy issue.
8. Use implementation science principles to carry out policy changes.

Translating evidence to practice and policy requires that attention be directed toward decreasing barriers to evidence adoption and enhancing factors that facilitate adoption. For instance, consideration must focus on communicating evidence in a timely and relevant manner, responding to the healthcare profession's or organization's needs, and presenting findings in a user-friendly manner easily understandable to decision-makers.

Good examples of translating evidence into policy do exist. Seat-belt laws that have been proved to save lives have been enacted in 49 states, the District of Columbia, and many U.S. territories; New Hampshire is the only state without such legislation (Brewer, 2020). Convincing evidence exists for wearing motorcycle and bicycle helmets to decrease injuries from accidents. Legislation for motorcycle helmets has been passed in 49 states but not always with the same requirements. Only 21 states require helmets for all riders, and the other 28 require helmets only for certain riders. Bicycle-helmet legislation has been passed only in 21 states; however, many localities have passed bicycle-helmet legislation for their communities. Tobacco-control legislation is similar in that legislation continues to be passed in many U.S. jurisdictions. However, the legislation's uptake or passage takes different formats due to local social, cultural, and economic factors. Nurses have made substantial contributions to the research evidence in many of these areas. The translation of injury-prevention guidelines for healthcare workers in the United States has also shown considerable uptake, most notably in organizations with better resources.

Professional associations have also participated in translating evidence to policy through the promulgation of position statements and clinical practice guidelines (CPGs). Professional associations bring together panels of experts to review, appraise, and synthesize evidence about a professional issue or disease or symptom management to make current practice recommendations to their membership and the healthcare community at large. These recommendations may be published in journals or posted on websites and have been adopted at all levels of policymaking (organizational, state, national). Safe patient handling and mobility is an example of how organizations are promoting policies based on evidence (see Chapter 2). The identification of this problem started with professional associations and moved through other policy development levels at the organizational, state, and national levels, involving both the private sector (e.g., businesses, nongovernmental organizations [NGOs]) and government agencies.

Federal Level

A widely cited example of the translation of nursing research to policy can be found in the inclusion of transitional care in the ACA. Strong evidence indicates that hospital readmissions can be significantly reduced, and the quality of care for patients can be improved by implementing a program that targets care transitions. Developed over a period of three decades by nurse scientist Mary Naylor and her team, the transitional care model (TCM), a translation of an evidence-based strategy into a practice-delivery model, uses advanced practice registered nurses (APRNs) with specialized training to care for older adults with multiple chronic conditions and support their family caregivers (Naylor et al., 2013). Testing the model has demonstrated significant and sustained outcomes, including avoiding hospital readmissions and ED visits for primary and coexisting conditions, improving health outcomes after discharge, enhancing patient and family caregiver satisfaction, and reducing total healthcare costs (Hirschman et al., 2015; Naylor et al., 2013).

Transitional care management includes discharge from acute care and long-term care hospitals, skilled nursing/nursing facilities, inpatient rehabilitation, and hospital observation status/partial hospitalization. It is covered through Medicare and insurance companies, as provided by the ACA (Centers for Medicare & Medicaid Services [CMS], n.d.; Maryniak, 2019; Nelson & Pulley, 2015). Policy established to support TCM includes two transitional care billing codes that can be used once in the 30 days after discharge. Specifically, Aetna has adopted the TCM to achieve better outcomes for its older adult enrollees with multiple chronic health problems. The AARP has recommended expansion of TCM services to its members. The National Quality Forum endorsed the deployment of evidence-based transitional care such as the TCM as one of 25 national preferred practices for care coordination.

The TCM is being replicated to determine the difference it makes on care outcomes in nine hospitals and five states (Penn Nursing (n.d.) www.nursing.upenn.edu/ncth/mirror-tcm/). The institutions involved are the Veterans Health Administration, Swedish Health Services, Trinity Health-Michigan, and the University of California San Francisco. Funded by Arnold Ventures and the Missouri Foundation for Health, successful replication of TCM "would provide convincing evidence that TCM could be used in hospitals nationwide to improve patient health and generate major healthcare savings" (University of Pennsylvania, 2020. Almanac. www.nursing.upenn.edu/live/news/1596-arnold-ventures-awards-6-million-grant-to-study).

In addition to trialing the effectiveness of models such as TCM's in new environments, it is also important to assess the impact of various reimbursement approaches and incentives for adoption. Monte Carlo methods for simulations that incorporated data from TCM studies and the CMS indicate that current reimbursement models provide little incentive for using the TCM; payer coverage of TCM costs and the economic attractiveness of adopting TCM would depend on the patient population receiving TCM services, readmission penalties, provider characteristics, and payment models (Rouse et al., 2019). The development of TCM, subsequent policy decisions, and data illustrating the need for fine-tuning policy decisions illustrate the ongoing nature of policy work.

State Level

States are pursuing various strategies for getting the research and analytical assistance they need (Pew Charitable Trusts, 2017), including the expansion of relationships with university-based health services research and policy analysis programs. A well-known and published translation of evidence to practice and policy at the state level was the establishment of nurse-staffing ratios in the state of California. After many unsuccessful attempts, Assembly Bill 394 was enacted in 1999 and implemented in 2004. This Bill was motivated by intense lobbying by nursing unions, media reports of poor patient outcomes related to insufficient RN numbers and by a small amount of research at the time that showed improvements in patient mortality, quality of care, and patient safety when RN staffing was adequate (Aiken et al., 1994, 2002).

As of July 2019, 14 states addressed nurse staffing in hospitals in law regulations—California, Connecticut, Illinois, Massachusetts, Minnesota, Nevada, New Jersey, New York, Ohio, Oregon, Rhode Island, Texas, Vermont, and Washington (deCordova et al., 2019)—but California remains the only state that legally stipulates required minimum nurse to patient ratios all times by unit type. Massachusetts has a law specific to ICU nurse-staffing ratios. The California staffing legislation has been the subject of many studies assessing its effectiveness. Following the state policy change, nurse staffing naturally improved, but it improved more so in safety net hospitals (McHugh et al., 2012); the RN skill mix did not decrease (McHugh et al., 2011); hospitals experienced more financial pressures (Mark et al., 2013), yet there is inconclusive evidence of improvements in patient care quality and safety (Spetz et al., 2013). Several states require some form of public reporting of staffing ratios. In New Jersey, a trend analysis revealed improved patient safety attributed to this disclosure (de Cordova et al., 2019).

The nation is facing an opioid epidemic, with overdose rates continuing to rise dramatically. One statewide intervention program, a collaborative of the North Carolina Medicaid authority, Community Care of North Carolina, and the Mountain Area Health Education Center began in 2013 by asking North Carolina counties to identify opioid-overdose reduction strategies relevant for their communities (Alexandridis et al., 2017). These strategies included community education, provider education, ED policies requiring additional checks before prescribing opioids, diversion control, support programs for pain, policies for naloxone distribution, and addiction treatment. Implementing this model in a pilot study in one county resulted in a 69% reduction in opioid overdoses. By 2014, 74 of 100 counties had implemented some intervention strategies, resulting in reduced overdose mortality rates (Alexandridis et al., 2017). As of January 2021, this initiative, Project Lazarus, had spread to 31 other states (Project Lazarus, 2021).

Local Level

On a local level and a public–private collaborative the city of Baltimore has an initiative called B'more for Healthy Babies (BHB, n.d.). The BHB is designed to improve the quality of care provided by physicians, nurses, social workers, and others who work with pregnant and postpartum women. This policy helps all home visiting programs in Baltimore to transition to evidence-based models of care. The BHB initiative is sponsored by the Office of the Mayor of Baltimore, the Baltimore City Health Department, and the Family League of Baltimore City, Inc., and HealthCare Access Maryland with catalytic funding from CareFirst BlueCross BlueShield and other donors. One major aspect of the program is an evidence-based strategy called "the BHB sleep initiative: Alone. Back. Crib. Don't Smoke" (www.healthybabiesbaltimore.com). The BHB sleep initiative has distributed culturally sensitive video materials to more than 120 sites to educate families on proper evidence to prevent crib deaths. Posters are used to target the message to different audiences to provide evidence for the initiative to the public (see Figure 5.1 for one message).

Although a direct correlation between the initiation of BHB and the drop in the infant mortality rate (IMR) cannot be made, the Baltimore IMR has dropped 32%, and sleep-related infant deaths in Baltimore City have decreased by more than 50% since the implementation of the BHB sleep initiative in 2009. However, in 2015, an African American infant was almost two times more likely to die than a White infant, indicating that additional work needs to be done in this community (see Chapter 14).

The BHB initiative has continued to expand its reach. The program also works to improve low-birth-weight delivery rates and maternal and infant outcomes (Harvey et al., 2016). Also, work that originated with the BHB program has expanded into the B'more Fit Coalition. This local partner works to shape policies related to nutrition, fitness, and wellness in the Baltimore area (Truiett-Theodorson et al., 2015).

Organizational Level

There are many examples of translation of evidence into practice and policy at the organizational level. These are often different types of translations because

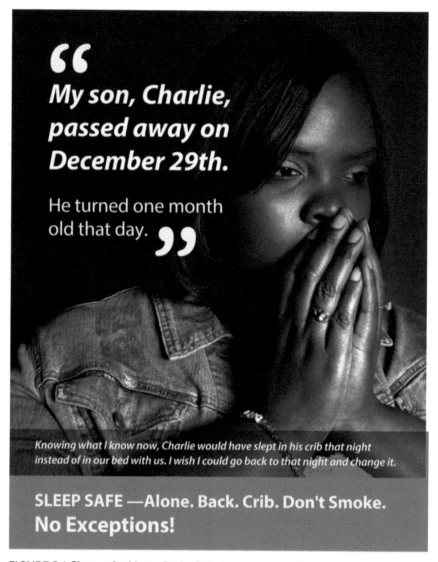

FIGURE 5.1 Sleep safe. Alone. Back. Crib. Don't smoke. No exceptions.

Source: Reprinted with permission from Baltimore City Health Department.

of the origins of their evidence. Clear evidence exists on the steps to take to minimize the chances of inpatients contracting a urinary tract infection (UTI) as well as the use of antibiotics to treat UTIs (Centers for Disease Control and Prevention [CDC], 2015). However, translating that evidence in organizations has offered specific challenges and great opportunities.

In Fairbanks, Alaska, the Denali Center is a 90-bed nonprofit nursing home (Health Compare, n.d.). In evaluating the organization's UTI metrics, nurses noted that the National Healthcare Safety Network criteria for symptomatic UTI (SUTI) were not met in 52% of 2018 cases, and antibiotics were ordered and given to 76% of these residents. Additionally, nursing acknowledged ownership for 60% of UTIs and identified that the problem stemmed from deficiencies in policies, including disparate documentation practices, confusion about the urinary catheter removal policy, and gaps in staff knowledge of this policy.

Denali Center nurses partnered with the American Association of Critical-Care Nurses' Clinical Scene Academy (American Association of Critical Care Nursing, n.d.-a). The goals were to improve Denali Center's UTI prevention and treatment policy, reduce SUTIs by 20%, increase compliance with a new organization policy to 80%, and decrease antibiotic use for asymptomatic UTIs by 44%. Significant policy changes include implementing and using three EBPs—a UTI Huddle form, staff education, and an order algorithm set. In 1 year, the Denali Center decreased its UTI rate from 0.75 in 2018 to 0.38 in 2019, a 49.3% reduction. The organization-level financial impact associated with the policy change is estimated at $124,137 per year (American Association of Critical Care Nursing, n.d.-b).

Another opportunity for translation at the organizational level is to ensure that policies and procedures are based on the best available evidence. This opportunity to question current evidence or seek new evidence arises when there is a need to develop a new policy or procedure or review current policies and procedures. Not all policies need to be reviewed with an extensive evidence-based protocol; it is necessary to consider other influencing factors, such as other initiatives that may occur, along with assessing the priority of the policy needing to be changed. This assessment may come from several sources (e.g., a policy analysis, quality data, new knowledge, staffing issues in implementing a policy).

Knowing how to find evidence and transform the evidence into policy are vital skills. Nurses with advanced education need to have these skills to guide and mentor others in finding evidence resources. For example, policy analyses performed by nursing PhD students Brooke Cherven and Courtney Sullivan provide much of the high-quality evidence used in the recent Association of Pediatric Hematology/Oncology Nurses' position paper on human papillomavirus immunization (Eshelman-Kent et al., 2018), and the World Health Organization Global Initiative for Childhood Cancer (Pergert et al., 2020).

Finding evidence can be a daunting experience regardless of one's background. Although numerous resources are available, all policy issues do not have adequate data for informing policy, and access to resources may be limited. When working in a clinical agency with electronic health records, access to the evidence used for the software's clinical decision-making tools may be available. A nursing program's library resources may vary from those where you are employed. Listing these resources is beyond this book's scope, but a good overview of resources can be found on many academic and hospital library home pages. A health sciences librarian at either a nursing program or a hospital can be an invaluable team member when searching for evidence. It is increasingly common for a librarian to be a team member for conducting systematic reviews. Resources and guidance in using them are often made available to the public by university libraries as illustrated in an example from the University of Rochester (see Tools for Nursing Research–Finding the Evidence at www.urmc.rochester.edu/libraries/williams/electronic_resources/NursingResearchEBP.cfm). However, there are numerous examples when healthcare practices are questioned in organizations, and the quality, quantity, and consistency of evidence are not available to make a practice change. In these cases, and many others, it is necessary for the organization to generate its own evidence to support practice decisions in the form of QI or research. Policy on the Scene 5.3 illustrates interprofessional collaboration and how answering one policy question may lead to another.

POLICY ON THE SCENE 5.3: NO VETERAN LEFT BEHIND: THE MISSION CONTINUES

Humanitarian organizations are another mechanism by which nurses can make their voices heard to influence policy based on evidence. In fact, these organizations may be able to assist in producing evidence for policy change. A recent example of this is the report produced by the Vietnam Veterans of America® (VVA, 2020) on the COVID-19-related deaths in state veteran homes, which are operated by the state and not the Veterans Health Administration. A small group of concerned nurses noted these high numbers of deaths and brought this issue to the VVA leaders (L. Schwartz, personal communication, August 13, 2020). The VVA's National Health Care Committee, led by the Honorable Linda S. Schwartz, PhD, RN, sought to produce the evidence needed to inform policy. Finding no repository of national data on COVID-19 deaths in the state veterans homes, they turned to the 50 state council presidents, and with the help of state Departments of Health or Veterans Affairs, the CMS, discovered 1,011 COVID-19 deaths in 47 of the known 162 homes over a 3-month period (VVA, 2020). This was followed by a Government Accountability Office report and testimony before Congress (VA Health Care, 2020). As a result, Congress has authorized $250 million for COVID-19 projects in state veterans homes, and the Veterans Health Administration is now required to report numbers of deaths in these state veteran homes (L. Schwartz, personal communication, August 13, 2020).

STRATEGIES FOR DISSEMINATION OF EVIDENCE

Carrying out evidence-based projects or QI is not complete if the work is not disseminated and the policy implications explicated. However, dissemination is often not given consideration, especially at the level of the little-p, until someone external to the project hears about it and encourages dissemination. Dissemination should be part of early planning for projects. Seasoned researchers know the value of developing dissemination plans from the earliest planning of a project and being cognizant of dissemination opportunities that may develop as a project develops. To effectively harness evidence for policy, there must be some method of dissemination.

Over time, researchers and others generating evidence to support policy have identified key determinants and strategies that can guide the translation of evidence to policymakers (Grimshaw et al., 2012; National Health and Medical Research Council, 2019). Four major elements that are basic to messaging in general and to researchers conveying messages about the evidence they have harnessed are knowing and selecting an audience, selecting dissemination techniques, understanding that context matters, and providing timely, relevant communication that is understandable, and practical. Although listed as separate elements, there is overlap. The type of audience you select influences what method you use to communicate your evidence. The immediacy of the evidence to a problem at hand is likely to influence how quickly and widespread you will want to convey your work.

Know Your Audience

Choosing dissemination strategies involves identifying and knowing the audience who needs to be involved in the translation. Identifying those with something to gain and something to lose is critical to the planning (Weston et al., 2013; also see Chapters 7 and 10).

At a minimum, evidence from projects needs to be shared across an organization, and broader audiences should be routinely sought out. As you strategically plan for dissemination, consider who within your organization should be informed about the project: patients, professional colleagues, staff, managers, and/or administration. Outside the organization, consider if your audience is local, national, and/or international; you also need to consider whom you should target. It may be that your results have bearing across a number of audiences, including lay audiences.

Often, you choose to disseminate your evidence to predetermined stakeholders who are decision-makers or influence the issue. Clinicians, administrators, researchers, and lay audiences may all be essential stakeholders. In policy analysis and, later, during the translation of evidence to policy, it is important to perform a stakeholder analysis. Stakeholder analysis identifies those who may positively or negatively influence your project's success, allows you to anticipate their influence, and provides you the opportunity to get the most effective support for the project and address barriers to implementation early in the translation process. There are key steps in any stakeholder analysis (see Chapter 6).

Early research is needed for understanding audiences and targeting interventions focused on the appropriateness and efficacy of specific interventions. It showed that there was a considerable lack of knowledge about which strategies work best for different audiences. Research on the translation of research into practice initiatives funded by the AHRQ indicates that the most commonly used intervention to translate evidence to the relevant audience was educational (Farquhar et al., 2002). However, educational materials (e.g., distribution of recommendations for clinical care, CPGs, audiovisual materials, electronic publications) and didactic educational meetings (e.g., lectures) have been shown to be the least effective ways to reach an audience (Bero et al., 1998).

Select Dissemination Techniques

Once you have determined who your audience is, it is important to consider what methods or communication methods will be used to disseminate your evidence. The audience and purpose are vital to knowing how you disseminate your evidence. There are numerous types of dissemination that should be considered, and several of these (e.g., press releases, white papers) are discussed in Chapter 10. Often, dissemination is not a singular act. If, for example, you have an article selected for a major publication or a premier research conference, you may want to consider submitting a press release to the local newsletter of an association or for work, as well as submitting the release to the local paper or even writing a letter to the congressional representative.

Researchers may only think of journal articles and peer-reviewed presentations for purposes of policy dissemination. However, these venues do not often reach policymakers, and the policy implications of the research are not often called for or discussed in articles. Thus, when choosing dissemination venues, consider which ones allow space and content to meaningfully discuss policy implications. Prioritize using venues that routinely consider policy implications of the research. Finally, consider whether the professional dissemination you have planned (e.g., poster, article) lends itself to its own publicity. Consider working with your marketing department to highlight work that has received acclaim by being accepted or by being published in a major venue.

To help in consideration of avenues for disseminating one's work, consider whether the evidence lends itself to the written or oral format or both. Often, a combination of dissemination modalities may be considered, and it is helpful to convey your findings. Besides formal posters at professional organizations, consider displaying a poster exhibited at a conference in a public spot at work so that colleagues and administrators, lay audiences, or students may be exposed to it. In addition, it is crucial to consider the use of social media platforms to disseminate work. Examples such as blogs, Twitter, Facebook, and other social networking programs may often reach a broader audience and augment traditional forms of publication. Exhibit 5.3 lists some examples of venues to consider for presenting evidence.

EXHIBIT 5.3 DISSEMINATION BEYOND ARTICLES

- Classroom presentations
- Fact sheets
- Newsletters and newspaper articles
- Pamphlets
- Posters
- Podcasts
- Professional and workplace presentations
- Public meetings (e.g., school board meetings, support groups)
- Reports (technical or research)
- Social media sites
- Town halls
- Webinar
- Webpages
- Workshops

Although we often think of dissemination as an external process, it is a strategy that can and should be used more widely within work settings. Too often, within a work setting, individuals are not aware of what others are working on, so efforts get duplicated and lost. Projects carried out on one unit have the potential to be incorporated across several others. The exposure to nurses and managers across units can help spread policy uptake. Effective strategies designed for disseminating and communicating evidence-based information to policy stakeholders are illustrated in Exhibit 5.4.

EXHIBIT 5.4 STRATEGIES FOR DISSEMINATION TO POLICYMAKERS

Strategy 1: Start dissemination plan at the beginning of the project.
Strategy 2: Consider the policy's stakeholders.
Strategy 3: Select essential messages tailored to audiences.
Strategy 4: Examine venues for dissemination.
Strategy 5: Develop materials applicable to the target audience.
Strategy 6: Analyze ways to ensure maximum accessibility.
Strategy 7: Implement the dissemination plan.
Strategy 8: Evaluate the plan's effectiveness.
Strategy 9: Treat dissemination as an ongoing responsibility.

Adapted from National Health and Medical Research Council. (2019, September 6). *Guidelines for guidelines: Dissemination and communication.* https://www.nhmrc.gov.au/guidelinesforguidelines/implement/dissemination-and-communication.

It is critical to recognize and understand the social, political, economic, historical, ethical, and legal contexts and other forces in the environment, both facilitating and constraining, that are present in any effort to integrate evidence into policy and practice. How do we increase the use of evidence for policymaking among healthcare professionals and nurses specifically? There are several strategies. First is attempting to understand how nurses and other health professionals receive, critique, and adopt evidence for practice and policy change. Busy professionals must have the evidence in easily digestible bits at their fingertips. Improvement and implementation science methods and techniques can help with this.

Second, identifying which organizational factors play a role in, and which detract from, facilitating translating evidence and innovations into practice and policy is important in the translation process. Facilitators include an organizational structure with open communication, strong involvement by senior leadership, effective clinical leadership and interprofessional team practice, organizational culture supportive of learning and inquiry, and resources, expertise, and infrastructure to support evidence acquisition, appraisal, change implementation, and management. Barriers that can hinder the uptake of evidence into practice or policy include not enough time, people, and other resources for implementation, poor access to research, and a lack of convincing evidence. Bach-Mortensen et al. (2018) recommend increasing internal research expertise, open access to journals, advisory groups, and expanding relations with researchers as system-level facilitators for implementing evidence-based policy and interventions.

Context also matters at the big-P level. Policymakers want to know about research findings and other evidence as well, that have policy implications for their constituents. The Policy on the Scene 5.2 provides an excellent example of context—the interaction of the COVID-19 pandemic, an active veterans group, news media, and rapid accumulation of evidence. When providing information about the evidence supporting a policy change, the communication should be in plain language and include the estimated number of constituents affected by the change.

Communicating Research So It Counts

Communicating research to other researchers is useful for knowledge development. However, it does not advance the healthcare field unless it is put to use by policymakers, practitioners, and other end users. In fact, research is just an interesting academic exercise unless its results are used for the betterment of society. It is incumbent on researchers to translate their findings in brief, concise "sound bites" of information that the lay public can understand and use.

Drawing from the policy and psychology fields, Cairney and Oliver (2017) have developed several recommendations to communicate research to policymakers. First, evidence needs to be communicated clearly and concisely, and tailored to your audience. Decision-makers are often besieged with information and have very little time to stay abreast of changes in current research or emerging evidence that could be of great use. Second, timing is important, and researchers should plan for windows of opportunity to deliver their message. Third, researchers need to become familiar with and engage with the real world of policymaking to better understand the political processes that will affect their influences. Networking and building alliances will go a long way to getting a message across.

Policymakers are busy human beings who often must make decisions rapidly, often with little or incomplete information. They do not have the cognitive reserve to comb through research papers or even systematic reviews to learn about research findings. They are interested in short, easily skimmed, and policy-focused information that presents the evidence rather than all the research methods. A one- or two-page documents, using the bottom-line-up-front principal, can be most effective.

A common dissemination tool specific to policy is a policy brief: a succinct presentation of an issue with policy options (usually including new evidence) geared to a specific audience. It is usually written for decision-makers and is often referred to as a two-pager. The policy brief attempts to make the issue understandable by presenting information on the problem, delineating policy options, and recommending the best option. The details of a policy brief and an example can be found in Chapter 10. For some decision-makers, a policy brief on the topic may be the first and only thing they read on the subject; for others, it may be the first effective compilation of evidence in a single accessible format, and for others, it may be entirely redundant. Benton et al. (2020) provide a template for, and an example of, a policy brief for the Nursing Now campaign.

Stories can be another means of effectively delivering a message. Patient safety initiatives have benefitted from emotionally laden stories of individuals who have been harmed by medical error. Podcasts, or short videos, may also be powerful ways of getting a message across.

Data supporting the importance of adopting new evidence into practice and policy can help propel decision-makers to act (Bradley et al., 2004). Data points or "killer numbers" would be selected for use in the messaging as appropriate. Today's dynamic environment requires that effectiveness data be included whenever possible. As many have experienced, if new evidence is going to be adopted, something else might have to be given up, such as an old way of doing things. Making the "business case" for the translation of evidence to practice and policy, such as any financial or administrative data to accompany the clinical evidence, might motivate an otherwise complacent decision-maker.

To convey the message, it is critical to have a well-thought-out and comprehensive communication plan that allows you to "tell your story." What communication media will be used? Will there be different messages for different media presentations? To increase the translation's success, you should know what is newsworthy in the environment (e.g., organizational, local, state, national; see Chapter 10).

The plan should design messages that fit the audience or different audiences. For example, a presentation to a large audience might include a PowerPoint presentation or a video. Equally important is the 30-second sound bite or elevator speech that is designed to be given in the 30 seconds that you have as you run into an essential stakeholder in the hallway or at a meeting.

When considering the message's development, a challenge arises to identify the key messages for different audiences and present them in the appropriate understandable format. Unfortunately, journal articles and research reports are written for researchers, not decision-makers. However, several formats are used to communicate evidence depending on the needs of the audience. As the message is crafted, it is important to inform, not inundate.

Too often, the dissemination of evidence into practice and policy is hampered by an inadequate presentation of the new information. The goal of translating evidence into practice and policy requires first that the new evidence be synthesized into usable information in a readable format for decision-makers. Several understandable and reader-friendly formats are used to communicate new research evidence to decision-makers, healthcare practitioners, and the public.

Evidence must be timely. The researcher should identify a window of opportunity for message delivery. Frequently, when evidence is needed, it is not readily accessible or available to those who need it. If the information is available, the evidence message is often not described in a way that resonates with those targeted to receive the message. Cairney and Oliver (2017) caution against delivering new information during periods of heightened emotion, such as an important political event when clear thinking or switching to new information may be difficult.

Fostering relationships with policymakers is important for obtaining their support. Individuals are more likely to hear a message and respond when delivered

POLICY SOLUTION	From the ICU to the State Capitol: Policy Change Starting at the Bedside

The Take It to the Street campaign employed multiple strategies to roll out its message from a health system to the larger community and across the state. The Just for Kids Critical Care Unit staff created statewide public awareness on nonaccidental pediatric head trauma. Pamphlets on proper ways to handle a crying baby were delivered to primary care offices. Presentations on the scope of nonaccidental trauma were made across the state. In addition, the staff used evidence to support their policy efforts. In a retrospective study using their unit-level data, the team identified bruising patterns in nonaccidental trauma patients that were indicative of risk for future child abuse (Pierce et al., 2010). This evidence was used to improve daily practice, resulting in the creation of bruising screening tools with automatic referrals to Social Services and the Pediatric Forensics Department for positive findings.

In 2010, Kentucky legislators introduced House Bill 285, which required mandatory education for pediatric abusive head trauma. The staff at Norton Children's Hospital were instrumental in getting the bill passed, making weekly trips to meet with legislators to share their patient stories and the evidence supporting the policy change.

What started as a few passionate individuals in the Just for Kids Critical Care Unit resulted in a major policy change across Kentucky. The hospital has seen an increase in child abuse referrals and a decrease in morbidity and mortality. The state has dramatically decreased its number one ranking in the United States for deaths of children from nonaccidental trauma. These individuals did an exceptional job of harnessing evidence in the policy process while ultimately saving lives.

by a known entity they trust. Towfighi et al. (2020) discuss building relationships between academia and the public using CTSA awardees' examples. They provide several examples of closing the gaps between research, public policy, and practice.

IMPLICATIONS FOR THE FUTURE

While harnessing evidence is not without controversy, it is expected that evidence use for all levels of policymaking will continue to be emphasized. As we move to the near future, when more nurses are prepared with the skills to advance research and better understand the processes of quality and EBP, as well as the potential interplay among all three, nurses can produce better-quality evidence to impact policy. Involving all nurses, as well as healthcare teams, in monitoring evidence related to policy is essential. It is not sufficient for us to defer QI to the "quality nurses," EBP to nurses who are members of an EBP internship or academy, or research to academics in nursing or to projects done while in school that are never applied to a real practice setting. A challenge that remains is integrating and using the evidence from these three processes more effectively and efficiently. Harnessing evidence is also important at the big-P level; therefore, nurses carrying out disciplinary or interprofessional research must consider the policy implications of research that they undertake as they design their work. We must be thoughtful and explicit when translating research for policy not only in how but also to whom we present the evidence.

In the future, more attention will be given to the difficult job of eliminating long-standing policies based on outdated information that could potentially harm patients. Many policies are based on evidence that may not be synthesized, evidence that is ignored because of cultural beliefs, outdated evidence carried over from outdated education, or the competition's adoption of a policy.

Furthermore, we need to be poised with the range of policy skills to use evidence; research evidence alone will not change policy. Communicating and disseminating evidence more quickly and more efficiently are critical to moving good practice from isolated practices and organizations to systems and regions and beyond. The lag time from evidence to viable policy must be decreased.

KEY CONCEPTS

1. Harnessing evidence involves locating evidence from various sources and using it at the right times and places in the policymaking process.
2. Institutionalization of research does not create a clear path to policymaking, as illustrated by the disconnect between research evidence and policies found in clinical settings.
3. Efforts have been instituted globally to ensure that decision-making in policy is informed by evidence.
4. Cultural differences between researchers and policymakers create challenges in translating evidence into practice.
5. The responsibility for ensuring the transfer of new research into policy and practice tends to be viewed as a unidirectional flow from researchers to policymakers.
6. Communication between researchers and policymakers has a vital role in translating research into policy.
7. Differences in understanding and use of research, EBP, QI, and translation research illustrate the complexity of harnessing evidence for practice and policy.
8. Translating research into policy involves communicating information about research in a useful and understandable manner.
9. Challenges in translating evidence into policy include decreasing barriers and enhancing facilitators of evidence adoption.
10. Translation of evidence into policy has been successful at the federal, state, local, and organizational levels.
11. Opportunities within organizations for translating evidence into policy include ensuring that current practices and policies are based on the best available evidence.
12. Carrying out research, EBP, or QI requires a comprehensive dissemination plan to harness evidence for policy.
13. Nurses need to be prepared in a wide range of skills to use data that have policy implications.

SUMMARY

The term *evidence-based policy* is used in the literature, yet generally relates to one type of evidence—that of scientific research. The literature and some organizations, including the WHO, use the term *evidence-informed policy* to reflect the need to consider different types of evidence and use the best available evidence when dealing with everyday problems and issues in the healthcare environment. Research and nonresearch evidence both play an important role in the translation of evidence to practice and policy. This chapter has presented the importance of context as critical to translation. When new evidence is generated or discovered, it is essential that not only the new evidence is evaluated on the quality and strength of that evidence but also that an organization must consider the "fit and feasibility" of the uptake and adoption of that evidence in that environment (organizational, professional, local, state, national). The fit and feasibility test considers things in the environmental context such as values, beliefs, norms, history, resources, infrastructure, legislation and regulation, politics, and the competency, skills, and knowledge of those involved. Translating evidence is not a linear process, and attention needs to be given to actively coordinating the dissemination to ensure that the evidence is implemented according to the plan.

END-OF-CHAPTER RESOURCES

LEARNING ACTIVITIES

1. Ask nurses employed in clinical positions in various settings about their knowledge and use of clinical guidelines available from specialty organizations and government agencies, such as the AHRQ or the CDC.

2. Locate resources for EBP at your place of employment and compare them to the resources for EBP at an academic institution.

3. Visit your specialty organization and review their process for standards/guideline creation and the level of evidence used in the process.

4. Visit your federal and state legislators' websites and identify one bill that they support or do not support that has healthcare implications. Write a letter to a legislator citing evidence for support or a lack of support of this piece of legislation.

5. Identify a policy in your organization (work or school) related to health or nursing education that should be changed. Discuss the level of evidence that is available to support the change.

6. Locate three research articles on a topic of interest to you and your organization. Evaluate the degree to which policy implications are discussed in each article. For each, briefly summarize policy implications that need further explication.

7. Discuss two or three policies that need changed in a healthcare organization. Describe the approach or combination of approaches (research, EBP, or QI) to change one of the identified policies.

E-RESOURCES

- AARP Public Policy Institute http://www.aarp.org/research/ppi
- AcademyHealth http://www.academyhealth.org
- Agency for Healthcare Research and Quality http://www.ahrq.gov
- Center for Economic and Policy Research (CEPR) http://www.cepr.net
- Cochrane Collaboration http://www.cochrane.org
- Commonwealth Fund http://www.commonwealthfund.org
- Dartmouth Institute for Health Policy & Clinical Practice https://tdi.dartmouth.edu
- Evidence-Informed Policy Network (EVIPNet) http://www.who.int/evidence/about/en
- Health Research and Policy Systems http://www.health-policy-systems.com
- Institute for Women's Policy Research http://www.iwpr.org
- JBI (formerly Joanna Briggs Institute): jbi.global
- Kaiser Family Foundation http://kff.org
- Office for Human Research Protections https://www.hhs.gov/ohrp/
- Patient-Centered Outcomes Research Institute (PCORI) https://www.pcori.org
- RAND Corporation http://www.rand.org/about/glance.html
- Robert Wood Johnson Foundation http://www.rwjf.org
- U.S. Department of Health and Human Services Office for Human Research Protections, Quality Improvement Activities FAQs https://www.hhs.gov/ohrp/regulations-and-policy/guidance/faq/quality-improvement-activities/

REFERENCES

Aiken, L. H., Clarke, S. P., Sloane, D. M., Sochalski, J., & Silber, J. H. (2002). Hospital nurse staffing and patient mortality, nurse burnout, and job dissatisfaction. *JAMA, 288*(16), 1987–1993. https://doi.org/10.1001/jama.288.16.1987

Aiken, L. H., Smith, H. L., & Lake, E. T. (1994). Lower Medicare mortality among a set of hospitals known for good nursing care. *Medical Care, 32*(8), 771–787. https://doi.org/10.1097/00005650-199408000-00002

Alexandridis, A., McCort, A., Ringwalt, C., Sachdeva, N., Sanford, C., Marshall, S., Mack, K. & Dasgupta, N. (2017). A statewide evaluation of seven strategies to reduce opioid overdose in North Carolina. *Injury Prevention, 24*(1), 48–54. https://doi.org/10.1136/injuryprev-2017-042396

American Association of Critical Care Nurses. (n.d.a). *AACN Clinical Scene Investigator (CSI) Academy.* https://www.aacn.org/nursing-excellence/csi-academy

American Association of Critical Care Nurses. (n.d.b). *Urinary tract infection (UTI) prevention with caution.* https://www.aacn.org/clinical-resources/csi-projects/urinary-tract-infection-uti-prevention-with-caution

Andermann, A., Pang, T., Newton, J. N., Davis, A., & Panisset, U. (2016). Evidence for health II: Overcoming barriers to using evidence in policy and practice. *Health Research Policy and Systems, 14*, 17. https://doi.org/10.1186/s12961-016-0086-3

Association of periOperative Registered Nurses. (2021). *Guidelines for perioperative practice: 2021 edition.* https://www.aorn.org/Guidelines

Attaran, A., Pang, T., Whitworth, J., Oxman, A., & McKee, M. (2012). Healthy by law: The missed opportunity to use laws for public health. *Lancet, 379*(9812), 283–285. https://doi.org/10.1016/S0140-6736(11)60069-X

Bach-Mortensen, A. M., Lange, B. C. L., & Montgomery, P. (2018). Barriers and facilitator to implementing evidence-based interventions among third sector organizations: A systematic review. *Implementation Science, 13*(103), 5–19. https://doi.org/10.1186/s13012-018-0789-7

Bauer, M. S., & Kirchner, J. (2020). Implementation science: What is it and why should I care? *Psychiatry Research, 283*, 112376. https://doi.org/10.1016/j.psychres.2019.04.025

Benton, D. C., Watkins, M. J., Beasley, C. J., Ferguson, S. L., & Holloway, A. (2020). Evidence into action: a policy brief exemplar supporting attainment of nursing now. *International Nursing Review, 67*(1), 61–67. https://doi.org/10.1111/inr.12573

Bero, L. A., Grilli, R., Grimshaw, J. M., Harvey, E., Oxman, A. D., & Thomson, M. A. (1998). Closing the gap between research and practice: An overview of systematic reviews of interventions to promote the implementation of research findings. *British Medical Journal, 317*(7156), 465–468. https://doi.org/10.1136/bmj.317.7156.465

B'more for Healthy Babies. (n.d.). *Sleep safe. Back. Crib. Don't smoke. No exceptions.* https://www.healthybabiesbaltimore.com/safe-sleep

Bradley, E. H., Webster, T. R., Baker, D., Schlesinger, M., Inouye, S. K., Barth, M. C., & Koren, M. J. (2004). Translating research into practice: Speeding the adoption of innovative health care programs. *Issue Brief (Commonwealth Fund), 724*, 1–12. https://doi.org/10.1111/j.1532-5415.2004.52510.x

Brewer, B. (2020). Click it or give it: Increased seat belt law enforcement and organ donation. *Health Economics, 20*, 1400–1421. https://doi.org/10.1002/hec.4140

Brownson, R. C., Royer, C., Ewing, R., & McBride, T. D. (2006). Researchers and policymakers: Travelers in parallel universes. *American Journal of Preventive Medicine, 30*(2), 164–172. https://doi.org/10.1016/j.amepre.2005.10.004

Cairney, P., & Oliver, K. (2017). Evidence-based policymaking is not like evidence-based medicine, so how far should you go to bridge the divide between evidence and policy? *Health Research Policy and Systems, 15*, 35. https://doi.org/10.1186/s12961-017-0192-x

Canadian Institute for Health Information. (2020). *Knowledge translation at CIHR.* https://cihr-irsc.gc.ca/e/29529.html

Caplan, N. (1979). The two-communities, theory and knowledge utilization. *American Behavioral Scientist*, 22(3), 459–470. https://doi.org/10.1177/000276427902200308

Carter, E.J., Mastro, K., Vose, C., Rivera, R., & Larson, E. L. (2017). Clarifying the conundrum: Evidence-based practice, quality improvement, or research? *Journal of Nursing Administration*, 47(5), 266–270. https://doi.org/10.1097/NNA.0000000000000477

Centers for Disease Control and Prevention. (2015). *Catheter-associated urinary tract infections.* https://www.cdc.gov/infectioncontrol/guidelines/cauti/

Centers for Medicare & Medicaid Services. (n.d.). *Transitional care management.* https://www.medicare.gov/coverage/transitional-care-management-services

Colby, D. C., Quinn, B. C., Williams, C. H., Bilheimer, L. T., & Goodell, S. (2008). Research glut and information famine: Making research evidence more useful for policymakers. *Health Affairs*, 27(4), 1177–1182. https://doi.org/10.1377/hlthaff.27.4.1177

Crowley, M., Scott, J. T. B., & Fishbein, D. (2018). Translating prevention research for evidence-based policymaking: Results from the Research-to-Policy Collaboration Pilot. *Prevention Science*, 19(2), 260–270. https://doi.org/10.1007/s11121-017-0833-x

de Cordova, P. B., Pogorzelska-Maziarz, M., Eckenhoff, M. E., & McHugh, M. D. (2019). Public reporting of nurse staffing in the United States. *Nursing of Regulation*, 10(3), 14–20. https://doi.org/10.1016/S2155-8256(19)30143-7

de Cordova, P. B., Rogowski, J., Riman, K. A., & McHugh, M. D. (2019). Effects of public reporting legislation of nurse staffing: A trend analysis. *Policy, Politics & Nursing Practice*, 20(2), 92–104. https://doi.org/10.1177/1527154419832112

Deming, W. E. (2000). *The new economics: For industry, government, education* (2nd ed.). MIT Press.

Devers, K. J. (2011). *The state of quality improvement science in health: What do we know about how to provide better care?* RWJF Brief. https://www.rwjf.org/en/library/research/2011/11/the-state-of-quality-improvement-science-in-health.html

Ebell, M. H., Sokol, R., Lee, A., Simons, C. & Early, J. (2017). How good is the evidence to support primary care practice? *British Medical Journal*, 22(3), 88–92. https://doi.org/10.1136/ebmed-2017-110704

Eccles, M. P., & Mittman, B. S. (2006). Welcome to implementation science. *Implementation Science*, 1, 1. https://doi.org/10.1186/1748-5908-1-1

Ellen, M. E., Lavis, J. N., Horowitz, E., & Berglas, R. (2018). How is the use of research evidence in health policy perceived? A comparison between the reporting of researchers and policy makers. *Health Research Policy and Systems*, 16, 64. https://doi.org/10.1186/s12961-018-0345-6

Eshelman-Kent, D., Cherven, B., & Landier, W. (2018). *Association of Pediatric Hematology/Oncology Nurses Position Paper on human papillomavirus immunization.* https://aphon.org/education/clinical-practice

Farquhar, C. M., Stryer, D., & Slutsky, J. (2002). Translating research into practice: The future ahead. *International Journal of Quality in Health Care*, 14(3), 233–249. https://doi.org/10.1093/oxfordjournals.intqhc.a002615

Graham, I. D., Logan, J., Harrison, M. B., Straus, S. E., Tetroe J., Caswell W., & Robinson N. (2006). Lost in knowledge translation: Time for a map? *Journal of Continuing Education for Health Professionals*, 26(1), 13–24. https://doi.org/10.1002/chp.47

Green, L. A., & Seifert, C. M. (2005). Translation of research to practice: Why we can't just do it. *Journal of the American Board of Family Practice*, 18(6), 541–545. https://doi.org/10.3122/jabfm.18.6.541

Grimshaw, J. M., Eccles, M. P., Lavis, J. N., Hill, S. J., & Squires, J. E. (2012). Knowledge translation of research findings. *Implementation Science*, 7, 50. https://doi.org/10.1186/1748-5908-7-50

Grinspun, D., Botros, M., Mulrooney, L. A., Mo, J., Sibbald, R. G., & Penney, T. (2018). Scaling deep to improve people's health: From evidence based practice to evidence-based policy. In D. Grinspun & I. Bajnok (Eds.), *Transforming nursing through knowledge: Best practices for guideline development, implementation science, and evaluation* (pp. 466–494). Sigma Theta Tau International.

Guerden, B., Adriaenssens, J., & Franck, E. (2014). Impact of evidence and health policy on nursing practice. *Nursing Clinics of North America*, 49, 545–553. https://doi.org/10.1016/j.cnur.2014.08.009

Hammersley, M. (2013). *The myth of research-based policy and practice*. Sage.

Harden, V. A. (1998). *A short history of the National Institutes of Health*. http://history.nih.gov/exhibits/history/index.html

Hartsfield, D., Moulton, A. D., & McKie, K. L. (2007). A review of model public health laws. *American Journal of Public Health, 97*(Suppl. 1), S56–S61. https://doi.org/10.2105/AJPH.2005.082057

Harvey, E., Strobino, D., Sherrod, L., Webb, M., Anderson, C., White, J., & Atlas, R. (2016). Community-academic partnership to investigate low birth weight deliveries and improve maternal and infant outcomes at a Baltimore city hospital. *Maternal and Child Health Journal, 21*(2), 260–266. https://doi.org/10.1007/s10995-016-2153-3

Hawkes, C., Smith, T. G., Jewell, J., Wardle, J., Hammond, R. A., Friel, S., Throw, A. M., & Kain, J. (2015). Smart food policies for obesity prevention. *Lancet, 385*(9985), 2410–2421. https://doi.org/10.1016/S0140-6736(14)61745-1

Holt-Lunstad, J. (2020, June 22). Social isolation and health [Health Policy Brief]. *Health Affairs*. https://doi.org/10.1377/hpb20200622.253235

Health Compare. (n.d.). *Denali Center, Fairbanks, AK*. https://www.healthcarecomps.com/nursing-homes/ak/025020/

Health Foundation. (2011). *Improvement science*. https://www.health.org.uk/sites/default/files/ImprovementScience.pdf

Hirschman, K., Shaid, E., McCauley, K., Pauly, M., & Naylor, M. (2015). Continuity of care: The Transitional Care Model. *OJIN: Online Journal of Issues in Nursing, 20*(3), Manuscript 1. https://doi.org/10.3912/OJIN.Vol20No03Man01

Institute of Medicine. (2009). *Leadership commitments to improve value in healthcare: Finding common ground. Workshop summary*. The National Academies Press. https://doi.org.10.17226/11982

Johns Hopkins Medicine. (n.d.). *Johns Hopkins nursing evidence-based practice model*. https://www.hopkinsmedicine.org/evidence-based-practice/ijhn_2017_ebp.html

KSPAN. (n.d.). *Child maltreatment*. www.safekentucky.org/index.php/menu-child-maltreatment

Lavis, J. N., Ross, S. E., Hurley, J. E., Hohenadel, J. M., Stoddart, G. L., Woodward, C. A., & Abelson, J. (2002). Examining the role of health services research in public policymaking. *Milbank Quarterly, 80*(1), 125–154. https://doi.org/10.1111/1468-0009.00005

Leuz, C. (2018). Evidence-based policymaking: promise, challenges and opportunities for accounting and financial markets research, *Accounting and Business Research, 48*(5), 582–608. https://doi.org/10.1080/00014788.2018.1470151

Loan, L. A., Parnell, T. A., Stichler, J. F., Boyle, D. K., Allen, P., VanFosson, C. A., & Barton, A. J. (2018). Call for action: Nurses must play a critical role to enhance health literacy. *Nursing Outlook, 66*(1), 97–100. https://doi.org/10.1016/j.outlook.2017.11.003

Lockwood, C., Aromataris, E., & Munn, Z. (2014). Translating evidence into policy and practice. *Nursing Clinics of North America, 49*, 555–566. https://doi.org/10.1016/j.cnur.2014.08.010

Mark, B. A., Harless, D. W., Spetz, J., Reiter, K. L., & Pink, G. H. (2013). California's minimum nurse staffing legislation: Results from a natural experiment. *Health Services Research, 48*(2 Pt 1), 435–454. https://doi.org/10.1111/j.1475-6773.2012.01465.x

Maryniak, K. (2019). *Transitional care model*. https://www.rn.com/clinical-insights/transitional-care-model/

McHugh, M. D., Brooks Carthon, M., Sloane, D. M., Wu, E., Kelly, L., & Aiken, L. H. (2012). Impact of nurse staffing mandates on safety-net hospitals: Lessons from California. *The Milbank Quarterly, 90*(1), 160–186. https://doi.org/10.1111/j.1468-0009.2011.00658.x

McHugh, M. D., Kelly, L. A., Sloane, D. M., & Aiken, L. H. (2011). Contradicting fears, California's nurse-to-patient mandate did not reduce the skill level of the nursing workforce in hospitals. *Health Affairs (Project Hope), 30*(7), 1299–1306. https://doi.org/10.1377/hlthaff.2010.1118

McKee, M. (2019). Bridging the gap between research and policy and practice. *International Journal of Health Policy Management, 8*(9), 557–559. https://doi.org/10.15171/ijhpm.2019.46

Melnyk, B., Fineout-Overholt, E., Stillwell, S., & Williamson, K. (2010). Evidence-based practice. Step by step: The seven steps of evidence-based practice. *The American Journal of Nursing, 110*(1), 51–53. https://doi.org/10.1097/01.NAJ.0000366056.06605.d2

Melnyk, B. M., Gallagher-Ford, L., Thomas, B. K., Troseth, M., Wyngarden, K., & Szalacha, L. (2016). A study of chief nurse executives indicates low prioritization of evidence-based practice and shortcomings in hospital performance metrics across the United States. *Worldviews on Evidence-Based Nursing, 13*(1), 6–14. https://doi.org/10.1111/wvn.12133

National Health and Medical Research Council. (2019, September 6). *Guidelines for guidelines: Dissemination and communication.* https://www.nhmrc.gov.au/guidelinesforguidelines/implement/dissemination-and-communication

Naylor, M. D., Bowles, K. H., McCauley, K, M., Maccoy, M. C., Maislin, G., Pauly, M. V., & Krakauer, R. (2013). High-value transitional care: Translation of research into practice. *Journal of Evaluation in Clinical Practice, 19*(5), 727–733. https://doi.org/10.1111/j.1365-2753.2011.01659.x

Nelson, J., & Pulley, A. (2015). Transitional care can reduce hospital readmissions. *American Nurse Today, 10*(4), 1–8. https://doi.org/10.1177/1941874414540683

Newhouse, R. P., Dearholt, S., Poe, S., Pugh, L. C., & White K. M. (2005). *The Johns Hopkins nursing evidence-based practice model.* Johns Hopkins Hospital & Johns Hopkins University School of Nursing.

Nowell, W. B., Curtis, J. R., & Crow-Hercher, R. (2018). Patient governance in a patient-powered research network for Adult Rheumatologic Conditions. *Medical Care, 56*(10, Suppl. 1), S16–S21. https://doi.org/10.1097/MLR.0000000000000814

Office for Human Research Protections. (2018). *45 CFR 46.* http://www.hhs.gov/ohrp/humansubjects/guidance/45cfr46.html

Patient-Centered Outcomes Research Institute. (n.d.). *PCORI 101.* https://www.pcori.org/assets/articulate_uploads/PCORI_1018/story.html

Penn Nursing. (n.d.). NewCourtland Center for Transitions and Health. https://www.nursing.upenn.edu/ncth/mirror-tcm/

Pergert, P., Sullivan, C. E., Adde, M., Afungchwi, G. M., Downing, J., Hollis, R., Ilbawi, A., Morrissey, L., Punjwani, R., & Challinor, J. (2020). An ethical imperative: Safety and specialization as nursing priorities of WHO Global Initiative for Childhood Cancer. *Pediatric Blood & Cancer, 67*(4), e28143. https://doi.org/10.1002/pbc.28143

Pew Charitable Trusts. (2017). *How states engage in evidence-based policymaking: A national assessment.* The Pew Charitable Trusts. https://www.pewtrusts.org/en/research-and-analysis/reports/2017/01/how-states-engage-in-evidence-based-policymaking

Pierce, M. C., Kaczor, K., Aldridge, S., O'Flynn, J., & Lorenz, D. (2010). Bruising characteristics discriminating physical child abuse from accidental trauma. *Pediatrics, 125*(1), 67–74. https://doi.org/10.1542/peds.2008-3632

Project Lazarus. (2021). States where components of the Project Lazarus model have been implemented. https://www.projectlazarus.org/partner-communities

Roller, C., Sedlak, C., & Draucker, C. (2015) Navigating the system: How transgender individuals engage in healthcare. *Journal of Nursing Scholarship, 47*(5), 417–424. https://doi.org/10.1111/jnu.12160

Rouse, W. B., Naylor, M. D., Yu, Z., Pennock, M. J., Hirschman, K. B., Pauly, M. V., & Pepe, K. M. (2019). Policy flight Simulators: Accelerating decisions to adopt evidence-based health interventions. *Journal of Healthcare Management, 64*(4), 231–241. https://doi.org/10.1097/JHM-D-18-00114

Sedlak, C. A., Boyd, C. J., & American Academy of Nursing Lesbian, Gay, Bisexual, Transgender, Queer (LGBTQ) Health Expert Panel. (2016). American Academy of Nursing on Policy Health care services for transgender individuals: Position statement. *Nursing Outlook, 64*(5), 510–512. https://doi.org/10.1016/j.outlook.2016.07.002

Sedlak, C. A., Roller, C. G., van Dulmen, M., Alharbi, H., Sanata, J., Leifson, M., Veney, A. J., Alhawatmeh, H., & Doheny, M. O. (2017). Transgender individuals and osteoporosis prevention. *Orthopaedic Nursing, 36*(4), 259–268. https://doi.org/10.1097/NOR.0000000000000364

Spetz, J., Harless, D. W., Herrera, C. N., & Mark, B. A. (2013). Using minimum nurse staffing regulations to measure the relationship between nursing and hospital quality of care. *Medical Care Research and Review: MCRR, 70*(4), 380–399. https://doi.org/10.1177/1077558713475715

Spruce, L., Van Wicklin, S., & Wood, A. (2016). AORN's revised model for evidence appraisal and rating. *AORN Journal, 103*(1), 60–72. https://doi.org/10.1016/j.aorn.2015.11.015

Titler, M. G. (2018). Translation research in practice: An introduction. *OJIN: The Online Journal of Issues in Nursing, 23*, 2, Manuscript 1. https://doi.org/10.3912/OJIN.Vol23No02Man01

Towfighi, A., Orechwa, A. Z., Aragón, T. J., Atkins, M., Brown, A. F., Brown, J., Carrasquillo, O., Carson, S., Fleisher, P., Gustafson, E., Herman, D. K., Inkelas, M., Liu, W., Meeker, D., Mehta, T., Miller, D. C., Paul-Brutus, R., Potter, M. B., Ritner, S. S., . . . Yee, Jr., H. F. (2020). Bridging the gap between research, policy, and practice: Lessons learned from academic-public partnerships in the CTSA network. *Journal of Clinical and Translational Science, 4*(3), 201–208. https://doi.org/10.1017/cts.2020.23

Truiett-Theodorson, R., Tuck, S., Bowie, J. V., Summers, A. C., & Kelber-Kaye, J. (2015). Building effective partnerships to improve birth outcomes, by reducing obesity: The B'more Fit Healthy Babies Coalition of Baltimore. *Evaluation and Program Planning, 51*, 53–58. https://doi.org/10.1016/j.evalprogplan.2014.12.007

University of Pennsylvania. (n.d.) *Arnold ventures awards $6 million grant to study replication of Penn Nursing's Transitional Care Model.* https://www.nursing.upenn.edu/details/news.php?id=1596

University of Wisconsin-Madison. (2021, November 9). *What Are the T0 to T4 Research Classifications?* UW Institute for Clinical and Translational Research. https://ictr.wisc.edu/what-are-the-t0-to-t4-research-classifications/

VA Health Care. (2020). VA needs to strengthen its oversight of quality of state veterans homes. Subcommittee on Health, Committee on Veterans' Affairs, House of Representatives, 116th international Congress. (testimony of Sharon M. Silas). https://www.gao.gov/assets/gao-20-697t.pdf

van de Goor, L., Hamalainen, R-M., Syed, A., Lau, C. J., Sandu, P., Spitters, H., Karlsson, L. E., Dulf, D., Valente, A., Castellani, T., & Aro, A. R. (2017). Determinants of evidence use in public health policy making: Results from a study across six EU countries. *Health Policy, 121*(3), 273–281. https://doi.org/10.1016/j.healthpol.2017.01.003

Vietnam Veterans of America® Subcommittee on the Aging Veteran Experience. (2020). *Leave no veteran behind . . . The mission continues. America's aging veteran population and the COVID-19 pandemic report.* https://vva.org/wp-content/uploads/2020/08/FINAL-SAVE-REPORT.pdf

Weston, M., White, K., & Peterson, C. (2013). Creating nursing's future: Translating research into evidence-based policy. Communicating Nursing Research Conference proceedings: Creating a shared future of nursing. *Research, Practice, and Education, 46*, 47–54.

Workman, T. A. (2013). *Engaging patients in information sharing and data collection: The role of patient-powered registries and research networks (AHRQ Community Forum White Paper, AHRQ Publication No. AHRQ 13-EHC124-EF).* Agency for Research Healthcare and Quality. . https://www.ncbi.nlm.nih.gov/books/NBK164513

World Health Organization. (n.d.). *Evidence-informed policy network.* https://www.euro.who.int/en/data-and-evidence/evidence-informed-policy-making/evidence-informed-policy-network-evipnet

World Health Organization, Europe. (n.d.). Evidence-informed policy making. https://www.euro.who.int/en/data-and-evidence/evidence-informed-policy-making

Yost, J., Thompson, D., Ganann, R., Aloweni, F., Newman, K., McKibbon, A., Dobbins, M., & Ciliska, D. (2014). Knowledge translation strategies for enhancing nurses' evidence-informed decision making: A scoping review. *Worldviews on Evidence-Based Nursing, 11*(3), 156–167. https://doi.org/10.1111/wvn.12043

CHAPTER 6

Setting the Agenda

LINDA K. GROAH AND AMY L. HADER

> *Things do not happen. Things are made to happen.*
> *—John F. Kennedy (1963)*

OBJECTIVES

1. Explain the importance of effective agenda setting in the policy process.
2. Discuss critical components of agenda setting.
3. Analyze effective strategies for advancing a policy agenda.
4. Describe methods for overcoming barriers to advancing a policy agenda.
5. Compare and contrast options for agenda setting at the organizational, local, state, and national levels.
6. Identify nonlegislative strategies to move an organizational, local, state, or national agenda forward.

Agenda setting is the first step, and some would argue the most important step, in the policy process. It is your navigation tool in your policy journey. It is an extension of the problem identification and prerequisite to successful policy development at all levels. Agenda setting is critical whether you are working on big-P or little-p issues. Agenda setting can seem a straightforward process; however, if you consider setting an agenda for a meeting and reflect on meetings that have gone in less than desirable directions, you can start to envision that agenda setting is an iceberg and only the tip is visible. Consider the complexities of agenda setting related to healthcare reform and current crises such as response to a pandemic at the national and state levels in the United States. Once you have identified a policy issue (see Chapter 4) and evaluated the available research (see Chapter 5), it is time to set the agenda.

This chapter discusses the importance of policy agendas and strategies for controlling and influencing the agenda-setting process. You are guided through the processes of agenda setting and the pivotal role that nursing plays in agenda setting. Consideration is given to variations in the agendas. The agenda-setting process is based on a variety of intersecting factors, such as the policy problem, the scope of the issue, the stakeholders, the timing, personal agendas, and public agendas. Agenda setting at the federal level, within key nursing organizations, and for key clinical issues are highlighted to showcase the critical role nurses must play in this process. Nurses' full understanding and control of agenda setting are foundational to the achievement of sustained power in policy. Knowing the basic

POLICY CHALLENGE | **Finding the Courage to Speak Out Against Surgical Smoke**

Melony Prince, MSN, RN, CNOR
Clinical Educator for Surgical Services, Littleton Adventist Hospital, Littleton, CO

The dangers of surgical smoke didn't hit home until a close colleague, Eva (pseudonym), confided in me about her battle from a career breathing in surgical smoke after a routine educational in-service on operating room safety. Eva closed the office door and shared her private battle recovering from multiple surgeries to have human papillomavirus (HPV) lesions removed from her nose and throat passages. This followed years of working with an obstetrical/gynecological physician who removed patients' HPV lesions using a laser without surgical smoke evacuation. Eva asked, "Will you please be my voice to protect others from what I'm going through?"

Taking up the challenge I began a journey to address the dangers of surgical smoke by educating surgical team members about its dangers. My first step included sharing published research in perioperative staff lounges and displaying posters from the Association of periOperative Registered Nurses (AORN) Go Clear Program™. Along with nurse and physician colleagues and champions we established surgical smoke[1] evacuation as the norm in 92% of surgeries at our facility.

We saw the value of moving the issue beyond our facility to the state level. Therefore, we began writing to legislators to educate them about the daily dangers of surgical smoke affecting nurses, surgeons, and patients. We also encouraged practice colleagues across Colorado to do the same as we believed nurses have a powerful voice in elections and that legislators know this.

After only 2 years of collaborative work by AORN and perioperative professionals across the state, Colorado Governor Jared Polis signed a bill into law in March 2019 requiring all healthcare facilities to have a policy requiring surgical smoke evacuation by May 2021.

---

[1] Surgical smoke is vaporization of substances into a gas form produced by surgical instruments including over 150 substances in dead and live cellular material, viruses, bacteria, and toxic compounds (Association of periOperative Registered Nurses, 2022).

concepts related to agenda setting is a prerequisite to appreciating its power. The Policy Challenge illustrates a turning point in agenda setting for a reoccurring workplace safety issue, surgical smoke.

AGENDA IDENTIFICATION

A problem or issue must get the attention of those who want to help make a change before the policy process starts. On any given day, numerous problems command and compete for attention. The repetition of a problem (e.g., frequency of personal protective equipment [PPE] shortages, musculoskeletal injuries, number of patient falls with injuries) or the scale and breadth of a problem (e.g., number of Americans without health insurance) are often seen as instrumental in shaping the agenda-setting process, but repetition and scale do not guarantee that an issue will make it to the top of an agenda. Understanding the definition of an agenda, the importance of an agenda, those who set and define an agenda, and levels of agendas are interrelated, and key concepts that are basic to getting an issue for an agenda identified.

What Is an Agenda?

An agenda is a complex process that involves laying out issues and solutions: "Social scientists define the agenda as the collection of problems—and the different understandings of causes, symbols, solutions, and other elements of public problems—that come to the attention of members of the public and their governmental officials" (Birkland, 2020, p. 211). This definition can be reworked more generically to encompass both the big-P and the little-p of policy: An agenda is a collection of difficulties or issues and their causes, representations (privately and publicly), and suggested resolutions that get the attention and consideration of policymakers locally, nationally, or internationally and within or across institutions, organizations, or governments. Thus, agenda setting is not solely applicable to government policy. In fact, nurses can and must be active in policy where they work, in their communities, and in their profession.

The agenda is the "list of things being discussed and sometimes acted upon by an institution, the news media, or the public at large" (Birkland, 2020, p. 207). Agendas influence events, news, and understanding. An agenda can be as simple as an identified issue and the proposed solution or as comprehensive as a descriptive series of problems that require solutions from varying vested individuals or groups (e.g., stakeholders in government, private sector, individuals, communities). For example, for a state nurses association, an agenda might include a list of legislation that has been introduced that has an impact on nursing, such as education and research funding, medical supply distribution, and overtime protections. It could also include a more comprehensive analysis of legislative and regulatory changes that need to take place within a state to remove scope of practice barriers such as telehealth and advanced nursing practice restrictions. Kingdon (2011) conducted hundreds of interviews with government officials and policymakers, yielding a comprehensive review of research on agenda setting. His findings indicated that context was important—timing, political climate, and other political realities—in the policymaking and agenda-setting process. In addition to an "accumulation" process, pressure may also build for an agenda to rise because of a sudden, sharp "focusing event" (Birkland, 2020; Kingdon, 2011). For example, the killing of George Floyd by a Minneapolis police officer, caught on camera for the world to see, along with numerous other videos, spotlight the long history of systemic racism in American society in a way that governments and all but the most avoidant can no longer deny.

For nurses considering or already engaged in policy work, it is important to stay mindful of current clinical and policy issues and at the same time we must continue to consider population healthcare needs, both as related to COVID-19 prevention, treatment, and vaccination policies and to the healthcare system and delivery flaws that were exposed in the response to the COVID-19 pandemic.

Importance of the Agenda

Many writers and speakers who are intent on urging readers and listeners to become more involved in the political process have used the saying, "If you are not at the table, you're on the menu." This quote is frequently used in Washington, DC, and bears repeating here. Individuals and organizations whose priority issues are not on the agenda stand little chance of influencing policy regarding their priorities; at worst, they may experience backward progress and lose ground on their issues. Agenda setting is about power. Power is exercised by determining what gets on the agenda and what is blocked from getting on the agenda.

A number of theories describe how power and its influence on activities such as agenda setting develop. Some researchers in the policy arena present an elitist theory, suggesting the power elite that dominate public decision-making are the same interests that consistently win, primarily those of business, the upper and middle classes, and Whites (Peters, 2019, p. 62). In contrast, the pluralist theory posits that competition among interest groups, each with their own expertise and agenda, help keep in check the balance among groups (Peters, 2019, p. 61). For example, the American Hospital Association usually has great power over legislative initiatives in the healthcare arena and very little sway when it comes to securities regulation. Within interest groups, grassroots efforts are often very effective (see Chapter 7).

"Agenda setting is crucial because if an issue cannot be placed on the agenda, it cannot be considered, and nothing can possibly happen in government" (Peters, 2019, p. 57). Nursing issues at the big-P level almost always lie within the policy issue category of healthcare. Your goals and action plan may vary from seeking legislative or regulatory changes to increased public awareness of a public health issue or even incremental policy changes within your healthcare facility. The national political climate, as well as interest groups and individual connections, all coalesce to inform your policy agenda and action plan. The COVID-19 pandemic has opened the world's eyes to the many reforms and improvements required of our healthcare system, including needed work on social determinants of health (SDOH). Nursing stands uniquely poised to advance this agenda because of the public's trust in the profession, the strength in its numbers, and nurses' everyday experiences witnessing the impact of SDOH on health.

Those Who Set and Define Agendas

All organizations and state and federal agencies and their subdivisions have mission statements and strategic plans that are routinely reviewed and updated. The partisan balance of Congress and other legislative bodies also influences the policies on an organization's agenda. The mission and strategic plans guide agenda setting at all levels and determine priorities for action. If an agenda is not linked to a controlling agency's mission and strategic plan, it is difficult, if not impossible, for the agenda to gain traction among key stakeholders. Understanding these connections among missions, strategic plans, and agendas is vital for nurses to move an agenda forward. Too often, an assumption is made that money, media, and power control agendas. Acceptance of this assumption (from elitist theory), can feed a sense of powerlessness that often leads to disillusionment about the ability to change policies, legislation, and regulation that have an impact. Rather, it is important to recognize who controls the agenda so that change efforts are not dissuaded but simply directed in the appropriate direction.

One example of the government's role in leading policy changes can be seen in the role of the Occupational Safety and Health Administration (OSHA) in sharps safety and preventing needlestick injuries. The year 2020 marks the 20th anniversary of the Needlestick Safety and Prevention Act and its amendment to OSHA's Bloodborne Pathogens Standard. These regulations cover sharps disposal practices, evaluation and selection of devices with sharps injury prevention features, PPE, education and training, record keeping for sharps injuries, hepatitis B vaccination, and postexposure follow-up. The standard has been effective in driving a significant reduction in needlesticks and blood and body fluid exposures, but it has not eliminated the problem. While OSHA plays a leadership role in enforcing the standards, it is the facilities and practice leaders within the facilities that must design, implement, evaluate, monitor, and improve the program. The Needlestick Safety and Prevention Act alone was not strong enough to have eliminated these injuries. An increasingly complex and changing healthcare environment requires renewed commitment at the facility level to needed surveillance and prevention. Facility leaders can use the support provided by government regulations to promote their safety programs. However, the effectiveness of an actual program requires local buy-in by both practitioners and facility administration, as the data show policies must be on the agenda of both those implementing and those enforcing in order to be fully effective at accomplishing an agreed-on goal, such as eliminating sharps injuries (International Safety Center, 2020).

Nurses specialty associations have well-established procedures for formulating their agendas. Some associations routinely seek and include members' ideas and concerns when developing their agendas. As membership organizations, they follow a democratic process that includes mechanisms to collect suggestions or mandates from the membership. The annual meetings of many associations include a process in which topics are debated and voted on to determine resource priorities for future actions. These topics often end up in policy agendas. Table 6.1 provides links to the policy agendas of several professional associations. Agendas may focus on a specific policy. Sometimes organizations may have a separate research agenda to address priorities for research.

Landmark reports can serve both as an agenda-setting function and as an agenda. Two seminal reports, *To Err Is Human* (Institute of Medicine [IOM], 2000) and *The Future of Nursing: Leading Change, Advancing Health* (IOM, 2011; now the National Academy of Medicine) brought national focus to the problems of patient safety, the frequency of medical errors, and the need for funding and support for nursing to be able to improve patient outcomes. These landmark reports serve as opportunities

TABLE 6.1: **POLICY AGENDAS OF SELECTED SPECIALTY NURSES ASSOCIATIONS**

ORGANIZATION	TYPE OF AGENDA	WEBSITE
AACN	Federal policy agenda	www.aacnnursing.org/Policy-Advocacy/About-Government-Affairs-and-Policy/Federal-Policy-Agenda
AANP	Advocacy center	www.aanp.org/advocacy/advocacy-center
ACNM	ACNM policy agenda	www.midwife.org/ACNM-Policy-Agenda
AORN	Policy agenda	www.aorn.org/government-affairs/policy-agenda
ENA	Public policy agenda	www.ena.org/government-relations/public-policy-agenda
NACNS	2016–2018 public policy agenda	www.nacns.org/advocacy-policy/public-policy-agenda/
NAPNAP	Health policy agenda	www.napnap.org/health-policy-agenda/
ONS	Policy priorities	www.ons.org/make-difference/ons-center-advocacy-and-health-policy/policy-priorities

AACN, American Association of Colleges of Nursing; AANP, American Association of Nurse Practitioners; ACNM, American College of Nurse-Midwives; AORN, Association of periOperative Registered Nurses; ENA, Emergency Nurses Association; NACNS, National Association of Clinical Nurse Specialists; NAPNAP, National Association of Pediatric Nurse Practitioners; ONS, Oncology Nursing Society.

for agenda setting and offer consensus support for nursing's specific policy issues. Looking forward, nursing groups seeking to advance specific agendas may also lean on the *State of the World's Nursing Report, 2020: Investing in Education, Jobs and Leadership* by the World Health Organization (WHO, 2020), which highlights the continued importance of nurses working to the full extent of their education and training. This WHO report recognizes the vital contributions of nursing to improving world health and recommends investing in nursing education, creating new nursing jobs, and strengthening nurse leadership. It will serve as both impetus and evidence for specialty nursing organizations as they set and advance their agendas.

Levels of the Agenda

Prior to Kingdon's (2011) extensive examination of political agendas and the policymaking process, Cobb and Elder (1972) examined the importance of the political agenda. Their work showcased the difference between issues or problems under discussion in society—which can be thought of as a systemic agenda or public problems—and institutional or organizational agendas. Birkland (2020) expands this concept to include four levels of increasing specificity: agenda universe, systemic agenda, institutional or organizational agenda, and decision agenda. The agenda universe consists of all ideas that could possibly be considered and discussed in a society or a political system. The systemic agenda or public problems are those worthy of public attention and within the scope of authority or legitimate jurisdiction of a government. When an issue elevates to active and serious consideration of decision-makers, it moves from the systemic agenda to the institutional agenda. Finally, the decision agenda narrows to include only those items that are about to be acted on; for government actors, these are often bills, court cases, and regulations. Without prominence on the institutional or organizational agenda, an issue is unlikely to make any meaningful headway through the political system (see Figure 6.1). Although any number of issues may be the important components of a nurses association agenda, the goal is to move an issue closer to the decision agenda so that desirable actions can be taken.

Often not discussed is the importance of an agenda in one's local environment and, in particular, the importance of nurses owning the policy agenda for their practice. For example, rather than becoming frustrated with the failure to move forward with a policy that implements an evidence-based practice (e.g., fasting times before surgery, prevention strategies for postoperative urinary retention, meal tray delivery, insulin administration times), nurses need to examine how to get their issue on the policy agenda of the group or groups that can best help implement the practice. While the previous discussion shows the importance of making it to the decision agenda for a legislature or court to act in healthcare, the same analysis is true at the institutional level. It is vital to show how the practice issue fits with the mission or strategic plan of the controlling institution, which usually means how your practice issue relates to safety outcomes, and/or cost. One nurse's efforts to implement practices designed to improve physical activity in schoolchildren required decision-makers' focus at the local school district and planning committee level (see Policy on Scene 6.1). Regardless of whether an issue requires attention at the legislative or regulatory level, within your healthcare institution, or even within a municipality or local civic group, an issue's prominence often directly correlates to the level of attention it receives from decision-makers and stakeholders. Identifying the systemic and, more important, the institutional agendas of the decision-makers you are trying to influence provides

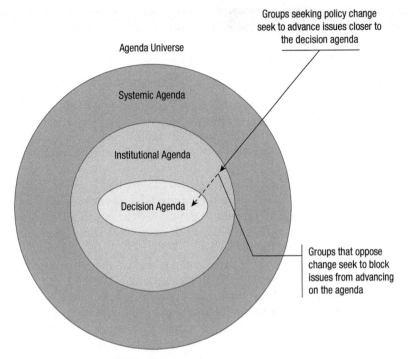

Groups seeking policy change
seek to advance issues closer to
the decision agenda

Agenda Universe

Systemic Agenda

Institutional Agenda

Decision Agenda

Groups that oppose
change seek to block
issues from advancing
on the agenda

FIGURE 6.1 Levels of the agenda.

Source: Reprinted with permission from Birkland, T. A. (2016). *An introduction to the policy process: Theories, concepts, and models of public policy making* (4th ed.). M. E. Sharpe.

the foundation for the development and refinement of your agenda so that your issue can rise to the decision agenda.

DEVELOPING AN AGENDA

Agenda development includes defining the problem and establishing the agenda. These are two intertwined and evolving processes. Articulating the problem provides the launching pad for establishing the agenda and controlling the solution.

Defining the Problem

> *A problem clearly stated is a problem half solved.*
>
> —*Dorothea Brande*

Conditions and problems can become agenda items, but there is a difference between them. Weather, illnesses, and poverty are conditions. Conditions become problems when someone decides to do something about them (Kingdon, 2011). Agenda setting is a process. Issues gain and lose attention in the spotlight every day. A "tractable" problem is one that can be effectively addressed by policy (Birkland, 2020, p. 222). For example, weather is not a tractable problem, but effective bridges and dams are. In addition to COVID-19 and all the systemic healthcare disparity, prevention, and delivery problems the pandemic exposed, widely accepted, ongoing policy agenda items in the United States are the problem of poverty, the

POLICY ON THE SCENE 6.1: FROM PASSION TO A POLICY AGENDA

Brea Loewit, MSN, RN, FNP, IBCLC
Lactation Consultant and Childbirth Educator, University Hospitals Portage
Medical Center, Portage, Ohio

Health policy is used to achieve specific health goals within a population on a local, state, or national level. Health policy gives clarity and direction to a specific problem with the goal of improving health outcomes. One public health issue that I feel passionate about is physical activity in schoolchildren. Remaining physically active has immense social, physical, and cognitive benefits for children. I am a parent of two elementary school children, and I know that if my kids stay physically active it gives balance to the demands of a school environment oriented meeting core curriculum goals and completing homework after school. I realized the issue became more acute in recent winter, with many inclement days that prevented children from going outside for recess.

When I started talking to stakeholders, I found there were no established physical activity time recommendations in the local school district and no contingency plans to provide physical activity alternatives during inclement weather. But I did identify opportunities for schools to meet physical activity guidelines within the existing policy, as well as areas for growth. I presented my findings and suggestions to the school board. My four recommendations were

- have an indoor recess plan in place for each elementary school building,
- implement the recommended 30 minutes of daily exercise as provided in Ohio's 2010 Healthy Choices for Healthy Children Act,
- develop a task force of Parent Teacher Association (PTA) members in each elementary school to help facilitate indoor recess, and
- revise and update the existing health and wellness policy.

These recommendations became the foundation for my policy agenda that was fueled by my passion. It provided me a vehicle for advancing my agenda to the school system. My presentation was well received and resulted in being invited to be on the planning committee for a new school in our district, where I could continue looking for opportunities to improve the health of children.

quality of our public education system, disaster preparedness after September 11, multiple devastating climate events, and the rash of mass shootings in recent years.

Issues pass through an "issue attention cycle" in which they are of high public concern for a brief period, and then enthusiasm wanes as the costs and difficulties of implementing real policy change emerge and the public moves on to new issues (Peters, 2019, p. 58). The environment, drug policy, and the women's and Black Lives Matter movements all have traded escalating and waning attention in recent years as the problems they present are not solvable by simple or quick fixes. In health policy, attention to the SDOH is on the rise; nurses can do their part to keep this at the forefront where it belongs.

A large part of agenda setting is defining the problem. For example, after the mass tragedies of September 11, 2001, in the United States, security for airline travel became a pressing issue. Everyone agreed on the importance of the issue of airline travel security. However, the finer points of how to increase travelers' security while balancing travelers' privacy were the subject of much disagreement. Whether to allow body scans, pat downs, profiling, and even liquids on airplanes became the subject of national debate. The next steps on the nation's agenda were framed largely by perceptions of the root of the problem. Did the problem lie in a failure to enforce existing rules, or were additional rules necessary to ensure nothing like September 11 could ever happen again to U.S. citizens? Should existing or new security measures for airline travel now be applied to other mass transit such as trains, subway systems, and buses? A person's reaction to and support for the agenda would depend, in large part, on the answer to these questions.

Another example of defining the problem can be seen in mass shooting incidents in schools. The absolute abhorrence and senselessness of these acts should focus policymakers' attention on the problem of school violence but have not, seemingly because there is a wide range of ways in which people explain the causes of school shootings: the ready availability of guns, the shortcomings of school security and school programs to detect and prevent violence, and the influence of popular culture (movies, music and video games; Birkland, 2020). (See https://ana.aristotle.com/sitePages/gunviolence.aspx). How we understand the root of the problem will inevitably shape how we perceive the solution. Using the example of COVID-19, nearly all agree that mass vaccination is the solution to the problem; however, while waiting for this solution, many did not agree on whether face coverings, social distancing, and closing schools and stores were effective solutions to the problem.

Those who describe the problem will also be in the best and most powerful position to define the solution (Birkland, 2020). A group must articulate its problem with the objective of swaying the right policymakers at the right time in the group's favor. Thus, it is important to have the right problem on the agenda. Individual and organizational or institutional stakeholders, including government agencies, are affected differently, depending on how a problem is defined. Focusing events, like the COVID-19 pandemic, may give new attention to old problems. For example, while telehealth has generally been understood as an effective strategy to improve access to care and evidence in favor is well documented, before the COVID-19 pandemic, telehealth was overly regulated and reimbursement was questionable, so it was of course infrequently used. Telehealth adoption dramatically improved out of necessity in response to the COVID-19 pandemic once the Centers for Medicare and Medicaid Services lifted restrictions, instituted payment parity, and waived potential penalties for Health Insurance Portability and Accountability Act (HIPAA) violations (Giese, 2020). The healthcare needs of the American people during the COVID-19 pandemic effectively thrust telehealth from the outer bounds of the agenda to the decision agenda, where policymakers acted fast to implement the solutions as defined by the telehealth providers.

An example of an ongoing policy problem for nurses working in intraoperative settings and other surgical team members is continuous exposure to surgical smoke. Surgical smoke is the result of human tissue contact with lasers and electrosurgical pencils commonly used for dissection and hemostasis during surgery. Ninety percent of all surgical procedures generate surgical smoke, and OSHA estimates 500,000 healthcare workers are exposed to surgical smoke each year (National Institute for Occupational Safety and Health, 2017). In addition to already known and documented health concerns related to the toxic gases and vapors in surgical smoke, including benzene, hydrogen cyanide, formaldehyde, bioaerosols, dead and live cellular material, blood fragments, and viruses—surgical teams now have the added concern of potentially inhaling the COVID-19 virus during surgical procedures on COVID-19-positive patients.

The problems associated with surgical smoke exposure have been with us for decades and hit surgical nurses the hardest because they spend the most time in the operating room. AORN, the professional membership association for perioperative nurses, has recently worked to implement solutions by claiming space on the decision agenda at both the institutional and legislative levels as shown in the Policy Challenge, providing a great working example of how a policy interest group such as a nurses specialty organization can work to highlight a problem for decision-makers and then showcase how the solution of evacuating the smoke at the source with cost-effective equipment solves the problem.

Nurses can also work on identifying similar problems at the state and local levels. Strategically, agenda setting evaluates the best approach and in what venue the issue should be first attempted. Some problems get addressed on a state-by-state basis first before their impact is recognized at the national level. Some problems may not gain traction at the state level until a handful of powerful institutions have first addressed the problem "voluntarily" and successfully, so the solution is readily apparent. The support of an issue at the local and state levels is often strategically planned before introduction at the federal level. The process can vary significantly, however. Sometimes a problem is identified by numerous organizations within and beyond nursing. Sometimes problems repeatedly fail to gain traction at the state level only to be recognized at the federal level.

Establishing the Agenda

There will always be competition among groups for policy makers' attention to their problems. Issues such as COVID-19 or federal budget negotiations that shut down the government affect nearly everyone in society and therefore will take precedence over nearly all other matters until solved. Issues with ramifications for greater numbers of people or important institutions may take precedence over issues with lessened societal impact but not necessarily and not as often as the public might like. Issues that may seem perfectly rational to some may not resonate as clearly with others. Immigration and gun control may be important one year only to slide off the radar the next year without any solution to the problems that thrust them onto the agenda in the first place.

The Gallup company has been routinely surveying Americans on the "most important problem facing this country today" for years. In 2009, a substantial majority of respondents (86%) cited economic problems, such as unemployment, the deficit, and taxes, as the most important problem (Gallup, n.d.). In 2017, 20% of respondents thought that government was the most important problem, and 17% thought healthcare was the most important problem (Swift, 2017). Contrast this with 2020, when the majority of respondents cited COVID-19, the government/poor leadership, and race relations/racism as more important problems than healthcare or the economy (Gallup, n.d.). Such polls can lend insight into groups looking to launch their issue onto policymakers' agendas. At any given time, people may be more or less receptive to proposed policy changes, depending on the nation's and policymakers' mood and preoccupation with other issues perceived to be more pressing. Solutions should be framed with the national mood in mind. In a time when government dissatisfaction is high, talking points for a bill that highlight the government's role in solving a nursing practice issue are less persuasive than talking points emphasizing how a bill authorizes and enables the profession itself to accomplish its stated goals. In contrast, if unemployment and economic concerns are high, nursing education and practice issues that involve government investment in education and job creation are ripe for the decision agenda.

Similarly, in the healthcare sphere, recent heightened public awareness of systemic racism across society has opened the door to conversations about SDOH and disparities in healthcare delivery, topics nursing has been aware of as problems for years but that have not previously been able to rise far enough on the agenda to see a marked investment in sweeping solutions.

Key influencers can work in favor of a policy issue gaining prominence on the agenda, but they can also work against it. For example, a president's role in agenda setting is interesting because the president and the executive administration are typically more involved in agenda setting than in developing the policy alternatives and solutions to the raised issues and problems (Birkland, 2020). A new government administration, new nursing leadership on your unit or at your healthcare facility, and even a planned accreditation visit can create new opportunities for issues to be presented to the decision-makers and potentially be placed on the agenda. Unpredictable events, such as weather-related disasters, a mass accident, or another local or regional tragedy, may also focus the public and decision-makers' attention on or off an issue without warning. COVID-19 essentially removed all other matters from any national healthcare agenda for 2020. Healthcare institutions' focus on the need for disaster response plans after mass tragedy events such as the Boston Marathon bombing and mass shootings in American workplaces, schools, and hospitals, as well as natural disasters, took a 180-degree turn toward needing an ICU response plan for COVID-19 patients in 2020.

Establishing agendas and public policies also usually requires a technology believed to be able to solve the problem (Peters, 2019, p. 69). For example, until the Keynesian revolution in economics explained reasons for economic fluctuations, people treated economic problems merely as conditions, like the weather and acts of God. Once people understood theories of economics and the government's role in driving change, economic management became a staple on government agendas (Peters, 2019). It is also common to have many issues of national importance in our country—even once understood as having a solution the government can provide—still take a backseat as budgets and availability of technological response waxes and wanes.

At the federal level, resources are allocated among competing federal agencies for their programs, the decisions of which are necessarily informed by the president's economic beliefs and policy goals (Peters, 2019). At the institutional level, budgets and financial constraints are similarly a leverage point with key executives and decision-makers. Obtaining funding for quality improvement projects within a healthcare institution can be as long and complex a process as seeking policy changes at the state and federal capitols.

At the local level, nurses' agendas are expected to address cost-effectiveness with their practice and policy development. One strategy in helping overcome this potential challenge is to provide data with sound cost–benefit ratio rationales when working for policies that may have financial implications. Although it may not be readily apparent, most policies and agendas have financial implications. For example, in creating an agenda to begin work on improving patient flow in the ED, you must consider not only the financial impact of the changes but also patient, employee, and physician satisfaction and the impact on other departments in offsetting costs.

STAKEHOLDERS

Careful consideration is necessary to determine whose interests and welfare should be considered in the agenda-setting process. Identification and inclusion of stakeholders are crucial in advancing a policy agenda. Stakeholders can be for an issue, against it, and even neutral. Including all stakeholders, regardless of their position, facilitates the broadest discussion and development of policy solutions. Stakeholders are the people, groups, and/or entities vested in the issue you are exploring or promulgating. Knowing the stakeholders is essential in helping define the problem and in setting the agenda. Stakeholders may include political parties, interest groups, the media, and the public and vary depending on the issue itself, the level, and the timing of the issue.

An example of stakeholders can be seen in the 2013 California Supreme Court decision, *American Nurses Association v. Tom Torlakson* (2013). The American Nurses Association (ANA) filed an amicus brief in support of California school nurses (Balestra, 2012). This controversial ruling allows trained school personnel to administer insulin in the California school system, which, in turn, had an impact on the policy agendas of key stakeholders. Strategies surrounding this issue are being refocused on how to promote safety for children under this ruling. Table 6.2 illustrates the diversity and complexity of interests of various stakeholders related to this policy agenda.

TABLE 6.2: STAKEHOLDERS AND INSULIN ADMINISTRATION IN SCHOOLS

STAKEHOLDER	INTEREST
Children with diabetes and their parents	Strong interest to have their healthcare needs addressed
Nurses in the school district	Interest by school nurses affected but a lack of desire by some to become involved
Teachers and staff in each school	Great interest in those with new duties but less interest in those whose duties remain the same
Principal and administrative staff in each school	Strong interest having been told to implement the plan with some potential ability to give input to the plan; interest in hiring fewer school nurses
State Department of Education	Strong interest to resolve issues to reduce costs to school districts
National Association of School Nurses	Strong interest and expertise
American Nurses Association	Strong interest and concern about implications for other practice arenas
American Diabetes Association	Strong interest to address its focused special interest
Local community	Strong interest but not a formed, cohesive group prepared to be involved
Local and state media	Not much interest, but if given the right information at the right time, could be very interested
Local politician	Indifferent but may change in an election year

As seen earlier, identifying the list of stakeholders can be a lengthy process. A complete analysis of all the stakeholders and their positions is necessary for setting effective policy agendas. Identifying the stakeholders is about not only knowing who your allies and opponents are but also strategizing about effective ways to capitalize on both. In the following pages, we describe how to use interest groups to advance your agenda and how to assess your opposition to overcome the obstacles they may present.

Including stakeholders can be strategic in terms of advancing the agenda. Sometimes, key stakeholders are included in the initial development of an agenda. Initially, for more controversial issues, groups may choose to start by including those who are primarily supportive of an agenda direction. This provides the group with the opportunity to examine its strategies, refine its arguments, gain support for an issue, and be sure that "everyone is on the same page." Subsequently, others may be invited to join when the initial group has gained a core sense of direction.

Importance of Interest Groups

Interest groups are often formed for common interests or purposes and to promote a cause. They may at some point decide that their mission and their needs will be met by influencing policy. Research has demonstrated that interest groups "often play a central role in setting the government agenda, defining options, influencing decisions and directing implementation" (Grossman, 2012, p. 172). Interest groups are credited with policy accomplishments in all three branches of government, influencing not only legislative changes but also court rulings, executive orders, and agency administrative decisions. In addition to being their own interest group for nursing, nurses can become part of additional interest groups by joining one. Types of interest groups include advocacy groups, consumer groups, community groups, business interest groups (e.g., chambers of commerce, corporations), academic groups, professional associations, unions, think tanks, and foundations. Interest groups may need to form coalitions to get a place on an agenda.

Interest Groups Aligned With Your Agenda

State nurses' and specialty nurses associations are professional interest groups typically open to registered nurses (RNs) and occasionally to other healthcare providers who support the association's mission. These associations can be a wise choice for enlisting support for a policy agenda. Partnering with your state nurses' and specialty associations is an important initial step in becoming an active and effective participant in setting the policy agenda. Registered nurse first assistants (RNFAs) in Minnesota partnered with their state nurses association in establishing reimbursement for RNFAs as a component of the Minnesota Nurses Association (MNA) policy agenda. Partnering with state nurses associations provides specialty nurses with a number of advantages to overcome challenges in setting their policy agenda. Another more recent example is the Rhode Island State Nurses Association's support for the first surgical smoke evacuation bill to be enacted in the United States; without the state nurses association's support, the specialty group for operating room nurses would have had a taller mountain to climb to convince stakeholders of the scale and breadth of the problem of surgical smoke (Evans, 2018). With state nurses associations' mission to represent all nurses, a partnership with nurses of specialty groups is logical to external constituencies, such as legislative bodies.

Diversity in interest group support, along with the traditional grassroots strategies, demonstrates the success of this approach. Expanding interest group support for your policy agenda involves not only determining who would naturally be aligned with your position but also identifying the advantages for interest groups with seemingly divergent goals. For example, natural potential allies in the surgical smoke evacuation initiative outside of healthcare providers are the American Lung Association and the American Cancer Society.

Keeping an issue on the agenda involves building and sustaining relationships to keep the agenda item from stalling and to realize success. Since Minnesota passed the RNFA-reimbursement bill in 1996, legislation has been introduced in 23 states and, as of 2021, has been enacted in 17 states, most recently in New York. That only 17 states have passed this legislation is in contrast with 41 states that passed legislation related to violence against nurses (see Chapter 1) illustrates how other issues can come to the forefront and how continued work is needed in moving an agenda forward. As of 2021, only three states, Rhode Island, Colorado, and Kentucky, enacted surgical smoke evacuation legislation. Many more states have introduced surgical smoke evacuation bills, but many states' legislative sessions were cut short by COVID-19 closures. New and different strategies or agenda modifications are needed to engage stakeholders as the political climate changes and problems rise and fall on agendas.

Professional associations can bring credibility and prominence to an agenda and enhance the potential for a policy agenda's success. Other kinds of interest groups in which nurses can find synergy and have an impact include business and industry groups. For example, a nurse responsible for directing an ambulatory surgery center might join, as a representative of the center, the local chamber of commerce to elevate the center's opportunity to have a voice in local business regulations that might affect it. Nurses in certain areas and specialties may also join other groups such as unions to advance their policy agendas.

Consumer groups may also have an impact on policy agendas. Consumer groups are often formed to champion causes framed as "in the public interest," such as consumer protection groups and "good government" organizations. Other examples of public interest groups include groups formed to speak for populations that cannot speak for themselves, such as children. These kinds of groups are often called on to respond to others' agendas on behalf of their constituents and intended beneficiaries. Consumer groups are often portrayed as counterpoints to the self-interested business, labor, and professional groups, but consumer groups do not exist solely to respond to the agendas of others. At times, consumer groups may have their own issue agendas.

Sometimes a group calling attention to an issue may not be an organized "group" at all. For example, on the day after the presidential inauguration in 2017, approximately half a million people took part in the Women's March in Washington, DC, with hundreds of thousands of others participating in their home cities, totaling 3.3 to 4.6 million nationwide (Waddell, 2017). More recently, the Black Lives Matter movement united millions across the United States in seeking social justice reform and representing the interests of Black communities nationwide.

Knowing the Opposition

Knowing groups that may be aligned with your policy agenda is not enough. It is equally important to consider your possible opposition as you advance your policy agenda. It is vital to try to understand early on what obstacles your group faces or may face in response to your policy initiatives. Early identification of barriers helps determine how best to work toward your objectives and keep your goals realistically attainable. Knowing the opposition involves identifying those who would oppose your agenda, as well as the specifics of their positions. Points to consider in determining the opposition and their positions are illustrated in Box 6.1.

BOX 6.1: ASSESSMENT OF THE OPPOSITION

- What is the nature of the opposition (e.g., finances, values, stereotypes)?
- Is the opposition proposing an alternative?
- Is the opposition from within your organization?
- Is the opposition coming from an individual or a group of individuals?
- Can you identify common ground with the opposition?
- Does the opposition answer to a constituency?
- How does the public view the opposition?
- Will swaying the opposition to a neutral position help your agenda?
- What are the financial resources of the opposition?
- To what extent is your agenda item important to the opposition?

Knowing and understanding the opposition allows you to identify competing interests. The information allows you to frame the issue, develop your arguments, and formulate strategies.

Unaligned Interest Groups

Some stakeholders or special interest groups may be unaligned with your policy agenda. It is just as important to identify groups that may have an interest in your policy agenda but that either are uninvolved or have taken a neutral position as it is to identify the opposition. Key decision-makers are interested in the positions of other organizations in relation to your agenda. When visiting a legislator, a nurse may be asked about the position of other groups. A legislator may want to gauge constituent interest in the issue. Although nurses cannot answer for other groups, nor should they, they should be aware of these positions to be prepared. While it is generally wise to avoid answering questions about the positions of other organizations, it is important to present as a team player and it may be wise to answer such questions along the lines of the following: "It is my understanding that the [powerful lobby group name] has some concerns about the bill and we have reached out to them directly in hopes of addressing those concerns."

Unaligned groups may be indicative of (a) internal disagreement about an issue, (b) private support for an issue when public expression of support may be politically incorrect for the organization, or (c) a belief that the issue is too far removed from the mission or focus of the group. Just because a stakeholder group is unaligned does not necessarily mean the group will stay unaligned. Likewise, it may be considered a victory when a stakeholder group moves from a position of active opposition to neutrality. Sometimes, large coalitions encourage a member organization that cannot fully support the focus of a coalition's policy initiative to simply remain silent on the issue.

Networking and Coalition Building

Influence is basic to agenda setting and should be taken into consideration, whether you are trying to influence others or others are trying to influence you. A number of factors are associated with success and/or failure of influence when setting an agenda. A person's status, for example, may play a role in others granting unconditional support and following; a well-respected nurse leader may get more support for an idea based on status. Three ways to build influence in support of your agenda are networking, building coalitions, and raising awareness of your issue.

Networking

Nurses seeking to advance a policy agenda should use a network. Building relationships is important so that they are in place when they are needed. You want to involve your network early in helping to create an agenda, foster engagement, and plan for the resources needed. Nurses can practice the art of networking every day in many ways—at work, at their children's schools and sporting events, at church, and even at the gym. Networking takes practice. Networking may be uncomfortable initially, but it really is just transferring communication skills into action.

Networking should include connecting with your legislators. Effective networking begins with simple steps. For example, legislators and their staff appreciate brief communications. This may include a note of thanks for a legislative position or a success attributable to their office. Legislators and their staff also may appreciate informational notes. For example, AORN and The Joint Commission promote a National Time-Out Day annually to highlight the importance of the "time-out" in preventing wrong-site, wrong-side, wrong-patient, and wrong-procedure surgeries. As part of this campaign, AORN asks its nurse members to write letters to the editor of their local newspapers explaining the key role perioperative nurses play in implementing the time-out and advancing patient safety in the operating room. When a letter is published, AORN urges the nurse to send an email about it to legislators with a personal note, as shown in Box 6.2. Simple personal notes like this are remembered, thus increasing the likelihood that a legislator and staff will remember an individual's name when that constituent later asks the legislator for support.

Persistence is often the key to success in networking with all contacts. Success does not happen with only one email or phone call. Networking needs to be a

---

BOX 6.2: SAMPLE LETTER TO LEGISLATOR OFFERING EXPERTISE

Dear [Senator or Representative name],

I thought you might be interested in this letter to the editor of [newspaper name] as an example of how complex healthcare has become and what perioperative nurses in your district are doing to improve patient safety in our operating rooms, ambulatory surgery centers, and catheterization laboratories. As an RN with many years of experience, I am available to assist and offer my expertise in these times of complex healthcare issues. I look forward to working with you and having ongoing conversations. Thank you for your service to our district and our country.

Sincerely, NAME, CREDENTIALS, CONTACT INFORMATION

habit, a way of interacting with people and using opportunities for putting forward an agenda. Having a wider network allows you to share your policy agenda with more people. A network takes time to build, but the reward is the expansion of your influence. Networking involves not only legislators but also nurses, community leaders, and members of the business community, as well as members of other professions (see Box 6.3 for tips on networking, and Chapter 11).

BOX 6.3: TIPS ON NETWORKING

1. Learn the person's name and repeat it later in the conversation.

2. Listen to the concerns of the individual and learn what is important to him or her.

3. Arrive early and stay late for meetings.

4. Volunteer for community or charitable events and legislative days.

5. Supplement your networking with an online professional network.

6. Introduce people to others who have common interests.

7. Follow up with a note, email, or phone call.

8. Keep messages about your policy agenda brief and to the point.

9. Share why your issue is important from your networking contact's perspective.

10. Be prepared with a description of your organization and its accomplishments.

11. Demonstrate knowledge and enthusiasm for your issue.

12. As appropriate, thank the individual for the meeting.

Coalition Building

Coalition building can be an effective tool for setting an agenda to influence a target audience. Coalitions can be official (formal) or unofficial (informal). Coalitions are alliances of organizations supporting a common policy goal, such as the Future of Nursing State Action Coalitions that have formed to advance nursing issues, the Nurses on Boards Coalition to promote nurses leadership in healthcare organizations, and the Immunization Action Coalition comprised of a wider group of healthcare professional groups. Coalitions marshal the energy of large numbers of people through organizations. The impact is greater when a coalition of several organizations supports a formal agenda than when separate organizations work alone. These partnerships demonstrate that organizations are not speaking from a narrow position of self-interest.

Nurse groups looking for other stakeholders not only should look to other groups such as state nurses associations, specialty nurses associations, and potentially aligned healthcare professional associations but also should reach out to business groups, patient safety groups, and other groups in the community whose agendas align. Nurses need to seek collaboration beyond the usual partners to develop coalitions. Just because a group has opposed a nursing initiative in the past does not mean that same group may not support a different initiative proposed by your nursing group. Hospital associations are often powerful voices at state capitals and may oppose a certain nursing agenda one year only to support it the next due to unrelated political pressures. Credible organizations take policy positions by issue, less often by "group." As consensus builds on your agenda, the merits of your solution should spread through the policy community.

Raising Awareness of the Agenda

Creating public awareness can also increase your group's chances of getting on a legislative agenda. Increasing public understanding of the scope of a problem increases your group's chances of regulatory, legislative, and other success. Numerous junctures and outlets exist for raising awareness of your agenda. Research studies, posters, protests, media campaigns, fundraising events, educational speeches, and informational flyers are all tactics that can be used to raise awareness of your interest group's policy agenda.

Social media is also an effective way to raise awareness of an issue. Social media facilitates the contributions of individuals in influencing agendas, which historically was missing in traditional constructions of agenda-setting models. With social media, any individual or organization can join and influence the communication dynamic. With social media's potential for vast reach stemming from one individual or one interest group, individuals, and groups with traditionally less power can stimulate the awareness of people, with the greater societal interest, in turn, pressuring powerful stakeholders to pay attention to an otherwise ignored issue.

Raising awareness of your identified policy agenda and your proposed solution can motivate people to support your cause or to actively join your interest group. This can cause a ripple effect so that others contact policymakers on your behalf and spread the word, creating an even greater awareness and, in turn, increasing the likelihood that your agenda will receive support from key policymakers (see Chapter 10). Raising awareness via social media and other mediums is important because the extent to which key stakeholders have knowledge and understanding of an issue matters not only to stakeholders taking positions but also speaks to the larger issue of priorities and agenda setting by key decision-makers.

Highlighting how your group's solution fits within the existing healthcare policy agendas to improve quality and safety while increasing access and cost-efficiencies is another media tip. As the most trusted health profession, when presented thoughtfully and with an eye toward the nation's current temperature and healthcare priorities, nursing's voice should be clearly heard in the offices of legislators and administrators. Nurses should have a powerful seat in redesigning the future of healthcare, particularly after the deficits in the system were exposed by the COVID-19 pandemic (Anders, 2020).

An important caveat about raising awareness is the need to speak with one unified voice. Cohesion among the group provides a distinct advantage in getting buy-in for an agenda. With numerous associations representing nurses, it is vital to speak with one voice to convince policymakers that an issue has support. An often-heard lament in the past is that nurses did not always speak with one voice. It does not take much to imagine the importance and power of over 4.3 million nurses speaking with a single, united voice.

FOCUSING THE AGENDA

An important step in agenda setting is focusing the agenda to maximize the influence of policy decisions. This includes assessing the most appropriate jurisdiction and determining whether legislative, regulatory, or judicial approaches would be most beneficial in advancing the agenda.

Jurisdiction

An important concrete step is determining who has jurisdiction over your identified issue. In other words, who is the decision-making body with the power to implement your agenda? Is legislative action necessary, or can the issue be remedied more expeditiously through a rulemaking process at an agency level?

At the state level, health policy issues may fall within the purview of the state's department of health. Issues relating to hospitals, ambulatory surgery centers, and other healthcare facilities often fall within the state agency responsible for licensing, certification, and/or oversight of such facilities. Scope-of-practice issues and other issues specific to licensed healthcare professionals fall under the state board with licensing authority, such as the board of nursing (BON) for RNs and APRNs and the board of medicine for physicians and, often, physician assistants. An effective way for nurses to influence healthcare policy and delivery in their state is to get to know their state BON. Many state boards rely on practicing nurses as clinical experts; when an issue comes before a board that relates to a certain specialty, board members reach out to their nursing friends and colleagues in that field for advice and guidance. Some nurses may find that they want to influence policy more directly by serving as a member of the BON or a state agency's advisory committee. Because state health departments tend to regulate hospitals and ambulatory surgery centers, another way for nurses to influence healthcare policy in their state is to get to know the department staff responsible for the agency's policy decisions in their area of practice.

Although we generally think of jurisdiction in relation to government entities, it is just as important to consider jurisdiction in relation to a healthcare organization, community group, or association. The goal is the same: to advance the agenda with the individuals or groups who have the power to make the decision. For example, nurses may complain to the materials management department about the ineffectiveness of a product rather than taking the issue to a nurse practice council, which might examine policy and safety related to the product's use and collect relevant data and evidence to make a change. Sometimes nurses, in frustration and without investigation of available channels and resources, ask a favorite physician or involve a patient to "complain" and hopefully get the intended change, as well as to champion an issue when the nursing department clearly has the primary jurisdiction. This "work-around" may create anger, stall progress on the agenda item, foster the status quo, perpetuate the myth of nurses being powerless, and create significant unintended consequences. Going through others who do not have the authority to handle the problem may backfire and is not often recommended.

Once you understand the jurisdictional context for your agenda, the next step in the process is venue shopping. "Venue shopping refers to the activities of advocacy groups and policymakers who seek out a decision setting where they can air their grievances with current policy and present alternative policy proposals"

(Pralle, 2003, p. 233). Venue shopping is a legitimate strategy for ensuring success as groups seek the branch or agency of government or institution to lobby or persuade to receive a sympathetic hearing (Birkland, 2020, p. 175). For example, for nearly 25 years, nurse practitioners (NPs) in Pennsylvania fought to obtain prescriptive privileges. When the first regulations were passed, they only applied to NPs collaborating with medical physicians, not osteopaths. This created a separate set of practice requirements based on which type of physician the NP was working with in a practice setting; very often, it was both in the same setting. The NPs were gearing up to go through the entire rulemaking process again with the osteopathic board, but instead, a legal ruling was made, also applying the regulations to collaborations with osteopaths. In this instance, changing the focus from creating a regulation to interpreting the existing regulation resulted in success for the NPs, allowing the agenda to move on to removing other practice barriers and gaining full practice authority for NPs; the most effective venue for this would be legislation.

Legislation

The first assumption that typically comes to mind when thinking of policy and advocacy work by an interest group is that the group is working to pass a new law. Not all agendas involve legislative activities. Legislation is often viewed as an ideal solution to a problem, and the passage of laws can be a very effective way to achieve the group's goals for the agenda. Legislation is often preferred over regulation because once a proposed solution is passed into law, it is less likely that the legislature or a new administration will later work to reverse the action, particularly as individuals and stakeholders begin their compliance efforts and the effect of the law becomes visible to society.

Another decision that needs to be made is determining which legislative body is the most appropriate for advancing your agenda. Consideration needs to be given to the likelihood of success in one legislative arena or another and the long-term implications for success. A critical mass of successes at the local or state level may be necessary before other jurisdictions will consider an agenda item. Cigarette smoke–free environments began with success in county and municipal jurisdictions before success could be achieved at the state level. For example, Chicago adopted a smoke-free policy before it was adopted by Illinois. Likewise, when working with national organizations, deciding where—which states and/or federal—to advance an agenda first can be strategic in terms of subsequent successes.

Regulation

Regulations made by state and federal agencies with rulemaking authority present opportunities for policy gains for interest groups. Agencies with directors who are appointed by the president or a governor are more accountable to the current executive administration's policy agenda, whereas agencies created by statute with staffing decisions made further outside the purview of a current administration might be more likely to attend to an issue not prominently on the current administration's agenda. The political leanings of an agency's leadership inevitably sway the agency's direction on rules, regulations, and other guidance. Elections have a direct influence on broad policy agendas and can, because of the appointment process, determine the partisan composition of agencies and Congress, which must approve many of a president's appointments (Birkland, 2020).

These appointed positions can be opportunities for nurses. For example, Mary Wakefield, PhD, RN, FAAN, who has a long history as a health policy activist, was named administrator of the Health Resources & Services Administration (HRSA) by President Barack Obama on February 20, 2009. The HRSA is a critical agency of the U.S. Department of Health and Human Services (DHHS). In this position, Dr. Wakefield's expertise was instrumental in expanding the use of RNs and improving services for the uninsured or underserved population while addressing severe provider shortages across the country. The nursing community supported Dr. Wakefield for the HRSA position and was pleased to see this major milestone for nursing. In 2015, Dr. Wakefield was appointed acting deputy secretary of the DHHS, becoming one of the highest ranking nurses in the federal government, a post she held until the Trump administration took office in 2017. It is the general practice for political appointees at the federal and state level to be replaced when the administration changes. In fact, with the change from the Trump administration to the Biden–Harris administration after the 2020 elections, Dr. Wakefield was tapped by the Biden–Harris administration to add the voice of nursing to the new administration's transition team.

Some legislation designates an agency to implement regulations to enforce the law. Laws governing nursing (e.g., state nurse practice acts) designate the state BON in most states as the implementing authority. Often, laws governing hospitals and other healthcare facilities designate the state department of health or another licensing body as the regulatory authority. The DHHS, within which the Centers for Medicare and Medicaid Services, the Agency for Healthcare Research and Quality, the Food and Drug Administration, the National Institutes of Health, and the Centers for Disease Control and Prevention reside, is often the federal regulatory authority for implementing federal healthcare laws.

The regulatory process is intended as a way for agencies with more expertise than legislators to add specificity to laws by providing implementation, interpretations, definitions, and compliance and enforcement provisions. For example, a nurse overtime law in a state may generally prohibit mandatory nurse overtime in hospitals. Further explanation of the prohibition and important definitions, such as definitions of *overtime* or *on call*, might then be provided by the state agency charged with oversight responsibilities for hospitals. Such rules and regulations can be adopted only by state agencies after a specific rulemaking process, typically set forth in a state's administrative procedure law. The specifics vary by state but, generally require agencies to publish proposed rules in advance and allow a specified period for public comment and possibly a hearing. Agencies are to consider all comments before issuing final regulations or rules.

Agencies can also take action that falls shy of regulation but still may have an enormous impact. Some agencies have the power to issue advisory opinions, reports, and other guidance that is outside of the rulemaking process. For example, state boards of nursing offer position statements, advisory opinions, and other guidance for the RNs licensed under their jurisdiction. This guidance is less formal than regulation but is nevertheless intended to guide the practice of nursing in a particular state and often does have the same practical effect as regulation.

Another example is when a state agency is charged with studying an issue and then publishing a report, either for the legislature or for another government body. For example, after a failed legislative initiative to mandate certification for surgical technologists in hospitals and ambulatory surgery centers, the Washington State Department of Health was asked to conduct a thorough review to examine the public policy impact of changing the surgical technology profession's scope of practice.

In September 2012, after collecting written comments and holding a hearing on the issue of requiring surgical technologists working in Washington hospitals and ambulatory surgery centers to hold and maintain national certification, the health department issued a 216-page comprehensive report that included the presentations from those who submitted comments and testified at the hearing. The report recommended against mandatory certification of surgical technologists with a detailed recommendation and its rationale for the Washington legislature (Washington State Department of Health, 2012). Similarly, the Washington State Department of Health issued a report on Midwifery Scope of Practice in 2013, recommending confirmation that licensed midwives' scope of practice includes medical aid to an infant up to 2 weeks old. These reports do not have the force of law or even regulation, and legislators are not bound to follow them though they often do.

Much healthcare policy also happens at the institutional level. How a hospital interprets and implements a practice, a state regulation, or a standard from The Joint Commission can vary. Nurses must establish channels to provide their expertise as institutions adopt and revise healthcare policies and directives. Even items such as continuing education programs, hospital newsletters, staff development initiatives, and serving on hospital committees and task forces offer opportunities for nurses to shape and influence healthcare delivery within their institutions.

One example of hospitals leading policy changes is in the area of healthy and sustainable food. Many hospitals across the nation are taking part in the healthy food initiatives focusing on both nutrition and food sustainability in response to a Healthy Food in Health Care program, an initiative of the Health Care Without Harm organization (Knudson, 2013). Hospitals are leading changes in communities by using their enormous purchasing power to favor local organic fruits and vegetables and healthy food from sustainable sources. Some healthcare systems have developed initiatives to reduce food insecurity in their communities. Examples of baseline policy actions facilities in the program might initially include taking a pledge or formally adopting a policy. Hospitals that have been successful in implementing change have used interprofessional teams, with nurses heavily involved and often leading the efforts.

Litigation

The legal system is another policy strategy used by interest groups to advance a cause or seek an intended outcome. In addition to resolving claims and disputes between individuals and corporations and adjudicating the innocence or guilt of persons accused of violating criminal laws, our American judicial system is used to establish, affirm, or clarify constitutional and statutory rights. Litigation initiated to accomplish policy outcomes is known as *impact litigation*. For example, in June 2012, in response to a challenge brought by many states' attorneys general, the U.S. Supreme Court upheld President Barack Obama's landmark healthcare reform legislation, the Patient Protection and Affordable Care Act (ACA) (*National Federation of Independent Business v. Sebelius*, 2012). The ACA has sustained numerous challenges since the 2012 ruling, with the next ruling expected in January 2021. *Brown v. Board of Education* (1954), the landmark case declaring state laws establishing that separate schools for Black and White students are unconstitutional, was a result of impact litigation. However, using litigation to enforce existing legislation or regulations can be very expensive. The American Civil Liberties Union (ACLU) is a well-known example of a funded interest group that uses impact litigation to accomplish its policy goals. The ACLU has more than 1 million members who financially support its work; its litigation efforts are paid for by member dues, contributions from individuals, and grants from private foundations. The

ANA and state and national specialty associations have impacted litigation that is important to the profession's agenda while protecting RNs and patients' rights and well-being.

Another way to use the legal system is to file amicus briefs in cases of interest to the group but in which the group is not actually a party. *Amicus curiae* means "friend of the court" in Latin. Interest groups may file amicus briefs with a court to provide information on the possible legal effects of a court decision and its potential impact on others who are not party to the litigation. For example, the ANA, the Louisiana State Nurses Association, and the Louisiana Alliance of Nursing Organizations filed an amicus brief to support the full scope of practice for certified registered nurse anesthetists (CRNAs). The focus of the brief was specific to CRNAs' interventional pain management (e.g., injection of local anesthetics).

Although the options for venues may vary with the issue and the particular locale, agenda setting is an important part of the policy process. The Policy Solution illustrates one route taken in a Colorado healthcare facility for addressing the hazards of surgical smoke. Other options or combinations of options may work better in other settings and may include different groups of stakeholders. It is to our advantage to think outside of the box in considering possibilities for setting the agenda.

| POLICY SOLUTION | Finding the Courage to be a Smoke Evacuation Advocate |

Melony Prince, MSN, RN, CNOR

While the policy solution for smoke evacuation would seem to end with the passage of legislation; it did not. These initiatives need to be extended with the passage of legislation in other states and moving other agendas or issues of concern to nurses forward. Nurses are encouraged to leverage their powerful voices to get legislators to listen and understand why no one should be forced to breathe surgical smoke or endure other workplace hazards and issues. These include sharing impactful stories, demonstrating the effectiveness of a solution that addresses the issue, and engaging in strategic partnerships. These tips can be adapted and applied to other legislative and policy initiatives. They are equally applicable when addressing a variety of issues within a healthcare organization, community settings, and regulatory bodies. Here are strategies that are most helpful:

1. **Share Stories**

   When you stand up to testify, share the stories of those you know or those you've read about in research articles and about real people, real nurses, and surgeons who are battling respiratory cancers and other illnesses linked to the exposure of surgical smoke. The story about Eva caught the attention of legislators and got them listening.

2. **Show Them How Smoke Evacuators Work**

   There was confusion during the discussion of the bill about the cost of smoke evacuation because some legislators thought incorrectly that smoke evacuation must be physically incorporated into the hospital's heating, ventilation, and air-conditioning (HVAC) system. Surgical smoke evacuator pens were brought to the floor. It was demonstrated how simple the pens were to use, which won over some initial skeptics.

3. **Don't Go It Alone**

   Understanding the details of getting a bill passed is too much for one nurse or even a group of nurses to tackle. In this example, help from AORN and its external support with a lobbyist on the floor and colleagues from around the state we were able to make change.

IMPLICATIONS FOR THE FUTURE

As you take steps to implement your agenda, you will begin to see political ramifications and responses. Nurses should capitalize on their unique professional talents to establish and advance their agenda. Nurses have the skills and courage to lead and influence health policy and development during the COVID-19 era (Anders, 2020). Nurses use their best attributes every day to manage conflict, cope with challenging personalities, and diffuse potentially explosive situations, all in the name of patient care and safety. It is well established that teamwork is essential for patient safety (Kalisch et al., 2009). Nurse advocates must draw on these same talents and skills as they engage in policy discussions at both individual and institutional levels. "Once a nurse is motivated to try to change or develop policy, and becomes engaged in the process, many of the basic approaches to work and problem-solvingdeveloped in nursing education and practice prove useful" (Gebbie et al., 2000, p. 314). Nurses are people of action, and their involvement in improving healthcare for all by serving as advocates is central to the nursing practice (Anders, 2020).

KEY CONCEPTS

1. Agenda setting is a complex process involving the laying out of problems and solutions so that the issue comes to the attention of the public and governmental officials.
2. Agendas are designed to influence events, news, and understandings.
3. The context of an agenda, timing, political climate, and political realities are important in the agenda-setting process.
4. Organizations, or groups within an organization, work to get their priority issue on the agenda to influence policy.
5. An organization's agenda needs to be linked to its mission and strategic plan to gain traction with key stakeholders.
6. Agendas have levels of increasing specificity: agenda universe, systemic agenda, institutional or organizational agenda, and decision agenda. Issues need to reach the institutional agenda to achieve progress toward a decision.
7. Nurses need to own the agenda for their practice, within their organizations, and within the profession.
8. Agenda development includes defining the problem and establishing the agenda.
9. Numerous internal and external factors influence whether an issue gains prominence on the agenda; these include a new administration, new leadership, unpredictable events, finances, public acceptance, opposition of powerful interests, or competing issues.
10. Knowing the numerous stakeholders and their varying degrees of support are invaluable in planning strategies for moving an agenda forward.
11. Interest groups, including associations, corporations, and consumer groups, may be supportive, neutral, or opposed to an agenda.
12. Understanding obstacles to an agenda facilitates designing a strategy to move an agenda forward.
13. Networking provides opportunities to build relationships with legislators, regulators, and key organizational and community leaders.
14. Coalitions provide an opportunity to expand influence in support of a common policy goal.

15. Raising awareness of an agenda either in the public arena or within an organization increases the chance of moving the agenda forward.

16. Speaking with a unified voice is important to the success of an agenda.

17. Focusing an agenda on a specific venue, such as legislative, regulatory, or judicial, can be strategic in maximizing successes.

18. Agenda setting is a process that can be used both in the public arena and within organizations to achieve important policy goals.

SUMMARY

Setting the agenda is a process that is in constant flux, and strategies need to change to reflect the dynamics of the situation. Policy changes rarely happen quickly. Advocates must be prepared, persistent, and patient in their approach to changes. Windows of opportunity may open and close over years or an even shorter time. Just when your group is about to close in on a regulatory success, a key agency personnel or elected official change may derail your efforts. Maintaining a long view is helpful and healthy. During times when your legislature is not in session or executives sensitive to your issue are not in office, do not sit idle.

Remain focused and monitor your policy-makers' agenda. Seize opportunities to raise your issue on that agenda. Keep your group and grassroots advocates engaged and prepared. Review and refine your messaging. Meet with public officials and legislators and their staff to educate them about your issue, even if you know this is not the year your issue will advance on the policy agenda. Stay committed to your group's mission and goals while continuing to redefine your policy issue as needed. Work to identify a solution in ways that stand the best chance of resonating with the largest number of policy-makers and stakeholders.

END-OF-CHAPTER RESOURCES

LEARNING ACTIVITIES

1. Determine the policy issues important to the governor in your state, your local representative, and one professional nursing organization. Describe the methods you used to obtain the information and critique the ease of access among the three sources.

2. Talk to a nurse leader or identify for yourself how a new agenda in management or in shared governance has been successfully or unsuccessfully introduced.

3. Identify the details of your state governor's agenda items that relate to healthcare. Compare those agenda items with the agenda of the nursing organizations with which you are involved and describe how you could frame your nursing organization's issues within the state executive's agenda.

4. Find fact sheets from various organizations, including a national organization, a state organization, and a consumer group, and identify strengths and weaknesses. Try to find fact sheets from opposing groups on the same issue and compare how the groups define the problem.

5. Find examples of press releases and other materials designed to increase public awareness of an issue. For example, the Coalition for Patients' Rights issues press releases and media stories designed to educate the public about the importance of the patient's right to choose providers. Can you find others?

6. Locate a health policy stakeholder's mission statement and/or strategic plan and identify how a practice issue that you believe needs to be on the agenda fits with the statement or plan.

E-RESOURCES

- Agency for Healthcare Research and Quality. Setting the agenda for research on cultural competence in health care http://www.ahrq.gov/research/findings/factsheets/literacy/cultural/index.html

- American Nurses Association http://www.nursingworld.org

- American Nurses Association. Gun violence https://ana.aristotle.com/sitePages/gunviolence.aspx

- American Nurses Association. Health system reform agenda https://www.nursingworld.org/practice-policy/health-policy/health-system-reform/

- Campaign for Action https://campaignforaction.org/

- Canadian Nurses Association. Nursing and the political agenda http://www.cna-aiic.ca/en/advocacy/nursing-and-the-political-agenda

- Immunization Action Coalition https://www.immunize.org/

- National Council for Research on Women https://www.2020wob.com/affiliate/national-council-research-women-ncrw

- Nurses on Boards Coalition https://www.nursesonboardscoalition.org/

- Oncology Nursing Society. Research Agenda of the Oncology Nursing Society https://onf.ons.org/onf/46/6/research-agenda-oncology-nursing-society-2019-2022

- World Health Organization. *Health service planning and policy-making: A toolkit for nurses and midwives, WHO Module 2: Stakeholder analysis and networks* https://apps.who.int/iris/bitstream/handle/10665/207061/9290611863_mod2_eng.pdf?sequence=5&isAllowed=y

REFERENCES

American Nurses Association v. Tom Torlakson. (2013). S184583 Ct. App C061150 Sacramento County Super. Ct. No. 07AS04631. http://www.cde.ca.gov/ls/he/hn/documents/anavtorlakson2013.pdf

Anders, R. (2020). Engaging nurses in health policy in the era of COVID-19. *Nursing Forum, 56*(1), 89–94. https://doi.org/10.1111/nuf.12514

Association of periOperative Registered Nurses. (2022). Guideline for surgical smoke safety. In *Guidelines for perioperative practice.*

Balestra, M. (2012). Amicus brief supports administration of insulin to students only by licensed nurses. *Journal of Nursing Law, 15*(1), 27–32. https://doi.org/10.1891/1073-7472.15.1.27

Birkland, T. A. (2016). *An introduction to the policy process: Theories, concepts, and models of public policy making* (4th ed.). M. E. Sharpe.

Birkland, T. A. (2020). *An introduction to the policy process: Theories, concepts, and models of public policy making* (5th ed.). Routledge.

Brown v. Board of Education. (1954). 347 U.S. 483. https://supreme.justia.com/cases/federal/us/347/483/

Cobb, R. W., & Elder, C. D. (1972). *Participation in American politics: The dynamics of agenda-building.* Allyn & Bacon.

Evans, G. (2018, November 1). Rhode Island passes landmark law protecting HCWs from surgical smoke. *Hospital Employee Health.* https://www.reliasmedia.com/articles/143416-rhode-island-passes-landmark-law-protecting-hcws-from-surgical-smoke

Gallup. (n.d.). *Most important problem.* https://news.gallup.com/poll/1675/most-important-problem.aspx

Gebbie, K. M., Wakefield, M., & Kerfoot, K. (2000). Nursing and health policy. *Journal of Nursing Scholarship, 32*(3), 307–315. https://doi.org/10.1111/j.1547-5069.2000.00307.x

Giese, K. (2020). Coronavirus disease's 2019 shake-up of telehealth policy: Application of Kingdon's multiple streams framework. *The Journal for Nurse Practitioners, 6*(10), 768–770. https://doi.org/10.1016/j.nurpra.2020.08.015

Grossman, M. (2012). Interest group influence on US policy change: An assessment based on policy history. *Interest Groups and Advocacy, 1*(2), 171–192. https://doi.org/10.1057/iga.2012.9

Healthy Choices for Healthy Children Act. (2010). *Ohio general assembly SB 210.* http://archives.legislature.state.oh.us/bills.cfm?ID=128_SB_210

Institute of Medicine. (2000). *To err is human: Building a safer health system.* The National Academies Press. https://doi.org/10.17226/9728

Institute of Medicine. (2011). *The future of nursing: Leading change, advancing health.* National Academies Press. https://doi.org/10.17226/12956

International Safety Center. (2020). *Moving the sharps safety in healthcare agenda forward in the United States: 2020 Consensus statement and call to action.* https://internationalsafetycenter.org/wp-content/uploads/2020/12/Moving_The_Sharps_Safety_In_Healthcare_Agenda_Forward_In_The_US.pdf

Kalisch, B. J., Weaver, S. J., & Salas, E. (2009). What does nursing teamwork look like? A qualitative study. *Journal of Nursing Care Quality, 24*(4), 298–307. https://doi.org/10.1097/NCQ.0b013e3181a001c0

Kingdon, J. W. (2011). *Agendas, alternatives, and public policies* (2nd ed.). Pearson.

Knudson, L. (2013). Healthier hospital food can affect health of patients and the planet. *AORN Journal, 97*(6), C1, C9–C10. https://doi.org/10.1016/S0001-2092(13)00474-2

National Federation of Independent Business v. Sebelius. (2012). 567 U.S. 519 132 S.Ct. 2566. http://www.scotusblog.com/case-files/cases/national-federation-of-independent-business-v-sebelius

National Institute for Occupational Safety and Health. (2017). *Health and safety practices survey of healthcare workers: Surgical smoke.* https://www.cdc.gov/niosh/topics/healthcarehsps/smoke.html

Peters, B. G. (2019). *American public policy: Promise and performance* (11th ed.). CQ Press.

Pralle, S. B. (2003). Venue shopping as political strategy: The internationalization of Canadian forest advocacy. *Journal of Public Policy, 23*(3), 233–260. https://doi.org/10.1017/S0143814X03003118

Swift, A. (2017, August 10). *Government, healthcare most important problems in the U.S.* http://news.gallup.com/poll/215645/government-healthcare-important-problems.aspx

Waddell, K. (2017, January 23). The exhausting work of tallying America's largest protest. *The Atlantic.* https://www.theatlantic.com/technology/archive/2017/01/womens-march-protest-count/514166/

Washington State Department of Health. (2012). *Surgical technologist certification.* http://www.doh.wa.gov/Portals/1/Documents/2000/SurgTechCert.pdf

Washington State Department of Health. (2013). *Midwifery scope of practice sunrise review. Summary of information and recommendations.* https://www.doh.wa.gov/Portals/1/Documents/Pubs/631045.pdf

World Health Organization. (2020). *State of the world's nursing report 2020: Investing in education, jobs and leadership.* https://www.who.int/publications/i/item/9789240003279

UNIT III

Strategizing and Creating Change

Building Capital: Intellectual, Social, Political, and Financial

LAUREN INOUYE AND COLLEEN LENERS

We in America do not have government by the majority. We have a government by the majority who participate.
—*Thomas Jefferson*

OBJECTIVES

1. Compare and contrast the types of capital used in policy and advocacy.
2. Understand the impact of capital on policy outcomes.
3. Explore competencies to successfully build capital, given an advocate's resources.
4. Examine the contributions and challenges of coalitions in developing political capital.
5. Discuss the critical role of lobbying and its impact on nursing.
6. Compare the phenomena of the "free-rider syndrome" and grassroots in relation to the impact on the nursing profession.

What does building capital truly mean, how does it shape policy, and to what extent is it important for nurses to engage in developing capital? At its core, capital is a necessary tool that can shape status, power, and reputation—in other words, influence. Capital can be developed in intellectual, social, political, and financial forms. For the individual, capital has ramifications on personal and professional life. For example, capital could be used to win the school board election or secure a promotion at work. Capital is necessary for state and national organizations to be effective in their mission. National organizations seeking to be leaders in health policy development and implementation may use all forms of capital to their advantage. Essentially, the more capital an individual, group, or institution controls, the more effective it is in influencing and shaping policy.

It is critical to understand not only how important it is to build capital, but also how to amplify the resources necessary to do so. Therefore, this chapter explores the individual nurse's role in developing personal capital, as well as how the individual nurse supports the growth of the profession's resources. Figure 7.1 illustrates the centrality of the nurse to the policy-making process.

Each type of capital is examined for its role in policymaking at the big-P level (e.g., federal or state policies) and little-p level (e.g., policies where you work and live). Nurses and the nursing profession have all the essential resources for maximizing the forms of capital to engage policymakers at the local, state, and national levels. The Policy Challenge highlighted here demonstrates the use of capital at the national level.

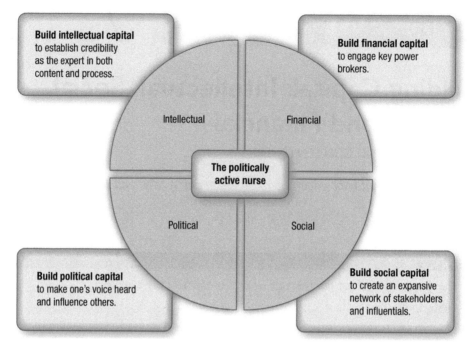

FIGURE 7.1 Creating capital for nurses' political engagement.

As we see in this Policy Challenge, nurses have multiple time points in their careers to maximize their capital to influence policies that would ultimately impact nursing and healthcare. This chapter explores the four types of capital (i.e., intellectual, social, political, financial), their interdependency, and ways that they can be maximized to advance healthcare policy. The introductory Policy Challenge and subsequent Policy Solution demonstrate how gaining political capital can accumulate from experience and challenging yourself to take opportunities when they arise.

| POLICY CHALLENGE | Gaining Political Capital by Being Part of a Team |

Colleen Leners, DNP, APRN, FAAN, FAANP
Director of Policy, American Association of Colleges of Nursing, Washington, DC

The routes to gaining political capital are varied. This Policy Challenge illustrates how one's professional experiences can be strategically used to develop political capital. I am a daughter of a nurse and grew up in a family in which politics was not discussed. My parents had differing political opinions and party affiliations, which taught me that there were two sides to every story. I obtained an associate degree in nursing and launched my career in the ED of a California hospital. I joined the U.S. Navy Reserves and became a nurse practitioner (NP) while still working in the civilian sector. My reserve duty varied as an NP from physical examinations to the care of mothers and children.

A turning point in my career came when I decided to join the U.S. Army so that I could apply my trauma and family medicine knowledge and expertise (my intellectual capital) to those serving on the front lines in Iraq. Leaving three children in the care of my mother, I deployed in 2005, worked in Tikrit, a battered city some 80 miles north of Baghdad, the Iraqi capital. The conditions were trying to say the least, even living in tents for short times. My responsibility was outpatient care in a combat support hospital, a role that included care and triage of mass casualties with oversight of a team of nurses, physicians, and other personnel. Working as a team was all important. One day a surgeon said to me, "I forgot you were a nurse." I responded that I forgot that he was a surgeon. I also worked off the base teaching emergency medical care. While off base, I provided care to people living in those areas. Informally, I provided advice and counsel to younger nurses, brand-new nurses, and personnel who were put in combat zones. These efforts resulted in my being awarded a Bronze Star. But in my heart, the real heroes are the ones who do not come home.

On returning to the United States, I had a persistent bad cough and was subsequently diagnosed with follicular lymphoma, most likely attributable to breathing air from open burning pits while in Iraq. I received a medical retirement. It was difficult to navigate the system and receive consistent treatment. Electronic health record interoperability between the health records of the Department of Defense and Veterans Affairs did not exist. If I was having difficulty with the system, how were enlisted personnel with no arms or legs and maybe a high school education going to manage? It upset me as a provider, a wounded warrior, and a veteran. This fueled my passion to make a difference for our soldiers and our veterans. It led me to apply for a Robert Wood Johnson Fellowship. I thought that my placement would be working directly with the Veterans Affairs Committee, but that was not to be.

See Policy Solution

INTELLECTUAL CAPITAL

Intellectual capital for nursing is the knowledge of an individual or the collective knowledge of a group that can be expended to influence policymakers to use or adopt suggestions, viewpoints, and solutions about healthcare and the healthcare environment. Nurses have the brainpower to effectively influence policy at both the big-P and little-p levels. They can also draw on a large body of research from nursing and other disciplines to support their policy initiatives (see Chapter 5).

Nurses in every type of position have intellectual capital that can be used to inform, communicate, and advance nursing and healthcare agendas. Nurses may not realize the extent of their intellectual capital when communicating with federal, state, and local officials, very few of whom have a healthcare background. These officials may have no practical context for what it is like to provide care to a patient, run a nurse-managed health clinic, or educate the next generation of nurses. Only nurses have this expertise.

Legislation may be necessary to improve access to care for individuals who use community clinics. For example, legislation designed to reimburse clinics for diabetes education might also include considerations related to the social determinants of health. Barriers may involve health literacy and accessible transportation that prevent patients from being able to self-manage their care. Nurses working with patients can provide these valuable insights to officials who oversee policy at the big-P and little-p levels in a variety of organizations. Policymakers rely on their expert constituents to provide them with the background across a broad spectrum of healthcare policies. Most of the time, officials and elected leaders do not reach out to an individual constituent for advice unless they have an established relationship (see Social Capital).

Social media is an important communication channel for constituents. According to 2015 data from the Congressional Management Foundation (CMF, 2015) 76% of surveyed federal legislative staff responded that they "agree" or "strongly agree" that "social media enabled us to have more meaningful interactions with constituents" (p. 10). In addition, 63% of respondents reported that they believe constituent communications will come in social media form more than email, phone, or other means in the next 5 to 10 years (CMF, 2015). Little did anyone know that the COVID-19 pandemic would rapidly accelerate the use of electronic platforms and social media as daily modes of communication between legislators, their staff, and constituents. In a June 2020 survey, 65% of House and Senate senior staff reported that their Representatives/Senators were videoconferencing with constituents "significantly more" than prior to the pandemic; 44% were conducting more virtual townhall meetings, and 26% were participating more in Facebook livestreaming and Q&A sessions (CMF, 2020).

The Big-P

In 2010, the Robert Wood Johnson Foundation (RWJF), in collaboration with Gallup, conducted a survey of over 1,500 healthcare thought leaders (e.g., from government and the healthcare sector) to ask their opinions about the role that nurses play and can play in policy (Khoury et al., 2011) The large majority reported that nurses should have a greater part in policy. Few nurses even today would argue that nursing's full intellectual power has been capitalized on in the policy arena. Change is needed as outlined in the updated *Future of Nursing 2020–2030: Charting a Path to Achieve Health Equity* report (National Academies, 2021). Nurses are called on to participate in formulating and implementing policies that will positively impact the health and social well-being of the most people.

Nurses and other leaders across the country believe that the science, experience, and skills unique to the nursing profession can drive positive transformations. However, policy can seem an elusive process to many individual nurses. As a result, this section first discusses some ways that individual nurses have capitalized on their unique skills at the level of the federal government.

The nursing profession is not in short supply of experts. From nationally and internationally renowned nurse researchers to the nurse practicing at the bedside, every nurse is an expert and can drive change from personal knowledge. A textbook example of a nurse using intellectual capital to inform policy change is Mary Naylor, PhD, RN, FAAN, professor and director of the New Courtland Center for Transitions and Health at the University of Pennsylvania. For years, Dr. Naylor demonstrated the successful use of advanced practice registered nurses (APRNs) to reduce readmission rates, known as the transitional care model. A similar model was adopted at the federal level. According to the Centers for Medicare & Medicaid Services Innovation Center (CMS Innovation Center), this program, the Community-Based Care Transitions Program, "tests models for improving care transitions from the hospital to other settings and reducing readmissions for high-risk Medicare beneficiaries" (CMS Innovation, 2013). This example illustrates how a nurse's expertise was used to shape national policy, but it may not be clear that vital to her success was her understanding of the policy process. Earlier in her career, Naylor had a W. K. Kellogg Foundation leadership fellowship with the Senate Committee on Aging. Many nurses carry out research, but they fail to tie their work to policy or are not savvy about the political process; thus, their research and expertise never achieve full fruition.

Therefore, it is important to understand that although expertise in an area is necessary, *intellectual capital* also refers to understanding the policy process and keeping abreast of policy issues. Congressional staff, nurse lobbyists, and medical lobbyists as groups have identified an understanding of the process as an essential strategy for moving an issue forward (Begeny, 2009). Understanding the intricacies of policymaking, like the timing of an issue, is vital to success. For example, if an intended goal is to increase funding for nursing education, knowing when to ask for increased funding or knowing when to support a request that has been made is vital. For example, requesting funding for federal programs must come during the time when Congress is developing its spending bills. A strong place to start learning this process and what is happening on the national agenda is through nurses associations (see Exhibit 7.1).

EXHIBIT 7.1 SELECTED RESOURCES FOR BUILDING INTELLECTUAL CAPITAL

Policy News From Nurses Associations
American Association of Colleges of Nursing's Washington Weekly: www.aacnnursing.org/Policy-Advocacy/About-Government-Affairs-and-Policy/Newsletters
American Nurses Association's Capital Beat: www.anacapitolbeat.org
Federal Agencies
Department of Health and Human Services Patient Protection and Affordable Care Act: www.healthcare.gov
Department of Health and Human Services: www.hhs.gov
Agency for Healthcare Research and Quality: www.ahrq.gov
Centers for Medicare & Medicaid Services: www.cms.gov
Health Resources & Services Administration: www.hrsa.gov/index.html
National Institutes of Health: www.nih.gov
National Journals, Nonprofit Organizations, and Think Tanks
Center for American Progress: www.americanprogress.org
Health Affairs: www.healthaffairs.org
Henry J. Kaiser Family Foundation: www.kff.org
Heritage Foundation: www.heritage.org
Robert Wood Johnson Foundation: www.rwjf.org
National Governors Association: www.nga.org/cms/home.html
Political Newspapers
Politico: www.politico.com
The Hill: thehill.com
Bloomberg Government: about.bgov.com
Association Toolkits
American Association of Colleges of Nursing AACN's Guide to Advocacy: August 2019 Edition: www.aacnnursing.org/Policy-Advocacy/Advocacy-Tool-Kit
American Association of Nurse Practitioners Federal Policy Toolkit: www.aanp.org/legislation-regulation/policy-toolkit
American Nurses Association Activist Toolkit: www.rnaction.org/site/PageServer?pagename=nstat_take_action_activist_tool_kit&ct=1&ct=1
Association of periOperative Registered Nurses Take Action Tools: www.aorn.org/community/government-affairs/advocacy-tools-and-resources
National Association of Clinical Nurse Specialist Legislative and Regulatory Toolkit: www.nacns.org/professional-resources/toolkits-and-reports/legislative-and-regulatory-toolkit
National Association of Neonatal Nurses Legislative Advocacy 101: www.nann.org/uploads/Advocacy_Fact_Sheets/Legislative_Advocacy_101.pdf

Nurses associations are rich with resources such as policy factsheets, newsletters, and web pages. Many associations send out monthly policy electronic newsletters that provide the most current actions occurring at the state and federal levels. Federal agencies, national journals, think tanks, and policy newspapers are all resources a nurse can use to build intellectual capital. These organizations and media sources report on what Congress is addressing and what healthcare topics are gaining or losing support. The importance of nurses associations is highlighted in the *Future of Nursing 2020–2030* report (National Academies, 2021) in its recommendation that nursing "nursing education programs, employers, nursing leaders, licensing board, and nursing organizations should initiate the implementation of structures, systems, and evidence-based interventions to promote nurses' health and well-being" (p. 13). Nurses have key roles to play through nursing organizations and other policy groups to advance nursing's future and its role in society.

To better hone both intellectual and political capital, consider getting help from lobbyists that nursing associations, universities, or healthcare systems can provide. Both types of lobbyists have an understanding about intellectual capital, often have relationships with congressional staff members, and can help arrange a meeting to discuss the issue at hand. They can assist in putting the research, data, and statistics into context for the legislator. Furthermore, when nurses' expertise is shared with their national or state associations, those organizations may use them as expert witnesses for a congressional or state legislative hearing.

Many state and specialty nursing associations also offer workshops in conjunction with what are referred to as *advocacy days* to learn the policy process. Advocacy days are events, usually a day long, held in a state or federal capital and sponsored by nursing associations. The event is educational and incorporates meetings with legislators and/or members of the governor's office. The goals are helping nurses understand the legislative process and providing them with proactive steps for advocating for their patients and practice. These events are open to nurses and nursing students and provide nursing associations the opportunity to brief their members and nursing students on the political climate and legislative requests.

Globally, nurses organizations are calling for nurses' increased leadership roles in advocacy and policy work; education for policy leadership and policy is critical (Turale & Kunaviktikul, 2019). Short-term programs are available for nurses and nursing students to develop their policy skills (see Exhibit 7.2). These programs are focused on helping nurses become stronger political leaders and expanding the grassroots capacity for the nursing profession by providing comprehensive health policy education and experiences. Attending these policy and advocacy programs opens the doors to endless possibilities. Aside from gaining information about the legislative processes that drive our federal government, the chance to network with other nurses and healthcare leaders is invaluable (social capital). It is important for nurses and nursing students wanting to become further involved in policy and advocacy to participate in opportunities that help build their knowledge base and professional experience because nurses are the best experts for their profession and can make a true and lasting impact.

EXHIBIT 7.2   OPPORTUNITIES TO BUILD INTELLECTUAL CAPITAL

For RNs   *American Nurses Advocacy Institute*   The ANA created the ANAI, a yearlong mentored program designed to develop nurses into stronger political leaders and expand grassroots capacity for the nursing profession and healthcare. To be considered, the nurse must belong to both the ANA and an SNA. On completion, each Fellow counsels the SNA in establishing legislative/regulatory priorities, recommends strategies for executing the advancement of a policy issue, and educates members about political realities, as well as assists in advancing the ANA's agenda.   www.nursingworld.org/practice-policy/advocacy   *The Alliance: Nursing Organization Alliance, Nurse in Washington Internship*   Open to any RN or nursing student (all levels of education) who is interested in learning about current issues in nursing and the legislative process. Each participant spends time meeting with his or her members of Congress while participating in the NIWI Annual Advocacy Days.   https://www.nursing-alliance.org/nurse-in-washington-internship
For APRNs   *AANP Health Policy Fellowship*   The AANP Health Policy Fellowship program provides AANP members with a comprehensive fellowship experience at the center of health policy and politics in Washington, DC. It is an outstanding opportunity for members with an interest in healthcare policy to promote the health of the nation and the advancement of NPs' ability to work within their full scope of practice.   www.aanp.org/legislation-regulation/federal-legislation/health-policy-fellowship
For Nursing Students   *American Association of Colleges of Nursing Student Policy Summit*   The SPS is a 3-day conference held in Washington, DC, and is open to baccalaureate and graduate nursing students enrolled at an AACN member institution. It is a didactic immersion program focused on the nurse's role in professional advocacy and the federal policy process (see Figure 7.2).   www.aacnnursing.org/Policy-Advocacy/Get-Involved/Student-Policy-Summit

AACN, American Association of Colleges of Nursing; AANP, American Association of Nurse Practitioners; ANA, American Nurses Association; ANAI, American Nurses Advocacy Institute; NIWI, Nurse in Washington Internship; NPs, nurse practitioners; SNA, state nurses association; SPS, student policy summit.

The Little-p

A nurse's individual expertise is vital to shaping policy change at every level, but nurses must be diligent to share this expertise. From the unit level to the hospital system level, the observation of one nurse could improve quality of care, save the healthcare system hundreds of thousands of dollars, improve the efficiency of care delivery, or develop a national policy standard. Yet, an exceptional idea never comes to fruition if it is not heard.

Empowered nurses can use their expertise to enact change in their organization (Bradbury-Jones, et al., 2008). On the contrary, if nurses do not feel empowered, feelings of frustration and failure emerge (Laschinger & Havens, 1996; Manojlovich, 2007). A thorough literature review conducted by Rao (2012) examined the concept of nurse empowerment over time. This analysis revealed that nurses have viewed empowerment through a lens that focuses on organizational

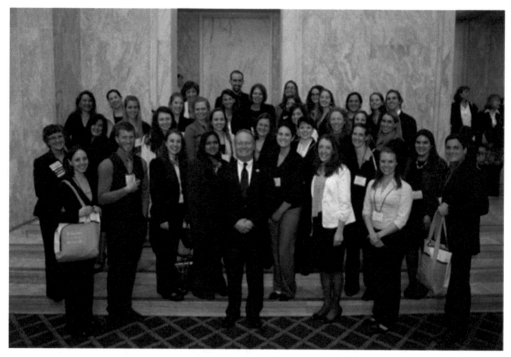

FIGURE 7.2 **American Association of Colleges of Nursing Student Policy Summit attendees, taking part in the association's advocacy day, are featured with the co-chair of the House Nursing Caucus, Representative David Joyce (R-OH; center).**

structure. According to Rao (2012), nurses rely "too heavily on rigid bureaucratic structures rather than their own professional power to guide practice. Limiting nurses in this way denies the professional power their role affords them and constrains their ability to achieve extraordinary outcomes" (p. 401). The first steps in many cases are recognizing one's intellectual capital and then overcoming the inertia and speaking out. At work, this process starts by regularly attending meetings and bringing forth issues that have policy implications, and nursing expertise can help guide these steps. Substantive policy changes often start when people see problems as they carry out their jobs. The policy may relate to an array of practice or clinical issues. Policy on the Scene 7.1 provides examples of how appointments can capitalize on nurses' intellectual capital.

POLICY ON THE SCENE 7.1: NURSES' APPOINTMENTS

In November 2020, President-Elect Joe Biden and Vice President-Elect Kamala Harris issued The Biden Plan to Combat Coronavirus (COVID-19) and Prepare for Future Global Health Threats. This plan outlines the incoming administration's proposal for how to combat the COVID-19 outbreak. The plan calls to "ensure that public health decisions are made by public health professionals and not politicians." Therefore, a COVID-19 Advisory Board was established to assist with the plans and policies to address the pandemic. The individuals selected to serve on this board included physicians and public health leaders. However, nursing was not represented, despite the intellectual capital that nurses bring to their roles combating COVID-19.

When the advisory board members were announced, it was clear to many nurses associations that the absence of nursing representation needed to be addressed. Therefore, a groundswell of professional nursing organizations, nursing coalitions, and individual nurses reached out to the Biden transition team requesting that a nurse be included. Additionally, nurses took to social media to raise awareness about the need for nursing representation, which they believed was necessary for formulating a truly interdisciplinary approach to problem-solving.

In late November, it was announced that Jane Hopkins, RN, MH, a registered nurse in Seattle, Washington, who emigrated from Sierra Leone, would be serving on the advisory board. Ms. Hopkins was serving on Washington state's COVID-19 Taskforce and Safe Start Advisory Board when she received the call from the Biden transition team asking her to serve. The outcome of securing nursing representation on this esteemed advisory board was the result of the transition team recognizing nursing's contributions, but it also stemmed from nurses wielding social capital.

SOCIAL CAPITAL

The second interdependent component is social capital. As noted, intellectual capital must be expended to be of benefit; it needs to be shared. Developing social capital is essentially relationship building. More specifically, relationships are built and nurtured with key decision makers at the state and national levels to influence policy change. For the nursing profession, social capital should be the most basic, intuitive, and strongest form of capital. Nurses create relationships with their patients, their patients' families, fellow nurses, managers, and so on. Contextually, it relates to the key elements that are necessary for a positive relationship, namely, honesty and trust. As is often repeated in this book but not always effectively capitalized on by nurses, the nursing profession consistently ranks highest among all others in ratings of honesty and ethics among the professions (Saad, 2020).

The Big-P

Social capital at the big-P level involves the development of relationships with appointed and elected officials. Members of Congress listen to the voices of their constituents. This is a reality that every lobbyist inherently knows well. It is constituents, not the registered lobbyists, who reelect legislators to serve another term. Therefore, the opinions of constituents are tremendously more relevant than any political wonk in the nation's capital. Even though many believe that and there is evidence that wealth plays an influential role in swaying policy, the value of constituents' opinions and support cannot be dismissed; however, constituents must make their opinions known.

To simply be a nurse constituent in the district of a member of Congress does not mean your voice will be heard among the other hundreds of thousands of constituents. You must be savvy. One of the best ways to accomplish this is to gain guidance from national or state nurses associations. If a nurse has an opportunity to directly communicate with a member of Congress, a nurses association's lobbyist could provide background on the member's political positions, information about what Congress is currently debating and what message would be most relevant, and talking points to help prepare for an interaction (see Chapter 10). This is the job of registered lobbyists: to prepare their members to be politically savvy through relationships or social capital. In relation to the big-P, political scientists have described these as *grasstops*.

Essentially, nursing needs to develop more grasstops. *Grasstops* are defined as leaders, such as those within an industry or field, who "usually know who within their sphere shares their interests and what other prominent leaders may be interested" (Gibson, 2010, p. 91). They also embody the social capital necessary to influence a member of Congress. "The member may listen to that person and no one else on a particular issue" (Gibson, 2010, p. 91). Many times, the grasstops are constituents who have supported members of Congress either politically (worked on a campaign) or financially (provided an individual donation to a campaign) or who are leaders in their industry (Goldstein, 1999).

An example of a grasstop is Tarik S. Khan, MSN, RN, FNP-BC, Pennsylvania State Nurses Association past president. Tarik is a nurse practitioner (NP) at Family Practice and Counseling, Philadelphia, Pennsylvania. He has a long history of advocacy and close relationships with legislators where he lives, where he works and where he grew up. During the COVID-19 pandemic, he has been working long hours in treating patients in his clinic. However, as an advocate for people with disabilities and the homebound, every night after work and on days off, he would spend up to 6 hours to rush leftover doses of COVID-19 vaccines to people who are homebound in the Philadelphia area and had no means of obtaining them. This garnered interviews with *People Magazine, The Philadelphia Inquirer*, MSNBC, *Good Morning America*, the *CBS Evening News*, and local television stations. He was also a panelist for a White House Virtual Forum on *Breaking Down Barriers for People who have Challenges Accessing COVID-19 Vaccination*. Tarik has over 15,300 followers on his Twitter feed, @InclusionPhilly. Tarik is one nurse who is making a difference through multiple strategies: caring for vulnerable populations, influencing legislators to understand the realities of healthcare delivery, and speaking out on nurses' issues through his association leadership. Tarik is at policy tables in his organization, his community, and at the national level. See Figure 7.3.

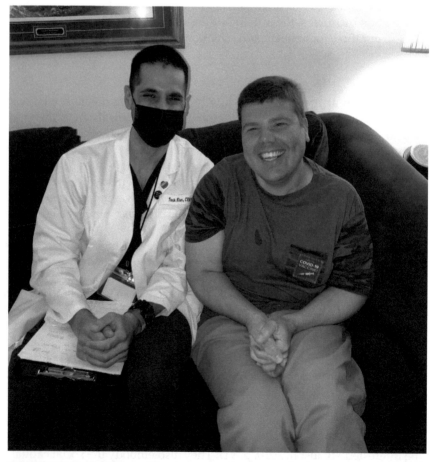

FIGURE 7.3 **Tarik Khan working to ensure the community has access to COVID-19 vaccines.**

To summarize, nursing can build its social capital by having individuals who are savvy (intellectual capital) and who have developed relationships with their elected representatives or staff: in other words, grasstops. The goal is to develop a meaningful relationship. That relationship helps the individual nurse be a valued and trusted resource to that member of Congress. At the core of social capital is developing a long-standing relationship.

Meaningful relationships can be nurtured through financial or personal volunteerism. If financially contributing to the campaign of a member of Congress is not feasible, consider volunteering to work on the campaign. If your political views do not align with your current members of Congress, work on the campaign of their opponent. Also consider being an ever-present voice in your legislators' offices, no matter their views or party affiliations. This activity can and has led to nurses becoming a major resource and influence on a legislator, a governor, or staff member.

Offering time and expertise is a significant determinant in one's ability to influence a member of Congress and staff. These relationships do not form overnight. Do not give up even when you are told no. Even when you have differing political leanings than the member of Congress, you can have the opportunity to educate the legislator or staff about issues that are important.

Relationship building takes tenacity, particularly when you are working with a congressional office that might not have the same viewpoint and may never support the issue at hand. This should never be a reason not to visit a member of Congress and staff and pass on the opportunity to educate them about the issue and its importance to their constituency. "No" does not always mean never.

Grasstop relationships are important in nursing, as exemplified in the Policy Challenge and Policy Solution in this chapter. The type of social capital that a high-level professional position in leadership or in politics provides is important in not only opening doors to the discussion of issues but also providing support that can sway the support of or defeat a project or legislation. Although discussed under the big-P here, there are grasstop advocates at the little-p level. As a chair of a local political party or a local board, you may have access to influencing to influence other opinion leaders.

The Little-p

Social capital can ensure policy change at the little-p level in many of the same ways as at the big-P level. The goal is developing relationships with individuals making the policy decisions and with individuals who have intellectual and social capital themselves. It is critical to identify who those individuals are and how you can connect with them. Often, at the big-P level, the individuals with whom you want to develop relationships may be obvious, and at the little-p level, it is sometimes less clear. At first, one may think of only the organizational hierarchy where you work as important in building social capital. Those relationships are vital. However, a good strategy is starting with your existing base of relationships and then broadening those relationships and networks. Consider all your acquaintances as potential opportunities to extend your social capital. As your network grows, it extends to people who do not necessarily think like you or do the same job as you. You will become less insulated in your views, friendships, and networks.

As discussed in the section Political Capital, there is power in numbers. Building a network of colleagues (nurses and nonnurses) who agree with the premise of the policy change can better solidify the chances of its implementation. Demonstrating that more than one individual supports the policy change can influence the decision. Establishing this network can sometimes be done easily. Talking during a shift or during an after-hours socialization are some ways to build your network. Oprah Winfrey popularized her "book club," and thousands began discussing literature. Take a cue from Oprah to create a "policy club," a network that can offer information and assistance.

Building social capital at the local level can be accomplished in many ways: attending continuing education programs provided by your employer, participating in district nurses associations or other nurses' groups, serving as a moderator for educational sessions, joining or participating in local organizations' social events or journal clubs, using break times to socialize with key leaders in your organization, or volunteering for your organization's community events. For example, one new graduate built social capital when she was asked by her nurse manager to volunteer for her hospital's community health fair a week before her employment start date because one of the volunteers had an emergency. The graduate had experience in organizing community events. She fulfilled an important need in making the event a success while building important social capital.

A particularly effective way of learning about social capital is from a mentor. Mentors can, formally or informally, help you by advising you through stories and exemplars of how they were successful and not so successful in relationship building. Nurse leaders, such as committee chairs, managers, or nurse executives, can serve as mentors. Successful nurse leaders embrace helping nurses with less experience; they often tell you they owe their success to a mentor or mentors. They believe in paying it forward.

Whether social capital is built at the national, state, or local level, the key is not necessarily quantity but quality. As your network grows, it is important to monitor and continually scan for changes in opinions, relationships, and opportunities to advance your social capital. Just as in building any relationship, it takes time and commitment to establish a trusted long-term relationship. A visit or phone call once a year is not enough. Consistent, regular communication is necessary. At the big-P level, consistently taking the time to send your legislators a new study or simply checking in and offering assistance establishes that necessary connection. Moreover, creating opportunities to connect with your network at the little-p level is also accomplished through consistent purposeful communications. Simple measures for maintaining a relationship yield a great return on the social capital investment and can ultimately assist in creating policy changes.

POLITICAL CAPITAL

Political capital is influence. It can take multiple forms: financial, social, and intellectual. For the context of this section, political capital is described as advocacy and "lobbying" efforts undertaken by nurses and the nursing profession.

Often when the term *lobbying* is heard, it may carry a negative connotation, depending on an individual's experience with the political process. *Lobbying*, used in the general sense, is promoting an agenda to influence specific decisions. However, there are precise definitions and regulations for lobbying at the federal and state levels that govern practices. The education of policymakers (e.g., providing information) and advocacy on an issue (see Chapter 2) are closely related but often misunderstood. The concepts of grassroots, free riders, and coalitions are introduced and clarified in relation to lobbying (see the section Financial Capital for the financial aspects of lobbying).

The Big-P

At the federal level, the Lobbying Disclosure Act (LDA) defines *lobbying contact* as any oral, written, or electronic communication to a federal official made on behalf of a client as specified in the LDA (Office of the Clerk, U.S. House of Representatives, 2017). Moreover, lobbying activities include "any efforts in support of such contacts, including preparation or planning activities, research, and other background work that is intended, at the time of its preparation, for use in [lobbying] contacts" (Office of the Clerk, U.S. House of Representatives, 2017, p. 5). Basically, any attempt to influence an official is considered lobbying. State laws also dictate what is considered lobbying (see E-Resources for the report by the National Conference of State Legislatures).

Not all attempts by nurses to contact their representatives should be considered lobbying, nor should these nurses be considered lobbyists. Because most nurses are not paid to lobby, they technically are not considered registered lobbyists; however, they are advocates and can share their intellectual capital with legislators.

Lobbyists work for a cause or, often, an association or firm, and are paid to "lobby" members of Congress. These individuals must file lobbying disclosure forms to legally engage in this process and are deemed registered lobbyists. There is also variations on what lobbyists can and cannot do under the LDA, depending on where they work. For example, the American Nurses Association (ANA) is a 501(c)(6) organization (trade association, defined under the tax code) that can lobby, have a political action committee (PAC),[1] and endorse candidates (see E-Resources, Internal Revenue Service). Many other nurses associations are considered a 501(c)(3) organization (nonprofit); because of this status, they can spend only a certain portion of their annual revenue on lobbying, and it cannot be a major component of the association's work; nor can they have a PAC or endorse candidates.

Money donated to candidates has a major impact at the big-P level. Notably, the *Citizens United* 2010 Supreme Court decision created controversy and confusion regarding the use of donated monies for political influence and the "Super-PAC" (*Citizens United v. Federal Election Commission*, 2010). Former chair of the ANA-PAC, Faith M. Jones, MSN, RN, NEA-BC, stated, "A PAC is not a PAC is not a PAC." The ANA-PAC is not a Super-PAC; it is a trade association PAC. The ANA-PAC is composed of nurses who are ANA members. Through their contributions to the ANA-PAC, these nurses participate in the political process and support candidates at the federal level who support ANA's legislative agenda. The ANA-PAC is bipartisan and supports candidates based on the candidates' stance related to issues important to nurses, regardless of party affiliation. Unique to a professional nurses association was the ANA-PAC's presidential endorsement process that was in place for many years until 2019. When endorsed presidential candidates win, it sometimes resulted in ANA members being appointed to key federal agencies and ANA leaders being invited to engage in policy discussions at the White House. However, despite not endorsing Trump's presidential bid in 2016, ANA Chief Nursing Officer Debbie Hatmaker, along with leadership from 12 other nurses associations, were invited to attend a roundtable with President Trump and White House officials in March 2020 to dialogue about protecting healthcare workers during the COVID-19 pandemic (see Chapter 10).

---

[1] A PAC is "an organization set up solely to collect and spend money on electoral campaigns. A type of organized interest" (Nownes, 2001, p. 231).

POLICY ON THE SCENE 7.2: FRONTLINE NURSES IMPACTING HEALTHCARE POLICIES DURING COVID-19 PANDEMIC

For over 50 years, the Title VIII Nursing Workforce Development programs, administered by the Health Resources & Services Administration, has provided essential support for maintaining a strong nursing workforce. The programs provide scholarships, loan repayment, and other financial support for nursing students, practicing nurses, and schools of nursing. The programs are designed to create a highly educated nursing workforce, increase recruitment and retention of individuals from disadvantaged and underrepresented backgrounds strengthen interprofessional education and practice, and ensure that access to nursing care is available to all communities, particularly those that are underserved.

Each year, Congress must determine how much funding, if any, these programs receive during the appropriations process. Title VIII is the largest dedicated source of federal funding specifically for nursing education. Even though this funding is modest compared with other health professions, In the 2018–2019 academic year, the Title VIII programs supported 26,126 nursing students and nurses received support from the bill (AACN, 2021). In order for the programs to continue receiving funding from Congress, they must go through a reauthorization process. Reauthorization confirms the authority of Congress to allocate discretionary funding for a specific period. It also provides an opportunity to make adjustments to the programs to make sure they are continuing to fulfill their mission. Prior to the passage of the CARES Act (P.L. 116-136), Title VIII had last been reauthorized in 2010 with the passage of the Affordable Care Act (111-148), meaning the programs were well overdue for reauthorization.

Title VIII passed the House at the end of 2019 with unanimous bipartisan support. Then, with the advent of COVID-19, the passage was delayed in the Senate. However, the pressures of the novel coronavirus (COVID-19) pandemic placed significant strains on the U.S. nursing workforce. The Nursing Community Coalition, composed of more than 60 national nursing organizations, recognized the opportunity to make the case for Title VIII reauthorization. Working with Congressional champions from both sides of the political aisle, including House Nursing Caucus co-chairs David Joyce (R-OH), Tulsi Gabbard (D-HI), Rodney Davis (R-IL), Suzanne Bonamici (D-OR), and Representatives Kathy Castor (D-FL), Doris Matsui (D-CA), David McKinley (R-WV), and Lauren Underwood (D-IL), who is also an RN, as well as Senate Nursing Caucus co-chairs Richard Burr (R-NC) and Jeff Merkley (D-OR), the Nursing Community coalition demonstrated how reauthorizing Title VIII would directly bolster the nursing workforce pipeline.

In March 2020, as the COVID-19 pandemic swept the nation, President Trump signed into law H.R. 748, the Coronavirus Aid, Relief, and Economic Security (CARES) Act, which included reauthorization of the Title VIII Nursing Workforce Development Programs. The $2 trillion stimulus package passed in an effort to address the economic impact of COVID-19 and included support for healthcare professionals on the frontlines of the public health crisis. The reauthorization continues funding for nursing workforce development programs through 2024.

This is an example of how political and intellectual capital are wielded to advance a critical issue. Political capital, or the long-standing working relationships that these nursing organizations hold with congressional champions, helped make sure that Title VIII reauthorization made it into the CARES Act (P.L. 116-136). Intellectual capital, or the ability for these nursing organizations to demonstrate how Title VIII programs will distinctly affect specific aspects of the nursing profession, is information that was vital to making the case for their reauthorization.

Grassroots

For the nursing profession, the single most powerful form of political capital is its grassroots. Using grassroots is powerful no matter the issue at hand. In grassroots efforts, numbers matter; this is why the RN workforce size is so important. There were 3,096,700 RN jobs in 2021 (Bureau of Labor Statistics [BLS], 2021a) as opposed to 752,400 physician jobs (BLS, 2021b). The RN workforce outnumbered the physician workforce by 412%. Consider the impact that nurses could make in their advocacy efforts compared with physicians. Political capital for nursing could be summarized in the long-standing adage: "power in numbers." The premise underlying this assertion suggests that numbers mean nothing if they are not maximized. In other words, the choice of the individual nurse plays a substantial role in building the profession's political capital. Engaging nurses as grassroots members can achieve this.

Moreover, each of the nursing organizations sent out multiple calls to action to their memberships to ramp up grassroots advocacy. When the Veterans Affairs (VA) department put out a request for public comment on whether to grant APRNs full practice in May and December 2016, nursing's response was swift. The first call for comments yielded 223,623 comments, of which a significant portion came from those in favor of granting full practice. The second call for comments yielded 38,831 comments, clearly, showing the public's interest in this proposed policy change. The department ultimately decided that NPs, certified nurse-midwives, and clinical nurse specialists could practice to their full scope. Certified registered nurse anesthetists (CRNAs) were not included in the final policy change, with the department citing a lack of evidence regarding anesthesia service needs. It should be noted that CRNAs faced heavy lobbying efforts stemming from the anesthesiology community, who did not want their professional counterpart to be granted full scope of practice. The VA sites across the country are in various stages of adopting full scope for the other three APRN roles. Grassroots efforts involve "using interest group members (or the public) to pressure congressional lawmakers to support a group's agenda" (Wilcox & Kim, 2005, p. 136). Grassroots can be in the form of letters/emails or social media campaigns, coordinated calls to Capitol Hill, or face-to-face meetings with members of Congress or their staff (Wilcox & Kim, 2005).

Many larger organizations use electronic databases to manage their grassroots advocacy communications. These platforms can be quite sophisticated and allow government affairs staff to target constituents based on a number of factors, such as whether their member of Congress sits on a particularly strategic committee or supports a particular bill. RNs who belong to national nurses associations benefit when their associations use these platforms to send messages to their memberships, often alerting them to take action. It is critical that memberships respond in a timely manner because these issues are often time-sensitive. Congressional offices take note of how much correspondence is sent on a certain issue and flag the issue if several constituents weigh in. This is another example of grassroots advocacy in the age of electronic communications.

As Goldstein (1999) suggests, "grassroots communications demonstrate to legislators that traceability has been established" (p. 39). Traceability suggests that a large constituent voice has been registered with the member of Congress through calls, emails, or other methods such as visits. The effectiveness of grassroots is often measured by the quality and quantity of output by the constituents (Kollman, 1998; Thrall, 2006; Wilcox & Kim, 2005). This is where nursing can excel and demonstrate its power in numbers.

Free-Rider Syndrome

With so much at risk, it is important to explore the reasons why nurses do not engage. Some may suggest time constraints, other competing priorities, or a lack of interest in policy work as factors. However, for nearly six decades, the political science community has described this as what Olson (1965) originally defined as the "free-rider syndrome." Free riders are individuals who avoid bearing any of the costs or burdens associated with the actions required to get a benefit. This is common, particularly in large groups.

With more than 3 million nurses in the workforce, the free-rider syndrome is not as easy to spot as in smaller groups. In small groups, it is easy to see when only a few individuals are doing the work and financially supporting the cause. As the group gets larger, members of the group do not notice if some are doing the work while others gain the benefits of that work. As an example, a nurses association sends an email action alert to its 10,000 members requesting them to tell their members of Congress to increase funding for nursing education. Normally, 100 responses would be considered robust. However, there are 100 U.S. senators and 435 members of the U.S. House of Representatives. With 100 letters, it is likely that some congressional offices did not receive a letter, some offices may have received only one or two, and others may have received 25. With 1% participating in this call to action, nursing education funds may not be increased as requested.

The explanation for this lack of participation is the free-rider syndrome: the fact that nurses rely on the large group to do their work and have excuses for their nonparticipation. Regardless of the explanation, lack of participation hurts the profession and ultimately hurts patients.

To achieve the desired outcome, quantity is necessary for grassroots advocacy. Numbers matter. and the only way to increase nursing's numbers are for the individual nurse to respond. The voice of each nurse does in fact make a difference; when nurses come together in coalitions, the impact intensifies.

Power of Coalition Building

For decades, coalitions have been an effective strategy for building political capital. Although the makeup, structure, and longevity of coalitions may vary, they demonstrate power in numbers. Coalitions are usually created to address an immediate issue (Nownes, 2001; e.g., passage of the ACA). Most nurses associations at the national and state levels are involved with some coalitions to advance policy agendas.

Coalitions provide credibility for the needs of organized interests. Credibility can be developed in two ways. First, organizations with a similar membership can form a coalition. For example, a coalition of all nurses associations could advocate for federal nursing appropriations or a piece of legislation. This demonstrates credibility because nurses are speaking with a unified voice. The RWJF and Gallup study (Khoury et al., 2011) pointed out that healthcare opinion leaders felt that one of the ways for the profession to make its voice heard was to speak with a unified message. Often, policymakers may become weary if only one organization promotes an issue (Nownes, 2001). Second, coalitions can reduce the level of conflict associated with an issue (Nownes, 2001). When conflict is minimal, an issue stands a better chance of being recognized and successfully moving through the policy process. As Price (1978) points out in his seminal work, an issue has a better chance of appearing on the congressional agenda if the degree of conflict among groups is low and public salience (or interest) is high.

Second, coalitions are extremely efficient because they allow organizations to pool their resources (Nownes, 2001). Pooling resources allows organizations to spend less than if they were advocating for the issue on their own (Hula, 1995). This is critically important to the nursing profession. As discussed in the section Financial Capital, nurses associations often do not have the same level of funding as other health professions associations. One of the advantages of creating coalitions is that they allow organizations to share resources in the forms of financial resources, lobbyists, expertise, and time.

Although coalitions may be effective, it is important to know that they do not always work. Olson (1965) warns that the assumption that groups of individuals with common interests usually work to further those interests is false and based on flawed logic. Just as in the case of grassroots efforts, coalitions can also fall victim to the free-rider syndrome." As organizations convene to work on an issue and as that group grows, members of the coalition quickly decide if the benefits outweigh the necessary contributions. In a coalition of 50 organizations, only five to 10 may do the work while the others benefit. If incentives are not in place for the five to 10 that do the work, they may not be willing to share their political capital. Although Olson points out that altruism is sometimes the case, it is not the norm. Knowing that Congress places significant weight on coalitions and their ability to speak with one voice, many organizations are actively pursuing coalitions. Coalition work is an opportunity to network (build social capital) with others who share similar views on an issue. However, a coalition must be strong enough to have members that become engaged and find value in its work. See Figure 7.4 for key components in coalition building based on lessons learned by the author.

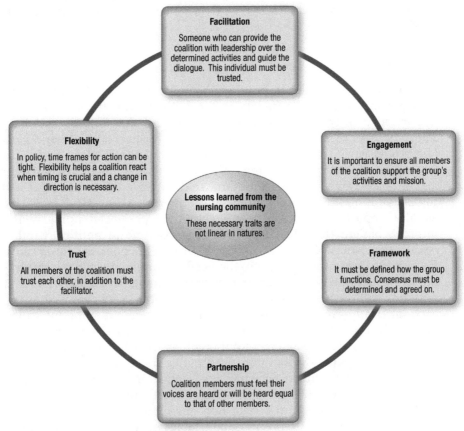

FIGURE 7.4 **Keys to building an effective coalition.**

One example of a strong collaboration within nursing is the Nursing Community Coalition (2020). Started circa 2002, the Nursing Community Coalition was a group of national nurses associations that came together once a year to discuss the unified funding request for the Nursing Workforce Development programs (Title VIII of the Public Health Service Act, 1944). For nearly 20 years, the Nursing Community Coalition has determined the funding request level for nursing education and advocated in a cohesive fashion to move this number forward. This forum has strengthened its power from a loosely affiliated group that came together once a year to a coalition that drafts letters to congressional appropriations; hosts virtual Lobby Days, receptions, and briefings on Capitol Hill; and visits with members of Congress who sit on the House and Senate Appropriations Committees. The coalition has, in recent years, become a more formalized structure that includes a Steering Committee and various ad hoc working groups. This has been done, in part, to address free-rider behavior. Currently, 63 national organizations belong to the Nursing Community Coalition, having grown from approximately 35 organizations. As mentioned earlier in this chapter, a major "win" of the coalition was the passage of Title VIII reauthorization.

Coalitions offer a prime opportunity to build political capital. However, not all coalitions are easily established or maintained. The common theme that has surfaced throughout this chapter is that all forms of capital are needed. When working in coalitions, trust (social capital) needs to be established and a common good must be identified. The ability of nurses to build coalitions as a form of political capital transcends across big-P and little-p. Coalitions can be effective tools for creating policy change at the unit, local, or state level. At the heart of coalitions is power in numbers.

The Little-p

In many respects, building political capital starts at the local level. It is not uncommon for elected officials to work their way through a number of appointed or elected positions before reaching the state or national level. The processes of big-P and little-p can and, by necessity, often do overlap. Grassroots work by its very definition starts at the local level. In addition, free riders exist across all settings. They do not attend meetings, are often critical of discussions and decisions, and seldom offer solutions or get involved to resolve issues. Just as coalitions are important at the big-P level, they are equally important at the little-p level. An experienced nurse working to improve patient flow illustrates a little-p example of political capital. This issue is problematic for many units (e.g., EDs, ICUs, postanesthesia care units). Each year, during the flu season, the need for timely discharges and transfers intensifies and becomes a major throughput issue. In anticipation of the flu season, a well-respected nurse convened a meeting with representatives from each unit. All agreed there was a need to recommend solutions to improve patient flow and formed a coalition, including staff from other departments. This group quickly assembled solutions that were implemented systemwide and in each department that improved patient flow and patient satisfaction.

Political capital is influence, which is essential for having an impact on policy. Nurses and the organizations that represent them must be strategic. Significant healthcare policy issues can benefit from the nursing perspective. When policy issues are identified, coalitions must be established, experts found, and resources pooled to achieve success.

FINANCIAL CAPITAL

Financial capital is often exemplified in the golden rule: He who has the money makes the rules (Nownes, 2001). Nurses may be quick to point out that, compared with other industries and professions in healthcare, nurses do not have the "gold" that would allow the profession's voice to resonate loudest. In many cases, this is true. According to the BLS (2021a, 2021b), in 2020 physicians' median pay was 2.7 times higher than that of RNs. This is clearly an important factor in the amount a nurse can contribute to a PAC or donate to candidates or causes. Nevertheless, financial resources are, without a doubt, a significant factor to organized advocacy and allow for a specific interest to be advanced.

The Big-P

At the federal level, it is believed that money is the driving force in achieving space on the congressional agenda. As Berry (1999, p. 85) points out, "space on the Congressional agenda is a precious commodity." A clear example is provided by ANA President Ernest Grant's testimony before the Senate Finance Committee on personal protective equipment (PPE) and the supply chain. Dr. Grant was the only health professional organization representative at the table to discuss PPE (see Figure 7.5).

Nursing's financial capital has not measured up to the capital of other healthcare professionals. Organizations' financial capital supports services such as professional registered lobbyists and provides resources to promote their agendas, such as studies to support an issue, expert analysis, and advocacy materials. Money also comes in the form of a PAC and individual contributions to members of Congress. Two forms of financial capital are lobbying and PACs.

Lobbying

As indicated earlier, lobbying serves to advocate, educate, and influence members of Congress. There are 11,722 registered federal lobbyists in the United States

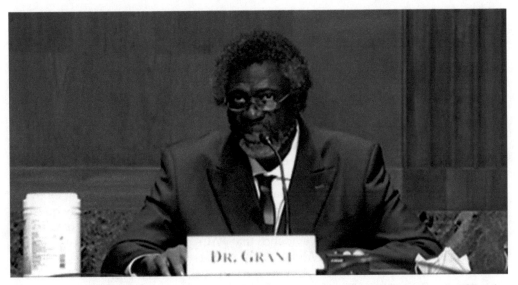

FIGURE 7.5 ANA President Ernest Grant testifying before the Senate Finance Committee on PPE and the supply chain.

working on issues from gun control to healthcare (Open Secrets, 2021). In 2020, "health professionals" organizations spent $67,898,289 on their lobbying efforts (Open Secrets, 2020). Comparatively, total healthcare industry spending in 2020 equaled $482,015,908. More than half of this was contributed by the pharmaceutical and health products sector (Open Secrets, 2020). The nursing profession spent a total of $4,335,652 in the 2020 election cycle (Open Secrets, 2020).

In Exhibit 7.3, the ANA spent $863,438 in contributions to political activity in 2020, whereas their physician counterpart (American Medical Association [AMA]), spent $15,245,000 (Open Secrets, 2020). The AMA spent 179% more on lobbying than the ANA (see Exhibit 7.3). This trend is not uncommon when comparing physicians' political spending with that of nurses.

EXHIBIT 7.3   LOBBYING DOLLARS SPENT IN 2020: TOP THREE NURSE AND PHYSICIAN ASSOCIATIONS

PROFESSION	LOBBYING DOLLARS SPENT IN 2020[a]
Nurses Associations	
American Nurses Association[b]	$863,438
American Association of Nurse Anesthetists	$270,000
American Association of Nurse Practitioners	$581,114
Total	$1,714,552
Physicians Associations	
American Medical Association	$15,245,000
American College of Cardiology	$1,510,000
American Academy of Family Physicians	$3,206,317
Total	$19,961,317

[a]Data compiled after every 2-year election cycle.
[b]Includes lobbying firms but not state associations.
(Open Secrets, 2020).

Political Action Committees

Some would argue that PACs hold much weight as a form of capital in helping secure space on the congressional agenda. Exchange theories suggest that lobbyists and legislators engage in unspoken agreements or trades (Austen-Smith, 1997; Morton & Cameron, 1992). As the theory suggests, the trade between a member of Congress and a lobbyist is an implicit trade that mutually benefits both parties and is typically identified as a political campaign or PAC contributions to a member of Congress for their vote on an issue. Exchange theories have been described as "vote buying," whereas others view this as "buying" a member of Congress's time (Stratmann, 1998). This suggests that PAC contributions are made so that lobbyists can discuss a specific issue with the hope of gaining "votes." Some may question the level of effectiveness between PAC contributions and the actions of congressional members, but there is evidence that PACs provide some level of access to legislators and their staff (Wright, 1990). As Berry (1999, p. 151) states, "interest group leaders believe that PAC donations are well worth it because the money is converted into more face time with legislators and key aides, and they think that this interaction increases the chances that these congressional offices will do something on the group's behalf."

For the context of this discussion, the assumption is that PACs, to a certain level, influence and build financial capital. More important, it is a quantifiable data piece that clearly illustrates the gap in nursing's political expenditures.

In comparing lobbying contributions among the top three nursing organizations and physician's organizations in the last presidential election cycle, it is clear to see that the physician organizations are raising and spending more (see Exhibit 7.4). The path for nursing to overcome the financial resources dilemma is clear. PAC activities are funded through contributions solicited from individual members. Numbers matter in achieving financial capital. Membership in national nursing associations is paramount. Individual nurses must determine where their money will be best spent, matching personal values and priorities.

It should also be noted that although the aforementioned information concerning PACs and lobbying relates to federal activity, trends are similar at the state level. At the state level, most nurse PACs and lobbying are done by state nursing associations. Unions representing nurses may also lobby at the state level. Therefore, nurses should consider joining not only national organizations but also state associations. This is important for APRNs for whom a unified voice at the state level is so critical to removing practice barriers. It is important for all nurses when unlicensed persons seek to represent themselves as "nurses" in states that do not protect the title "nurse" or "RN." There are numerous issues addressed at the state level that require an ongoing and vigilant presence at the statehouse that benefits from the use of PACs and lobbying efforts. These same principles can be applied at the local level such as in the case of a school board, city council, or township board.

The Little-p

Money speaks at all levels. Although financial capital at the big-P level receives a lot of attention, the financial impact at the little-p level is often not fully realized. Contributions locally are just as important as at the national and state levels. Your personal contribution of time or money will be acknowledged and may lead to opportunities for influencing policy within your community. Personal donations are strategic and can lead to future board appointments. Often there is the expectation for board members to support foundations and special events, causes, and programs. However, financial capital is not just about what you contribute. It is important to realize the opportunities that exist to fund and support your cause or policy. Foundations, hospital auxiliary boards, and alumni groups can be solicited for financial support.

The first essential step a nurse can take to maximize the profession's political capital is joining the organizations that advance the voice of nursing at the national and state levels. Second, knowing the importance and significant gap in nurses' financial-political capital, nurses should consider contributing to a PAC, to a member of Congress, or to both.

IMPLICATIONS FOR THE FUTURE

Nursing has remarkable potential to build and expand its capital. This is true of each individual nurse, as well as state and national nursing associations. However, the cornerstone of achieving this potential is the ability of individual nurses to

EXHIBIT 7.4 NATIONAL NURSE AND HEALTH PROFESSIONALS ASSOCIATIONS: TOP CONTRIBUTORS TO FEDERAL CANDIDATES, PARTIES, AND OUTSIDE GROUPS

CONTRIBUTOR	TOTAL CONTRIBUTIONS	TO CANDIDATES AND PARTIES			TO OUTSIDE SPENDING GROUPS
		Total	Democrat	Republican	Total
Nurses Associations[a]					
American Association of Nurse Anesthetists	$866,000	$866,000	46.5%	53.5%	$0
American Nurses Association	$350,423	$350,243	67%	33%	$0
American Association of Nurse Practitioners	$163,000	$163,000	49.1%	50.3%	$0
American College of Nurse-Midwives	$50,676	$50,676	74.3%	25.77%	$0
Oncology Nursing Society	$10,022	$9,995	98.8%	0%	$0
American Academy of Nursing	$6,013	$6,013	100%	0%	$0
Total	**$1,446,134**	**$1,445,927**			
Health Professionals[b]					
American Society of Anesthesiologists	$2,140,474	$2,140,449	50%	50%	$0
American Dental Association	$1,879,921	$1,755,412	40.6%	59.4%	$125,105
American Optometric Association	$1,530,180	$1,530,180	48.9%	51.1%	$0
American Association of Orthopaedic Surgeons	$1,525,099	$1,527,099	38.3%	61.3%	$0
American Medical Association	$1,405,119	$1,390,835	55.1%	44.5%	$13,223
American College of Emergency Physicians	$1,164,293	$1,164,293	52.4%	47.6%	$0
Total	**$9,645,086**	**$9,508,268**			

[a]Nurses: Top Contributors to Federal Candidates, Parties, and Outside Groups (top six nurses associations; includes individual donors who identify with groups). The Center for Responsive Politics. https://www.opensecrets.org/industries/contrib.php?cycle=2020&ind=H1710

[b]Health Professionals: Top Contributors to Federal Candidates, Parties, and Outside Groups (Top Six Health Professional Associations; Includes Individual Donors Who Identify With Groups). The Center for Responsive Politics. www.opensecrets.org/industries/contrib.php?ind=h01

Gaining Political Capital by Being Part of a Team

Colleen Leners, DNP, APRN, FAAN, FAANP

The military taught me to be part of a team, as well as it was the mission that was most important. Now, one of the first things that I learned in my Robert Wood Johnson Fellowship is that people on Capitol Hill were not interested in my neutrality. I was very pointedly advised that I needed to declare my political affiliation. My placement was with Senator John Thune (R-SD). It was the year that Senate flipped to Republican control. Senator Thune was a member of the Finance Committee, which has jurisdiction over Medicare, Medicaid, and other health programs. I had the opportunity to work on issues related to the healthcare needs of not only veterans but also rural and urban communities. Since the senator was from South Dakota, we worked particularly hard to address the needs of the Native American communities. I realized that we could not just make changes to improve life for one segment of the population, without making changes that impacted everyone. My experience had primarily focused on a single-payer healthcare system in the military and was thrust into examining policy in a much more complex environment. I wrote memoranda based on current research, took calls from veterans, and during peak times, worked many 12-hour days. A highlight of the year was taking a weeklong tour of South Dakota reservations and talking with community leaders to gain insights into the special needs of the Native American communities. We worked very hard to get 12 bipartisan health-related bills passed out of the Senate, and four were passed into law; I witnessed that in the Senate, it is not as partisan as it appears that many senators will work together to get bills passed that affect their communities.

My policy work reached into new arenas. As was true in the military, I saw the importance of working together to achieve a common goal. I took advantage of opportunities to advance nursing's positions. For example, when full practice authority for CRNAs was being debated, questions were raised about the quality of CRNAs' outcomes. I pointed out the inconsistencies of the arguments to restrict CRNA practice and related that I had worked with CRNAs deployed to Iraq who practiced when their patients had massive trauma with no blood pressure! This experience and their education and training would certainly prepare them for whatever surgeries they had to do stateside.

I realized to pay attention to economic evaluations. Although a nursing lens is valuable, nurses need to use an economic lens on a much more regular basis and speak specifically to the economic impact of our work. One area where nurses can benefit is paying attention to "reach back" amendments. These new paragraphs are inserted at the end of a bill change funding amounts that were specified earlier. In addition, associations can provide economic data to legislators. For example, the AACN has provided such data for nurse education funding.

My advice to nurses beginning to develop political capital is that the very first thing you must do is to vote and be involved in your community. When we address a specific need of a population, remember that there will be an impact on ALL populations and be cognizant of unintended consequences. We are all working as a team and that the best work is accomplished when we are focused on how to achieve our goals. My passion for working with wounded warriors enhanced the work I did in my fellowship year and that, in turn, prepared me to continue my policy and advocacy work at the American Association of Colleges of Nursing. Do not hesitate to take a well-thought-out stance on an issue. Our patients, our friends, our neighbors, those who have fought for our country, and our communities deserve nothing less from us. As of this writing, 23 states, two territories, and the District of Columbia allow full practice authority for APRNs. This is not just a win for nursing but also for the residents of these locations. However, like many policy initiatives, work is still needed so that the residents of the remaining 27 states can have better access to care.

understand that their voices and resources (i.e., money, time, expertise) are necessary for the greater good of the profession, as well as patients, families, and communities. Although many of the themes outlined in this chapter relate to capital focused on national advocacy, they translate to the work of each nurse. If one's goal is to change a standard in the hospital setting, how can relationships, coalitions, resources, and expertise be maximized?

Over the decades, nursing has made epic strides as a profession. Nurses are trusted and respected by the public, but they must make their voices heard, and heard in unison. It was evident in the Financial Capital discussion that significant work is essential for nursing to be comparable with the lobbying efforts of other national health professions. This is within our reach by using our expertise and dedication to the patient.

KEY CONCEPTS

1. Nursing's capital must be grown and cultivated.
2. Nurses must value and appreciate the importance of the individual voice in building capital.
3. At the heart of the profession is patient advocacy. This innate trait should be used to improve the health of the nation at every level.
4. Nurses must not be intimidated or hesitant to offer their valued contribution to those in power. Nursing's expertise is a commanding form of capital.
5. Nurses must view political awareness and engagement as a professional responsibility.
6. Whether social capital is built at the local, state, or national level, the key is not necessarily quantity but quality.
7. For nursing, coalitions offer prime opportunities for building political capital.
8. Nurses must invest in their nursing associations to ensure that they have the resources to build the profession's capital.
9. Building capital is obtainable and necessary for every nurse because all politics are local.
10. If nurses do not build all forms of capital, policy changes will occur without the profession's insight.

SUMMARY

If nursing wants a seat at the table when healthcare policy decisions are being debated and made, then it must invest in the efforts to obtain that seat. As Dr. Anthony Fauci, director of the National Institute of Allergy and Infectious Diseases who helped lead the Trump administration's response to the COVID-19 pandemic described the collaboration between private and federal stakeholders said, "I don't think we've ever seen it to this extent in the relationship between the industry and the federal government." He recognized that in order for a timely and effective development and rollout of a vaccine to occur, the sharpest minds, the most influential, the most trusted, and the most well-resourced entities would need to join forces. In other words, intellectual, political, social, and financial capital will directly shape a successful response. The nursing profession and individual nurses must insert their own capital into formulating policies that will result from this response, such as mass public education about the safety and efficacy of the vaccine and ensuring proper distribution.

END-OF-CHAPTER RESOURCES

LEARNING ACTIVITIES

1. Identify your local, state, and federal legislators. Select one whom you want to visit. Identify the key points that you will discuss at the visit. Plan for a 10-minute visit and for a 20-minute visit. Consider how your visit will vary if you talk to a staffer or the legislator. Then make a visit to the office and report on the highlights of the visit.

2. Determine when your state and national nurses associations are hosting their advocacy days and the process to register. Be sure to familiarize yourself with the advocacy materials before attending.

3. In your work environment consider inviting a leader to coffee. Ask for recommendations and advice for becoming politically active. Specifically inquire about their pathways in policy and mentors.

4. Follow your legislators on social media, such as Twitter, for an easy way to stay up to date on their issues. Challenge yourself to connect with them.

5. Develop a list of strategies for convincing classmates of the importance of supporting a nurses association and its PACs at the state or national level.

6. Reread the sections on "free riders" and "grasstops." Consider whether you know people in either category. Develop talking points to challenge one "free rider" to join an advocacy effort with you.

7. Investigate the funding received by your state from the Title VIII Nursing Workforce Reauthorization Act.

8. Make sure you and your nursing colleagues are registered to vote and have a voting plan (knowing where to vote, knowing deadlines to vote for primary and general election, etc.)

E-RESOURCES

- American Nurses Association. Political Action Committee https://ana. aristotle.com/SitePages/pac.aspx

- Coalition for Patients' Rights http://www.patientsrightscoalition.org

- Future of Nursing Campaign for Action https://www.campaignforaction.org

- Internal Revenue Service. Lobbying http://www.irs.gov/ Charities-&-Non-Profits/Lobbying

- National Conference of State Legislatures http://www.ncsl.org/research/ ethics/50-state-chart-lobbyist-report-requirements.aspx

- Nursing Community Coalition http://www.thenursingcommunity.org

- Open Secrets http://www.opensecrets.org/pacs/pacfaq.php

- Public Affairs Council http://pac.org

REFERENCES

Aiken, L. H., Clarke, S. P., Sloane, D. M., Sochalski, J., & Silber, J. H. (2002). Hospital nurse staffing and patient mortality, nurse burnout, and job dissatisfaction. *Journal of the American Medical Association, 288*(16), 1987–1993. https://doi.org/10.1001/jama.288.16.1987

American Association of Colleges of Nursing. (2021). *Title VIII nursing workforce development programs* [Fact sheet].

Austen-Smith, D. (1997). Interest groups: Money, information and influence. In D. C. Mueller (Ed.). *Perspectives on public choice* (pp. 296–321). Cambridge University Press.

Begeny, S. M. (2009). *Lobbying strategies for federal appropriations: Nursing versus medical education* [Doctoral dissertation, University of Michigan]. University of Michigan Library Deep Blue Documents. http://hdl.handle.net/2027.42/64641

Berry, J. M. (1999). *The new liberalism: The rising power of citizen groups*. Brookings Institution Press.

Bradbury-Jones, C., Sambrook, S., & Irvine, F. (2008). Power and empowerment in nursing: A fourth theoretical approach. *Journal of Advanced Nursing, 62*(2), 258–266. https://doi.org/10.1111/j.1365-2648.2008.04598.x

Bureau of Labor Statistics. (2021a). *Occupational outlook handbook: Registered nurses.* https://www.bls.gov/ooh/healthcare/registered-nurses.htm

Bureau of Labor Statistics. (2021b). *Occupational outlook handbook: Physicians and surgeons.* https://www.bls.gov/ooh/healthcare/physicians-and-surgeons.htm

Centers for Medicare and Medicaid Innovation. (2013). Community-based care transitions program. http://innovation.cms.gov/initiatives/CCTP

Citizens United v. Federal Election Commission. (2010). 558 US 310. http://en.wikipedia.org/wiki/Citizens_United_v_Federal_Election_Commission

Congressional Management Foundation. (2015). # *Social Congress 2015.* https://www.congressfoundation.org/projects/communicating-with-congress/social-congress-2015

Congressional Management Foundation. (2020). *The future of citizen engagement: Coronavirus, congress, and constituent communications.* https://www.congressfoundation.org/storage/documents/CMF_Pubs/cmf_citizenengagement_covid-19.pdf

Federal Register. (2016). *Medicare program; merit-based incentive payment system (MIPS) and alternative payment model (APM) incentive under the physician fee schedule, and criteria for physician-focused payment models.* https://www.federalregister.gov/documents/2016/11/04/2016-25240/medicare-program-merit-based-incentive-payment-system-mips-and-alternative-payment-model-apm

Gibson, J. (2010). Persuading Congress: How to spend less and get more from Congress. TheCapitol.Net, Inc.

Goldstein, K. M. (1999). *Interest groups, lobbying, and participation in America*. Cambridge University Press.

Hula, K. W. (1995). Rounding up the usual suspects: Forging interest group coalitions in Washington. In A. J. Cigler & B. A. Loomis (Eds.), *Interest group politics* (4th ed., pp. 239–258). CQ Press.

Khoury, C. M., Blizzard, R., Wright Moore, L., & Hassmiller, S. (2011). Nursing leadership from bedside to boardroom: A Gallup national survey of opinion leaders. *Journal of Nursing Administration, 41*(7–8), 299–305. https://doi.org/10.1097/NNA.0b013e3182250a0d

Kollman, K. (1998). *Outside lobbying*. Princeton University Press.

Laschinger, H. K. S., & Havens, D. S. (1996). Staff nurse work empowerment and perceived control over nursing practice: Conditions for work effectiveness. *Journal of Nursing Administration, 26*(9), 27–35. https://doi.org/10.1097/00005110-199609000-00007

Manojlovich, M. (2007). Power and empowerment in nursing: Looking backward to inform the future. *OJIN: Online Journal of Issues in Nursing, 12*(1), 2. https://doi.org/10.3912/OJIN.Vol12No01Man0

Morton, R., & Cameron, C. (1992). Elections and the theory of campaign contributions: A survey and critical analysis. *Economics and Politics, 4*, 79–108. https://doi.org/10.1111/j.1468-0343.1992.tb00056.x

National Academies of Sciences, Engineering, and Medicine. (2021). *The future of nursing 2020–2030: Charting a path to achieve health equity*. The National Academies Press. https://doi.org/10/17226/25982

The National Institute for Lobbying & Ethics. (2017). *What is lobbying?* https://lobbyinginstitute.com/what-is-lobbying

Nownes, A. J. (2001). *Pressure and power: Organized interest in American politics*. Houghton Mifflin.

Nursing Community Coalition. (2020). *Core principles*. https://www.thenursingcommunity.org/core-principles

Office of the Clerk, U.S. House of Representatives. (2017). *Lobbying disclosure act guidance*. https://lobbyingdisclosure.house.gov/ldaguidance.pdf

Olson, M. (1965). *The logic of collective action: Public goods and the theory of groups*. Harvard University Press.

Open Secrets. (2021). *Lobbying*. https://www.opensecrets.org/federal-lobbying/

Open Secrets. (2020). *Top industries*. https://www.opensecrets.org/lobby

Patient Protection and Affordable Care Act of 2010. (2010). Pub. L. No. 111-148. 124 § 119-1025.

Price, D. E. (1978). Policy making in congressional committees: The impact of "environmental" factors. *American Political Science Review, 72*(2), 548–574. https://doi.org/10.2307/1954110

Public Health Service Act of 1944. (1944). Pub. L. 78-410, Title VIII.

Rao, A. (2012). The contemporary construction of nurse empowerment. *Journal of Nursing Scholarship, 44*(4), 396–402. https://doi.org/10.1111/j.1547-5069.2012.01473.x

Rosenstone, S., & Hansen, M. (1993). *Mobilization, participation, and democracy in America*. Macmillan.

Saad, L. (2020, December 22). *U. S. ethics ratings rise for medical workers and teachers*. Gallup. https://news.gallup.com/poll/328136/ethics-ratings-rise-medical-workers-teachers.aspx

Stratmann, T. (1998). The market for congressional votes: Is timing of contributions everything? *Journal of Law and Economics, 41*, 85–113. https://doi.org/10.1086/467385

Thrall, A. T. (2006). The myth of the outside strategy: Mass media news coverage of interest groups. *Political Communications, 23*, 407–420. https://doi.org/10.1080/1058460097689

Turale, S., & Kunaviktikul, W. (2019). The contribution of nurses to health policy and advocacy requires leaders to provide training and mentorship. *International Nursing Review, 66*(3), 302–304. https://doi.org/10.1111/inr.12550

Tversky, A., & Kahneman, D. (1981). The framing decisions and the psychology of choice. *Science, 211*, 453–458. https://doi.org/10.1126/science.7455683

Wilcox, C., & Kim, D. (2005). Continuity and change in the congressional connection. In P. S. Herrnson, R. G. Shaiko, & C. Wilcox (Eds.), *The interest group connection: Electioneering, lobbying, and policymaking in Washington* (2nd ed., p. 129–140). CQ Press.

Wright, J. R. (1990). Contributions, lobbying, and committee voting in the U.S. House of Representatives. *American Political Science Review, 84*, 417–438. https://doi.org/10.2307/1963527

CHAPTER 8

Transforming Policy With Innovation

TIM RADERSTORF, TAURA L. BARR, MICHAEL ACKERMAN, AMY JAUCH, AND
BERNADETTE MAZUREK MELNYK

Creativity is thinking up new things. Innovation is doing new things.
—Theodore Levitt

OBJECTIVES

1. Examine the reciprocal nature of the relationship between innovation and policy.
2. Compare and contrast the difference between innovation and invention and their relationship to policy advancement.
3. Describe the strategic significance of innovation for the development of policy.
4. Analyze the different approaches utilized to evaluate and improve innovation.
5. Compare and contrast organizational supports for the structure and culture of innovation.

Innovation in a policy book. Why? At first glance, it may seem like an unlikely marriage of dichotomous topics. One focuses on setting rules, the other focuses on rewriting them. However, by the end of this chapter, you will see that these two topics are deeply entangled with one another. New policy is often the by-product of innovation, and innovation is often the by-product of new policy.

Our changing world and the increasing demands for healthcare across our country and the globe require dramatic strategies that change how we deliver healthcare while providing quality health services. Innovation has the potential to change the prevailing paradigm of how various aspects of care can be delivered. Nurses who understand how innovation can be applied to healthcare and nursing practice can make substantial improvements in the access to care and the quality of care. The central position of nurses in healthcare provides the potential for nurses to be the leaders in innovation given the right resources and the right climate for change.

As nurses, the essence of our work is about innovation, change, and creating policies to support the expected work of patient care excellence. Nurses work with patients to change and improve their state of health on a continual basis. When, for example, a new technology or treatment is initiated, it is often the nurse in direct care who is the first to see the unforeseen impact to patients and nurses as they carry out new work and recognize the need for policy change. The numerous redesigns of workflow that occur when moving from paper to electronic documentation is one example of how policy with a little-p is implemented. In this chapter, innovation, theories, structures that support innovation, advances in technology, entrepreneurship, the relationship between policy and innovation, and future opportunities are addressed.

Learning to embrace both change and innovation is necessary to successfully navigate events and, ultimately, thrive in our ever-changing world. Successful advocates have mastered the competencies of embracing change and innovation. Having an appreciation of the nature of theories of change and innovation provides a foundation for nurses to assume an active role in the policy process. What is also important to understand is that the multifaceted nature of change and innovation makes it nearly impossible to focus on all aspects of change simultaneously.

POLICY CHALLENGE | **COVID-Inspired Innovation**

Innovation and COVID-19 went hand in hand by dire necessity. Witnessing what nurses were doing, people across the world have a greater appreciation of the role of nurses. People saw the efforts of nurses to bridge the divide between technology and caring for the dying by using devices to connect loved ones. The realities of practice led to a spate of innovations by nurses in efforts to meet the nearly impossible and relentless demands of nursing practice in the midst of the COVID-19 pandemic. This is highlighted by De Bode (2021), who contrasts the innovation in healthcare about things, the discovery of a molecule, or the use of a robot with innovation in nursing, which reflects the complex relationship between patients and technology: "Nurses have created new methods of COVID care on the fly. . . . Nurses' stories of rapid improvements in care, communication and logistics reveal the deep unexpected role of trust in innovation as well as how changes instituted in the pandemic could shape healthcare for years to come" (p. 51).

Examples of innovations in care, communication, and logistics have been widely disseminated in media outlets, nurse and organizational networks as well as the published professional literature. High-profile examples of innovation in care include the placement of equipment, such as intravenous pump, and ventilator consoles outside of patient rooms and supervision and implementation of turning and oxygenation protocols. Innovations in communication ranged from the very simple use of markers on windows for messaging with staff and families and the use of electronic devices (e.g., cell phones, tablets) for critical conversations and observations. The latter example was especially poignant when it was used for end-of-life care. Logistic innovations included modifications to the usual clustering of care, equipment, and rooms to ensure quality care and safety for patients and staff.

These creative innovations, borne of necessity, cause us to think about policy and how we might envision the future. Should these innovations become embedded in practice? Should some of the tried and presumably true practices be discarded in the face of better information or a shifting paradigm? Which of these innovations are candidates for being slated into the permanent way of doing things in nursing and healthcare by being memorialized through organizational policy or regulation or legislation at the state and/or federal level or adopted globally as a standard of care? Which of these innovations when incorporated into policy have the potential to make substantive improvements in access, cost, quality, and safety, the experience of care, and the work environment?

These innovations have changed the delivery of healthcare. In some instances, temporary revisions have been made to policy. The challenge is to evaluate their effectiveness and safety over the long term to determine how to harness the best innovations in policy for improvement in healthcare delivery and policy.

Thus, our attempts to understand change and innovation are necessarily limited and incomplete—but necessary in the evolution of effective change and health-care policy creation. To be sure, the change expert will integrate multiple facets of change to increase understanding of the concepts and processes involved in change and innovation.

Innovation can be defined as the process of implementing new products, services, or solutions that create new value (Melnyk & Raderstorf, 2021). It can also include alternations in established practice or policies. The word *innovation* has taken on a variety of meanings. Many believe that the words *innovation* and *innovate* are used so often they have lost their meaning. Quite often, *innovation* is used interchangeably with creativity because being innovative implies that one is creative. Innovation is sometimes confused with *invention*. They are not the same. An invention is a novel idea, which may even be patented, but does not mean that it has been implemented. Whereas innovation is carrying it out in practice. The innovation cycle is like the nursing process and includes the following steps: empathy, define ideate, prototype, and test (Leary, 2020). The nursing process and the innovation cycle are similar and are further detailed under Innovation and Entrepreneurship later in this chapter.

Complexity of Innovation and Change

Innovation and change can be examined from numerous nuanced perspectives. It is important to understand the similarities and differences among innovation, types of innovation (disruptive, frugal), and an iterative model for innovation. While innovating may lead to the creation of new value, it's important to understand that being innovative does not mean that you must create a new widget or gadget. It can involve a new process, care delivery model, educational strategy, or policy. The approach or process can be innovative, especially when adding value to an existing product or service. In this case, it is not the product or service that is novel; these products or services currently exist. It is the new utilization or process of applying an existing product/service that brings the new value and this something is applied innovatively.

As nurses, the essence of our work requires an understanding of the nature of innovation and change. Policy revision or development can result. While *change* and *innovation* are not synonymous, there are common characteristics to consider when planning and implementing policy change and innovation. These essential characteristics of a change or innovation process—alteration type, agency type, time, level of impact, predictability, and driver—should be determined for any anticipated policy change or innovation. It is helpful to reflect on these common characteristics of change and innovation as one examines nurses' innovation. See Exhibit 8.1.

Nurses have a long history of being inventive, innovative, and making change that may lead to policy. Nurses' inventions to meet specific patient needs were often the innovations highlighted in the literature. The *American Journal of Nursing* at various times in its history had columns devoted to invention with titles such as "Improvising," "The Trading Post," "Ideas that Work," and "Creative Care Unit"; however, with the passage of time, the focus on invention diminished with the development of nursing research to provide the scientific foundations for nursing care (Gomez-Marquez & Young, 2016). It is widely recognized that clinicians should be encouraged to develop their creativity not only in high-resource countries but in low- and medium-resource countries as well. With the

EXHIBIT 8.1 COMMON CHARACTERISTICS OF CHANGE AND INNOVATION

CHARACTERISTIC	KEY FEATURES
Alteration	Both change and innovation involve a modification of the present way of doing things. Change can be an event of moving an item from one position to another. Innovation adds qualifiers to the movement and includes benefits, irreversibility, and nuance.
Human agency	Range from one individual to groups to organizations.
Time parameters	These include the rate of change, when change will occur, and the extent of the change whether episodic or continuous.
Level of change	This refers to the size of the units of change and innovation.
Predictability of the change or innovation	Both planned and unplanned changes can occur simultaneously at differing levels of an organization. Planning includes the degree to which change can be choreographed, scripted, or controlled. Unplanned change can be driven by choice or the unexpected that can lead to a desirable or undesirable direction.
Driver of change or innovation	Four drivers of change include life cycle, teleological, dialectical, and evolutionary. Life-cycle change and innovation occur in sequenced stages. Teleological drivers emphasize social construction and the cycle of goal formation, implementation, and modification. Dialectical drivers involve balancing opposing forces while emphasizing discussion, confronting conflict, and determining the best option. Evolutionary change is one of repetitive sequences of variation, selection, and finally retention emphasizing competition for scarce resources.

Source: From Poole, M. S., and Van de Ven, A. H. (Eds.). (2004). *Handbook of organizational change and innovation.* Oxford University Press; Porter-O'Grady, T. & Malloch, K. (2015). *Leadership in nursing practice. Changing the landscape of healthcare* (2nd ed.). Jones & Bartlett.

development of nursing research and the emphasis on evidence-based practice (EBP), the focus on "newness" has been on innovations that lead to improved care outcomes. An innovation based on research evidence is illustrated by the pioneering work of Dorothy Brooten, PhD, RN, FAAN, who tested a model of nurse-managed transitional care for very low-birth-weight infants discharged from the hospital. This model was expanded to other high-risk populations including patients with heart failure, women with unplanned caesarean sections (Brooten et al., 2002).

Consumers consistently seek opportunities to add new value. People often jump at opportunities to engage with innovations to save time and money or provide entertainment. For instance, the Amazon Dot is a voice-activated device that brings information to the end user. When these devices first arrived on the scene, they introduced the ability to obtain information, manage appliances in the home, and be alerted to deliveries by just talking to the device in natural language. The Dot also introduced novel services that brought value to the end users, such as reminders (e.g., medication), the option to make online purchases, and the ability to turn homes into "smart homes." Clearly, the new value was seen by end users, with more than 100 million Dots being sold in a little over a year. Taken a step further the integration of sensor technology, with smart in-home sensor systems, are a strategy that can be used by nurses to improve health and detect and manage disease in populations across the life span (Ward et al., 2020).

The emergence of ridesharing or the development of services, such as Uber and Lyft, is considered to be a "disruptive" innovation. It changed how people use transportation. It filled a void in that it upended the prevailing paradigm for car services. The void, often in underserved markets, fills a need. However, there is also a void in policy as it became evident that the existing practices and policies didn't address potential challenges for keeping riders safe and protecting the rights of workers. Features of "disruptive" innovation include simplicity, convenience, accessibility, and affordability (Dyer et al., 2011). Because of one or more of the highly desirable features of the innovation, it ultimately displaces the prevailing way of doing things. A common example in healthcare is establishing retail clinics staffed by nurse practitioners (NPs), which has improved access to care for many.

"Frugal" innovation is not necessarily about making a profit but is about the ability to do more with less to meet the needs of many people and accelerate change and improve health globally. Frugal innovation is often linked with a "Jugaad" mindset. *Jugaad* is a Hindi word that describes "an innovative fix; an improvised solution born from ingenuity and cleverness" or more simply a makeshift solution. The solution is affordable and has quality and sustainability (Wylie, 2012). Frugal innovation often means bringing resources to underserved populations. It has particularly taken hold in India and is being emulated by Western businesses and CEOs. An example of a frugal innovation is a fetal heart monitor that uses microphone technology instead of ultrasound (Radjou & Prabhu, 2013). The development of "open-source" ventilators designed to mitigate the impact of limited resources, such as a regular supply of electricity, pressurized oxygen, tubings, and suction, can facilitate equity across the world by providing access to these critical resources (Dave et al., 2021). Low-cost frugal innovations can, in turn, be scaled to improve health in the United States by (a) changing delivery settings and providers, (b) facilitating communication between healthcare providers and patients, (c) addressing health-seeking behavior, and (d) using leaner processes and simpler organizational structures (Bhatti et al., 2017). Elements of frugal and disruptive innovations may overlap. Both types are important in improving the health of populations.

The Novation Dynamic (see Figure 8.1) represents the complex relationships among innovation, renovation, and exnovation (Ackerman et al., 2020). *Novation* comes from the Greek word *novare*, which means to make new (Lexico, n.d.). Viewed as dynamic as opposed to *linear* or on a continuum, healthcare leaders must adapt to the ever-changing needs of the system. This has tremendous policy implications, whether it be internal policy or public policy. Innovation fills the gap between what is known (the current evidence or practice) and what is needed and currently does not exist. Because nurses provide direct care, they have intimate knowledge of what is working and not working in practice and policy. Filling these gaps is essential for healthcare systems to move forward. More often than not, innovation occurs at a pace much quicker than policy, and thus, policymakers must pay keen attention to the environment and innovation landscape. Very often, work-arounds are a sign of these gaps that may be harnessed for innovation.

Renovation refers to adjusting or making incremental change. It is in renovation that process and quality improvement takes place. Renovation is different from innovation in that renovation takes what currently exists and makes adjustments. The gap that exists is the lack of achievement of goals and/or objectives of the current system. Renovation is typically a "looking-backward" approach to solving problems as opposed to innovation as a more "forward-looking" process.

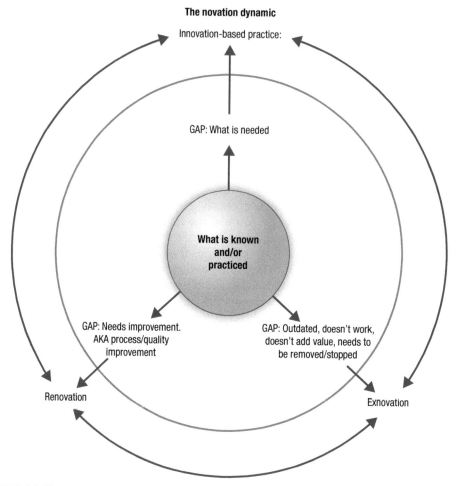

FIGURE 8.1 The novation dynamic.

Exnovation, or deimplementation, is a necessary step in the Novation Dynamic. Exnovation requires an examination of what is outdated, does not work, or brings no value followed by its elimination. The healthcare system is filled with examples of tasks or requirements that have never been questioned regarding their value. Oftentimes, new initiatives are created and very little time or effort is spent examining what can be eliminated with the implementation of the new initiative. Exnovation requires a simultaneous look at policy to assure there is alignment with the change.

Innovation and Entrepreneurship

Used so commonly together, it is easy to think that innovation and entrepreneurship are synonyms. While there is synergy between the two concepts, understanding the differences between them will help leaders better utilize each when the time is right. As discussed earlier, *innovation* can be boiled down to creating new value. And in that same venue, *entrepreneurship* is defined as creating new value in the hopes of generating profit. In this light, all entrepreneurship hopes to encompass innovation, but not all innovation leads to entrepreneurship.

In healthcare, it can be challenging for clinicians to come to grasp entrepreneurship's desire for profit. After all, nurses typically didn't enter the profession for money. But it is important for clinicians to recognize that in healthcare, *profit is an artifact of impact*. Think about it. How many products, services, or other solutions in healthcare are delivered at either no cost to the patient or no cost to the health system? The answer is zero. Thus, to be truly impactful in healthcare and reach patients across the world, finding a way to be entrepreneurial, to sell products, services, or solutions is the only path forward. But that's great news! There is a path forward for one to have an immense impact, and it is something that should be embraced by healthcare professionals around the globe.

Nurses are already trained to be entrepreneurial thinkers. The entrepreneurial mindset is taught in nursing school; it is just known as something different: the nursing process. Compare the linkages between steps of the nursing process and a model of entrepreneurship: Morris's Entrepreneurial Concepts (Melnyk & Raderstorf, 2021; Morris et al., 2013). See the well-known ADPIE steps of the nursing process on the left and the detailed descriptions of Morris's Entrepreneurial Concepts on the right in Figure 8.2.

Even at a surface level, it's clear that the entrepreneurial concepts parallel the nursing process with shocking similarity. And that means that nurses have already been trained how to think like an entrepreneur. And with those tools in hand, the next step is to identify opportunities for impact.

Developing a Structure and Culture of Innovation

The development of innovation requires a blend of structural and cultural elements in order to be successful. It is not uncommon for organizations to put immense focus on building a strong culture of innovation. While building a strong culture of innovation is essential for the success of an organization, it is important to note that the culture of innovation relies heavily on the organization's structure of innovation. Attempting to build a culture of innovation without a solid structure will cause efforts to innovate to ebb and flow, disappear and reappear, and ultimately not be

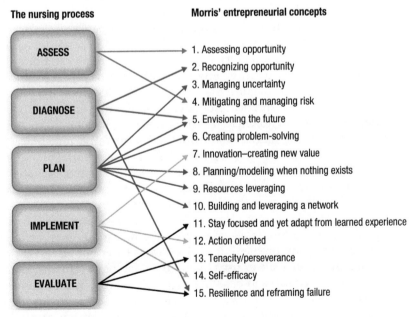

FIGURE 8.2 Comparison of the nursing process with Morris's entrepreneurial concepts.

Source: © Tim Raderstorf, DNP, RN, FAAN

sustainable for the organization and cause it to stagnate. Remember, the structural components of innovation are built into the system and do not change when people enter or leave the system. Structural components include resources both tangible and intangible. Broad categories of structure that should be considered when building a foundation for innovation include policy; incentives, rewards, and seed money; roles and titles; workflow and reporting structures; work-life support; governance and committees, and education and training opportunities. Each of these elements has a number of components that will enhance innovation. For example, work-life support can include breaks, protected time for planning and working on projects, and structured opportunities for networking.

It is essential that once in place, the structural components of innovation remain constant. They must be built into the system and not leave the organization with the departure of individuals. For example, many organizations have early adopters, that is, people who are excited about innovation and seek out opportunities to improve their organization. Sometimes, these people are in executive roles; other times, they are frontline staff members exploring ideas that may or may not capture the attention of managers or administrators. These people impact the culture of innovation; they are champions of innovation. See Policy on the Scene 8.1.

POLICY ON THE SCENE 8.1: COOLING VEST: LITTLE-P EXAMPLE WITH CONSEQUENTIAL IMPACT

Jill Byrne, PhD, RN, CNOR, Lecturer, Case Western Reserve University
Cleveland, Ohio

Early in our nursing careers, we learn the importance and benefit of advocating for the needs and care of patients. Whether advocating is learned or intuitive behavior, we are advocating for the best interests of human beings to improve health and well-being. Almost three decades into my nursing career, I began to observe a relationship among the appearances of sweat-soaked scrub clothing, surgeons demanding that I decrease the ambient temperature in the operating room, and an increase in incivility among the surgical team while performing surgery.

Perioperative recommended practice and standards address normothermia in surgical patients as a quality metric. This is especially important for pediatric and fragile, elderly patients. Environmental factors that contribute to surgical team temperature can include the ambient room temperature, personal protective equipment (PPE), and heat from overhead lighting and some operating room equipment. These environmental factors make it challenging to simultaneously meet the needs of the surgical team and the perioperative patient.

The surgical team was suffering from thermal discomfort, fatigue, and dehydration, and I knew that I needed to advocate for their well-being so patients remained safe and the surgical team was able to perform their job optimally. My solution to this clinical challenge was the design and development of a disposable cooling vest that I created for surgical team. The six-pocket cooling vest is lightweight and designed to be worn under a sterile surgical gown and is an innovative approach to solving a common problem. It demonstrates that "not all nursing innovations take place on a large scale or use advanced technology" (Thomas et al., 2016 para. 16). The positive changes in behavior and well-being of my colleagues who wore the cooling vest were immediate and dramatic. It was evident that the cooling vest is a sustainable innovation that addresses the needs of the surgical team while protecting the needs of the surgical patient.

In accordance with the diffusion of innovations theory, an innovation must be communicated over time among members of a social system (public, professional, organizational) and adopted by stakeholders in order to be sustainable (Rogers, 2003). Roger's theory is applicable to the innovative evidence-based research necessary to design and support healthcare policy that protects individuals who wear PPE from the detrimental effects of heat stress. My journey in disseminating this innovation to influence public policy has taken me across the country and allowed me to meet thousands of individuals who share a common goal of improving the well-being of healthcare workers. I have communicated with leaders in healthcare at public and professional conferences and events nationally and internationally over the last decade about thermal comfort during surgery. I completed the first national study to examine the thermal comfort, body temperatures, cognitive performance, and perceptions of exertion and fatigue of surgeons with and without a cooling vest while performing surgery in real time (Byrne & Ludington-Hoe, 2021).

As a nurse leader, I believe I have the professional responsibility to play an active role in the education and development of healthcare policy to improve and innovate nursing practice. Each perioperative setting establishes the guidelines and policies that follow the Association of periOperative Registered Nurses (AORN) recommended practice and standards for room temperature. The adoption and use of the cooling vest is an example of a little-p policy to keep patients safe and facilitate surgical team performance.

It is important to provide support to innovation champions. If they were to leave the organization, their influence on the culture of innovation would leave along with them. So, a structural approach to harness the impact of these champions would be to create job titles and job responsibilities that ensure the individuals who take these roles are required to engage in innovation behavior. By creating these roles and responsibilities, the organization creates a structure of innovation that lives beyond the actions of any one individual. When someone leaves the organization, that person is backfilled with another individual who still has the roles and responsibilities of the innovation champion. Thus, the culture of innovation continues to thrive, bolstered by the strong structure it rests on. There are many ways beyond formal job titles and roles/responsibilities to create a structure of innovation.

Hackathons are a structural element originating in the technology space with a facilitator that brings people of diverse backgrounds together to compete in brainstorming innovative solutions to a specific problem in a shortened time frame. An award-winning example is the use of a global positioning system to help nurses locate needed equipment (Thomas, 2020). Hackathons can be set up within an organization or by external groups committed to supporting innovation. External groups that have coordinated hackathons include the American Nurses Association (ANA), Johnson & Johnson, Microsoft, and the Society of Nurse Scientists, Innovators, Entrepreneurs and Leaders.

Culture is a way of life for an organization. It encompasses norms, values, attitudes, and behaviors of an organization's people. It's easy to confuse structural components for cultural components. Culture is much greater than the sum of its parts. It includes everything about an organization: "all the practices, processes, habits, values, structures, incentives, and naturally people" (Nieminen, 2020).

The culture of an organization influences individuals' beliefs and behaviors. Therefore, building a culture of innovation within an organization encourages and supports people to think and be innovative. However, building a culture of innovation is challenging in healthcare because healthcare is highly regulated, and healthcare organizations have a long history of using blame to address errors. There are considerable consequences to the risks associated with failure, and time is regulated and monitored leaving little room for dialogue and the development of strategy. It has taken years for healthcare organizations to recognize that reducing error required a systems approach. Efforts to improve quality and safety require innovation in order to achieve its goals. "If we avoid embracing innovation, we'll miss the opportunity to use emerging technologies that support optimal patient care, minimize error, enable decision support, and ultimately relieve potential burden on nurses and other caregivers" (Sensmeier, 2019, p. 2).

The interplay of structure and culture is evident in policy, incentives, education, innovation centers, and partnerships. Policy sets the framework for innovative behavior. This area may often be overlooked by organizations, so it is incredibly important for leaders to recognize how team members engage with and interpret policies that impact engagement within organizations. If organizational policy is often being circumvented by staff, understanding the need for the "work-around" could lead to opportunities for policy innovation. Work-arounds are created for efficiency, saving time, or possibly addressing inequities in the healthcare system. If a work-around solves a problem, there should be open discussion about how a need is not being addressed and possible policy solutions to address the problem. Organizations can create opportunities for team dialogue by creating a culture where there are no negative repercussions for speaking up, engaging in humble inquiry through listening and asking questions, avoiding making assumptions, and developing rapport (White et al., 2019). Encouraging staff to identify policy flaws and solutions within organizations is challenging. The culture should support the establishment of policies to encourage staff to identify potential areas for improvement. Policies should support staff members in identifying flaws in care delivery that impact safety and quality. When staff members present creative solutions to problems, organizations need to have policies that clearly define intellectual property allocation for innovations created by staff to foster an engaged innovation workforce.

Incentives influence how people direct their behavior. It is important to note that not all incentives take a monetary form. An incentive can be an increase in wages or the sharing of royalties that result from monetizing an innovation, but incentives also include seeing patients thrive and succeed or receiving a note of recognition from a supervisor. Different incentives have differing values for different people. With incentives taking so many different forms, it is important for organizations to consider how they structure the incentives within the organization and how those incentives drive the behaviors that make the organization successful. National programs to incentivize innovation in nursing include the awards given by the ANA (www.nursing-world.org/practice-policy/innovation/events/awards/) and Johnson & Johnson (www.jlabs.jnjinnovation.com/quickfire-challenges/johnson-johnson-nurses-inno-vate-quickfire-challenge-improving-access-care). Incentives can drive motivation to make short-term behavior change but often do not sustain behaviors.

An educated workforce is another key element to successfully structuring innovation. It is important for leaders, both formal and informal, to understand the core concepts of innovation. Universities, including nursing schools, are incorporating innovation into their programs. There are a growing number of programs in higher education that help prepare leaders of innovation in healthcare. The American Association of Colleges of Nursing (AACN, 2021) emphasizes the integral role of nurses in innovation in its essential domain for systems-based practice. There is also an immense opportunity for impact on organizational innovation when employees understand how to navigate the organization's innovation ecosystem.

Efforts placed on educating employees should focus on the resources available, the incentives for engagement, and how engaging in innovation behaviors aligns with the organization's mission, vision, and values to maximize impact. However, education alone does not guarantee retention. Thus, any educational program should be combined with mentoring and coaching to ensure the individual can actualize the educational offerings and create an attainable plan for their organization.

Partnerships are another structural component of innovation that can both catalyze the innovation efforts of an organization and enhance the organization's reputation as a leader of innovation. Building policies into the organizational structure that make it clear and easy to engage with external partners are key steps to building the collaborative innovation culture. An example of partnerships in healthcare innovation has been shown among IBM, Scripps, and Geisinger Health System to leverage artificial intelligence and the electronic health record to predict heart failure in hospitalized patients (Ng et al., 2016). Together, everyone elevates their level of impact.

Innovation centers are virtual or physical locations where an organization's members can meet to develop solutions to problems affecting their teams. The brilliance of an innovation center is that it provides a formidable structure of innovation, creating a tangible location for innovation work. Centers of innovation may contain high-tech tools for prototyping, like laser cutters and 3-D printers, but the true value of the innovation center is that, through its presence alone, the organization has issued a commitment to the structure of innovation that becomes embedded throughout the organization.

The functioning of an innovation center is determined by each organization's policies. This is illustrated by the Center for Healthcare Innovation and Wellness at The Ohio State University College of Nursing which houses The Innovation Studio. See Figure 8.3 and Policy on the Scene 8.2.

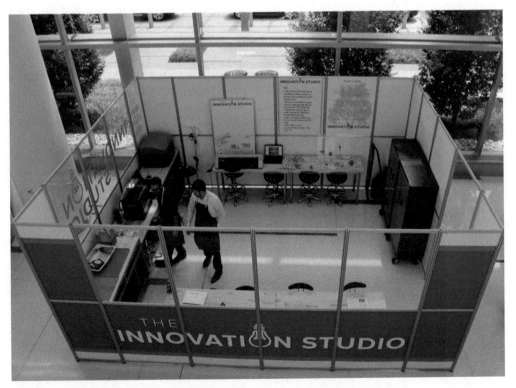

FIGURE 8.3 The innovation studio at The Ohio State University College of Nursing.

Source: © Tim Raderstorf, DNP, RN, FAAN

POLICY ON THE SCENE 8.2: INNOVATION STUDIO

The Innovation Studio at The Ohio State University is made up of two maker-spaces, one stationary location located in the center of campus, and one movable makerspace that travels to different high-traffic locations. A makerspace is a physical location that hosts a variety of prototyping tools and encourages the turning of ideas into actions. With the goal of democratizing innovation, the Innovation Studio has developed a model to help every student, faculty, and staff member at The Ohio State University turn their ideas into actions. Their movable makerspace makes five tour stops throughout the calendar year, staying at each location for about 7 weeks at a time. During these residencies, the Innovation Studio staff engages with individuals and teams that showcase an interest in innovation. They ask participants, "What are the things you love the most about your job? What are the things you can't stand about your job? What do you wish your boss would fix for you?" And with those questions answered, the Innovation Studio team encourages participants to solve a problem in one of those areas.

Working alongside the Innovation Studio team, participants begin work on their ideas and develop a 5-minute presentation to deliver during the Innovation Studio Pitch Day that occurs on the last day of every tour stop. The Innovation Studio takes a truly unique and impactful approach to structuring their Pitch Day by committing to the funding of every team. As long as the team's pitch improves the health and well-being of one person and is delivered by a team of two or more Ohio State University students, faculty, or staff with different educational/professional backgrounds, *every* team receives at least one round of funding to initiate their project. After the first round of funding, teams are given a milestone to achieve and are encouraged to return to the next pitch day to demonstrate their progress and ask for their next round of support from the Innovation Studio. Teams continue in this cycle of achieving milestones to receive ongoing support until their project finds success or failure.

The innovation studio model leverages all of the components of structural innovation listed above. Through its policies, the innovation studio fosters interprofessional collaboration. The innovation studio hosts educational programs, teaching frontline workers how to use three-dimensional (3-D) printers, design their own computer-aided design (CAD) drawings, and learn how to program simple sensors. More importantly, it serves as an educational platform on how to navigate innovation within the organization. It also partners with the university technology commercialization office to ensure that innovations with commercial potential receive the resources they need to bring these ideas to consumers.

Lastly, the Innovation Studio leverages its own policy to develop incentives, which have been dubbed "Inspirational Capital." Inspirational capital is a tool used to encourage teams to continue to turn their ideas and action and push beyond barriers. Inspirational capital can take the form of cash or grants, but it can also take the form of access to technology, equipment, and prototyping tools, or connections to collaborators or mentors who can help the team find success. The Innovation Studio has found the most impactful form of inspirational capital, is its policy that funds every team pitching an idea. By funding every team, the innovation studio is able to say to all who engage that it believes in the team and their ideas and that the organization wants everyone to bring their ideas forward and engage in the culture of innovation.

Evidence and Innovation: A Balancing Act

It is well known that EBP and decision-making lead to a higher quality and safety of healthcare in addition to a reduction in costs. EBP is a problem-solving approach to the delivery of care that incorporates the best evidence from well-designed studies with a clinician's expertise and a patient's preferences and values (Melnyk & Fineout-Overholt, 2019). Key steps in EBP are conducting a search to answer a clinical question and critically appraising the body of research. However, there are times when huge gaps in evidence exist for a problem as well as the implementation of its solution. These are areas where innovation is desperately needed to creatively solve challenges in healthcare.

The challenge is striking the balance between innovation and evidence. Evidence and innovation are conceptualized within a dynamic relationship (Porter-O'Grady & Malloch, 2021, p. 108). Using evidence can be paradoxical in that it involves a systematic review of research to find out what works, a look back at completed research. Looking back may prohibit looking forward, a necessary component of innovation. In this case, translation of research into practice, or the implementation of change is the challenge of innovation. It is important for people who are conducting research and implementing the use of evidence in practice and policy to capitalize on opportunities for innovation and change. The lag between the results of research and implementation into practice is well known. Likewise, there is a lag between the innovation and its widespread adoption into practice.

For example, Henrik Kehlet initiated enhanced recovery programs in the 1990s (Melnyk et al., 2011); in 2001 there was an Enhanced Recovery After Surgery (ERAS) Study Group and by 2010, the ERAS Society was established (ERAS® Society, 2016). Since 2010, the ERAS literature has exploded. There is a large body of evidence to support the implementation of ERAS protocols. The policy on the scene not only illustrates the use of evidence but also illustrates the lag in adoption of innovation and sustaining it. The innovation for ERAS is not only its implementation, but its expansion to different types of surgeries, settings, and organizations. See Policy on the Scene 8.3 for an illustration of this process.

Facilitators and Barriers to Change and Innovation

Building a structure of innovation provides the foundation on which a culture of innovation can thrive. Barriers and facilitators can be subtle and overt and render the policy process either effective and impactful or can dismantle it. Understanding the significance of both facilitators and barriers to change and innovation further supports the advancement of new ideas. Regardless of the best preparation and planning, resistance to change and innovation occurs. Individuals often state they are supportive and want to participate in innovation or changing; however, their participation does not happen. Likewise, an organization may proclaim innovation as part of its mission, but in reality, the status quo is maintained. Generally, resistance to change occurs when there is a perceived threat to safety and security. Some barriers or resistors to change and innovation are covert and difficult to uncover. Examining resistance is a critical part of the change and innovation process. There are similarities among the facilitators and barriers to change and innovation among individuals and within organizations.

Understanding individual facilitators and barriers are foundational to identifying the work needed to support innovation and change. Many of these are then multiplied at the organizational level when individuals with various expectations for innovation and change collaborate within the same environment.

POLICY ON THE SCENE 8.3: PARADIGM SHIFT: PROTOCOL FOR PATIENTS HAVING SURGERY

Angela Milosh, DNP, CRNA, Program Director
School of Nurse Anesthesia
Cleveland Clinic
Cleveland, Ohio

There is a paradigm shift evolving in the policies and practices for the management of patients having surgery with a goal of reducing surgical stress, optimizing physiologic function, and facilitating recovery. An example is the approach to perioperative care, called Enhanced Recovery After Surgery, (ERAS), a patient-centered, evidence-based practice used by practitioners to reduce postoperative opioid use, length of stay, and cost of care while enhancing patient recovery. ERAS requires significant coordination and collaboration among many stakeholders at multiple points in the perioperative environment. The best adherence is typically seen when the implementation is under the control of a single discipline, rather than the complex postoperative environment (Byrnes et al., 2020).

The ERAS protocol at our facility includes the use of opioid-sparing techniques through a comprehensive pain management pathway. The use of opioids during the perioperative period is associated with a number of side effects, including respiratory depression, nausea and vomiting, impaired gastrointestinal function, urinary retention, impaired mental status, and an increased risk for developing opioid dependence. In the United States, there is an epidemic of opioid abuse that often starts with a surgical procedure. The ERAS pain management pathway includes a multifaceted approach to reducing opioid consumption during the intraoperative and postoperative period, thereby reducing the risk of long-term opioid use and dependence.

This comprehensive pain management plan begins prior to admission for surgical procedures and extends past the point of discharge from the surgical facility. Components of the plan include patient education, modification of the standard fasting protocol, the use of major and minor nerve blocks, and the use of nonopioid analgesics. Patients are involved in the preoperative education process to help set realistic expectations for surgical recovery and pain management. An oral carbohydrate beverage is consumed up to 2 hours prior to surgery, helping reduce anxiety, pain perception, and nausea and vomiting. Preoperatively, patients take oral medications, which may include acetaminophen, gabapentinoids, cyclooxygenase (COX) inhibitors, and anti-emetics. They may receive a major or minor nerve block to block pain impulse transmission, often for 24 hours or more. Intraoperatively, they may be given non-opioids that reduce pain perception, including ketamine, lidocaine, or magnesium. Postoperatively, the patients will begin nutritional intake as soon as possible and will utilize staggered schedules of nonopioids as the first treatment for pain, before introducing opioid analgesics. These medications may include acetaminophen, ketorolac/ibuprofen, COX-inhibitors, gabapentinoids, and muscle relaxants.

The demonstrated success of ERAS in promoting positive patient outcomes has led many facilities to adopt specific protocols and pathways for surgical subspecialty populations, which have been incorporated into facility-wide policies. These pathways have shown particular success in patient populations whose disease process and treatment may include increased opioid use, such as spine, colorectal, and orthopedic surgical procedures. The benefits have included increased patient satisfaction, reduced cost of care, reduced length of stay, and more rapid return to baseline function.

Competing commitments are often cited examples that can create conflict and frustration and become a barrier. These competing values often make it difficult to understand which side of the policy debate an individual will eventually choose.

Facilitation of innovation and change results from multiple factors including knowledge and understanding of the intended purpose, expected personal or professional investment, and an active role in the processes. Facilitating change and innovation results when goals and values are mutually supported, and the personal impact of the change or innovation is acceptable to the individual. There is nothing more frustrating than learning about an intended change or innovation that will impact one's work after it has been formulated and proposed.

Working in a supportive professional environment enhances openness and creativity. Change and innovation can arouse emotions and passionate pleading for one choice or another. When one's choice is sustaining the current reality, barriers to considering and adopting new ways are quickly raised. Fear of what the change might result in as well as avoidance of risk-taking contributes to resistance. These barriers to change and innovation are most often related to personal comfort with the current situation. Personal baggage includes everything from once-valid beliefs and practices that have outlived their usefulness to misinformation and misconceptions that have been accepted or even embraced without much examination, thought, or evidence.

Leadership within an organization is critical to the success of change and innovation. It includes accountability and the allocation of resources to the processes supporting change and innovation. Leaders set the agenda and contribute to openness in the culture for innovation. Facilitating change and innovation occurs when there is stakeholder engagement, the sharing of knowledge and ideas, and team building. Strategies to decrease resistance include using sound principles of team building, working to understand the rationale, resolving competing commitments that result in resistance, and allowing adequate time for discussion and collaboration. Change and innovation need to be aligned with the mission of the organization. It is then possible to create the structures and work processes to establish a supportive culture critical to successful innovation. See Exhibit 8.2 for common barriers to change and innovation at the individual and organizational level.

EXHIBIT 8.2 BARRIERS TO INNOVATION AND CHANGE

Fear
Lack of leadership
Short-term thinking
Lack of resource/capacity
Lack of collaboration
No time
Lack of focus
Lots of ideas, no delivery to market
No clear process
Lack of urgency

Source: Data from Gower, L. (2015, September 7). *10 barriers to innovation.*
https://www.lucidity.org.uk/the-ten-barriers-to-innovation/

Leveraging Policy to Guide Innovation

Policy can either encourage or obstruct innovation. The political environment has a profound impact on innovators. Throughout history, scientists and artists were controlled by the political establishment, and not following requests could have dire consequences. An example of how creativity was stifled can be found in the work of Michelangelo. While best known for his frescoes of the Sistine chapel, Michelangelo thought of himself primarily as a sculptor. Constrained by the political establishment, he left many of his sculptures unfinished as he had little time for them after addressing the pope's requests.

Although the times have changed, similarities remain today. Money, resources, policies, and governments drive innovation. Scientists and innovators follow funding opportunities and regulatory pathways, often shifting entire programs to meet requests for applications or adapt to obscure regulatory frameworks. On a positive note, policies can be highly supportive of innovation. However, in some instances, innovation is stifled because of regulations that either make it impossible or near impossible to bring a product to market with the thought of commercialization only arising after the research and discovery (R&D) phase is complete. Consequently, there is a need for work in policy to simultaneously be forward thinking and yet be coordinated within current organizational structures.

When it comes to policy and regulation, the United States has historically been considered the most innovative economy in the world, yet work needs to be done for the United States to keep its lead seat at the table. Its leadership in innovation has been established by a strong alliance between government, academia, and private business, which did not happen randomly but was purposely united during and after World War II to accelerate technology development. This innovative partnership model gave life to many of America's most influential private corporations, fueled primarily by government funding and policymakers who continued to reinforce funding for R&D. Over the course of many decades, these policies resulted in 50% of the gross domestic product (GDP) being attributed to innovation (U.S. Chamber of Commerce Foundation, 2015). Unfortunately, over the last few decades, government funding for academic research has decreased significantly. Although the overall U.S. investment in research has grown, the proportion of R&D funded by the federal government has declined; this is concerning because this funding is important for the development of basic research (National Science Foundation, 2020). This decrease in government funding has primarily been felt as a growing U.S. innovation deficit. The freedom to create and explore is critical to marketplace innovations; therefore, the less that is spent on exploration, the less it can be expected to be seen in the marketplace. Reversing these policies, or at least equalizing them, is a critical step for the United States in remaining a world leader in innovation. Advocacy and education of both policymakers and the public are the best places to start. Increased funding will not occur until scientists and innovators speak up and clearly articulate why reenergizing government-funded research is necessary. There is also an urgent need to translate research findings into real-world settings at a much faster rate than currently exists.

As a result of the need for using research in the real world, innovation policy needs to address both the invention of novel ideas and their translation into products and services. Policies are merely goals that policymakers create for society's development. These goals are based on current needs and potential future trends. When it comes to innovation, there are certain concerns that need to be taken into consideration. These include inventor rights and ownership, public and private partnerships, federal regulations governing the path to implementation (e.g., Food and Drug Administration [FDA], Centers for Disease Control and Prevention), funding, training, and resource development, public education and interpretation, and end-user evaluation. Many opportunities exist in each of these categories to make innovation easier and more attractive to corporations and investors. In addition, federal regulations, although necessary, are often restrictive and need to be balanced to allow for creativity and exploration while also protecting the public. Beyond these challenges, there is a tremendous opportunity to educate the public and eliminate the spread of misinformation and the distrust in the scientific community. This challenge may be the steepest given the current political environment.

One of the most difficult challenges in the life of any innovation is the well-known "valley of death," which is the period between idea conception to market adoption (Klitsie et al., 2019), a concept also used to address the time between research and its translation into practice. The speed with which an innovation is adopted depends on numerous factors like the competency and training of the team, operational efficiencies, and governmental policies. Government policies tend to focus primarily on idea generation and funding for research but not so much on idea implementation and commercialization. Policymakers need to address matters of technical viability, market/user research, and business case development. Research needs to examine these issues at the start of their program, as opposed to at the end of it. All innovators should have a lens toward policy, sustainability, and commercialization, or else one runs the risk of investing money in programs that are not commercially or politically viable. This is an area where government funding can be greatly improved.

The Global Trade and Innovation Policy Alliance (GTIPA) is a network of 33 groups from 25 economies throughout the world that believe innovation is critical to their success. In a cross-country study about innovation, the GTIPA found that many high-performing innovative economies have generous R&D tax credits, investment incentives, and collaborative tax credits; unfortunately, that is not the case with the United States (Information Technology & Innovation Foundation, 2019). The U.S. federal government is significantly underinvesting in R&D compared to its peers. This results not only in a slowing growth of innovation but also in forcing scientists and innovators to stop their programs or leave their professions altogether. On the flip side, there is an opportunity in the business sector to pick up the slack. Since the government is under-supporting research, maybe it is time for big corporations to step in and secure our future. There is no other alternative funding source. The future of innovation in the United States lies with our ability to be innovative ourselves.

Using Laws and Regulations to Support Innovation

Legislation and regulation can be leveraged for innovation. Therefore, monitoring bills related to one's area of interest can be beneficial. However, with an overwhelming number of legislative bills introduced each year in the U.S. Congress, monitoring legislation related to one's area of interest can take extensive amounts of time. The 116th Congress (2019–2020) introduced 1,816 bills that were classified by subject as health policy, yet only 18 became law (Library of Congress, n.d.). The Library of Congress offers the ability to create an account on the Congress. gov website. Once an account is created, searches can be saved with alerts created based on the search criteria or based on a specific piece of legislation. This is a good way to get notifications concerning federal legislation that can impact one's area of interest and provide an opportunity for innovation.

Following legislation provides insights on the pulse of changes lawmakers are seeking within an industry. The real opportunity for innovation may exist in exploring the regulations promulgated from legislation once passed. Federal agencies, such as Centers for Medicare and Medicaid Services (CMS), Health and Human Services, the FDA, and OSHA are given authority to create, adapt, or remove regulations for the implementation and compliance with the law. With the scope and breadth of the Patient Protection and Affordable Care Act (ACA), a large number of rulemaking activities ensued as the ACA is credited with triggering 265 rulemaking activities (Haeder & Yackee, 2020). Typical rulemaking activity from legislation may not be as robust as with the ACA, but this is a good source of information when seeking inspiration for innovation or implementation of innovation.

To be informed about the rules and rulemaking process, the National Archives and Records Administration's Federal Register (federalregister.gov) is a helpful tool. The Federal Register provides the public the opportunity to review proposed and enacted rules, review the public notices to provide feedback on proposed rules, and participate in the rulemaking process. Searches of the website can be narrowed by a specific term or to a specific regulatory agency and you can have alerts sent directly to your email or Really Simple Syndication (RSS) feed. The proposed rule section of the Federal Register will give insight to the regulatory agency's vision for compliance, enforcement, or other aspects of existing or new rules. While one can go to individual regulatory agency's websites and search "proposed rules," using the Federal Register can be a more efficient way to navigate proposed policies that can inspire innovation. States have similar mechanisms for informing the public about proposed rules and regulations. For example, the *Pennsylvania Code and Bulletin* is Pennsylvania's publication for its code and the bulletin is for proposed rules and regulations (www.pacodeandbulletin.gov/). California's official repository for regulations is the California Code of Regulations (ccr.oal.ca.gov/).

When looking to leverage policy to guide innovation, it is important to engage those who are immersed in policy at the local, state, or federal level. Many healthcare organizations and professional associations have staff who monitor federal and state health policy changes and proposed changes. Connecting with a department or individuals whose job is to monitor health policy at the state and/or federal level is probably one of the most effective ways to keep informed on policy changes that can spur innovation.

Consider the length of the actual times in which legislative bodies are in session and the available time frames for which changes can be submitted. Fitting change processes into legislative schedules requires significant collaboration and teamwork prior to the start of the session; being strategic and timely in this work is essential. Ensuring that key stakeholders are knowledgeable and able to support the proposed change cannot be accelerated without some anticipation of a loss of support.

The COVID-19 pandemic resulted in a loosening of restrictions for APRNs. For example, in response to the need to provide medical care for residents of long-term care (LTC) facilities, Ontario allowed NPs to work as medical directors in LTC and act as the "Most Responsible Provider" (McGilton et al., 2021). If these changes can be made at a time of high stress for organizations in delivering healthcare services, it seems logical that policies can be created and/or modified to retain these innovations. Another example of a policy change inspired by the COVID-19 pandemic is illustrated in Policy on the Scene 8.4.

The Affordable Care Act as an Exemplar for Innovation Opportunity

Innate opportunities for innovation occur when laws or regulations are created or modified. The passage of the ACA provided multiple opportunities for

POLICY ON THE SCENE 8.4: POLICY IS A GAME CHANGER

Intravenous (IV) insulin infusion therapy is the established standard for patients with hyperglycemia in ICUs. It is one of the more time-consuming aspects of critical care nursing. The required hourly point-of-care glucose testing and regular insulin titrations. Caring for these patients utilized a tremendous amount nursing care time that was also disruptive for the patients. As the number of patients with COVID-19 and their acuity increased, clinical staff were faced with finding solutions to provide safe care and manage the workload. Ironically, the technology to provide continuous glucose monitoring (CGM) was approved as a safe standard of care only to be used for patients outside hospitals.

One interprofessional team led by Eileen R. Faulds, PhD, MS, RN, FNP-BC, CDE, an endocrinology NP, explored how COVID-19 impacted patients with diabetes. The interdisciplinary team recognized many patients with COVID-19 had preexisting diabetes that required high doses of insulin and steroids and that they often became septic.

During COVID-19, the Food and Drug Administration (FDA) adjusted some protocols and revised policies that permitted clinicians more readily to change and innovated new practices. Simply stated, the FDA allowed for the use of CGM in all settings but provided little guidance for how CGM should be implemented in the new settings.

The CGM technology allows for glucose values to be transmitted up to 10 feet from the patient. Thus, the team revised guidelines and the CGM protocol so that it could be implemented in ICUs. The interprofessional team's primary aim was to provide safe appropriate glucose testing that maintained patient safety, minimized workload, and decreased disruptions to patients. The team used a rapid cycle review approach to develop an innovative protocol. It confirmed the validity of the CGM devices with each patient by comparing point of care (POC) and CGM values. Once two consecutive POC/CGM pairs, taken 1 hour apart, were within 20% then the CGM could be used for hourly glucose testing and IV insulin titration. Once initial confirmation was obtained, POC/CGM values were compared every 6 hours. The CGM's protocol allowed POC glucose testing to be reduced from 24 to just four times a day without negatively impacting care.

The FDA policy change has been a game changer. It permitted the team to innovate while managing the patient's hypoglycemia care needs, saving time, and minimizing unnecessary disruptions to patients. This clinician-led innovation was shared with the CGM manufacturer to disseminate the protocol nationally. Twelve known health systems have adopted the new guidelines. This innovative protocol, without compromising patient safety, also had the benefit of reducing COVID-19 exposure risks (Faulds et al., 2021). By developing a new policy, the team was able to scale their innovation for valuable impact.

www.endocrinepractice.org/article/S1530-891X(21)00017-3/fulltext

innovation within the U.S. healthcare system. These include the establishment of the Consumer Operated and Oriented Plan Program (CO-OP), designed to foster the creation of qualified nonprofit health insurers to offer competitive health plans for individuals and small groups (CMS, n.d.a), and State Innovation Waivers, allowing states to establish innovative ways to provide access to healthcare provided that coverage is comparable and does not increase the federal deficit (CMS, n.d.b). Furthermore, the ACA opened the door to innovation in quality reporting, medication therapy management, determining the value of health plans, and reimbursement. While the ACA is considered landmark legislation because of the fundamental changes to healthcare it set to achieve, it does not take landmark legislation to leverage enacted legislation to guide innovation. In addition, the regulations promulgated from the legislation provided other opportunities for innovation and also, commercialization.

The ACA provided for the implementation of many new practices to help incentivize organizations to improve healthcare systems and to involve patients more directly in their care. Value-based purchasing that resulted in financial penalties for hospitals that failed to meet quality-of-care indicators, such as readmission rates for select patient populations, were among the new incentives.

Prior to the ACA, there was little incentive in policy to do anything about high hospital readmission rates. However, Kathy Bowles, PhD, RN, FAAN, FACMI, and her research team at the University of Pennsylvania were working on a decision support tool to identify which patients are most likely to benefit from post-acute care (PAC) services (Bowles et al., 2008). Their data indicated that patients who were at high risk had multiple comorbid conditions and that they took multiple medications, making placing them at high risk for poor discharge outcomes; fewer than half of the patients received PAC, and that was linked to high readmission rates. With the support of the National Institute of Nursing Research, Dr. Bowles was able to develop and test an expert-based clinical decision support tool dubbed the "Discharge Decision Support System" or D2S2 (Bowles et al., 2009). Dr. Bowles put it this way: "We had a nice tool that nobody really cared about" (K. Bowles, personal communication, December 1, 2020). Hospitals were not interested in their solution, so it was shelved and forgotten about by everyone, except the team. However, the passage of the ACA changed everything. Dr. Bowles knew that she had a solution that would result in two key outcomes: improving the lives and outcomes for patients PAC and saving hospitals money by reducing readmission penalties required by the ACA.

Dr. Bowles reached out to her organization's Technology Transfer Office and informed them that the time was right for disseminating the D2S2 tool. Dr. Bowles and Eric Heil, a student member of her team, co-founded RightCare Solutions, with Eric becoming the company's chief executive officer of the company (Bowles & Heil, 2014). A digital version of the decision support tool that could be integrated into the electronic health record was developed.

Over the next few years, RightCare Solutions raised funds through research awards, National Institutes of Health small business grants, and venture capital investment. Dr. Bowles continued to conduct research demonstrating the value of the D2S2 platform (Bowles et al., 2014, 2015) leading to its installation in more than 30 hospitals. Without a change to policy and subsequent commercialization, the work may have remained shelved, missing the opportunity to impact the lives of many patients. Subsequently, a second-generation decision support tool called Discharge Referral Expert System for Care Transitions (DIRECT), which not only identifies those who need PAC but also recommends the level of care, home-health or facility-level care, was developed.

Commercialization is not easy and its complexity can grow along with the company. The purchasing cycle in healthcare is longer than most industries, resulting in an extended period between first contact and receiving payments. Inventors often have to give up control of the destiny of their invention. Although rewarding to see one's work launch, and make a difference, the product development and marketing approaches may evolve in unexpected ways making you feel a loss of control. It is not only stressful but also extremely exciting and rewarding. The commercialization path is not for everyone and those who engage should enter with their eyes wide open, be patient, and be persistent.

A crucial issue for innovation, whether COVID-19 related or not, is the evaluation of current, retrospective, or prospective outcomes about innovation itself and existing or potential policies. Evaluation methods could be challenging but should be tailored to the issues, innovations, and policies under review. One size does not fit all as there are a large variety of initiatives across settings, with varying degrees of complexity and urgency. For example, one can use a cost–benefit analysis or one of the environmental scan methods (see Chapter 4) or a structure, process, outcome approach (see Chapter 12). No matter the methods used, data is essential.

One area of innovation and policy that is receiving much attention and is accumulating information is digital health, which includes categories such as wearable devices, mobile medical apps, telehealth and telemedicine, mobile health, health information technology, and personalized healthcare (FDA, 2020). In a scoping review, it was found that the largest and strongest body of evidence related to digital health was for applications of telehealth (Gunasekeran et al., 2021). While there were data for other applications, the others had design weaknesses that the authors critiqued as needing more practical evaluation. See Figure 8.4.

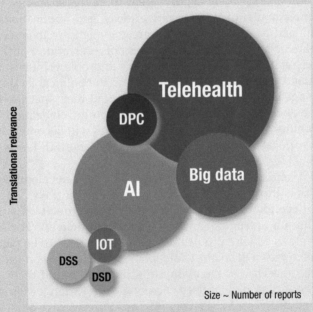

FIGURE 8.4 Bubble plot of translational relevance and strength of evidence.

AI, Artificial Intelligence; DPI, Digital Platforms for Communication; DSD, Digital Solutions for Data Management; DSS, Digital Structural Screening; IOT, Internet of Things

Source: Reprinted with permission from Gunasekeran, D. V., Tseng, R. M. W. W., Tham, C., & Wong, T. Y. (2021). Applications of digital health for public health responses to COVID-19: A systematic scoping review of artificial intelligence, telehealth and related technologies. *NPJ Digital Medicine, 4*(4), 40. https://doi.org/10.1038/s41746-021-00412-9

Based on this type of evidence, one innovation in policy supported by the ANA (2021) is the Connect for Health Act, S-1512/HR-2903. Key provisions include

- removing the Medicare originating site and rural area restrictions,
- allowing telehealth to be used to recertify patients as eligible for hospice benefits,
- working to prevent telehealth fraud and abuse, and
- permanently allowing federally qualified health centers and rural health clinics to furnish telehealth services as distant site providers.

While telehealth is not new, the innovation in the proposed is its extensive patient access and scope.

IMPLICATIONS FOR THE FUTURE

Innovation, change and policy formation, and modification are inextricably linked. They are rarely the result of linear approaches or even sequential dynamics in which their stages are logically determined. Organizations will need to pay more attention to the creation of structures and cultures that foster innovation. Educational institutions and healthcare organizations will provide dedicated resources and programming to facilitate the innovation process to teach nurses innovation and change theories, divergent thinking; strategies for the development and implementation of innovative ideas, and applications to policy. This will, in turn, lead to nurses playing a greater role in innovation. It will require that nurses are not only open to the process of innovation but that they develop competencies related to shepherding change and policy. Nurses will need to not only understand organizational dynamics and the political landscape for innovation and change but also be knowledgeable about their specific rights and issues related to the development of inventions and commercialization. It is anticipated that opportunities to develop these competencies will become increasingly available and incorporated into educational preparation at all levels and continuing education.

The digital landscape will play a key role in the development of innovation and as well as in the growth of collaboration across the globe. As society becomes increasingly dependent on technology, it will be used to solve problems to improve specific healthcare outcomes as well as healthcare delivery. For technology to be used effectively in solving problems, the end users need to be part of the process. This is where nurses will be most valuable, not only as the end users of technology themselves but because of their communication skills and their unique perspective in understanding patient needs across a wide variety of settings and circumstances as well. Nurses will be recognized as a rich resource of ideas and solutions ripe for further innovation. Learning how to translate the prototype for an idea into a workable solution that can be scaled up to serve a larger population will be increasingly important. It is the nursing lens that will help nurses to imagine these solutions.

The changing digital landscape will also impact policy formation and change. Social media will continue to present opportunities for innovative and dynamic opportunities for connection. Throughout the globe, overwhelming political, social, and economic circumstances have been both challenged and reacted to through predominantly online media mechanisms. Digital realities have created a whole new set of challenges and opportunities for democratic action, decision-making, discourse, cooperation convergence, and social revolution. The breadth of connections and interaction creates an entirely different social construct, diminishing the two-dimensional value of borders, boundaries, limited access, and human communities. The universality of the human condition and human interaction has emerged as the critical centerpiece of these digital tools whose most widely used purposes are connection, communication, linkage, networking, convergence, and relationship. Groups with diverse memberships are more productive. There must be an increase in opportunities for people from diverse backgrounds to work together. This diversity will have greater potential for the development of disruptive and frugal innovations that can significantly improve the lives of people across the globe.

The acceleration of innovation and change will inevitably impact the need for policy formation, evaluation, and modification. In order to more effectively harness innovation and change, policies will need to be examined closer to the development of the innovation and change. For example, as seen with infertility treatments and genomics, it may be difficult to imagine the possible ramifications and solutions. The COVID-19 pandemic and the need to address new problems of great magnitude led to the development of a variety of solutions with or without the accompaniment of appropriate policies or careful deliberation before their implementation. This phenomenon is likely to be repeated in a world with more disasters and unexpected events that impact health and healthcare delivery. Nurses, representing the largest healthcare professional workforce are ideally suited to be at the policy tables that address long-term solutions that facilitate the implementation of innovations, their sustainability, widespread adoption, and potential commercialization.

KEY CONCEPTS

1. Nurses' work is about innovation, change, and creating policies to support the expected work of patient care excellence.

2. Innovation can involve a new process, an invention, a care delivery model, an educational strategy, or a policy.

3. Healthcare leaders need to respond to the changing needs of healthcare systems through a complex process that includes innovation, renovation, exnovation, or the "Novation Dynamic."

4. Nurses are trained to be entrepreneurial thinkers as illustrated by the similarities between the steps of the nursing process and Morris's Entrepreneurial Concepts.

5. The development of innovation needs a supportive structural and cultural environment that includes champions, incentives, innovation centers, and opportunities for partnerships.

6. The need for innovation has to be balanced with the use of evidence to creatively solve challenges in healthcare.

7. Failure and mistakes engender opportunities for innovation.

8. Money, resources, policies, and governments have a powerful influence on the innovation process.

9. Policies supportive of innovation need to address not only the invention of novel ideas but also their translation into products and services.

10. Innovators should have a lens toward policy, sustainability, and commercialization.

11. Monitoring legislation and regulation is important for identifying opportunities for innovation created by shifts in policy.

12. The passage of the ACA led to changes in policy that supported the creation of innovative practices and delivery models.

13. The COVID-19 pandemic resulted in innovation and the revision of policies, which will require evaluation for long-term sustainability.

SUMMARY

The combination of policy and innovation may be one of the most powerful tools available to healthcare professionals. Whether using policy to create innovation, or innovation to create policy, the opportunity for impact is exponential. Nurses are critical stakeholders in the innovation and change process. Developing policy that works requires that nurses be knowledgeable about processes involved in innovation and change. The pragmatic lens of nurses that is grounded in understanding the needs of patients and the needs of the workforce in delivering care ideally suits them to be leaders in designing structures and developing cultures that enhance innovation. The future is filled with opportunities for nurses to be innovators.

END-OF-CHAPTER RESOURCES

LEARNING ACTIVITIES

1. Review the results of an online hackathon and critique one of the innovative outcomes for applicability to policy and one of the following areas: practice, education, or research.

2. Find descriptions of three nursing innovations in the literature and/or internet and identify possible policy implications of implementing the innovation on a sustained basis.

3. Identify a COVID-19 inspired innovation, determine whether the innovation should be continued in the post-COVID era. Analyze policies that would need to be implemented and/or modified in order to sustain the innovation.

4. Initially, work individually to identify a problem or a hassle that is faced by patients, or nurses in delivering their care. Then, work in a team of three to five people evaluating each of these problems and then decide on one that can be best addressed by the group.

5. Examine a historical nurse figure who developed a key innovation and describe its implication for policy.

6. Search "nurse" or "nursing" in the Federal Register or the regulatory bulletins/notices on a state's website. Identify proposals and/or rules that may have a significant impact on how RNs or APRNs deliver care. Determine whether the proposed rules are supportive of patient care and/or nursing practice.

7. Distinguish the differences between the elements of structure and culture in the workplace or educational setting that can be modified to support the innovation process.

8. Examine an organizational policy that is outdated. Analyze why it doesn't work, or no longer provides value. Develop an action plan to address the policy change that is needed.

9. Identify the kind of preparation and revision to educational programming and the policy changes that would be needed to facilitate the ability of NPs or clinical nurse specialists to serve as LTC medical directors.

E-RESOURCES

- About Hackathons https://sonsiel.org/news-about-hackathons
- Agency for Healthcare Research and Quality: Will it work here? Decisionmaker's Guide to Adopting Innovations https://www.ahrq.gov/innovations/will-work/index.html
- American Academy of Nursing Edge Runners https://www.aannet.org/initiatives/edge-runners
- American Nurses Association Enterprise Innovation https://www.nursingworld.org/practice-policy/innovation/
- American Nurses Foundation Reimagining Nursing Initiative https://www.nursingworld.org/foundation/programs/rninitiative/
- The CMS Innovation Center https://innovation.cms.gov/
- Design Thinking for Health https://www.nursing.upenn.edu/innovation/design-thinking-for-health/
- Duke University School of Nursing Health Innovation Lab https://hil.nursing.duke.edu/

- Johnson & Johnson Nurses Leading Innovation https://nursing.jnj.com/nursing-news-events/nurses-leading-innovation/

- Johnson & Johnson Nurse Innovation Hackathons https://nursing.jnj.com/nurse-innovation-hackathons

- InventR.N. Nurse-Led Teams Innovating for Dignity, Capability, & Health Equity https://www.inventrn.org/

- See You Now Podcast https://nursing.jnj.com/see-you-now-podcast

- Society for Nursing Scientists, Innovators, Entrepreneurs, and Leaders (SONSEIL) sonsiel.org

- Walker, R.: The "E" in Stem should stand for Empathy. TEDTalk. https://www.youtube.com/watch?v=dW2QoNiYWJ8

REFERENCES

Ackerman, M. H., Guilano, K. K., & Malloch, K. (2020). The Novation dynamic: Clarifying the work of change, disruption, and innovation. *Nurse Leader, 18*(3), 232–236. https://doi.org/10.1016/j.mnl.2020.01.003

American Association of Colleges of Nursing. (2021). *The essentials: Core competencies for professional nursing education.* https://www.aacnnursing.org/Portals/42/AcademicNursing/pdf/Essentials-2021.pdf

American Nurses Association. (2021). *2022 ANA innovation awards.* https://www.nursingworld.org/practice-policy/innovation/events/awards/

Bhatti, Y., Taylor, A., Harris, M., Wadge, H., Escobar, E., Prime, M., Patel, H., Carter, A. W., Parston, G., Darzi, A. W., & Udayakumar, K. (2017). Global lessons in frugal innovation to improve health care delivery in the United States. *Health Affairs, 36*(11), 1912–1919. https://doi.org/10.1377/hlthaff.2017.0480

Bowles, K. H., Chittams, J., Heil, E., Topaz, M., Rickard K., Bhasker, M., Tanzer, M., Behta, M., & Hanlon A. (2015). Successful electronic implementation of discharge referral decision support has a positive impact on 30- and 60-day readmissions. *Research in Nursing and Health Care, 38*(2), 102–114. https://doi.org/10.1002/nur.21643

Bowles, K. H., Hanlon, A. L., Holland, D. E., Potashnik, S., & Topaz, M. (2014). Impact of discharge planning decision support on time to readmission among older adult medical patients. *Professional Case Management, 19*(1), 29–38. https://doi.org/10.1097/01.PCAMA.0000438971.79801.7a

Bowles, K. H., & Heil, E. (2014). From unmet clinical need to entrepreneurship: Taking your informatics solution to market. *Studies in Health Technology and Informatics, 201,* 315–320. https://doi.org/10.3233/978-1-61499-415-2-315

Bowles, K. H., Holmes, J. H., Ratcliffe, S., Liberatore, M., Nydick, R., & Naylor, M. D. (2009). Factors identified by experts to support decision making for post-acute referral. *Nursing Research, 58*(2), 115–122. https://doi.org/10.1097/NNR.0b013e318199b52a

Bowles, K. H., Ratcliffe, S. J., Holmes, J. H., Liberatore, M., Nydick, R., & Naylor, M. D. (2008). Post-acute referral decisions made by multidisciplinary experts compared to hospital clinicians and the patients' 12-week outcomes. *Medical Care, 46*(2), 158–166. https://doi.org/10.1097/MLR.0b013e31815b9dc4

Brooten, D., Naylor, M. D., York, R., Brown, L. P., Munro, B. H., Hollingsworth, A. O., Cohen, S. M., Finkler, S., Deatrick, J., & Youngblut, J. M. (2002). Lessons learned from testing the quality cost model of Advanced Practice Nursing (APN) transitional care. *Journal of Nursing Scholarship, 34*(4), 369–375. https://doi.org/10.1111/j.1547-5069.2002.00369.x

Byrnes, A., Mudge, A., & Clark, D. (2020). Implementation science approaches to enhance uptake of complex interventions in surgical settings. *Australian Health Review, 44*(2), 310–312. https://doi.org/10.1071/AH18193

Byrne, J., & Ludington-Hoe, S. M. (2021). Theory of heat stress management: Development and application in the operating room. *Journal of Advanced Nursing, 77*(3), 1218–1227. https://doi.org/10.1111/jan.14668

Centers for Medicare and Medicaid Services. (n.d.a). *Consumer Operative and Oriented Plan Program.* https://www.cms.gov/CCIIO/Programs-and-Initiatives/Insurance-Programs/Consumer-Operated-and-Oriented-Plan-Program

Centers for Medicare and Medicaid Services. (n.d.b). *Section 1332: State innovation waivers.* https://www.cms.gov/CCIIO/Programs-and-Initiatives/State-Innovation-Waivers/Section_1332_State_Innovation_Waivers-

Dave, C., Cameron, P., Basmaji, J., Campbell, G., Buga, E., & Slessarev, M. (2021). Frugal innovation: Enabling mechanical ventilation during coronavirus disease 2019 pandemic in resource-limited settings. *Critical Care Explorations, 3*(4), e0410. https://doi.org/10.1097/CCE.0000000000000410

De Bode, L. (2021). Innovating "in the here and now." *Issues in Science and Technology, 37*(2), 50–55. https://issues.org/nurses-covid-innovation/

Dyer, J., Gregorsen, H., & Christensen, C. M. (2011). *The innovator's DNA: Mastering the five skills of disruptive innovators.* Harvard Business Review Press.

ERAS® Society. (2016). *ERAS/about/history.* https://erassociety.org/about/history/

Faulds, E. R., Jones, L., McNett, M., Smetana, K. S., May, C. C., Sumner, L., Buschur, E., Exline, M., Ringel, M. D., & Dungan, K. (2021). Facilitators and barriers to nursing implementation of continuous glucose monitoring (CGM) in critically ill patients with COVID-19. *Endocrine Practice, 27*(4), 354–361. https://doi.org/10.1016/j.eprac.2021.01.011

Food and Drug Administration (FDA). (2020). *What is digital health.* https://www.fda.gov/medical-devices/digital-health-center-excellence/what-digital-health

Gomez-Marquez, J., & Young, A. (2016, May 12). *A history of nursing making and stealth innovation.* Institute of Medical and Engineering Science. https://papers.ssrn.com/sol3/papers.cfm?abstract_id=2778663

Gower, L. (2015, September 7). *10 barriers to innovation.* https://www.lucidity.org.uk/the-ten-barriers-to-innovation/

Gunasekeran, D. V., Tseng, R. M. W. W., Tham, C., & Wong, T. Y. (2021) Applications of digital health for public health responses to COVID-19: A systematic scoping review of artificial intelligence, telehealth and related technologies. *NPJ Digital Medicine, 4*(4), 40. https://doi.org/10.1038/s41746-021-00412-9

Haeder, S. F., & Yackee, S. W. (2020, August 4). Regulation, delegation, and the Affordable Care Act. *The Regulatory Review.* theregreview.org

Information Technology & Innovation Foundation. (2019, June 13). *National innovation policies: What countries do best and how they can improve.* https://itif.org/publications/2019/06/13/national-innovation-policies-what-countries-do-best-and-how-they-can-improve

Klitsie, J. B., Price, R. A., & De Lille, C. S. H. (2019). Overcoming the valley of death: A design innovation perspective. *Design Management Journal, 14*(1), 28–41. https://doi.org/10.1111/dmj.12052

Leary, M. (2020, November 20). The innovation cycle and the nursing process—they go together. *American Nurse.* https://www.myamericannurse.com/the-innovation-cycle-and-the-nursing-process-they-go-together/

Lexico. (n.d.). Novation. In *Lexico Online Dictionary.* https://www.Lexico.com/en/definition/novation

Library of Congress. (n.d.). *Congress.gov.* https://www.congress.gov

McGilton, K. S., Krassikova, A., Boscart, V., Sidani, S., Iaboni, A., Vellani, S., & Escrig-Pinol, A. (2021). Nurse practitioners rising to the challenge during the Coronavirus Disease 2019 pandemic in long-term care homes. *The Gerontologist, 61*(4), 615–623. https://doi.org/10.1093/geront/gnab030

Melnyk, M., Casey, R. G., Black, P., & Koupparis, A. J. (2011). Enhanced recovery after surgery (ERAS) protocols: Time to change practice? *Canadian Urological Association Journal, 5*(5), 342–348. https://doi.org/10.5489/cuaj.693

Melnyk, B. M., & Fineout-Overholt, E. (2019). *Evidence-based practice in nursing and healthcare: A guide to best practice* (4th ed.). Wolters Kluwer.

Melnyk, B. M., & Raderstorf, T. (2021). *Evidence-based leadership, innovation, and entrepreneurship in nursing and healthcare: A practical guide for success.* Springer.

Morris, M. H., Webb, J. W., Fu, J., & Singhal, S. (2013). A competency-based perspective on entrepreneurship education: Conceptual and empirical insights. *Journal of Small Business Management, 51*(3), 352–369. https://doi.org/10.1111/jsbm.12023

National Science Foundation. (2020, January). *The state of U. S. science and engineering 2020. Executive summary.* https://ncses.nsf.gov/pubs/nsb20201/executive-summary

Ng, K., Steinhubl, S. R., deFilippi, C., Dey, S., & Stewart, W. F. (2016). Early detection of heart failure using electronic health records: Practical implications for time before diagnosis, data diversity, data quantity, and data density. *Circulation. Cardiovascular Quality and Outcomes, 9*(6), 649–658. https://doi.org/10.1161/CIRCOUTCOMES.116.002797

Nieminen, J. (2020). *Innovation culture—The ultimate guide.* https://www.viima.com/blog/innovation-culture

Poole, M. S., & Van de Ven, A. H. (Eds.). (2004). *Handbook of organizational change and innovation.* Oxford University Press.

Porter-O'Grady, T., & Malloch, K. (2015). *Leadership in nursing practice. Changing the landscape of healthcare* (2nd ed.). Jones & Bartlett.

Porter-O'Grady, T., & Malloch, K. (2021). Evidence-based practice and the dynamic of innovation: A model for advancing practice excellence. In D. Weberg & S. Davidson (Eds.). *Leadership for evidence-based innovation in nursing and health professions* (2nd ed., pp. 103–140). Jones & Bartlett Learning.

Radjou, N., & Prabhu, J. (2013). *Frugal innovation: A new business paradigm.* Insead Knowledge. https://knowledge.insead.edu/innovation/frugal-innovation-a-new-business-paradigm-2375

Rogers, E. (2003). *Diffusion of innovations* (5th ed.). Free Press.

Sensmeier, J. (2019). Cultivating a culture of innovation. *Nursing Management, 50*(11), 6–12. https://doi.org/10.1097/01.NUMA.0000602800.19443.68

Thomas, K. (2020, June 25). Nurse innovators present winning ideas at Hackathon. *Daily Nurse® The Pulse of Nursing.* https://dailynurse.com/nurse-innovators-present-winning-ideas-at-hackathon/

Thomas, T. W., Seifert, P. C., & Joyner, J. C., (2016). Registered nurses leading innovative changes. *OJIN: The Online Journal of Issues in Nursing, 21*(3), 3. https://doi.org/10.3912/OJIN.Vol21No03Man03

U.S. Chamber of Commerce Foundation. (2015). *Enterprising states. Executive summary.* https://www.uschamberfoundation.org/enterprisingstates/assets/files/Executive-Summary-OL.pdf

Ward, T. M., Skubic, M., Rantz, M., & Vorderstrasse, A. (2020). Human-centered approaches that integrate sensor technology across the lifespan: Opportunities and challenges. *Nursing Outlook, 68*(6), 734–744. https://doi.org/10.1016/j.outlook.2020.05.004

White, B., Walker, J., & Arroliga, A. C. (2019). Avoiding organizational silence and creating team dialogue. *Proceedings (Baylor University. Medical Center), 32*(3), 446–448. https://doi.org/10.1080/08998280.2019.1593707

Wylie, I. (2012, December). *Jugaad innovation: How to disrupt-it-yourself.* https://www.thinkwithgoogle.com/future-of-marketing/management-and-culture/jugaad-innovation/-

CHAPTER 9

Implementing the Plan

MARIANNE BAERNHOLDT AND ASHLEY BRYANT LEAK

We've learned that quiet isn't always peace
And the norms and notions of what just is
Isn't always justice
And yet the dawn is ours before we knew it
Somehow we do it
—Amanda Gorman, January 20, 2021

OBJECTIVES

1. Assess the leadership necessary for implementing the plan.
2. Appraise collaborations with key stakeholders and groups.
3. Identify the resources needed in implementing the plan.
4. Review and refine the strategies for carrying the plan forward.
5. Communicate the plan.
6. Carry out steps of an action plan that will impact policy processes and outcomes.
7. Evaluate and adjust the plan.
8. Assure sustainability is in place for the plan.

Implementing a plan is a pivotal step in the policy process. Having a plan and giving careful thought to the phases of the plan, as well as to who the key stakeholders will be at each phase, are integral to the success of the plan. The plan and the details depend on the particular policy issue and the environment for bringing that policy issue forward in either the big-P or the little-p arena. This chapter is designed to help you develop the knowledge and competencies necessary to successfully activate an advocacy plan.

Implementing the plan at both the big-P and the little-p levels are natural extensions of nursing knowledge and skills. Firsthand knowledge acquired from day-to-day practice, such as developing new models of care delivery, obtaining resources within an organization, coordinating, negotiating, and doing conflict resolution, as well as advocating for patients, families, and communities, help position nurses effectively to carry out plans. The stakeholder and group work help identify the policy alternatives to be considered and to verify the level of policy work (i.e., little-p or big-P) needed. Will the work involve writing a new policy or altering or finessing new policies? Are you faced with implementing a policy that you have little say in developing? Different components are important for the successful implementation of a plan. In this chapter, we discuss leadership strategies for implementing the plan, evaluating it, handling unexpected events, and adjusting and sustaining the plan. This Policy Challenge is focused on addressing health equity by doing.

POLICY CHALLENGE | **Addressing Health Equity in the Community**

Angelo Moore, PhD, RN, NE-BC, Program Manager and LaSonia Barnett, MA, Senior Program Coordinator, Duke Cancer Institute Office of Health Equity, Durham, NC

In such a critical time in society in which structural and institutional racism are at the forefront, we need to take a look, review, and evaluate the impact past and current policies contribute to health inequities especially among historically marginalized and under-resourced Black, Indigenous, and people of color (Bailey et al., 2020). Disparities in cancer predated the COVID-19 pandemic and will continue to persist if concerted efforts are not put in place to address social determinants of health that have been ignored for many years (American Association for Cancer Research, 2020).

African American men (AAM) and Jamaican men of African descent have the highest rates of prostate cancer with a persistent prostate cancer burden and disparity gap for AAM compared with Caucasian men. Factors contributing to this gap: literacy, jobs held, access to care, healthcare affordability, stigmatization by healthcare professionals, and mistreatment of African American physicians contribute to the mistrust of the healthcare system by AAM. My early research (Angelo Moore) indicated that interpersonal treatment accounts for a significant portion of the variability in patient satisfaction. One must understand how history has influenced the lack of trust in the healthcare system for many historically marginalized groups (Jones, 2018). It is imperative for these communities to receive health information from trusted sources. Therefore, efforts to create a supportive environment where healthcare providers focus on patient-centered care creates the trust necessary to help AAM make informed decisions about treatment in a timely manner.

See Policy Solution

LEADERSHIP

Leadership is an important factor in the success of implementing a plan. In this chapter, Formal and informal leadership and empowerment are described, followed by examples of how leadership is used in professional organizations, empowerment through coalition, and networking with policymakers' allies. Leadership belongs to us all. We are all leaders and we're leading all the time, well or poorly (Lowney, 2005). Leadership comes from within and is anchored in an understanding of who one is and what one cares about. Leadership includes understanding one's strengths, weaknesses, values, and worldview and acting accordingly. A leader engages or empowers others using a positive attitude. Leadership is a way of living and an ongoing process of self-development. As the external environment and personal circumstances change, a leader will continue to learn about themselves and the world.

Individuals holding formal leadership positions such as "president" or "unit manager" have important roles in implementing plans. To implement a plan, one has to align with the formal and/or informal leadership. This is a critical driver for tailoring the plan, which capitalizes on the strengths of the setting and influences a particular course of action. Each setting has unique considerations that can be harnessed in the implementation of the plan. In some settings, you may have access to both formal and informal leaders with a wide variety of expertise, whereas in other settings, access may be limited. In some settings, formal team leadership is strong and cohesive, but it may be less so in other settings. No matter the setting, leadership is vital to change and so is leaders' ability to empower others.

Empowerment is an interpersonal process in which adequate information, support, resources, and environment exist, enabling the formulation of increased personal ability and effectiveness to set and achieve organizational goals (Hawks, 1992). In the context of patient care, this is translated as the extent to which nurses possess the power to influence those around them to deliver safe, effective care. Empowerment should be the standard and not a luxury (Linnen & Rowley, 2014). Organizations can empower nurses through a collaborative governance structure as an umbrella for the decision-making process. Such a structure makes interdisciplinary clinicians central to patient care and part of the decisions with outcomes such as fostering self-growth and organizational development (Ives Erickson et al., 2003). Hospitals with Magnet® accreditation have organizational structures that promote empowerment.

Research examining Magnet hospital outcomes has demonstrated the value of creating empowering social structures that enhance nurses' abilities to take ownership and leadership for enhanced practice (Nascimento & Jesus, 2020; Petit Dit Dariel & Regnaux, 2015). Nurses empowered in this manner feel free to question policy, investigate problems, offer solutions, participate in decisions, and enable others to do the same. By engaging other nurses in the work of an organization, nurses can further hone their problem-solving skills to address and implement important unit and organizational policy changes related to patient care and nurses' work. Nurses with organizational power use research to close the gap between evidence and practice by raising awareness of the importance of problems (e.g., sleep and rest, falls, nurse fatigue) and then finding solutions to change unit (hospital) policies and practices. The success of little-p initiatives then feeds the cycle of leadership, empowerment, and policy change.

Professional Associations Provide Leadership

Professional and specialty associations can provide indispensable leadership when advocating issues, especially when it comes to implementing plans. They may, for example, be a source for (a) practice, clinical, and policy guidelines or (b) support and staff assistance for pursuing a policy issue. Professional associations enable nurses to articulate values, integrity, practice recommendations and standards, and social policy and to demonstrate advocacy and self-regulation (Matthews, 2012).

Since its beginning, the American Nurses Association (ANA) has led and coordinated the development of position statements and the documents that express those ideas and beliefs, facilitate stakeholder meetings, analyze issues, and develop potential solutions to help with advocacy. It is just as important to understand that the ANA uses a deliberative and democratic process to develop the documents advocating its positions. This democratic process allows nurses a voice in the development of guiding the policy documents so vital to advocacy. Publications such as the *Code of Ethics for Nurses* (ANA, 2015), *Nursing's Social Policy Statement* (ANA, 2010), and *Nursing: Scope and Standards of Practice* (ANA, 2021), as discussed in Chapter 2, not only provide a wealth of information to its members, the nursing community, and the public but also can provide direction when implementing a plan and can help validate why a policy is needed.

The ANA is unique as a nurse association because it has an affiliate partnership in every state. Each partnership aligns with ANA to carry out legislative advocacy efforts. The ANA focuses on national issues, whereas the individual state nurses associations and their respective districts provide leadership for nurses working on projects at the state or community level. The state nurses' associations often work to change state laws and local issues specific to their members. The majority of these constituents or partnerships have websites, linked from the ANA (www.nursingworld.org/membership/find-my-state), where current advocacy of a group can be found. Nurses' policy engagement can be enhanced with education supported by partnerships among leaders of nurses' organizations, academia, and practice settings (Perry & Emory, 2017). As can be seen in Policy on the Scene 9.1, state nurses associations also have to implement or update their policies to stay relevant and grow interest in the organization.

Other nursing organizations also provide leadership opportunities and member services, such as specialty-specific standards, education and/or annual conferences, and membership meetings, that can help determine policy. Some dedicate resources to formulate position statements, develop formal policy agendas, engage their members in advocacy, and provide specific resources to enable members to take action on specific issues. Larger organizations may have staff members in various roles related to lobbying or government relations. Increasingly, many provide members with toolkits with actionable items that enable members to easily participate in the implementation of an advocacy plan. Eight such examples are found in Exhibit 9.1. These toolkits show a small but diverse sampling of the available resources.

EXHIBIT 9.1   PROFESSIONAL ASSOCIATIONS ADVOCACY TOOLKITS

ORGANIZATION	NAME OF TOOLKIT	LINK
American Association of Critical-Care Nurses	Alarm Management	www.patientsafetysolutions.com/docs/April_16_2019_AACN_Practice_Alert_on_Alarm_Management.htm
American Association of Nurse Practitioners	Support for Running a Practice and Managing a Business	www.aanp.org/practice/practice-management
American Nurses Association	Well-Being Initiative	www.nursingworld.org/practice-policy/work-environment/health-safety/disaster-preparedness/coronavirus/what-you-need-to-know/the-well-being-initiative/
American Psychiatric Nurses Association	Undergraduate Education Faculty Toolkit	https://www.apna.org/undergraduate-education-faculty-toolkit/
Association of Women's Health, Obstetric and Neonatal Nurses	POST-BIRTH Warning Signs Implementation Toolkit	https://www.awhonn.org/education/hospital-products/post-birth-warning-signs-education-program/
National League for Nursing	Public Policy Advocacy Toolkit	https://www.nln.org/professional-development-programs/teaching-resources/toolkits/advocacy-teaching/toolkit-home
National Association of School Nurses	Naloxone in Schools Toolkit for School Nurses	https://www.nasn.org/advocacy/professional-practice-documents/position-statements/ps-naloxone
Oncology Nursing Society	Health Policy Toolkit	https://www.ons.org/make-difference/ons-center-advocacy-and-health-policy

Beyond advocacy support and help to individuals or groups, active involvement in an association or a professional organization can help empower nurses and the organizations that employ them. Healthcare organizations benefit from supporting nurse managers' and staff nurses' involvement in professional organizations. Nurses can develop leadership competencies, which, in turn, can be very productive for the organization. Being involved in organizations, boards, and committees is a strategy for influencing their direction and implementing plans to address issues pertinent to the mission of the group. Organizational change as illustrated in Policy on the Scene 9.1 can provide valuable leadership experiences in change management that can be applied to one's workplace.

POLICY ON THE SCENE 9.1: IMPLEMENTING CHANGE WITHIN A STATE PROFESSIONAL ORGANIZATION

Megan P. Williams, EdD, MSN, RN, FNP, Clinical Associate Professor, University of North Carolina at Chapel Hill School of Nursing, Past NCNA President 2013–2015

Professional associations are nonprofit organizations that engage individuals of a particular profession and represent the interests of the profession. "The associations help provide a professional *home* to people who identify with the profession and help them engage with those who feel part of the same identification" (Agarwal & Islam, 2016, p. 2). During the period, between 2000 and 2010, the North Carolina Nurses Association (NCNA), the ANA's state nurses' association, grappled with the best way to stay relevant and grow membership. In the early 2000s, social media was growing in popularity and provided an easy and convenient way for professionals to find each other and network.

In late 2011, the NCNA embarked on a journey to evaluate the association's governance structure. The overall goal was to revamp the association's structure to boost and diversify member engagement opportunities. Although minor adjustments had been made, the NCNA organizational chart reflected the structure implemented in the mid-1990s. The first step in the change process was to complete a needs assessment of the NCNA members. Through surveys and interviews, key drivers for change were identified, including declining volunteer interest in current opportunities, increased time pressures on nurses, changes in volunteer preferences, and new and evolving technology to support alternative engagement approaches. Following the needs assessment, the board appointed an Emerging Governance Models Taskforce, and the task force began meeting to review information about emerging governance models. An important decision by the association was to enlist a consultant to provide expert facilitation. The consultant's focus was to lead the task force through a discussion of the survey and interview data and help identify emerging themes. That process resulted in the following recommendations:

1. Reduce the size of the board of directors
2. Implement a leadership development committee
3. Replace the House of Delegates with a Member Forum to allow participation of all members
4. Redesign district structure into a regional structure with more centralized financial and operational support

The next step in the change process involved listening. The task force presented the recommendations to the board and membership and focused on gathering feedback. The task force met to review the feedback and ask, "Are there new ideas identified that we should consider?" A central theme emerged from this work: *valuing each NCNA member's talents and expertise*. With this central theme identified, the task force then updated the recommendations and planned a communication strategy. The recommendations were communicated through informational webinars and a virtual Issues Forum. The final step of the change process was to ask the full membership to vote. After almost 2 years, a Special House of Delegates was called in the spring of 2013 and through engaged and thoughtful discussions, the final recommendations were approved.

Following any organizational change, an evaluation of the change is necessary. In 2018, the NCNA board of directors reviewed the governance changes made and identified that the reduction in board size had inadvertently also minimized board diversity. In addition, the evaluation of the NCNA's governance changes was measured in membership growth and increased member engagement. The NCNA had a 6.6% growth rate in membership for a total of more than 7,700 members in 2020 and had seen year-over-year growth for more than a decade. In addition, 4,162 attendees took advantage of the NCNA's continuing education opportunities over the previous year and in direct response to members changing needs, the NCNA offered 24 virtual programs in 2020 and is active on social media platforms with a total of 14,667 followers. North Carolina has a history of being first in nursing and NCNA continues to move Nursing Forward (NCNA's political action committee [PAC]) as a strong and responsive professional organization.

Empowerment Through Coalitions and Alliances

Coalitions and alliances may be created for an advocacy plan when there is a specialized need to bring together representatives from diverse constituencies. Nurses, other healthcare professionals, and consumer groups may form temporary or informal coalitions or groups to advance an issue. A council or ad hoc task force might band together to address a specialized issue. One example can be found in the alliances formed for the 53 million family caregivers who provide daily unpaid care to adults and children; the majority of that help is given to adults older than age 50 (National Alliance of Caregiving [NAC] & AARP Public Policy Institute, 2020). The Caregiver Advise, Record, Enable (CARE) Act passed in most states and requires hospitals to help with care transition from hospital to home, with an emphasis on medical caregiver tasks, such as medication administration. As often happens, legislation and regulation alone are not enough for a successful policy. Often, additional support is necessary for effective implantation of a policy and, to that end, a new organization, The Home Alone Alliance, was created (Reinhard & Young, 2017). This private–public and not-for-profit organization is working to increase the education of nurses, who often are responsible for teaching caregivers and may be unpaid caregivers themselves. Thus, Home Alone Alliance worked to partner with the *American Journal of Nursing* to launch videos and articles to educate nurses about common caregiver questions. As you read and hear more about caregiving, remember that as a nurse, you can contribute to the work of this coalition. See Exhibit 9.2 for some action strategies for involvement in this legislation.

Nursing Now is another example of a coalition. It created a 3-year global campaign to improve health, promote gender equality, and support economic growth by elevating the status and profile of nursing. Nursing Now's campaign launched in 2018 and culminated in 2020 (World Health Organization ([WHO], 2021). The campaign was designed to coincide with the WHO's declaration of 2020 as the International Year of the Nurse and Midwife, which was later extended through 2021.

EXHIBIT 9.2 ADOPTION AND IMPLEMENTATION STRATEGIES FOR THE CARE ACT

- Stay up-to-date about legislation in your state.
- Establish an awareness event in local, community, or statewide healthcare settings to highlight the work of caregivers and the status of the CARES Act. This day could be part of a statewide public education campaign.
- Use social media applications (e.g., Facebook, Twitter, Instagram, LinkedIn) to increase community awareness.
- Work with legislators to visit caregivers in their homes to observe issues of caregiving firsthand.
- Become active in organizations supporting caregiver advocacy (e.g., AARP, National Alliance for Caregiving) to learn ways to volunteer and engage in initiatives.

Source: Adapted from Glazer, G., and Ali, A. A. (2017). Legislative: Family Caregiving Act: Healthcare impact and nurses' role. *OJIN: Online Journal of Issues in Nursing, 23*(1). https://doi.org/103912/OJIN.Vol23NoO1LegCo101

The coalition among the Burdett Trust, the International Council of Nurses (ICN), and the WHO had five foci for the campaign:

1. Ensuring that nurses and midwives have a more prominent voice in health policymaking.
2. Encouraging greater investment in the nursing workforce.
3. Advocating for more nurses in leadership positions.
4. Encouraging research that helps determine where nurses can have the greatest impact.
5. Sharing examples of best nursing practice (Nursing Now, n.d.).

The global coalition set up national Nursing Now groups. In 2019, the ANA, the U.S. Public Health Service Chief Nurse Officer, the University of North Carolina at Chapel Hill, School of Nursing, and the University of Washington School of Nursing, launched Nursing Now USA (www.nursingnow.org/usa/). Nursing Now's final report indicates that nurses are vital to change, the improvement of health, and the transformation of healthcare and that, in order to improve population, governments need to invest in nursing (Holloway et al., 2021).

Networking Policymaker Allies

Take the time to strategically identify where to focus efforts and how to choose issues that are important, the profession and for which a nurse would be a respected, knowledgeable advocate. Consider who potential allies are, ask why the policy you advocate for (or would like to prevent) has not been adopted, and decide whether if one has the interest and stamina to see the issue through to its conclusion. Integral to any plan are opportunities to have direct interactions with lawmakers, policymakers, and key decision-makers. Key strategies are visiting with leaders in your workplace or legislators or having them visit your unit or facility to see the real people (e.g., patients, nurses) impacted by the problem.

Visiting legislators and providing testimony can be one component of leadership needed to implement a plan. Because building new relationships takes time, capitalizing on existing relationships is key, just as it is in delivering patient care. As part of this process, it is important to identify any existing personal connections with important opinion leaders and public policy decision-makers; a nurse who is active in their town government, worked on a campaign, or went to school with a legislator's child has an entrée that can add credibility. Getting to know the decision-makers, educating them about issues, solving the inevitable constituent patient care and employment questions that arise, and alerting them to breaking news—good and bad—at your institution are excellent ways to foster these relationships. Invitations to visit and see your unit or institution can also be extremely effective.

Extending invitations, for outside visitors often is a routine responsibility of the CEO and/or chief nurse officer/executive (CNO/CNE). Finding ways to showcase and highlight advocacy work might include invitations to shadow a nurse on an inpatient unit, explanations on how patient acuity is calculated for staffing, observation of surgical procedures, or tour services unique to your organization (e.g., an interprofessional approach to a particular disease, a specialized cancer treatment, or cutting-edge technology).

Another aspect of strategically building allies is attending meetings or special events that are held by those you want to enlist in your plan. In public policy, this might mean attending events held by a policymaker in their home office, in public meetings, or at the state or national level. You can attend as an individual, but more political influence can be gained if you are part of an organized group that attends the event (see Chapter 7). The obvious advantage of these events is efficiency; it is an opportunity to highlight your plan on your policy maker's turf. The visit also helps convey a consistent message, and the common experience creates some accountability among the leaders who attend. An event can also help with communication because often, public events are great opportunities for publicity.

STRATEGIES FOR IMPLEMENTING THE PLAN

An advocacy or policy plan can take many forms, depending on the issue addressed and desired goals, whether it is a public policy or a policy change within an organization. Nurses advocating for a policy are going to need to make who, what, when, and where decisions to make the best use of strategy to move an issue forward. Exhibit 9.3 compares strategic and nonstrategic methods of advancing an issue.

EXHIBIT 9.3 COMPARISON OF APPROACHES FOR ADVANCING AN ISSUE

	STRATEGIC	NONSTRATEGIC
Who	Shared governance nursing council or nurse manager	Complaints to the chief surgeon or chief of medicine
What	Targeted issue focused on a doable solution or discrete problem	Huge laundry list of all the ills associated with the problem
When	A time when related reports indicate the issue is a problem that, when solved, could improve outcomes or when a precipitating event occurs	Same time as when a major change initiative is introduced, or 3 months after national publicity on a topic
Where	Privately or in a small group	In front of other staff members or the person's supervisor

Success in implementing policy is contingent on the development and activation of a plan specifically targeted using proven strategies. Some of these strategies may be the culmination of years of efforts to achieve the desired change. For example, efforts to reduce tobacco use included (a) policies and funds to promote education about the hazards of smoking in schools, (b) workplace smoking-cessation programs, and (c) smoke-free environments. Each of these required the support of different constituencies and strategies tailored to achieve the policy action. Goal refinement, framing the issue, targeting an audience, applying influence, addressing resources, and presenting the plan are important parts to consider when strategizing on how to implement a plan.

Goal Refinement

As an ongoing process, goal refinement involves specifying the "what" as illustrated in Exhibit 9.3. Although initial problem identification and agenda setting might be more laborious and intense, it is essential to continue to modify and refine advocacy goals. You need to determine what and the extent you want to change a particular policy goal while considering the context of the environment. For example, in 2020 President-Elect Joe Biden announced his 13-member COVID-19 task force that included physicians and public health experts but no nurse. In several opinion pieces, nurses strongly encouraged Biden to add a nurse to the task force. One nurse, Theresa Brown, started a petition on Change.org and used social media to get the word out. Within weeks she had more than her goal of 5,000 signatures—and Biden added a nurse to the task force. She termed the petition "the Little Petition that Could."

There is always uncertainty with policy, but at some point, you need to make the decision to move forward or wait strategically for another time. There is no perfect time, even when a window of opportunity exists. As new information becomes available or as the circumstances change, the plan may need refinement. Implementing the plan should be based on the best available evidence, and consideration needs to be given to the fact that you may need to change course and revise strategies and/or goals.

Finally, you have to consider the potential opposition. Barkhorn et al. (2013) developed a framework for assessing an advocacy plan that includes conditions for a successful policy campaign. The framework conditions include considering (a) what route your advocacy plan will take (e.g., legal, legislation), (b) whether there is a window of opportunity, (c) what solutions and benefits are possible, (d) if you have a flexible master plan that is readily communicated, (e) if advocates can deliver on the resources needed, (f) if and when allies can help win over policymakers, (g) whether the relevant community will support the policy, (h) how you can employ champions to overcome any opposition, and (i) if the way is clear from the organization behind you to implement the solution.

Strategic Framing of an Issue

Once you have identified goals, that it is the right time, and the potential opposition, it is time to frame your issue in a way that provides the greatest likelihood of advancing your targeted agenda and attaining your goals. The policy issue should be framed within the context of existing policy agendas when possible. Framing the issue is not just for legislative audiences. Regulators, executive agency staff, judges, potential jurors, executives, and the public are not listening only to the problems and solutions on policymakers' agendas; many may have their own policy agendas, or they might be more receptive to the agendas of others, depending on how they understand the problems as described.

How we construe the problem is "linked to the existing social, political and ideological structures at the time" (Birkland, 2011, p. 71). Advocates must frame their issue to maximize the likelihood that it will be important to stakeholders and within the context of their values to motivate people to action. For example,

Americans have generally and historically valued individualism, freedom, and free enterprise over socialism and, some would say, community. Nurses seeking to define an issue that requires public attention should not only highlight how their solution advances patient safety, improves access to care, and/or achieves cost efficiencies in delivering healthcare but might also take heed of how the traditional American values may or may not be consistent with your group's proposed solution. For example, a proposal for staffing legislation might resonate with legislators and the public if it is framed from a patient-safety perspective rather than as a labor issue, which is a key reason that 14 states (CA, CT, IL, MA, MN, NV, NJ, NY, OH, OR, RI, TX, VT, and WA) currently have regulations in place for staffing, albeit with very different stipulations (www.nursingworld.org/practice-policy/ nurse-staffing/nurse-staffing-advocacy).

Framing an issue is an ongoing process. Although consistency in messaging is needed, one needs to be mindful of the changing context for an issue. Framing an issue involves focusing on a specific aspect of it to highlight a particular feature. Framing within an existing issue strengthens the priority for it within a given political context. This was witnessed during the drafting and implementation of the provisions of the Patient Protection and Affordable Care Act (ACA). Policy solutions designed to improve patient safety, access to care, and cost-effectiveness are received more positively than initiatives that do not address any of these goals. See Exhibit 9.4 for examples of how an issue can be framed.

EXHIBIT 9.4   FRAMING AN ISSUE

BROAD TOPIC	IMPACT ON HEALTH	STRATEGIC FRAMING
Climate change	Health consequences of global warming	Weather-related disasters, emerging infectious diseases
APRN scope of practice and full practice authority	Access to care	Uninsured in a local community, antitrust issues impacting APRNs; removal of collaborative agreements and provider neutral language
Nurse shortage	Not enough nurses for growing demand for complex care	Patients are not receiving adequate care
School nurse–student ratios	Healthy children, allergies, preventative and screening services	Higher educational attainment of school children
CRNAs as sole providers	Access to obstetrical, surgical, interventional diagnostic, trauma stabilization, and pain services	Closure of rural hospitals
Federally funded clinics	Access to care for disadvantaged populations	Lack of preventive care for disadvantaged populations and overutilization of emergency care

APRN, advanced practice registered nurse; CRNAs, certified registered nurse anesthetists.

Although framing is designed to have issues resonate with key policymakers, it is necessary to ensure that members of the team advancing a policy agenda are prepared with key facts. This important strategy is accomplished with the creation of talking points to provide easily remembered and succinct information about the proposed policy change. Talking points may be made on an informal basis when preparing for a meeting, or they may be more formal, such as when preparing nurses to visit legislators. Organizations and associations may prepare talking points for general distribution to the public and legislators, with more detailed backgrounders so that individual nurses can quickly learn the salient facts and answer potential questions (see Chapter 10).

Targeting an Audience

Identifying the best audience for a policy issue goes hand in hand with framing an issue and is the "who" of being strategic. Although framing an issue is designed to make the policy goal resonate with the audience, targeting the audience is a careful and strategic analysis of the key decision-makers and those in a position to influence the key decision-makers. Thus, targeting the audience involves strategizing to highlight an issue for a particular constituency in a way that motivates decision-makers to take action. In a hospital setting, it might be a chairperson of a committee, a department head, or a board member. In the regulatory arena, it might be an administrator of an agency. In Congress, a state legislature, or a city council, it might be the chairperson of a committee for a bill. In the community, the target audience might be members of key agencies or community boards. Framing an issue for a group means individualizing approaches. Federal legislators may be different from states. Legislators collectively may have different demographic characteristics than their constituents do. For example, the 116th Congress had the greatest number of women and Black, Indigenous, Latinx, and people of color (BILPOC). As of 2020, it is the most racially and ethnically diverse in history, and more openly Lesbian, Gay, Bisexual, Transgender and Queer (LGBTQ) lawmakers will serve than ever before. Even with this progress, the numbers are widely discrepant of the share of BILPOC and LGBTQ people in the United States.

Targeting an audience involves learning about its characteristics and being strategic about the location and timing of a presentation. This information can be obtained through direct interaction, such as when making visits to a legislator's office, and consultation with colleagues and policymakers. Examination of websites and other publicly available information about the decision-maker provides information about positions and values. For example, a legislator's website can provide information about legislative committee memberships and expertise. Other sites can provide information on specific votes cast for certain bills. Very often, legislators have had contact with health professionals and nurses through their own illnesses or experiences with family members. This information can be used to develop messages that take advantage of these important details. The when and where of targeting an audience depend on the current milieu for the issue and other issues on policymakers' agendas. For example, something seemingly simple might be the placement of an issue on an agenda for a meeting, whether it is part of another agenda item or it stands alone. Location factors might include whether members of an audience are on their home turf or a meeting is public or private.

Nurses seeking policy changes locally or within their healthcare organizations also need to be mindful of the ideologies and biases of the decision-makers. Kingdon (2011) indicates that policy solutions must be "acceptable in the light of the values held by members of the policy community" (p. 143). Acknowledging the impact on patient quality and safety helps advance strategies. When selling the need for a new policy designed to improve patient safety to the chief financial officer of a healthcare facility, nurse leaders need to speak to the financial impact, including the bottom line that can be realized from the new policy (e.g., reduced readmissions, which are not paid for by Medicare; fewer costly medication errors).

When seeking adoption by staff, nurse leaders need to frame the policy as advantageous to them and patients. For example, a new handwashing policy needs to include support from leadership, a facility-wide campaign, knowledge of staff traffic patterns, availability of sinks, and education for multidisciplinary teams and patients so that it will more likely be implemented by members of the team. Policy on the Scene 9.2 shows how strategies for implementing a plan can come together quickly when there is a concerted effort among decision-makers and the policy community, in this case staff nurses and administrators in a hospital.

POLICY ON THE SCENE 9.2: WORK-RELATED FATIGUE: EVIDENCE-BASED POLICY DEVELOPMENT IN A HEALTHCARE SYSTEM

Cheryl A. Smith-Miller, PhD, RN-BC, Nurse Scientist; Nancy Havill, PhD, CNM, Nurse Scientist; Center for Nursing Excellence—University of North Carolina Medical Center, Chapel Hill, NC

Fatigue negatively affects clinician health and well-being as well as patient safety. While individual lifestyle choices and personal circumstances influence workplace fatigue, administrators and leaders have a responsibility to mitigate fatigue and overwork. Numerous workplace factors contribute to fatigue including, but not limited to, long hours, overtime, shift work, a lack of time for breaks, heavy patient loads. Policy changes can be difficult to implement even with strong evidence that nurse fatigue is dangerous to patients and nurses, and costly to healthcare systems and society.

The inability to take lunch breaks, a common problem for nurses, was a constant source of stress for our staff. Although breaks are outlined in law and written into workplace policies, the hospital's policy was inconsistently followed. It was a typical practice for nurses to forgo breaks during their 12-hour shifts, a common long-standing phenomenon across the country. The nursing department was presented with the challenge of developing recommendations for policy change in order to reduce work-related fatigue among clinical nursing staff at a Magnet-designated institution. A study team was convened consisting of Nursing Practice Council members, a doctorate in nursing practice (DNP) student and an experienced researcher to tackle this practice issue.

The changes that the nursing department eventually incorporated into a house-wide policy began with a literature review focused on reasons for clinician fatigue (Smith-Miller et al., 2014) and concluded with the findings of a five-unit intervention study using a participatory-action framework (Blouin et al., 2016; Smith-Miller et al., 2016). While policies can be easily changed their adaptation can be stalled when members of the target community are excluded from the planning and development. However, a more inclusive approach, such as that promoted by shared governance, actively solicits input regarding planning and development and can positively influence adherence and nurse engagement.

Before any policy changes were made, the prevalence of work-related fatigue among nurses and assistive personnel was established using surveys. Based on the literature review a study team was developed consisting of Practice Council members, a DNP student, and an experienced researcher. The team identified scheduling as a key issue. Staff nurse focus groups were held and an assessment of scheduling practices across the health system was done. The lack of consistent scheduling policies across the institution was striking. The intervention components and evaluation plan were presented to the Practice Council for feedback and the Nursing Research Council provided final review and approval. The steps used to address this policy development within our healthcare system included the following:

1. Invitations to participate were issued to nurse managers of the units with the highest level of fatigue. Although nurse managers accepted the invitation participation was not assured until the clinical nurses on each unit also approved.
2. Research team members attended unit staff meetings to explain the intervention components and the expectations and obligations.
3. Nursing staff on each unit agreed to engage in the components as written and offered suggestions about how to most effectively implement the interventions.
4. The components were implemented on five clinical units and included duty-free breaks, limiting consecutive work hours/shift duration, limiting the number of consecutive shifts, and requiring 48-hours between night-to-day rotations.
5. Unit leadership monitored scheduling and shift length while unit champions and Practice Council members supported duty-free break efforts.

The use of focus groups at the beginning and end of the project was critical to staff engagement. Framing the activities as a study in which nurses were involved rather than a policy mandate, engaged the nurses and empowered them to provide peer-to-peer reminders about taking duty-free breaks and leaving the unit "on time." The duration of the intervention was 3 months, which allowed for shifts in work habits and unit cultures. The interventions resulted in positive changes in nurse fatigue, fostered teamwork, and reduced unit costs by reducing overtime. The study results demonstrated the feasibility of the intervention components and the value of using evidence, a participatory-action framework, and shared governance strategies in developing and standardizing policy and increasing staff engagement.

Applying Influence

Nurses who are active policy advocates and who have significant accomplishments have learned to recognize that they can effectively influence policy development and implementation. A myriad of factors impact policy. To make sense of the complexity of influence that pervades the policy process, one can look at how the development of advocacy skills can be enhanced with the development of leadership, as discussed earlier in this chapter, and an understanding of the process of influence.

Influence is the ability of an individual to sway or affect another person or group (Adams & Ives Erickson, 2011). The Adams Influence Model (AIM) provides a framework for understanding how various factors, attributes, and processes support nurses to influence and impact individuals and/or groups and thus can be used to inform the implementation of a policy (Adams & Natarajan, 2016). The AIM highlights the relationship between two parties. The first party is the influence agent (e.g., the nurse with knowledge and skill of healthcare) who seeks to influence a decision. The second party is the influence target, likely the policy-maker (including legislators, staff, or other political leaders or groups), who is the focus of the effort and has a role in setting the ultimate policy. Both the agent and the target possess the same influence factors and attributes, although these may be titrated in different amounts for the agent and target depending on the issue.

As Exhibit 9.5 illustrates, five factors are in play in any effort to influence policy: (a) authority, (b) communication traits, (c) knowledge-based competence, (d) status, and (e) use of time and timing. By considering these elements, nurses can develop a well-organized plan for working on and implementing a plan to form a policy. It amounts to finding the right spokesperson with the appropriate knowledge and authority, who communicates clearly, consistently, and effectively at the right moment(s) in time. Very often, nurses do not believe that they have the power to use influence, but as shown in Exhibit 9.5, nurses' attributes do align to influence policy. As a result of this alignment, nurses are in an ideal position to use influence in policy development and to be successful at it. Although nurse leaders have a long history of being influencers, the expansion of this concept as part of the role of all nurses is in its early stages; having an understanding of the role of the nurse as influencer will inspire more nurses to harness their capacity as change agents and team decision makers to improve the health of their patients and the population (Gentry & Prince-Paul, 2021). Ultimately, it is the entire social system and the organizational culture that need to be considered in developing strategies to influence policy direction.

EXHIBIT 9.5   AIM INFLUENCE FACTORS AND ATTRIBUTES

FACTOR	ASSOCIATED INFLUENCE ATTRIBUTES	ALIGNED NURSE ATTRIBUTES FOR INFLUENCING POLICY
Authority	Access to resources Accountability Responsibility	Extended education Understanding of patient experience Accountability for care delivery
Communication traits	Confidence Emotional involvement Message articulation Persistence Physical appeal Environment	Experience in communication in challenging situations involving patients and their families
Knowledge-based competence	Aesthetic knowledge Empirical knowledge Ethical knowledge Personal knowledge Sociopolitical knowledge	Empirical knowledge (science, nursing) Personal experience Capacity to envision needed improvements Commitment to ethical and moral judgment Understand the role of socioeconomic status on access to healthcare
Status	Hierarchical position Informal position Key supportive relationships	Highly respected and trust Expertise in relationship building
Time and timing	Amount of time to sell an issue Timing to deliver the issue	Experience in selecting actions based on competing priorities

AIM, Adams Influence Model.

Source: Adapted from Adams, J. M., and Ives Erickson, J. (2011). Understanding influence: An exemplar applying the Adams Influence Model (AIM) in nurse executive practice. *JONA: The Journal of Nursing Administration*, 41(4), 186–192. https://doi.org/10.1097/NNA.0b013e31821l8736

If reflecting on one's day, both personally and professionally, one can think of many times when one was successful and unsuccessful in using influence. Using Exhibit 9.5, consider which factors and attributes were used successfully or unsuccessfully. Furthermore, consider how these same factors and attributes worked in some situations and not others or even evolved over time. The power to influence is a key tool in the policy process and is explained in more detail in Chapter 7.

Assessing Resources

The ability to implement policy depends on the resources and support available for carrying it out. Regardless of the environment, whether it be a healthcare organization, a professional association, an informal group, or a community setting, it is necessary to assess resources. This includes identifying resources that are readily available, as well as those that need to be acquired. The assessment of resources includes people and manpower, data, and economic resources.

People and Manpower

Although the power of one person can never be underestimated, the availability of people as resources and the sheer manpower to implement an advocacy plan are primary determinants of the level that your policy can be implemented (i.e., little-p or big-P) and the success of that implementation. Manpower can be paid or unpaid, and the assessment of that manpower needs to include an examination of the expertise of volunteers, staff members of organizations, and any other individuals who could contribute to the plan.

Volunteer expertise includes determining who is interested in the issue and potential sources of volunteers. A state, for example, may have several nurse practitioner groups, based either on region or on specialization, as well as a statewide practitioner organization. When an issue involves prescriptive privileges, individuals from all of these groups are key to success. Other APRNs may wish to join because advancing a cause for one advanced practice group may benefit all advanced practice groups in terms of political capital (see Chapter 7).

Having quick access to volunteers for quick response and help is often critical. The ANA, for example, has an RN Action Center (ana.aristotle.com/SitePages/HomePage.aspx). To learn more about ANA's advocacy efforts in Washington, DC, and beyond, nurses can sign up for the latest updates and get involved in advocacy campaigns. Due to the ANA's tireless advocacy on Capitol Hill, the Title VIII Nursing Workforce Reauthorization Act (S. 1399/ H.R. 728) was included in the Coronavirus Aid, Relief, and Economic Security (CARES) Act reauthorizing nursing workforce development programs through fiscal year 2024. These workforce development programs are the largest source of federal funding for nursing education, particularly in rural and medically underserved communities. Consider becoming a volunteer that the ANA, your state nurses' association, or your specialty organization can call on for advocacy efforts when a quick turnaround is needed.

Included in assessing volunteer expertise is ensuring that individuals understand the dynamics of the policy issue being advanced in the action plan. For example, if an organization wants to take responsibility for systematically evaluating proposed legislation (e.g., endorsement or opposition), then members need education and guidance for making those decisions. To facilitate the process, the group might create talking points or a background document for the issue, or they might also organize regional town halls to raise awareness of an issue. The strategies used to assess volunteer expertise depend on the information that is available to an organization, which might include a member database, a speaker's bureau, or some other systematic way of gathering information. Larger organizations have the capacity to conduct member surveys or obtain systematic feedback on an issue. Smaller groups, of necessity, use more informal means, such as networking, email, or social media (e.g., Facebook, Twitter), to obtain information. It is important that the volunteer activities match the organization's mission, as well as the volunteer's interests.

Manpower can also include staff employed by organizations or associations. Staff members may include nurses who have direct experience with the issue or ancillary staff, such as secretaries or administrative assistants, who can be released to devote time to an issue. In addition, some workplaces employing RNs may want nurse management or staff with direct care responsibilities related to an issue to help with a community, state, or even national policy. That involvement then requires consideration of the need to have protected time for such activities. Advancing a policy issue, for example, might be a component of a clinical nurse specialist's regular job duties, but obtaining input, particularly on a substantive level, may require a further provision of time for activities. Many agencies have guidelines for staff involvement in volunteer activities tied to their work role.

Consideration should be given to marshaling the forces of other types of volunteers who are willing or have the capacity to support the activation of a plan. This might include family members who have connections to media outlets, students, family members of volunteers with computer or webpage skills, or people who might be willing to provide short-term service for the plan. Individuals who teach at universities and colleges may be able to provide introductions to faculty members who place students in internships or externships in fields such as communications, computer science, business, and media. Universities and colleges may have volunteer offices that serve as a clearinghouse for students desiring to be involved in community service.

Data

Data are important in any policy endeavor. Data may take the form of findings from research, evidence-based projects, or quality improvement processes in providing the foundation for a policy position or background information that can support the plan. Data can be used to help with the issue itself, as emphasized in Chapter 5, or data can be used for implementing the plan as described here. Data sources can include research on priorities, demographic characteristics, and other details in support of implementing an issue.

Demographic data are important, for example, in explaining, analyzing, and predicting nursing workforce needs. Publicly available big data are needed to fully understand the nature and complexity of the nursing workforce. These needs and gaps in the availability of nursing workforce data were identified by the Institute of Medicine (IOM, 2011), now the National Academy of Medicine (NAM), report, *The Future of Nursing: Leading Change, Advancing Health* recommendation that nursing workforce data collection be improved. The report included recommendations on reconceptualizing nurses' roles within the context of the entire workforce; the nursing shortage; societal issues; and current and future technology. Recommendations related to education included expanding nursing faculty, increasing nursing school capacity, and redesigning nursing education. Recommendations related to healthcare delivery focused on attracting and retaining well-prepared nurses across a variety of practice settings. The subsequent progress report indicates that data regarding the makeup of the workforce are an ongoing need (National Academies, 2016). The nursing workforce continues to be a global issue that was exacerbated by the COVID-19 pandemic. *The Future of Nursing 2020–2030: Charting a Path to Achieve Health Equity* report includes the workforce as a key area for strengthening nursing so that nurses can better address health inequities and improve health (National Academies, 2021; nam. edu/publications/the-future-of-nursing-2020-2030/).

For decades, the National Sample Survey of Registered Nurses (NSSRN) provided demographic data about RNs every 4 years from 1977 to 2008. The surveys restarted in 2018. However, data are needed at both the state and the national levels. State data were used to "tell stories" about the nursing workforce that helped inform policy discussions with legislators (Fraher, 2017). The state data provided information about care access, the proportion of nurses with baccalaureate degrees, workforce diversity (and match to the state's population), and career trajectories of RNs and LPNs (Jones et al., 2018). Data can also be obtained from the National Nursing Workforce Study and U.S. Census Bureau's American Community Survey (ACS). The former is conducted every 2 years and is funded through a partnership between the National Council of State Boards of Nursing (NCSBN) and the National Forum of State Nursing Workforce Centers (NCSBN, 2021). The ACS is conducted continuously, thus providing constantly updated social, economic, housing, and demographic data that can be used for policy decisions by communities (Spetz, 2013; U.S. Census Bureau, 2017).

Data may include not only characteristics about nurses but also information about the impact of an issue or the number of people affected, often a key to policy implementation. Ensuring that one has the right and the latest data can facilitate the development of information and other support materials in implementing the advocacy plan. A hospital, for example, may examine its own pressure injury rate compared with national benchmark data from the National Database of Nursing Quality Indicators (NDNQI) or may consult its own workers' compensation cases for nurses with back injuries to make the case for purchasing ceiling lift equipment. At the community level, hospitals are required to complete community assessments every 3 years as part of their federal reporting requirements. These documents, which are usually available online, provide rich information about the community, which can be used for making the case for implementing a specific program and/or policy change.

Economic Resources

Economic resources require a realistic appraisal of what will be needed for implementing the advocacy plan. This includes supplies, materials, and personnel time, both paid and unpaid. Organizations typically budget financial resources to implement advocacy programming, and when additional resources are needed, they can sometimes divert resources from other priorities or seek external funds. Healthcare organizations may have resources to finance a policy initiative. Some organizations, such as a professional association or a nonprofit organization, may not have significant financial assets. However, they may be able to obtain financial assistance through community organizations designed to assist nonprofits with their business processes or join a coalition that will have greater combined resources. Although large foundations such as the Robert Wood Johnson Foundation (RWJF) or the Kellogg Foundation may fund major initiatives, smaller foundations may be a resource for policy initiatives or pilot projects that have policy implications in their own communities. Local affiliates of national organizations (e.g., March of Dimes, Susan G. Komen for the Cure, American Heart Association) and hospital foundations or auxiliaries are some resources to consider.

Equally important to finding funding for policies is determining the economic costs of implementing the policy plan given the competing funding for and rising costs of healthcare. Economic evaluations of interventions associated with policy should always be addressed. A variety of tools can be used for this evaluation and can include one or more of the following: cost–benefit analyses, cost-effectiveness analyses, cost–utility analyses, or cost avoidance (Zalon & Ludwick, 2018). For example, an interdisciplinary group of practitioners used cost avoidance to convince a health system to fund a free clinic for patients between 40 and 65 years of age with five or more comorbidities. The money it cost to set up and run the clinic was saved in less than 3 years in a decrease in uncompensated emergency department visits and inpatient care for this population.

Knowing the challenges to achieving success in implementing or changing policy can make the task appear quite daunting. One strategy for strengthening your position and increasing the likelihood of success is to propose a pilot project with the suggested policy change. This would allow you to collect data. More realistically, a pilot would provide you with preliminary information about the policy and challenges, foreseen and unforeseen, in implementing a policy. This information may lead to a revision in the policy or to a strategy for getting it implemented.

Presentation of the Plan

Once the details of the plan have been developed, it is time to enact the actions and procedures to put the policy into practice. To roll out the plan, it is necessary to build momentum and create stories and education that can be taken on the road so that the plan is understood when communicated.

Building Momentum

Building momentum pushes an issue into the policy limelight, much like the tipping point described by Gladwell (2000). For example, in Thomas et al. (2020), her team builds on the momentum of sustaining telehealth beyond COVID-19. During COVID-19 when physical distancing was essential, there has been a rapid uptake of telehealth in clinical practice. As a result, the COVID-19 pandemic has led to a heightened awareness of the necessity of continuing to use telehealth after the pandemic. The article recommends the following strategies for telehealth sustainability: develop a skilled telehealth workforce, empower consumers, reform funding arrangements, improve the digital ecosystems, and integrate telehealth into routine clinical workflows. Another way to build momentum is to capitalize on current events and news stories that relate to the policy. News and events can help draw attention to problems and sometimes can be used as tipping points for some action, but they cannot be counted on to sustain the momentum of a plan.

Creating Narratives

Any advocacy plan includes enhancing the visibility of an issue. Nurses can bring their real-world experiences to bear in the discussions through the creation of narratives. Although media strategies are critically important, nurses need to be adept at developing narratives that make issues real and understandable across a spectrum of audiences (see Chapter 10). Encouraging nurses to share their stories about their clinical practice and its impact are effective means of empowering nurses to become advocates for their patients and for the profession at all levels of policy.

A clinical narrative is a first-person story that describes a specific situation. Narratives help us understand practice through reflection by making it visible, uncovering hidden aspects of the practice, and sharing with the larger community clinical knowledge, caring practices, and the complex environment in which we practice. In healthcare organizations, narratives can be used to strengthen nurses' abilities to voice their concerns and speak up about extraordinary situations. They are used to make the case for a policy initiative by serving to inform and influence colleagues, members of other disciplines, management, board members, and the public. As it happens, the way in which a nurse communicates through a narrative is also an extremely effective way of communicating in the policy arena—by telling an important first-person story in a clear and concise way that the uninitiated can easily understand. Narratives can be used external to a health organization, as when talking with a reporter, visiting a legislator, or framing testimony for a legislative hearing. We are increasingly seeing the use of narratives in books about clinical practice in nursing, medicine, and other healthcare disciplines. The prestigious health policy journal, *Health Affairs*, has a long-running column, "Narrative Matters," designed to capture the stories of patients, families, and their caregivers, and nurses have shared their narratives in this column. Berendonk et al. (2020) share one example by providing poignant insights about the challenges of persons living with dementia in institutional care settings.

Characteristics of situations that make good clinical narratives and may be included in advocacy plans are listed in Exhibit 9.6. These characteristics, derived from the work of Benner et al. (2011), can be used to select compelling narratives for policymakers.

EXHIBIT 9.6   ELEMENTS OF GOOD NARRATIVES

- Portray excellence in nursing
- Describe practice breakdowns, errors, or moral dilemmas
- Raise issues and problems
- Illustrate differences made by nurses
- Provide opportunities for learning new perspectives
- Etch into memory

Source: Benner, P., Hooper-Kyriakidis, P., & Stannard, D. (2011). *Clinical wisdom and interventions in acute and critical care: A thinking-action approach* (2nd ed.). Springer.

In writing the narrative, provide the context for the reader and include details such as time of day, the setting where it took place, and what occurred. The focus should be one's thoughts, using *I* rather than *we*. The narrative gives the reader insight into the practice, and it also provides the opportunity to *reflect* on practice—what the nurse did and why. The story that is told is the right one for that person at that time. For many nurses, the idea of writing a narrative is paralyzing. They worry that their story is not enough: It is not extraordinary enough, it is not long enough, and it is not perfect. Presentation skills can be learned. Education and practice help participants understand how to organize clear messages and hone their delivery skills.

Nurse leaders can create an environment that is not judgmental, that values and respects practice at all levels, and that offers encouragement and support as nurses share their narratives. Encouragement and support from managers and administrators for the voice of nurses is critical. Giving this support individually, in public, and verbally and in writing is vital. Not only does it reassure nurses, but also it may help inspire others to help or to work on narratives for their own projects. See Chapter 5, as many of the same techniques discussed there can be used for disseminating narratives.

Telling one's story is not without its caveats. Suzanne Gordon and Bernice Buresh, both journalists who have written extensively about issues in nursing, indicate that nurses need to be more vocal and visible by telling their stories in a way that represents nurses as knowledgeable and competent. In their classic book *From Silence to Voice*, Buresh and Gordon (2013) take nurses through a step-by-step process of developing and refining narratives to more effectively capture the realities of nurses' work and showcase their expertise and credibility. A touching narrative from Brown (2016), *The Shift: One Nurse, Twelve Hours, Four Patients' Lives*, shares the life of a nurse caring for four patients with cancer during a 12-hour shift.

Communication

Communication is essential throughout the process of implementing the plan. It was discussed briefly in the AIM Model (see the section Applying Influence) and also discussed in the section Creating Narratives and in greater detail in Chapter 10. The ability to deliver a clear and consistent message is important in all settings and circumstances and is especially important for a nurse who is advocating for policy. The goal of communication as discussed here is to emphasize its role in mobilizing staff, members of organizations, and the public to carry out all phases of the activation step. Communication includes the management of internal and external relationships, as well as messaging.

Free or inexpensive resources, such as community bulletin boards, radio or television talk shows, email list servers, and public service announcements, can be used to get your message out. A town hall or well-publicized event can also be used to communicate important messages about a policy issue. Town halls are open forums that are opportunities to provide information about an issue to the community while allowing for dialogue with key stakeholders. The degree of formality of a town hall depends on the overall goal and the way it is being used to advance a particular policy. Often, the forum is a panel discussion, followed by questions from the audience. With advertising savvy, a town hall or workplace forum draws additional supporters who are interested in and supportive of your positions or proposed policy.

EVALUATION

Once a policy is in place, do take time to celebrate but remember that the work is often never fully realized. Often, policy work is ongoing. Any number of examples throughout the book point out the need for the long view for policy and advocacy.

Dealing With the Unexpected

In any advocacy plan, there may be an unexpected turn of events or unintended consequences. For hospitals, these may be sentinel events; for APRNs, it may be a report of less-than-desired outcomes; for anesthesia providers, it may be a lapse in infection-control practices, leading to a potential widespread outbreak of disease; or for nurse educators, it may be a loss of accreditation status. These events require an immediate response and transparency. The public wants and needs to be assured that something is being done about the situation and that your organization's staff will provide safe care. Transparency provides information and helps restore trust. An organization's commitment to transparency and continuous improvement is critical in times of turmoil and uncertainty. For example, the COVID-19 pandemic led to managing unexpected challenges due to a low capacity of ICU beds and personal protective equipment (PPE). With limited PPE, including gowns, gloves, and face shields, nurses were asked to change policies and reuse their PPE. Working under such conditions was challenging and left nurses frustrated knowing that they were "breaking" regular safety precautions. This policy and safety challenge illuminated the importance of strategies for optimizing the supply of PPE with a focus on operational processes.

In the legislative or regulation process, there are often many ups and downs. Even when a plan successfully ends in legislation, the passage of a law is only the beginning of the regulatory process, and then there is an evaluation of the law's outcomes. In the legislative process, a bill may be passed but not funded, or the regulations may fall short of the full vision of the policy planners. Certainly, the many twists and turns that led to the passage of the ACA and the subsequent twists and turns that have followed its passage clearly illustrate how the unexpected can occur. Passage of the ACA shows the importance of the long view, no matter whether you supported or opposed the law. Equally important to the long view is appreciating what can be gained by looking historically at legislation, a point made in the important work on the topic of unintended consequences in 2001 by the IOM. The discussion of consequences broadly focused on several general policy areas: "Medicaid, Assessing Risks and Regulating Benefits, Delivery System Restructuring" (IOM, 2001, p. 2). Several reasons for unintended consequences were identified. Time was the first lesson learned. How long a bill takes to pass and to be written into regulation is one example of how timing can impact consequences. Sometimes, it is just a matter of time before the unintended consequences can be learned. A second lesson was that policy is born of politics; that is, factors such as reelection and the need to act can lead to unintentional outcomes such as imperfect legislation. The third and last lesson was that politics often overrides science, an important lesson receiving much attention today.

Staffing is a common but complex problem across healthcare settings today and has been the subject of much debate, study, and policy work. It serves as a good example of unintended consequences. In a study by Chen and Grabowski (2015) of nursing home minimum staffing in California and Ohio, the researchers found that adopting minimum staffing standards led to some improvements but also unintended consequences. In these staffing regulations, all direct-care staff (e.g., RNs, LPNs, certified nursing assistants [CNAs]) were treated the same and the indirect-care staff (e.g., housekeeping, activity workers) were overlooked. Thus, the state changes had the unintended impact of reducing direct care staff skill mix because of a lower ratio of professional nurses to CNAs.

ADJUSTMENT AND SUSTAINABILITY

The leaders responsible for implementing a plan need to work to maintain interest in and efforts to support it. It usually takes years of effort to achieve policy goals and is often not very direct. Persistence is important. With many issues and efforts to move forward, it usually takes years of effort and success to achieve policy goals. The path may be circuitous or not very direct, but persistence is important. A single policy achievement is only one step of the process. Incrementalism is a credible strategy for achieving sustainable results. At times, achieving only small steps is possible. Today, full practice authority is a reality for APRNs in most states, a situation that was not a possibility when these roles were first conceived years ago. When implementing a plan, there is constant consideration of the pros and cons for possible solutions or compromises. Often, the implementation of a policy provides the first opportunity to learn if it will be effective in the manner it was conceived.

Sustaining interest involves creating interest among key legislators, stakeholders, and decision-makers. These strategies can include maintaining contacts with key leaders, sending newsletters or updates, and developing press releases on the topic (see Chapters 7 and 10). In general, you can work on expanding your influence by meeting new people and building coalitions. Networking never ends.

Keeping interest involves having the supporters of your plan engaged in continuing the work. Transparency in sharing information and providing your team members with progress updates is essential. As with any issue, some individuals who were once leaders will drop out, and new leaders will emerge. It is important that your plan includes consideration to succession planning and ongoing leadership development to ensure that the policy agenda continues.

Finally, any advocacy plan needs periodic revision and regrouping through an evaluation process. This may be accomplished formally, with an evaluation tool, or informally, depending on the nature of the plan. This provides necessary information about your stakeholders, your organization, the external environment, and the impact of your plan. Having the newest information and the latest information empowers you and your team members as your plan is refined and implemented. Although it is important to deliver a consistent and preferably unified message, the plan may need revision, depending on new circumstances. Being strategic at the big-P or little-p level requires constant shifting and gauging, environment, concerns of your patients and colleagues, and concerns and challenges faced by key policy decision-makers. It is an iterative process and is most successful when the people who are most affected by the issue are involved.

POLICY SOLUTION | Addressing Health Equity in the Community

Angelo Moore, PhD, RN, NE-BC, and LaSonia Barnett, MA

To address mistrust of the healthcare system and the need to improve cancer education and screenings, the Duke Cancer Institute Office of Health Equity developed and implemented a Community Health Ambassador program. The following steps outline the implementation of the program:

1. Assess the Need of the Program
   a. Reviewed North Carolina cancer incidence and mortality rates
   b. Met with community stakeholders and determined needs
   c. Identified target populations (African Americans, Latinx, Native Americans/Indigenous people, Asian Americans, refugees, and other smaller marginalized groups)
   d. Determined there was low participation of target populations in clinical trials
2. Develop Course Content
   a. Used evidence-based guidelines:
      i. Cancers—American Cancer Society
      ii. Hypertension—American Heart Association
      iii. Diabetes—American Diabetes Association
   b. Focused on top priority cancers related to target populations (prostate, breast, lung, cervical, and colorectal)
   c. Incorporated common comorbid chronic diseases
3. Determine Teaching and Delivery Modalities
   a. Considered educational and health literacy levels of potential Community Health Ambassadors and community members
   b. Determined the best location and delivery methods for transferring information and knowledge

4. Implement
   a. Developed selection criteria for faith-based and community-based organizations and Community Health Ambassadors
   b. Created logistical processes for selection, course dates and times, registration, communication, delivery of course materials, and virtual platform
   c. Developed evaluation tools
   d. Launched program
5. Evaluate Program Outcomes

The course was initially developed face-to-face teaching. However, due to COVID-19 restrictions and precautions, it was modified and conducted virtually for a 4-hour training session. We interviewed all potential participants to ensure that they had a passion for working with individuals from these targeted populations. The program launched in the latter part of July 2020, and we trained 34 Community Health Ambassadors through October 2020 representing 18 counties (seven rural) in North Carolina.

Since the launch, cancer education has been provided to thousands of English-speaking and Spanish-speaking community members who then have gone to receive cancer screenings for the very first time. The program created a network of individuals who share best practices with each other, collaborate on activities, and provide cancer education to community members that healthcare organizations do not have the ability to reach including in rural areas which have high cancer incidence and mortality rates, limited healthcare facilities and resources, and increased transportation barriers to care. The Community Health Ambassadors are helping community members gain access to healthcare systems and services with the assistance of Community-Facing Patient Navigators within the Office of Health Equity at Duke. Importantly, this program has the potential to help address the health inequalities that currently exist in our community.

"I'm optimistic that things will change; things will get better. You have to be.
Or else people will lose the motivation to want to change. I don't say much, I'm a doer."
Angelo Moore, PhD, RN, NE-BC.

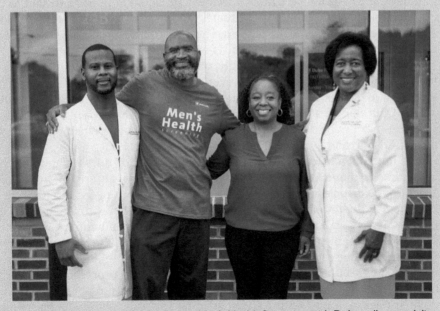

FIGURE 9.1 Dr. Moore (second from left) at a Men's Health Screening with Duke colleagues, Julius Wilder, MD, PhD; Nadine Barrett, PhD; and Marva Price, DrPH, FNP, FAANP, FAAN.

IMPLICATIONS FOR THE FUTURE

Nurses have unique professional skills for implementing an advocacy plan. Therefore, a greater involvement by nurses at the grassroots level is needed. Resources are increasingly limited, and plans need to be creative, strategic, well thought out, and anticipating desired and unintended consequences. In some instances, establishing or joining coalitions certainly adds resources, support, and credibility, particularly when the coalitions include other healthcare professional and consumer groups. State nurses' associations had greater visibility with efforts to advance 2011 *Future of Nursing* (IOM, 2011) recommendations. The next round of recommendations from the latest *Future of Nursing 2020–2030* report (National Academies, 2021) focuses on the importance of nurses in addressing health inequities and the need to do more for nurses to help them to support others (National Academies, 2021).

In response to the 2011 recommendations, state nurses associations established networks and partnerships that provided an ideal infrastructure for supporting these initiatives. The Campaign for Action has state action coalitions working with advocates from the community including representatives from interest groups, health organizations, businesses, and education to advance nursing's role in building healthier communities (campaignforaction.org/our-network/state-action-coalitions/). It is often members from the state nurses' association who are leading these efforts. State-based affiliates of specialty nurses' associations also have greater opportunities for visibility through partnerships and coalitions.

Greater emphasis should be placed on mentoring recent graduates, involving them in policy through (a) shared governance at their place of employment, (b) professional associations, and (c) community organizations to lead advocacy plan efforts. Many recent graduates have been involved in service-learning. This means that they are accustomed to providing service. However, nurses who have had service-learning experiences may not have necessarily thought about service as a means to influence policy. In addition, many recent graduates of undergraduate, graduate, and doctoral programs have been involved in projects related to policy change, but on graduation, the graduates' enthusiasm was not marshaled for further engagement in the policy process. These graduates are an ideal resource when organizations seek to vitalize their advocacy efforts.

Advocacy plans in an increasingly wired society will involve greater use of technology and social media. However, attention will need to focus on how to include individuals living in remote areas and those who do not have internet access. Data analytics will increasingly become part of advocacy plans. Therefore, strategies need to be designed for seamless data collection when plans are developed, initiated, and evaluated.

The implementation of many policies important for nursing and health policy will be implemented at the state level. Often, laws and regulations must be enacted in a critical number of states before they capture the attention of policymakers at the national level. As organizations make improvements in certain policies, it may take time for the value of these improvements to achieve widespread recognition and then be adopted, as we saw with the Magnet Recognition Program. Likewise, when new programs, laws, or regulations are established, it may take months to years for related policies and procedures to be implemented. The contributions and knowledge of nurses need to be maximized, but so do their roles in implementing and sustaining advocacy plans to enhance nursing practice and promote the health of the public.

KEY CONCEPTS

1. Implementing a plan is a pivotal step in the policy process.

2. Informal and formal leadership is important for implementing a plan.

3. The environment for implementing a plan can be a healthcare organization, a professional association, or an entirely new group developed for the specific policy issue; each has unique features to be considered in plan activation.

4. Shared governance provides opportunities to address policies and serve as a vehicle for implementing a plan.

5. Participating in a professional association enables nurses to activate plans in an organized and systematic manner and provide resources, toolkits, and infrastructure for activities.

6. New structures and/or coalitions may be created to energize support for an advocacy plan.

7. Implementing the plan involves the use of multiple strategies, including refining goals, framing an issue, targeting an audience, and applying influence.

8. Resources that need to be assessed for an advocacy plan include people and manpower, data, and economic resources.

9. Rolling out the plan includes creating narratives and building momentum and communication.

10. Strategies to build momentum include marshaling forces to advance a policy position, visiting legislators or key policymakers, seeking out organizational leaders, attending policy maker's events, and bringing policymakers to your organization.

11. Evaluating the plan includes dealing with the unexpected, including unintended consequences. These require an immediate response, frequent communication, and transparency to restore trust.

12. Sustaining an advocacy plan may take years and include numerous refinements and reiterations as implementing the policy or related policies unfolds.

SUMMARY

Nurses, long champions for their patients and communities, must now become champions and indeed experts in implementing plans for advocacy. Consistently involving nurses and widening the circle of involved nurses are key to implementing an advocacy plan. Each environment—workplace, professional associations, or the larger community at the state, national, or international level—has its own unique circumstances and challenges in implementing an advocacy plan. The establishment of a new policy, law, or regulation may only represent the initial phases of a plan that addresses a critical issue.

Consistently articulating the importance of advocacy from within the profession and equipping nurses with practical tools facilitate the activation of an advocacy plan. The AIM provides a useful framework for understanding, articulating, and using influence to help nurses gain the knowledge needed to advance healthcare policy issues and successfully persuade key decision-makers. Involving professional organizations and advocacy groups provides nurses with the additional competencies and confidence to advance policy goals.

Understanding the environment, assessing resources, and being strategic and systematic in the rollout are all critical to an advocacy plan's success. Activating a plan is not a single activity but is an ongoing process that needs to be sustained through constant refinement, involving those directly impacted by a policy and engaging decision-makers. It involves ongoing work, an ability to respond to the unexpected, and a tolerance for ambiguity as policies are moved forward.

END-OF-CHAPTER RESOURCES

LEARNING ACTIVITIES

1. Write a personal narrative to use to support a policy at your work, locally in your community, or for a state or federal legislative action. Include it in your portfolio.

2. Identify an issue you support at the big-P level, identify the target audience, and then examine websites and other publicly available information to determine the accuracy of the information and credibility of the source.

3. Select an issue at the big-P level and identify groups that would be good strategic partners or members of coalitions to advance a policy position and explain why these groups should be involved.

4. Select an issue at the little-p level and determine how the members of the task force should be selected to oversee the issue. Identify the people who should be on the task force and what roles need to be represented and provide the rationale for your selections.

5. Examine one of the toolkits listed in Exhibit 9.1, identify personal talking points that you can speak to, and review them with a colleague where you work.

6. Describe the strategies you would use for implementing a plan to implement a policy change for an issue. Include who, what, when, and where (see Exhibit 9.3).

7. Describe how you would communicate to stakeholders in your organization about a new policy plan.

8. Identify how your state nurses association, specialty nurses association, or state action coalition plans to address the recommendations of the Future of Nursing 2020–2030 report.

E-RESOURCES

- American Association of Nurse Anesthesiology. Substance Use Disorder Workplace Resources www.aana.com/sudworkplaceresources

- American Heart Association. How to Schedule and Conduct a Successful Meeting With Your Elected Officials http://www.youtube.com/watch?v=Q320LHS847w

- American Nurses Association. Action Center http://www.rnaction.org

- American Nurses Association. Policy and Advocacy http://www.nursingworld.org/MainMenuCategories/Policy-Advocacy

- Campaign for Action http://campaignforaction.org

- Community Preventive Services Task Force. (2020). *Guide to Community Preventive Services. Cancer Screening: Interventions Engaging Community Health Workers – Breast Cancer.* https://www.thecommunityguide.org/findings/cancer-screening-interventions-engaging-community-health-workers-breast-cancer

- Frameworks Institute http://www.frameworksinstitute.org

- Illinois Education Association. Tips for Talking to Legislators http://www.youtube.com/watch?v=8TtAe-_rs5U

- National Association of Clinical Nurse Specialists (NACNS). Coalitions http://nacns.org/advocacy-policy/coalitions

- Oncology Nursing Society. Center for Advocacy and Health Policy https://www.ons.org/make-difference/ons-center-advocacy-and-health-policy

- Prevention Institute. Prevention and Equity at the Center of Community Well-Being http://www.preventioninstitute.org

- Rising Voices. Featured Guide: Social Advocacy Toolkit for Activists and Non-Profits https://rising.globalvoices.org/blog/2012/05/28/featured-guide-social-advocacy-toolkit-for-activists-and-non-profits/

- Robert Wood Johnson Foundation. Nurses & Nursing http://www.rwjf.org/en/topics/rwjf-topic-areas/nursing.html

- UNICEF. Advocacy Toolkit: A Guide to Influencing Decisions That Improve Children's Lives http://www.unicef.org/evaluation/files/Advocacy_Toolkit.pdf

- Video for Change Toolkit https://toolkit.video4change.org/what-is-impact-toolkit/

Additional e-resources can be found in Exhibit 9.1

REFERENCES

Adams, J. M., & Ives Erickson, J. (2011). Understanding influence: An exemplar applying the Adams Influence Model (AIM) in nurse executive practice. *JONA: The Journal of Nursing Administration*, 41(4), 186–192. https://doi.org/10.1097/NNA.0b013e3182118736

Adams, J. M., & Natarajan, S. (2016). Understanding influence within the context of nursing: Development of the Adams Influence Model using practice, research, and theory. *Advances in Nursing Science*, 39(3), E40–E56. https://doi.org/10.1097/ANS.0000000000000134

Agarwal, N. K., & Islam, M. A. (2016). How can professional associations continue to stay relevant? knowledge management to the rescue. *Proceedings of the Association for Information Science and Technology*, 53(1), 1–10. https://doi.org/10.1002/pra2.2016.14505301028

American Nurses Association. (2010). *Nursing's social policy statement: The essence of the profession*.

American Nurses Association. (2015). *Code of ethics for nurses with interpretive statements*.

American Nurses Association. (2021). *Nursing: Scope and standards of practice* (4th ed.).

American Association for Cancer Research. (2020). *AACR cancer disparities progress report 2020. Achieving the bold vision of health equity for racial and ethnic minorities and other underserved populations*. https://cancerprogressreport.aacr.org/disparities/

Bailey, Z. D., Feldman, J. M., & Bassett, M. T. (2020, December 16). How structural racism works—Racists policies as a root cause of U.S. racial health inequities. *The New England Journal of Medicine*. Advanced online publication. https://doi.org/10.1056/NEJMms2025396

Barkhorn, I., Huttner, N., & Blau, J. (2013, Spring). Assessing advocacy. *Stanford Social Innovation Review*. https://ssir.org/articles/entry/assessing_advocacy#

Benner, P., Hooper-Kyriakidis, P., & Stannard, D. (2011). *Clinical wisdom and interventions in acute and critical care: A thinking-action approach* (2nd ed.). Springer.

Berendonk, C., Blix, B., Hoben, M., Clandinin, D., Roach, P., & Compton, R. (2020). A narrative care approach for persons living with dementia in institutional care settings. *International Journal of Older People Nursing*, 15(1), e12278. https://doi.org/10.1111/opn.12278

Birkland, T. A. (2011). *An introduction to the policy process: Theories, concepts, and models of public policy making* (3rd ed.). M. E. Sharpe.

Blouin, A. S., Smith-Miller, C. A., Harden, J., & Li, Y. (2016). Caregiver fatigue: Implications for patient and staff safety, Part 1. *JONA: The Journal of Nursing Administration, 46*(6), 329–335. https://doi.org/10.1097/NNA.0000000000000353

Brown, T. (2016). *The shift: One nurse, twelve hours, four patients' lives.* Algonquin Books.

Buresh, B., & Gordon, S. (2013). *From silence to voice: What nurses know and must communicate to the public* (3rd ed.). ILR Press.

Chen, M. M., & Grabowski, D. C. (2015). Intended and unintended consequences of minimum staffing standards for nursing homes. *Health Economics, 24*(7), 822–839. https://doi.org/10.1002/hec.3063

Fraher, E. P. (2017). The value of workforce data in shaping nursing workforce policy: A case study from North Carolina. *Nursing Outlook, 65*(2), 154–161. https://.doi.org/10.1016/j.outlook.2016.10.003

Gentry, H., & Prince-Paul, M. (2021). The nurse influencer: A concept synthesis and analysis. *Nursing Forum, 56*(1), 181–187. https://doi.org/10.1111/nuf.12516

Gladwell, M. (2000). *The tipping point.* Little, Brown.

Glazer, G., & Ali, A. A. (2017). Legislative: Family caregiving Act: Healthcare impact and nurses' role. *OJIN: Online Journal of Issues in Nursing, 23*(1). https://doi.org/10.3912/OJIN.Vol23No01LegCol01

Hawks, H. J. (1992). Empowerment in nursing education: Concept analysis and application to philosophy, learning and instruction. *Journal of Advanced Nursing, 17*(5), 609–618. https://doi.org/10.1111/j.1365-2648.1992.tb02840.x

Holloway, A., Thomson, A., Stilwell, B., Finch, H., Irwin, K., & Crisp, N. (2021). *Agents of change: The story of the Nursing Now Campaign.* Nursing Now, Burdett Trust for Nursing. https://www.nursingnow.org/wp-content/uploads/2018/01/NursingNow-final-report.pdf

Institute of Medicine. (2001). *Unintended consequences of health policy programs and policies: Workshop summary.* National Academies Press.

Institute of Medicine. (2011). *The future of nursing: Leading change, advancing health.* National Academies Press.

Ives Erickson, J., Hamilton, G., Jones, D., & Ditomassi, M. (2003). The value of collaborative governance/staff empowerment. *JONA: The Journal of Nursing Administration, 33*(2), 96–104. https://doi.org/10.1097/00005110-200302000-00006

Jones, C. P. (2018). Toward the science and practice of anti-racism: Launching a national campaign against racism. *Ethnicity and Disease, 28,* 231–234. https://doi.org/10.18865/ed.28.S1.231

Jones, C., Toles, M., Knafl, G., & Beeber, A. (2018). An untapped resource in the nursing workforce: Licensed practical nurses who transition to become registered nurses. *Nursing Outlook, 66*(1):46–55. https://doi.org/10.1016/j.outlook.2017.07.007

Kingdon, J. W. (2011). *Agendas, alternatives, and public policies* (2nd ed.). Pearson Education.

Linnen, D., & Rowley, A. (2014). Encouraging clinical nurse empowerment. *Nursing Management, 45*(2), 44–47. https://doi.org/10.1097/01.NUMA.0000442640.70829.d1

Lowney, C. (2005). *Heroic leadership. Best practices from a 450-year-old company that changed the world.* Loyola Press.

Matthews, J. H. (2012). Role of professional organizations in advocating for the nursing profession. *Online Journal of Issues in Nursing, 7*(1), 3. https:/doi.org/10.3912/OJIN.Vol17No01Man0

Nascimento, A., & Jesus, E. (2020). Nursing work environment and patient outcomes in a hospital context: A scoping review. *JONA: The Journal of Nursing Administration, 50,* 261–266. https://10.1097/NNA.0000000000000881

National Academies of Science, Engineering, and Medicine. (2016). *Assessing progress on the Institute of Medicine report on the future of nursing.* National Academies Press.

National Academies of Sciences, Engineering, and Medicine. (2021). *The Future of Nursing 2020–2030: Charting a Path to Achieve Health Equity*. The National Academies Press. https://doi.org/10.17226/25982

National Alliance of Caregiving, & AARP Public Policy Institute. (2020). *Caregiving in the U.S. 2020*. https://www.aarp.org/content/dam/aarp/ppi/2020/05/full-report-caregiving-in-the-united-states

National Council of State Boards of Nursing. (2021). *National nursing workforce study*. https://www.ncsbn.org/workforce.htm

Nursing Now. (n.d.). *Who we are*. https://www.nursingnow.org/who-we-are/

Petit Dit Dariel, O., & Regnaux, J.P. (2015). Do Magnet®-accredited hospitals show improvements in nurse and patient outcomes compared to non-Magnet hospitals: A systematic review. *JBI Database of Systematic Reviews and Implementation Reports, 13*(6), 168–219. https://doi.org/10.11124/jbisrir-2015-2262

Perry, C., & Emory, J. (2017). Advocacy through education. *Policy, Politics and Nursing Practice, 18*(3), 158–165. https://doi.org/10.1177/1527154417733438

Reinhard, S. C., & Young, H. M. (2017). Nurses supporting family caregivers. *American Journal of Nursing, 117*(5), 58–60. https://doi.org/10.1097/01.NAJ.0000516385.05140.b0

Smith-Miller, C. A., Harden, J., Seaman, C. W., Li, Y., & Blouin, A. S. (2016). Caregiver fatigue: Implications for patient and staff safety, Part 2. *JONA: The Journal of Nursing Administration, 46*(7–8), 408–416. https://doi.org/10.1097/nna.0000000000000366

Smith-Miller, C. A., Shaw-Kokot, J., Curro, B., & Jones, C. B. (2014). An integrative review: Fatigue among nurses in acute care settings. *JONA: The Journal of Nursing Administration, 44*(9), 487–494. https://doi.org/10.1097/nna.0000000000000104

Spetz, J. (2013). The research and policy importance of nursing sample surveys and minimum data sets. *Policy, Politics and Nursing Practice, 14*(1), 33–40. https://doi.org/10.1177/1527154413491149

Thomas, E., Haydon, H., Mehrotra, A., Caffery, L., Snoswell, C., Banbury, A., & Smith, A. (2020, September 26). Building on the momentum: Sustaining telehealth beyond COVID-19. *Journal of Telemedicine and Telecare*. Advanced online publication. https://doi.org/10.1177/1357633X20960638

U.S. Census Bureau. (2017). *American Community Survey: Information guide*. https://www.census.gov/content/dam/Census/programs-surveys/acs/about/ACS_Information_Guide.pdf

World Health Organization. (2021). *Health workforce*. Nursing Now Campaign. https://www.who.int/hrh/news/2018/nursing_now_campaign/en/

Zalon, M. L., & Ludwick, R. (2018). Health economics. In J. J. Fitzpatrick, C. Alfes, & R. Hickman (Eds.), *Encyclopedia of clinical nursing* (pp. 216–218). Springer.

CHAPTER 10

Influencing Public Opinion and Health Policy Through Media Advocacy

JESSICA KEIM-MALPASS AND KIMBERLY D. ACQUAVIVA

> *If you don't exist in the media, for all practical purposes, you don't exist.*
> —Daniel Schorr, Commentator, National Public Radio

OBJECTIVES

1. Design a media strategy to influence policymakers and/or public opinion on a current policy issue.
2. Develop written communication—specifically, letters to the editor, press releases, op-eds, and policy briefs—to convey a clear message to policymakers and the public.
3. Use at least one social media platform to influence policymakers and/or public opinion on a policy issue.
4. Tailor messages to meet the needs of different audiences.
5. Engage strategically with print, broadcast, and digital media to disseminate a clear message about a policy issue.
6. Use a combination of media to accelerate and amplify a message about a policy issue.

Media advocacy can be a powerful tool for influencing public opinion and health policy. Before using a tool safely and effectively, the tool must be identified in one's toolbox, one needs to know when and how to use it, and understand both the power and perils associated its use. This chapter provides guidance about various tools in the media advocacy toolbox and how (and when) to use each. The chapter also focuses on how to communicate one's message to different audiences to influence opinions on policy issues and how to use media to amplify nursing's voice in policy arenas. To influence public opinion and shape policy, nurses must use media to communicate clear, compelling messages relevant to health and the advancement of the profession.

The term *media* is used more often than the phrase "the media" because nurses should think about media as tools for use rather than as a faceless monolith they need to persuade. Nurses are not passive actors subject to the whims of an amorphous entity known as "the media" to amplify their messages. On the contrary, nurses have the power to amplify their own messages. The key is knowing how and when to use different types of media. This chapter focuses on the skills needed to do this effectively.

NURSES AND MEDIA ADVOCACY

This book teaches nurses how to create or change laws and policies to promote health, improve healthcare, and advance nursing. Why is it essential for nurses to use media in advocating for laws and policies? Individually and collectively, nurses can use media to advocate for little-p and big-P policy changes. As nurses, we have an obligation to express opinions and advocate for policies that benefit patients, families, populations, communities, and the profession. Advocacy means speaking up—media is our megaphone.

Advocacy is not new for nursing: nurses have always embraced patient advocacy (see Chapter 2). Historically, however, nursing has been woefully ineffective at media advocacy. In 1997, the landmark Woodhull Study on Nursing and the Media found that fewer than 1% of articles in news magazines referenced a nurse, and nurses were referenced in less than 4% of 2,101 health articles from seven leading U.S. newspapers (Sigma Theta Tau International Honor Society of Nursing, 1997). Twenty years later, after the study was replicated, little progress was made: Only 2% of the health policy article quotes identified nurses as the source, nurses' quotes were primarily on the nursing profession, and nurses were only identified in 4% of photos in accompanying articles (Mason et al., 2018). Their conclusion? "Nurses remain invisible in health news media, despite their increasing levels of education, unique roles, and expertise" (Mason et al., 2018, p. 10).

POLICY CHALLENGE 10.1	The American Nurses Association and the 2020 Presidential Election

In 2018, at the direction of its Membership Assembly, the American Nurses Association (ANA) president at the time (Pam Cipriano) convened a task force chaired by Virginia (Ginna) Trotter Betts to examine the ANA's Presidential Endorsement Policy, a nonpartisan policy that had been in place since 1984 (Betts, 2020). The task force examined the political landscape carefully and determined that (a) associations of healthcare professionals refrain from endorsing presidential candidates, (b) presidential candidates value large financial contributions and personal efforts to host lucrative fundraising events more than symbolic endorsements, (c) the Supreme Court's *Citizens United* case and subsequent influx of money into politics has had a major impact, (d) presidential candidates are less responsive to questionnaires and interview requests from the ANA and its political action committee (PAC), which were an integral part of the ANA's endorsement process, (e) the ANA membership had become more evenly split between Republicans and Democrats, and (f) it is not necessary for the ANA to endorse a presidential candidate in order to take a position on a political or policy issue (Betts, 2020). The task force ultimately recommended that the ANA move away from endorsing presidential candidates and, instead, focus on supporting ANA members in political engagement (Betts, 2020). Taking these recommendations into consideration, 87% of the delegates in ANA's Member Assembly, the organization's highest governing body, voted to rescind the presidential endorsement policy in 2019 (Betts, 2020; Myers, 2019).

While the ANA's process to evaluate policy alignment between the organization and presidential candidates had a long history of nonpartisanship, the organization's history of consistently endorsing Democrat candidates led to tension within the membership (Myers, 2019). Had it not been for the contentious campaign and election in 2020, and the prominence of critical issues impacting health and of importance to nursing, this policy decision might not have been so controversial. Nurses wanted their voices heard, and they took to social media and grassroots activity.

The time has come for nurses to step out of the shadows and up to the microphone. By using media to influence public opinion and health policy, nurses can use their expertise to realize the vision for an improved healthcare system in which nurses are leading change.

Types of Media

Media are "means of mass communication" (Oxford Lexico, n.d.) that can be grouped into three general categories: print, broadcasting, and internet media. Print media is by far the oldest, the first newspaper was printed in Strasbourg, Germany in 1605 (American Printing History Association, n.d.). Today, print media includes newspapers, magazines, books, billboards, brochures, and flyers. Broadcasting media arrived in 1917 when the University of Wisconsin's radio station 9XM began the first voice broadcast (Everhart et al., n.d.). Today, broadcasting media includes television, radio, and movies/films. Internet media is the newest arrival, with its meteoric rise to prominence beginning around 1990 to 2000. Today, internet media includes social media platforms, video streaming, websites, and blogs, among others.

Before the 21st century, the favored approach in mass communications was broadcast media, in which a single broadcast was created for an audience with a delay in public response. Media outlets were few, so sources could be leveraged to deliver health-promotion campaigns and reach large audiences (Institute of Medicine [IOM], 2002). Regardless, the problem with broadcast models was that the approach was relatively ineffective in targeting specific populations with minimal audience engagement (IOM, 2002).

The ubiquitous nature of internet media and smartphone technology has transformed people's media use in interacting with the world around them (Bird, 2011), the media landscape has changed as well; with the rise of multidirectional user-generated content, individuals now have the opportunity to both consume and produce content. Internet media has overtaken print and broadcast media in terms of both speed and reach, with social media platforms facilitating the exchange of real-time, user-generated content about ongoing events. Unbridled by traditional reporting ethics or publishing formalities and scripting, social media users may post incorrect or harmful information, or they may post accurate, thought-provoking content that inspires, educates, and/or persuades. Social media is neither good nor bad—like every other type of media, its value depends on the quality of content being disseminated.

Public Opinion

Public opinion is a social construct—a representation of what "the public" thinks about an issue (McGregor, 2019). Because "the public" is not a homogeneous body of individuals, accurately representing what the public thinks is wholly dependent on defining the "public" and the methods are used to ascertain their opinions. Before one can design a media strategy to influence public opinion, one needs to decide what is meant by "public opinion" and how it should be measured. Public opinion polls serve as a gold standard for measuring public opinion. The world's largest collection of public opinion poll data can be accessed through Roper iPoll (n.d.). Sentiment analysis using social media platforms like Twitter is another way to measure public opinion, but it is much less precise than opinion polls using rigorous sampling methods.

Media Advocacy

Using media to have one's message heard, advance opinions about issues, and influence policy decision-makers is considered media advocacy. When a nursing or healthcare issue is promoted, the goal is to educate the public, influence policymakers, and shape public viewpoints. Media advocacy combines mass communication with community advocacy. By using a range of media with purposeful strategies, groups can evolve episodic news stories into reframed public health issues. When children were dying from drunk driving accidents, a far-reaching media advocacy campaign shone a spotlight on the dreadful effects of drunk driving, eventually resulting in stiff laws and long prison sentences for offenders. Effective media advocacy addresses gaps in power and resources to effect changes that improve health and healthcare (Dorfman & Krasnow, 2014). Media advocacy requires building skills for using media as a tool to pursue social change and shift power within a community.

The Political Context of Media Advocacy and Nursing

Understanding the political context of media advocacy is essential for being successful. When newspapers and television stations run stories about an issue, that coverage can exert a powerful influence over public opinion. Historically, policymakers used press releases to capture the journalists' attention in hopes of generating positive coverage. Policymakers are attentive to media coverage because their constituents pay attention and are influenced by what they see and hear. The presidential election of 2016 and its aftermath, however, caused a shift in public and policymaker confidence in mainstream media, with partisan divides and general concern that some news is "fake" with no way to decipher fact from fiction (Easley, 2017).

Thanks to social media's ubiquity, policymakers are no longer simply the subject of media coverage. Now they have the power to generate their own coverage to influence public opinion without having to persuade journalists to deliver their message. Policymakers can use social media to speak directly to their constituents and hear their opinions in real time. Theoretically, social media's removal of mainstream media as an intermediary should have increased public confidence in the information being received from policymakers. This is not what happened, however. Unlike journalists who are required to follow a rigid set of ethical guidelines when reporting a story, policymakers are generally free to say whatever they want on social media. Policymakers who are federal employees have to follow the Hatch Act (U.S. Office of Special Counsel, n.d.), but the act imposes no constraints on the veracity of a policymaker's social media posts.

Without journalists fact-checking statements of policymakers before reporting them, information can flow directly from policymakers to the public—and that information is not always accurate. This was witnessed during Donald Trump's term as president, with President Trump making 30,573 false or misleading claims during the 4 years of his presidency (Fact Checker, 2021). In the 48 hours following Election Day in 2020, the social media platform Twitter tagged eight of President Donald Trump's tweets with warning labels, stating, "Some or all of the content shared in this Tweet is disputed and might be misleading about an election or other civic process" (Robertson, 2020).

Although social media may facilitate disseminating incorrect information from policymakers to the public, it also facilitates the dissemination of information from nurses to policymakers. This provides nurses with unprecedented policymaker access. Nurses can interact directly with local, state, and federal elected officials on social media and can shape policy through their strategic engagement with policymakers.

HOW TO DESIGN A MEDIA STRATEGY

In order for media advocacy efforts to be successful, one needs to design a media strategy. This is a detailed plan for influencing policymakers and/or public opinion on a current policy issue. Planning the approach to media advocacy involves a number of steps and strategies to get the desired outcome.

In designing a media strategy to influence public opinion on a particular issue consider whose opinion is the target of the strategy and how one wants to influence it. Research the current opinion and the sources for that information. A simple way to begin is to fill in the blanks of the "Media Strategy Planner" in Exhibit 10.1. The steps in the Media Strategy Planner will help develop a plan for communicating messages efficiently and effectively so that the message is understood and amplified.

Media campaigns are used to spread a message quickly to a large audience. Campaign messages may include providing public health information and advisories, asserting viewpoints, or declaring pro or con positions on current issues. Social media may also be used to generate immediate attention to raise awareness or garner support for a cause or policy. Simple techniques such as having a letter or editorial published can capture media attention. The more media coverage, the more potential influence is gained. Targeting multiple means of exposure for media coverage garners the attention of policymakers from local to national elected officials. For local or state issues, media can help publicize opinions, information, or events. Maintaining contact with local reporters, as well as radio and television personalities, helps familiarize them with one's expertise and content and can lead to coverage of one's issues on a regular basis.

Media advocacy involves not only planned activities to initiate a policy change but also activities arising as a result of current events. A multipronged approach can garner widespread publicity and support. Media advocacy can be used for different types of situations or health policy initiatives. Media advocacy combines mass communication with community advocacy.

HOW TO USE PRINT AND BROADCAST MEDIA FOR ADVOCACY

Whether one wants to contact the media as an individual or as a representative of a group, first, become familiar with the type of media believed to be helpful in conveying the message. For local issues, knowing the interest and track record of the print and broadcast media coverage of public health issues are important. Become acquainted with the reporters and, if possible, cultivate relationships that can lead to more longitudinal coverage of an issue. If the reach is to Congress, contacting newspapers and media outlets that cover politics and access a broader audience is beneficial.

Organizations should maintain an updated media contact list. When holding events, maintain a sign-in list and follow up with media representatives to thank them for attending. National directories are available for a fee to locate media outlets. Media directories are available by state, which can be easily found by typing "media directory" and the state into a search engine. Professional associations can also be a resource.

It is also important to seek community resources and establish relationships before a pressing issue becomes news. Get to know the local newspaper editorial staff, talk radio personalities, and television broadcasters. Healthcare organization public relations (PR) and marketing staff may be less familiar with how to promote nursing stories, so it is important to familiarize them with issues important to nurses, as well as nursing interest stories. For example, invite the organization's PR staff to attend events such as nursing research presentations, awards ceremonies, advancement celebrations, and community service days. Request a consistent person assigned to cover nursing events to avoid a repetitive learning curve. PR staff members make excellent partners, are familiar with writing guidelines, and usually have already established relationships with local media representatives. Because their job is to make an organization look good in the public eye, you can make their job easier by being a resource and alerting them to newsworthy stories. As you work with the media, it is essential to make yourself available in a timely manner to reporters seeking information, interviews, or quotes; this helps journalists respond to tight deadlines. These stories do not always have much lead time. Remember, you are responding on the record, so your comments can be used and quoted. Being prepared when a hot issue breaks allows for immediate coverage and premier positioning of nursing's response. If you initiate the media contact, your message must be clear and concise. Using personal experiences makes examples more compelling and easily understood.

Message Development

Whenever you communicate with a member of the media, you must explain why an issue is important, what is at risk, why the reader/listener/viewer should care, and why that reader/listener/viewer should act. The more closely you can align the message with others who share your values and concerns, the more support you will engender. Being prepared with a plan is the starting point for advocating an issue. The Media Strategy Planner (Exhibit 10.1) will help you develop your message and align it with your target audience.

Professional associations provide a wealth of background information for their members such as fact sheets, issue briefs, policy analysis, and talking points. These

EXHIBIT 10.1 MEDIA STRATEGY PLANNER

Group	I want to change the opinion of _____.
Issue	I want to change their opinion about _____.
Current Opinion	Currently, their opinion is _____.
Evidence	I know this is currently their opinion because _____.
Desired Opinion	I want their opinion to be _____.
Message Problem → Impact → Value Proposition → Dangers of Inaction → Call to Action →	_____ is a pressing concern because It affects [xyz community] in the following ways:_____. Addressing this problem will have numerous benefits:_____. If this problem continues to be ignored, the consequences could be _____. You can be part of the solution by_____.
Media	The group I am trying to influence can best be reached through . . . (print, broadcast, internet).
Timeline	I want to change the opinion of this group by the following date: _____.
Resources	I have the following resources available to implement this media strategy: (staff, volunteers, money, other).
Evaluation	I will assess whether their opinion has changed by _____.

may be combined into a comprehensive resource, allowing one to be prepared when planning outlining goals and objectives, and crafting an effective message. Knowing the overall goal of the actions you are taking on an issue allows you to identify appropriate audiences and the most effective types of media to reach them. Your goal may be to introduce a new issue and ask others to join in the action. Or you may want to express a position or opinion about a current issue in your community or on a state or national agenda. Your plan to develop a clear and simple message includes the steps in Exhibit 10.2.

EXHIBIT 10.2 STEPS TO DELIVERING A SUCCESSFUL MESSAGE

1. State your goal clearly.
2. Identify your audience(s.)
3. Define your issue—the issue must draw attention and be considered "newsworthy."
4. Include only one main message with no more than three underlying themes of support.
5. Limit your message to 30 seconds or less so that it is memorable.
6. Frame your statements so that your message connects to the greater public's interest.
7. Be strategic when proposing a solution.
8. State the support sought.
9. Compel the audience to be concerned about your issue.
10. Use humanizing examples and/or analogies.
11. Match your message and language to the audience.
12. Repeat your message frequently and consistently in all communications.
13. Evaluate the effectiveness of your message.

Developing a Case Statement: Tell Your Story

A simple compelling story often captures attention. Telling your story starts with facts building on what your audience knows and believes. Case statements are often used in fundraising circles and involve a simple compelling story capturing the essence of your values, as well as what you are trying to address with policy. Try to establish a personal connection, one inspiring an emotional attachment from the audience. In developing a case statement, make sure that the message does not reinforce population or group stereotypes. Drawing the lines and explaining your side helps define what is at stake. Define actions wanted to solve a problem. Linking problems to solutions, and explaining how the audience can help, advances an agenda.

Talking Points

Talking points focus a message on facts, which in turn educates media sources, stakeholders, and the public. This short list of arguments succinctly summarizes arguments for or against an issue. Advocating for pending or new legislation routinely calls for concise communication to express opinions to lawmakers and to educate the media and the public. Many nursing organizations equip members with talking points on current issues, particularly for planned lobbying events. Examples are issues highlighted by the American Organization for Nursing Leadership (AONL) on the advocacy portion of its website (AONL, 2020).

The "Pitch": Getting a Story Heard

Getting a story heard can be achieved with a succinct, powerful, 25- to 35-word description of the subject and position, answering what the issue is about, who is the target of the issue, why anyone should care, why the position is different, and one's qualifications are for making the pitch. Otherwise known as an *elevator speech*, it is an ideal way to pitch newsworthy information (see Chapter 2). An elevator speech should be able to be shared with someone in an elevator in less than a minute, and when the doors open and when exiting the elevator, the listener will be left with a clear understanding of the message and why it matters. Brevity is key to getting messages across. The pitch can be made in writing, in person, or via telephone. When pitching the story, follow these rules: (a) Introduce yourself, your credentials, and your affiliations; (b) inform them of your story idea; (c) ask if it is a good time to talk; (d) offer your brief description of what, who, and why; and (e) confirm follow-up plans. Avoid jargon to enhance clarity.

Written pitches by letter or email should be no more than one page. Present the issue concisely and establish relevance and timeliness to the audience. Include a simple description of the story and provide names of contacts, their details, and resources. Other preparations include compiling supporting documents and talking points, and determining who is available to be interviewed. However, when working with television stations, plan on no more than 15 to 30 seconds of coverage and prepare recommendations for video coverage to support the story. Be clear about one's identification, and one's credentials. It is important to identify whether one is acting as an individual, as a concerned citizen, or as an official spokesperson of an organization or group.

Reporter Calls/Emails

When a local issue breaks or if the organization is on the critical path of a story line, being prepared for reporters to call or email puts one in a prime position to respond. Reporters are looking for access and information, not an adversarial relationship. Some due diligence is essential for preparing ideas and being sure to anticipate the request of the reporter and the timeline for responding. Understanding the reporter's interest and familiarity with the subject, as well as the priority for the story, provides clues about the amount of information needed. Information to gather from the reporter is reviewed in Exhibit 10.3. Touch base with the organization's media relations office before agreeing to being interviewed by a reporter. Some organizations have specific requirements for how employees interact with the media, so it is always a good idea to check with the media

EXHIBIT 10.3   QUESTIONS TO ASK BEFORE AGREEING TO AN INTERVIEW

Questions to Ask the Reporter
- What is the overall focus of the story?
- What are you hoping an interview with me will add to the story?
- Am I being asked to speak as an individual nurse or as a representative of my organization?
- Who have you interviewed already? Who are you still hoping to interview?
- What is your deadline?
- How would the interview be conducted—by phone? Videoconference? In a TV studio? At a radio station? Is it being recorded?
- When/where will the story run/air?

Questions to Ask Yourself
- Do I have the expertise and experience to do this interview?
- Do I have my organization's permission to speak on its behalf, or will I need to make it clear in the interview that I am speaking as a private citizen?
- What background information is available that I can share during the interview?

relations office before doing an interview. Depending on the organization's size, the media relations office may offer to help with crafting talking points before the interview. Reporter calls and emails can turn into the start of an ongoing, mutually beneficial relationship. Respond promptly and politely to interview requests, even if the response is to decline the interview.

Sound Bites

A short 10- to 20-second statement comprises a sound bite that can be developed or that the media may distill from longer stories. Sound bites should support the proposition. They can be promulgated as short quotes that can be used repeatedly in conversations, in interviews, or on social media. Anticipating what might be used in a negative perspective is helpful as well; try to avoid providing ammunition for the opposition. Sound bites can also be pulled from written statements with a memorable phrase that creates an emotional connection between the issue to the intended audience. Shorter social media messages are prime vehicles for conveying poignant and pithy phrases.

PRESS RELEASES AND ADVISORIES

Press or news releases are intended to convince reporters to cover a story. Reporters scan news releases to gauge interest in potential stories. Bloggers, policy experts, and the public also pay attention to press releases for basic information on issues. This section includes techniques for writing releases and provides examples of press releases that can provide additional and correct misinformation.

Inverted Pyramid

Widely used for more than a century, many news writers use the inverted pyramid guide as depicted in Figure 10.1 in response to readers' desire for fast-paced delivery of information that holds their interest. In this style, the most

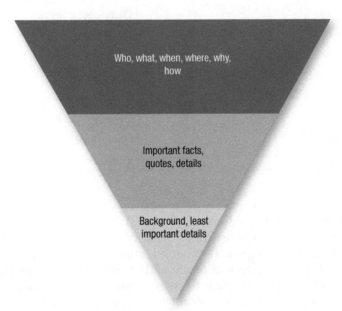

Who, what, when, where, why, how

Important facts, quotes, details

Background, least important details

FIGURE 10.1 Journalism inverted pyramid.

important information is provided up front. The content covers the five Ws and one H: who, what, where, when, why, and how. The amount of content diminishes as do the sizes of the three areas of the pyramid. Alternatively, presenting a story that is idea-driven or reported in chronological order may be appropriate for more human-interest stories rather than breaking news.

Writing a Press Release

The standard format for a press release provides quick access to all the information a reporter needs and indicates how to get in touch with the author. To grab a reporter's attention, start with one or two strong leading sentences and be convincing about the issue's news value. Address who and what in the first sentence. Throughout the story, address when, where, why, and how. Follow the introductory paragraph with one that begins to communicate feeling; using a quote helps personalize the message. The concluding paragraph typically includes a quote. Above all, information must be credible and defensible. Once the entire release is written, devise an eye-catching headline. It can have up to 10 words, and subheadlines are acceptable. Purposeful inclusion of positive or negative words can shape a reader's opinion of the story. A sample list of positive and negative words in Exhibit 10.4 illustrates the power of adjectives; the same impact applies to oral presentations.

EXHIBIT 10.4 POSITIVE AND NEGATIVE OPINION WORDS

POSITIVE WORDS	NEGATIVE WORDS
Acclaimed	Abysmal
Appealing	Angry
Beneficial	Callous
Courageous	Despicable
Distinguished	Difficult
Effective	Disastrous
Flourishing	Dishonest
Generous	Expensive
Impressive	Ill-conceived
Knowledgeable	Terrible
Quality	Tired
Respected	Unhappy
Successful	Unpleasant
Transformative	Weak

Nurses associations actively disseminate press releases on a variety of topics throughout the year to address issues from responses to tragic events; notable events and funding awards; congratulatory accolades; expressions of positions on issues of major import at the local, state, or national level, depending on the organization's scope and reach; and recognition of major legislative victories. Important items to consider when issuing a press release include using letterhead, detailed contact information, catchy headline, release date, location (city, state) and lead sentence, powerful introductory paragraph, quotes, organizational tagline, more (if going to a second page) and ### to indicate the end. See Exhibit 10.5 for a sample.

Nurses associations use press releases to inform, influence, and connect with key stakeholders. In response to the growing concerns about the rising opioid

EXHIBIT 10.5 ANA PRESS RELEASE

ANA President Condemns Racism, Brutality and Senseless Violence Against Black Communities

Jun 1st 2020

MEDIA CONTACTS:
Shannon McClendon
301-628-5391

shannon.mcclendon@ana.org
Keziah Proctor
301-628-5197
keziah.proctor@ana.org

SILVER SPRING, MD - The following statement is attributable to American Nurses Association (ANA) President Ernest J. Grant, PhD, RN, FAAN:

"As a nation, we have witnessed yet again an act of incomprehensible racism and police brutality, leading to the death of an unarmed black man, George Floyd. This follows other recent unjustified killings of black men and women, such as Ahmaud Arbery and Breonna Taylor, to name a few.

Protests have erupted in cities across the country and the world in response to a persistent pattern of racism in our society that creates an environment where such killings occur. Justice is slow and actions to ensure real change are lacking.

As a black man and registered nurse, I am appalled by senseless acts of violence, injustice, and systemic racism and discrimination. Even I have not been exempt from negative experiences with racism and discrimination. The Code of Ethics obligates nurses to be allies and to advocate and speak up against racism, discrimination and injustice. This is non-negotiable.

Racism is a longstanding public health crisis that impacts both mental and physical health. The COVID-19 pandemic has exacerbated this crisis and added to the stress in the black community, which is experiencing higher rates of infection and deaths.

At this critical time in our nation, nurses have a responsibility to use our voices to call for change. To remain silent is to be complicit. I call on you to educate yourself and then use your trusted voice and influence to educate others about the systemic injustices that have caused the riots and protests being covered in the news. The pursuit of justice requires us all to listen and engage in dialogue with others. Leaders must come together at the local, state, and national level and commit to sustainable efforts to address racism and discrimination, police brutality, and basic human rights. We must hold ourselves and our leaders accountable to committing to reforms and action.

I have a deeper moral vision for society, one in which we have a true awareness about the inequities in our country which remain the most important moral challenge of the 21st century. This pivotal moment calls for each of us to ask ourselves which side of history we want to be on and the legacy we will pass on to future generations."

(continued)

EXHIBIT 10.5   ANA PRESS RELEASE (*CONTINUED*)

The American Nurses Association (ANA) is the premier organization representing the interests of the nation's 4 million registered nurses. The ANA advances the nursing profession by fostering high standards of nursing practice, promoting a safe and ethical work environment, bolstering the health and wellness of nurses, and advocating on healthcare issues that affect nurses and the public. The ANA is at the forefront of improving the quality of healthcare for all. For more information, visit www.nursingworld.org.

crisis in the United States and the legislation paving the way for nurse practitioners to prescribe medication-assisted treatment (MAT), the American Psychiatric Nurses Association (2017) issued a press release announcing the offering of two free online courses to prepare advanced practice registered nurses (APRNs) to be able to meet requirements to prescribe MAT for opioid use disorders, desperately needed care in communities across the country. When President Donald Trump signed the Substance Use-Disorder Prevention that Promotes Opioid Recovery and Treatment (SUPPORT) for Patients and Communities Act (H. R. 6) into law, the ANA (2018) issued a press release to express the organization's "gratitude to the professional nursing organizations and diligent congressional leaders that worked with [them] to pass SUPPORT with the key nursing provisions" (para. 2).

An important initiative for advancing evidence-based practice is the Choosing Wisely® campaign of the American Board of Internal Medicine Foundation. The American Academy of Nursing (AAN) is an active partner in this initiative and, in turn, has engaged other nurses associations to identify evidence-based recommendations to help patients make the best decisions about their care. In 2017, the AAN announced its fourth set of specialty recommendations in collaboration with the American Association of Neuroscience Nurses in a press release building the Academy's list to "Twenty Things Nurses and Patients Should Question" (AAN, 2017). In 2018 the list was further expanded to "Twenty-Five Things Nurses and Patients Should Question" (AAN, 2018).

In 2020, the ANA issued close to 40 press releases about a wide range of topics including the coronavirus, violence against nurses, the CARES Act, systemic racism, the Patient Protection and Affordable Care Act (ACA), and personal protective equipment (PPE) shortages. Recent releases can be viewed on NursingWorld (www.nursingworld.org/news/news-releases), a site that is updated regularly.

Press Advisories

Press advisories alert the media to a pending event. For example, an organization may want to invite the press to cover an upcoming conference. A hospital or nursing school may want to alert the press to a release of research findings or innovations important to improving care. The announcement should be brief but arouse interest without exposing the whole story. Be sure to include the sponsor (who), subject (what), time (when), place (where), and relevance (why), as well as contact information. A press advisory may also ask media representatives to respond if they are planning to cover the event. If more than a week's advance notice has been provided, plan to send a follow-up message 1 or 2 days before the event. Email is a common way to send both press releases and advisories.

When sending information to media sources via email, limit the text to 500 words, or approximately five paragraphs. Avoid sending the key information only in an attachment. Place a short headline in the subject line of the email using the most important attention-grabbing words. Include URL links to additional information sources. Mirror the format of a press release. Both the advisory and the email should begin with contact information followed by the headline and then the body of the release. Do a test of email because formats may change with transmission. When sending to multiple media representatives, place the names as blind copies so that addresses are not shared without permission. Releases and advisories sent at slower business times receiver greater attention. Aim for late morning.

Nurses rarely have difficulty establishing credibility. Despite the portrayal of inaccurate stereotypes on television and other entertainment, the mainstream media recognizes and respects nurses' expertise. Academic degrees, certifications, and job titles convey a certain status and should be used when contacting the media. When representing an organization, pick an appropriate leader or spokesperson.

MESSAGE DELIVERY

Effective message delivery includes knowing the target audience and their interest in the story, as well as ways to deliver a message using a specific medium. Each of these media—written, voice, or visual—requires specific strategies to enhance policy impact.

Knowing the Audience and When the Story Is of Interest

Knowing the right medium for reaching the target audience guides media strategies. If taking the message to a broad audience, it may need to be tailored in several different ways to reach different groups. Questions to bear in mind for any audience include: What is important about this issue that should make others care? Of what interest is this to the targeted audience? What will capture the attention of this audience? Is it a friendly audience or one that bears convincing? What actions can I expect or request the audience to pursue? Is the timing right? The reporter's or the target's response to a conversation can reveal if or when one has piqued their interest.

Policymakers

Local policymakers often fulfill public duties on a part-time basis but their contact information can usually be located online. Reaching state and national policymakers usually requires initial contact with their staff. Response times may vary. Federal officials have a chief of communication and dedicated communications staff, as well as issue-specific staff. Many have someone assigned to cover healthcare issues. The more potent the message, the greater the likelihood policymakers will take note and listen. Successfully getting on the public's agenda also almost guarantees getting on a policymaker's agenda. The messages are synergistic for focusing attention on health issues and concerns that affect large constituencies. The typical vehicles for delivering messages to policymakers include letters, emails, opinion editorials (op-eds), background papers, blogs, press releases, and published articles, all of which can be made available to the individual and staff.

The Public

Broadcast media (both television [news and nonnews] and radio), newsletters, newspapers, bulletin boards, and social media will reach the public. Offering nursing's response to time-sensitive current events or weighing in on a larger debate, can bring attention to nursing's interest in and viewpoints about public health issues, as well as the welfare of the public and nurses. Although most consumers have interest in nursing's message, it may be only situational and, thus, calls for aiming the message for broad appeal. Nurses should also weigh in on current events that relate to public health and well-being to solidify nursing's role of advocacy in the eyes of the public. Issues such as obesity, substance use disorders, gun violence, and legalization of marijuana have struck a chord, and nurses, as opinion leaders, can provide a viewpoint that shapes local sentiment and brings the perspective of a trusted professional. The mass shootings targeting the gay community at the Pulse Nightclub in Orlando in June 2016, where 49 people lost their lives, sparked outrage in the healthcare community and the public at large. The ANA's Membership Assembly joined the public outcry by issuing a declaration in support of meaningful gun-control legislation to protect society, including repeal of the legislation that blocks Centers for Disease Control and Prevention (CDC) research on gun violence and encouraging dialogue to stop hate and violence (ANA, 2016).

Sometimes issues of broad interest to the public present opportunities for nursing engagement. TIME's Up is an antisexism, antiharassment movement that has garnered widespread public attention. An outgrowth of the TIME'S Up movement was TIME'S Up Healthcare, "a new affiliate which aims to drive new policies and decisions that result in more balanced, diverse and accountable leadership; address workplace discrimination, harassment and abuse; and create equitable and safe work cultures within all facets of the healthcare industry" (ANA, 2019, para. 1). The ANA was among the first organizations to partner with TIME'S Up Healthcare, announcing its support to the national effort in a statement that expressed "the rate of violence against registered nurses and other healthcare workers has reached epidemic proportions. The ANA, through our #EndNurseAbuse campaign, works to raise awareness about the abuse that nurses routinely experience on the job and to address workplace cultures that prevent greater reporting of these incidents. We are proud to support Time's Up Healthcare's goals to make the workplace safe and respectful for all" (ANA, 2019, para. 11).

Public service announcements (PSAs) are also an effective way to spread messages at no cost to the organization. The announcement must benefit the community; most often, it is used to announce a nonprofit community event or service. The announcement can be in written form or presented in an audio or visual format. If transmitted electronically, radio or television coverage is typically a short spot less than 1 minute in length. Like press releases, the PSA includes the typical who, what, where, when, and why.

Journalists

Often, nurses seek to deliver messages to print and broadcast media through journalists. Press releases, letters to the editor, op-eds, email communications, interviews, and media events target health and general interest media with the intent having the story published or broadcast. Multiple channels increase the odds of successfully disseminating the issue and opinions. Journalists also rely more on social media as information sources. Despite a plethora of criticism of mainstream media from public officials, journalists remain the top vehicle for coverage of our issues and enable message delivery across a variety of platforms.

PUTTING MESSAGES INTO WRITING

As previously discussed, communication about an issue written in one's own words or expressing the position of an organization is a simple tool that can deliver a powerful message. Written communication can be sent to multiple media sources at the same time to maximize coverage.

Letters to the Editor

Newspapers and journals accept letters offering commentary on other published articles or issues of current interest. Letters are also used to respond to criticism, offer a different view on a recently covered topic, correct inaccuracies, or add interesting content to a recent story. A letter to the editor is simple and focuses on one key point. Plan on a short letter of approximately 150 words succinctly describing one's ideas; check editorial specifications because limits may vary. If referencing a previous article, include a brief explanation so readers connect the current letter with the original. Send letters quickly and in close proximity to the event or article being addressed. Include complete contact information for follow-up.

When nurses and other groups across the country were involved in advocacy for APRNs to gain full practice authority within the Veterans Affairs (VA), the ANA secured a letter to the editor in the *Washington Post* (Cipriano, 2016), as seen in Exhibit 10.6. The use of a high-profile letter to the editor on this issue is an example of effective media advocacy.

EXHIBIT 10.6 ANA PRESIDENT'S LETTER TO THE WASHINGTON POST EDITOR SUPPORTING FULL PRACTICE AUTHORITY FOR APRNs IN THE VA

Proposed VA rule is about providing better care to veterans, July 22, 2016

The July 19 *Washington Post* article "Battle Over VA Plan for Veterans' Care Builds" framed nurses' efforts to provide our nation's veterans with direct access to high-quality patient care as a turf battle between physicians and nurses. This is not about doctors versus nurses but about how we can work together to meet the pressing care needs of veterans. The proposed VA rule that would grant APRNs full practice authority states that "APRNs would not be authorized to replace or act as physicians or to provide any healthcare services that are beyond their clinical education, training, and national certification." Veterans service organizations, consumer groups, and more than 80 members of Congress support this change because the research is clear: Nurses consistently deliver exceptional care with high patient satisfaction when allowed to work to the full extent of their education and training. To provide quality care to veterans, all healthcare professionals must work together as a team.

Pamela F. Cipriano

Silver Spring, Maryland

The writer is president of the American Nurses Association[1].

ANA, American Nurses Association; VA, Veterans Affairs.

---

1. Pam Cipriano was ANA president when this was written. She is now the president of the International Council of Nurses.

Opinion Editorials

Op-eds appear *opposite* the editorial page in a newspaper and aim to evoke an emotional response from the reader. The targeted opinion piece opens with a strong statement or argument and offers a clear point of view. Op-eds can be used to persuade public sentiment or to defend a policy position. They are more successful when they are written about current issues that appeal to readers with an urgency for understanding and action. In March 2017, Mary Wakefield, former acting deputy secretary of the U.S. Department of Health and Human Services, sent an op-ed to five newspapers across North Dakota as the U.S. House of Representatives was preparing to vote on their American Health Care Act (AHCA). The *Grand Forks Herald* (Wakefield, 2017) and others published her editorial, which highlighted facts about the AHCA that revealed stark contrasts in benefits provided under the ACA. Most notable was her clear articulation of facts and emphasis on her perspectives as a nurse. Because of her stature as a highly regarded policy expert, others took notice, spawning dialogue on the issues she raised.

When a coalition of more than 700 nurses signed a letter and published it as an opinion piece in *Newsweek* titled "We Are Nurses, America's Most Trusted Profession. And We Support Biden," it sent a powerful message ("Over 700 Signatories," 2020). Accompanying that message was an equally powerful visual—a photo montage of the nurses who endorsed the letter (Vogel, 2020).

Tips for a successful op-ed are displayed in Exhibit 10.7. Be sure to check the publication's policies and submission guidelines. Contacting the editor to introduce oneself and the topic in advance may increase the likelihood of publication. For local publications, a strong association with a local angle increases editorial appeal.

EXHIBIT 10.7 KEY POINTS FOR GETTING AN OP-ED PUBLISHED

- Provide author's credentials and expertise.
- Develop a catchy title.
- Incorporate data/statistics, expert testimony, or other resources.
- Describe a personal story or analogy.
- Create an engaging flow of ideas.
- Close with a strong final sentence culminating the argument/position.
- Limit reading time to under 5 minutes; 700–800 words.

op-ed, opinion editorial.

Organizational Policy-Oriented Newsletters and Electronic Communications

Many different types of nursing groups use newsletters and email blasts to electronic mailing lists as effective vehicles for reaching specific target audiences. Hardcopies are less common, giving way to electronic ones that arrive quickly and at a lower cost, with links to additional information. Newsletters, in general, can be read asynchronously at someone's leisure, making them more effective than media such as radio, television, and some websites, where content is updated and older coverage may be available for only a brief period.

The content must match the target audience's interests and include items that are newsworthy. Newsletter contents should also follow the inverted pyramid style of an effective headline followed by the five Ws and H and then the supporting information in descending order from most to least important. Newsletter articles and email update designs should focus on a primary issue with a persuasive argument or point of view that creates interest. Ensure the accuracy of the content to earn the audience's trust.

Content delivered electronically requires some additional preparation, including addressing visual display differences for electronic inbox formats, offering other versions such as HTML, and offering an opt-in process for receiving the newsletter. Sending frequent electronic editions can increase one's reputation as a top-of-mind source of information. The same format can be used to send special messages highlighting a release of distinct urgent information.

The ANA *SmartBrief* is an example of an opt-in electronic member newsletter. It addresses newsworthy items with URL links to retrieve in-depth information. It offers optimized mobile or inbox email versions. ANA members can sign up to receive this daily collection of handpicked news sources for current trends and issues; it is also offered to nonmembers for a small subscription (www2.smartbrief.com/getLast.action?mode=sample&b=ANA).

Policy Briefs, Backgrounders, and Tip Sheets

A policy brief succinctly states a position. The target audience is policymakers who seek facts and arguments about an issue from trusted sources. A brief, as its name implies, is concise and quickly conveys the important policy facts and implications, poses questions for policymakers to consider, and proposes arguments substantiating one's position on the issue. An effective policy brief is persuasive and well organized. The contents of a policy brief are addressed in Exhibit 10.8.

EXHIBIT 10.8   CONTENTS OF A POLICY BRIEF

- Introduction
- Overview
- Statement of the problem or objective
- Argument or thesis
- Clear statement of position
- Recommendations (placed at the beginning)
- History and relevant background
- Analysis
- Critique of arguments, alternate viewpoints, and quality of evidence
- Citation of evidence that supports your thesis and recommendations
- Conclusion
- Argument
- Call for action
- Summary statement

Issuing a policy brief on an emerging or a critical issue positions an organization as an opinion leader. One of the recurring issues plaguing nursing is workforce shortages. COVID-19 increased and exacerbated the global nursing shortage. In a recent policy brief on the nursing shortage, the International Council of Nurses (n.d.) lays out the facts, contributing factors, impact, and strategies for addressing the problem. With links to other pertinent documents and supporting information, it is a resource to nurses, the media, and others interested in understanding this complex issue.

When a policy brief is designed primarily to persuade policymakers to introduce or sponsor a bill, it is called a *legislative brief*. In 2018, the AACN issued a legislative brief regarding the Title VIII Nursing Workforce Reauthorization Act

(S.1109/H.R. 959). At the top of the legislative brief, AACN's call to action is stated clearly: "Request: Cosponsor & Pass S. 1109" (AACN, 2018). Like other types of policy briefs, a legislative brief should use a combination of text and visuals to convey a clear, compelling message.

A media backgrounder addresses one topic and is written without bias. It usually includes a fact sheet with statistics, a timeline of related events, contact information, and a description of sources. Backgrounders should be no more than three or four pages, with facts in an easily identifiable format, such as bulleted notes, so one can easily identify salient points. Longer papers, such as white papers, reports, or analyses, are not expected to generate rapid responses but to lay the groundwork and stimulate discussion for policy changes. Tip sheets providing either facts at a glance or an exhibit expanding on a policy brief are helpful materials in adding depth to formal statements. Consistent updates of media backgrounders, tip sheets, and fact sheets advance an ongoing agenda by having information ready when new developments occur or when an organization wants to refresh coverage of their position.

DELIVERING MESSAGES—VOICE AND VISUALS

Live presentations provide opportunities for powerful message delivery. Recording a presentation—whether through video or audio alone—allows rebroadcasting and making it available to remote audiences.

Images

Visual images can help transmit a message that words alone cannot convey. The availability of portable, high-quality still and video cameras has made the use of visual images an integral part of messaging today. Photographs are commonly used in newsletters, on websites, and in social media, as well as supplied to print media outlets. In the absence of live footage, television stations may also use still photos.

Obtaining permission with a signed photography/videography release form is essential for using pictures of individuals not associated with the organization. A professional photographer owns the copyright to photos and must grant permission to place images on a website or reuse photos. In addition to any required fees, the photo must be attributed. When choosing photos, give careful thought to issues of diversity and inclusion. Select photos that represent the diversity of the nursing workforce, as well as the diversity of the patients, families, and communities that nurses serve.

Speeches

Speeches at scheduled meetings may get the attention of a reporter with an advance promotion of a well-known or important presenter or the announcement of breaking news. Reporting controversial expert knowledge or revealing important findings also helps guarantee coverage. As with press conferences, advance materials enable the reporter to judge the importance of covering the meeting. Typically, nursing media representatives cover a limited number of national meetings, but regional, state, and local meetings draw fewer reporters in the absence of a high-profile speaker or topic.

Speakers need to be asked for permission to record presentations for later use. Speakers can be asked to sign a consent/release form describing how the presentations will be used and shared and whether the presentation will be publicly posted, or placed on the organization's intranet. It is important to note whether there is a charge for viewing the presentation and the opportunity to earn continuing education credits. A signed consent/release form will help to ensure that an organization is on the same page with speakers regarding how their recorded presentations will be used.

Setting aside time after a presentation for an invited speaker to talk with the press can provide a personal angle and more in-depth content for a reporter. Speakers may or may not have honed their interview skills, therefore, work with the interviewer to limit the subject matter to what was presented at the meeting and a specific area of expertise. Having the organization's spokesperson in attendance also allows for an additional perspective to represent the organization in the event that there is a discrepancy between the speaker's comments and the organization's; it is important to provide a distinction between the two.

Organizations want to have experts ready for interviews of all types (live or taped, radio or television, print coverage). When a hot topic emerges, have the organization's most compelling spokesperson available and prepared for impromptu or scheduled interviews. Many organizations maintain a speaker or media contact list or advertise a speaker's bureau. Remember to keep expertise and contact information up to date.

Interviews

During an interview with the reporter, ask clarifying questions before providing answers. It is important to never argue but to stick to one's message. If it is a negative story, additional preparation may be necessary, but in general, taking time to prepare thoughtful responses is valuable. Getting back to the reporter within the designated time frame is respectful of their deadlines. Never repeat a negative statement or question to prevent its inadvertent association with the organization. Sometimes when reporters are working on a tight deadline, they will be open to getting responses to questions via email instead of over the phone or on camera. When giving written answers to a reporter's questions, write out answers exactly as wanted in print. The advantage of giving a written rather than a verbal response to a reporter's questions is that provides time for thought on wording the message.

Radio interviews, often done by phone, are usually short, less than 5 minutes; questions are direct and predictable; these can be shaped by talking with the radio show host in advance or sending in questions in advance (Fitch & Holt, 2012). Television and video add emotional intensity. Television is part show and part content. Like radio, interviews can be live or taped. If live, be prepared to respond to an emerging critical issue. If taped, there is typically more time to prepare and stage the interaction. Timely topics include connections to a current news story or a new development in healthcare or one's organization. Maintaining readiness and being available are critical to getting radio or television coverage as new topics and changes emerge. Scheduling appearances on live talk shows can reach a broad audience. Research the host's questioning style and audience. Different media offer different approaches for transmitting messages. Using multiple forms of media allows for wider dissemination.

Preparing for an Interview

Securing a coveted interview carries the responsibility of keen preparation. Do homework. Determine the reporter's questions in advance and understand the key areas of interest. Know what type of work the reporter has recently covered. For radio and television, know the name of the host, show, station, and any other guests on the same appearance. Listen in advance to anticipate the style of the interviewer, pace, format of the show, audience or call-in questions, and length of the segment. Print journalists often request permission to tape the conversation to retrieve details at a later time. Before the interview, review previous statements and talking points on the topic, be clear on positions, and rehearse messages, including sound bites, personal stories, anecdotes, and answers to anticipated questions.

Remember, anything said can be repeated on television, radio, or the newspaper, so being well prepared is key. Offer a fact sheet with sound bites and have additional background information prepared. When working with a reporter, know the deadline. Offer a list of questions to be covered, and ask if the reporter will also provide a set of anticipated questions. It may be beneficial to establish the setting and time frame that works best so that the spokesperson is prepared and relaxed, taking into consideration any deadlines or schedule constraints. Advice for successful message delivery in an interview is presented in Exhibit 10.9.

EXHIBIT 10.9   IN THE HOT SEAT: POINTERS FOR A SUCCESSFUL INTERVIEW

- Keep your responses short, clear, and crisp.
- State your main message as succinctly as possible and follow it with supporting points.
- Use simple language and no jargon or acronyms.
- Remain calm.
- Never get defensive or angry.
- Be comfortable with pauses between questions.
- Resist urges to fill the silence.
- Don't be afraid to say, "I don't know."
- Politely correct any inaccuracies on the part of a reporter/interviewer.
- Redirect the focus of a negative question by saying something like, "The real question is . . ." and return to your main message on the issue.

Appearing on Camera

Television adds the dynamic of conveying appearance, voice, and overall impression with an audience. A successful on-camera interview appearance requires attention to appearance and actions. It is important to dress professionally and wear something that makes one feel confident. Jewelry should complement the delivery of the message rather than distract from it. For example, if someone tends to nod a lot when speaking with someone, avoid wearing dangling earrings. A good example of distracting jewelry can be found in *The Woodhull Study Revisited* press conference at the National Press Club. One of the authors of this chapter (Acquaviva) wore bright-colored, dangling earrings that shook every time she moved her head. Instead of her message taking center stage, her jewelry did (GW School of Nursing, 2018).

Clinical attire such as scrub suits and laboratory coats are worn only in settings reflecting patient contact or in settings that are in immediate proximity to the event being covered, such as a disaster response or an in-hospital press event. However, during a pandemic such as COVID-19, wearing a mask on camera if one is in close proximity to others is essential. When ANA President Ernest J. Grant appeared on camera with President Trump in 2020 in an event recognizing National Nurses Day, he and other nursing leaders present were widely criticized on social media because they were not wearing face masks. Criticism also came during the event itself from a reporter who asked President Trump, "Mr. President, what kind of message does it send that you're surrounded by nurses who are not doing social distancing, who are not wearing masks? What kind of a message is that?" President Trump responded, "Well, I can't help that. I mean, look, I'm trying to be nice. I'm signing a bill and you criticize us." Later in the question and answer session, Sophia Thomas, president of the American Association of Nurse Practitioners, followed up by saying, "To answer your question earlier, we're all COVID-19-free. We were all tested. So, we're not socially distancing, but we're all negative. And we wouldn't do anything to harm our President, obviously" (The White House, 2020). Although Grant and other nurses attending the White House event believed they had a valid reason to forego wearing a mask, not everyone who saw the picture of the mask-less nurses in the Oval Office would have taken the time to read the transcript of that meeting to know the backstory. When appearing on camera, always pay careful attention to optics.

If an interview will be conducted using videoconferencing (e.g., Zoom, Skype), pay attention to the background in front of the camera. Whenever possible, make plans for children and pets to be in another room. If a child or pet wanders in front of the camera during the interview, do not panic—smile warmly and continue on as if nothing is amiss. Viewers will relate more positively than if one snaps impatiently at the interruption. Conveying the message is important, but in order to do that effectively, viewers need to perceive the speaker as someone who is trustworthy. An unflappable nurse inspires confidence.

When appearing on television, show energy and enthusiasm, make purposeful eye contact, maintain good posture, use gestures appropriately, and speak clearly. Practice interviewing skills by videotaping one's performance. Look for positive motions, animation, comfortable posture, and good eye contact. Do not speak too quickly; listen for clear enunciation of each word. Media training like that provided by nurse leaders and media experts Barbara Glickstein and Diana Mason is a worthwhile investment to hone camera skills. Glickstein and Mason offer group training called "Nurse Media Labs," as well as individual coaching.

Press Conferences and Briefings

Press conferences, also called *news conferences*, are planned for the release of a significant story or development. The more prestigious the organizer or the more compelling the issue, the greater response from the media. Nursing and healthcare organizations, schools, and other groups may be tapped to participate in press events organized by lawmakers or others to address key issues. When the U.S. Senate was facing the initial introduction of the Better Care Reconciliation Act, Senators Debbie Stabenow, Jeff Merkeley, and Maggie Hassan worked with the ANA and provided a press event that was livestreamed from the Capitol. The ANA president and two other ANA nurse leaders presented statements humanizing the effects of the proposed bill that would decimate health benefits and put healthcare and insurance out of reach once again for many Americans. An Associated Press photo of the ANA president holding a placard with the ACA's Essential Health Benefits was circulated widely in print media and internet reports the following day. The press event was recorded on YouTube and can be viewed at www.youtube.com/watch?v=k84KkcZuZiw.

Press conferences are not always complex, but all require a compelling story and careful planning. In addition to respected speakers, audiovisuals can be used to not only help tell the story but also seize the audience's attention and emotions. Both positive and negative visuals can evoke a response. The palm-sized preterm infant, the injured accident patient saved from the clutches of death, and the handcuffed perpetrator of a crime are powerful symbols of the human condition. When possible, include other participants such as children, heroes, or favorite personalities in the press conference to draw in the audience.

The selected venue must support space for video cameras and reporters, adequate sound and lighting, access to electrical outlets, and open space at the rear of the room for additional cameras. A podium and front table to accommodate all speakers sets the stage for the conference. Be careful that the venue is not so large that chairs remain empty because empty chairs send an inaccurate message of a lack of interest. Popular venues include press clubs, hotels, public buildings, and settings that highlight or complement the topic, such as a clinic, hospital, neighborhood, or other location within easy access of media offices.

Schedule the event to avoid any major national, state, or religious holidays or conflicting popular local or regional events. The same schedule restraints affecting reporters apply to press conferences. The best times are late morning (10 a.m.–12:00 noon); Tuesdays, Wednesdays, and Thursdays are less busy.

Several days prior to the event, email or fax a media advisory to secure greater participation. Be sure to have extra printed materials available. Preparing presenters is fundamental to any public speaking. Maximize coverage of events by quickly posting video or audio and pictures on the organization's website and reuse materials in other publications.

Specially planned briefings give journalists background information on issues to be covered and establish one as a trusted source of information on an issue that captures the public's attention. The content can be used to identify an emerging issue, update any key developments on an issue, or present organizational policies and positions. Briefings are usually informal and offer the chance to build relationships and rapport with media representatives. Keeping a briefing small allows reporters to ask questions meaningful to their media outlet. Briefings can also be held virtually to allow more convenient participation of nationwide press representatives. Press conferences and briefings require careful planning, execution, and follow-up. Whether one is a seasoned PR professional or a volunteer, following the tips in Exhibit 10.10 helps ensure a successful event.

EXHIBIT 10.10 TIPS FOR A SUCCESSFUL PRESS CONFERENCE

Initial planning
- Identify target media outlets/individuals.
- Choose a strategic date and time.
- Write the press advisory.
- Select an accessible, familiar location.
- Identify and secure speakers.
- Schedule speaker lineup.
- Schedule an American Sign Language interpreter.

Groundwork
- Pitch the event; send press advisory 1 to 2 weeks in advance.
- Contact media outlets to determine attendance.
- Prepare media kit materials:
  - Press release
  - Background information
  - Speaker biographies
- Prepare on-site visuals (charts, photos, and slides) and precheck all equipment.
- Confirm event venue setup.

(continued)

EXHIBIT 10.10 TIPS FOR A SUCCESSFUL PRESS CONFERENCE (*CONTINUED*)

The event
- Record the list of press in attendance.
- Collect information from press representatives for postevent needs.
- Distribute press release and/or full media kits on arrival.

Same-day follow-up
- Post press release and related material on the website.
- Post video and provide links.
- Follow up with response to reporters' additional needs.
- Summarize coverage for future reference.
- Provide appropriate written and verbal acknowledgments.

Tracking
- Collect inventory of all media coverage.
- Prepare final summary for archives.

Source: Adapted from Fitch, B., and Holt, C. J. (Eds.). (2012). *Media relations handbook for government, associations, nonprofits and elected officials* (2nd ed.). TheCapitol.Net.

Crisis Communications—When Bad News Happens

Tragedy, disaster, and wrongdoing all capture media attention. It is disheartening when the story implicates one of our own. Nursing's darker side becomes newsworthy when, for example, a nurse strays from the contract with society and intentionally inflicts harm or when negligence or when human error results in a sentinel event or near miss. All too often, reporters use the generic *nurse* without accurately identifying the person's qualifications believed to have done harm or acted in a way unbecoming to a law-abiding professional.

When bad news happens, organizations must be truthful, admit to mistakes, and express remorse. Aim for full disclosure. The public and the organization want to get facts straight and move on to repair and healing. Most negative stories are 1-day events. If prolonged, a multiday event or one spanning months and years can be trying for any organization and requires effective PR management. Handling negative stories is part of the PR professionals' skill set. It is unpleasant and embarrassing to have to deal with patient abuse or harm, safety violations, or illegal behavior. If surprised by a negative issue raised by a reporter, remain calm and suggest needing time to check facts before responding. While gathering facts, plan the strategy, which may include a brief written statement or interview. Sometimes, an independent third party is effective as a spokesperson who can defend the organization. If the group is truly in crisis management mode, a crisis communication plan is essential and varies based on the magnitude of the blunder.

When an organization experiences a crisis, leaders must inform their internal constituents, as well as keep media channels open. It is important to generate a response quickly and be prepared to define the event, say what is being done to address it, and let others know whether help is needed. Top leaders must be visible. In addition, identify a team of individuals capable of interacting with the media. Anticipate questions and prepare talking points. Integrate social media into a plan to keep constituents informed with frequent updates. Remember, the organization's values and ethics are judged by these responses.

HOW TO USE INTERNET MEDIA FOR ADVOCACY

Websites

An internet website address (URL) serves as the organization's anchor for information. Maintaining current information in various formats, including stories, news updates, videos, photographs, and links to other resources, secures an organization's position as a source of information. Reporters, policymakers, colleagues, competitors, and the public use organizational websites to gather insights about what the organizations have to offer in terms of expertise, influence, and opinions. Many organizations have online communities that provide not only information but also interaction through message boards, surveys, blogs, and links to other resources. The ANA Community is one such example (community.ana.org/home). If the organization provides clinical care, patients and families use its website as well. The vast majority of U.S. hospitals have interactive tools on their websites to facilitate interaction with patients (Huang et al., 2020).

Websites have become a mainstay for accessing health information for patients, healthcare professionals, and public health officials. Although many consider access to health information a positive force for public health and disease knowledge/management, not all websites and not all website searches are created equally. Dunne et al. (2013) note that websites containing inaccurate or biased information may precipitate unintended consequences of misinformation and that most internet search engine strategies rely on the number of hits a website receives and the readability of content but do not account for the accuracy of the information presented. The authors further note that search engine optimization, or providing guidance in tailoring results, can be a critical factor in delivering trusted health resources and that such search practices should be considered by professionals or groups to deliver quality information to the public.

The ubiquitous nature of the information available on the internet and the proliferation of social media have accelerated the importance of media literacy, which used to be focused primarily on recognizing legitimacy and bias. More developed critical thinking skills are required to recognize bias and satire, discern real news from news that is fabricated or distorted, and evaluate reliable sources (Kiley & Robertson, 2016). Political friction over alternative facts and accusations of fake news has further fueled concerns because fabricated information can spread in a matter of seconds over social media before it is corrected. Nurses can help provide legitimate information when the public is at risk from misleading reports intended to fool readers by expressing extreme views as fact. Tactics may include reiterating positions that have been debunked, presenting partial truths with a spin to appeal to a specific audience, and designing sources of information to look legitimate when they are not. The best advice is if a story seems shocking, be sure to read carefully past the headline, investigate sources, and look for other corroboration of information from credible sources. A growing number of organizations such as FactCheck.org and Snopes.com provide fact-checking.

Social Media

The internet has made possible rapid communication, collaboration, and connection with others on a real-time basis. Much of that communication, collaboration, and connection takes place through social media. Social media platforms offer tools to participate in active dialogue through user-generated content and sharing of personal and professional information. More and more organizations are finding social media to be an important adjunct to the more static website-based information for the distribution of professional content. Given the diverse preferences for communication among generations, social media helps reach segments of audiences that may not follow traditional sources such as print materials.

Social media has changed the entire landscape of communication and is an essential component of PR. Whereas PR used to be the vehicle to manage a message, it is now the means to facilitate an ongoing conversation in a 24/7 world. The use of social media tools by healthcare organizations has grown rapidly. Many hospitals, associations, consumer groups, and healthcare businesses use social media platforms, such as Facebook and Twitter, placing icons on their webpages to link visitors to their websites. Businesses may also use LinkedIn, a professional networking site, to provide news and updates about their work, as well as encourage ongoing connections.

The digital media revolution has taken hold. Multiple platforms are being used with a shift to user engagement and user-generated content. Current and emerging tools are making information and interactive communication available from single sites where video, livestreaming, the ability to toggle to social media links, chats, messaging, and more traditional static information that reside together on a single site. Already, social media sites have formed partnerships to provide livestreaming from traditional television sites, impacting immediate access to news that reaches a mobile multigenerational audience. Rapidly evolving technology makes information portable and device-agnostic, allowing the public to choose how and when they receive information, whether from smartphones while on the go or from the comfort of watching television at home.

The possibilities for policy applications are endless. Nurses can use these techniques to reach coworkers, student groups, public gatherings, or association members. When planning strategies to promote a policy, nurses are challenged to consider new methods that increase the reach to target audiences locally, nationally, and even globally. Nurses looking to the future will consider technology changes an essential component. Facebook, Twitter, blogs, Instagram, TikTok, video-streaming sites, and Quick Response (QR) codes are some of the current popular free tools that have revolutionized real-time information sharing with the public.

Facebook

Started in 2004, Facebook (now Meta) connects people with other individuals or businesses (Facebook for Business). Boasting more than one billion users, Facebook businesses are sharing news, photos, and promotions with their followers. The primary use of Facebook in healthcare is for casual connection and information sharing because it makes posting messages, photos, and videos easy. It is also useful to advertise events. However, many hospitals, as well as nurses' associations, have Facebook pages and use it to engage with their communities.

Twitter

Twitter, considered a microblogging service, is a vehicle for connecting with other people and sharing timely news, opinions, and updates. Twitter with more than 186 million active daily users (Goldsmith, 2020) focuses on the message. Opinions containing as many as 140 characters and posted as blast communication, photos, and links can be sent. Regular media sources use Twitter as an additional means of drawing attention to stories and people and connecting with audiences on the go. When clicking a button to follow a Twitter account, one becomes a "follower."

Twitter posts are sourced in major search engines, allowing access to real-time information, and can be data mined with stored searches through the use of either search terms or hashtags. As is true with other blogs, one must consider the value of the source. Some popular nursing Twitter feeds include the ANA Government Affairs, *NursingWorld* (Twitter.com/nursingworld), and *American Nurse* (Twitter.com/myamericannurse). International and national nursing and health conferences disseminate specific hashtags for attendees to use while at the conference to network with other health professionals and disseminate research findings. The use of Twitter among scholars and clinicians has been shown to promote engagement in research (Salzmann-Erikson, 2017; Sinnenberg et al., 2017) and education (Diug et al., 2016). As Acquaviva et al. (2020) note, "social media platforms (e.g., Twitter, Facebook, Reddit, Instagram, and TikTok) now provide scholars with a significant platform for engaging in and disseminating scholarship. . . . Each of these social media platforms has greater academic and nonacademic reach than all of the medical and nursing journals in the world combined" (p. 1).

Rapidly sharing information on critical issues (e.g., drug safety alerts, potential epidemic developments, emerging disasters) is another benefit. Healthcare providers can also tweet about new care developments or reminders about self-care. Using Twitter for health policy is burgeoning, as are applications for using Twitter in health-related research (Keim-Malpass et al., 2017). Twitter is an ideal medium to help understand sentiments (overall negative or positive stance) of various communication and messaging tactics.

Instagram

Instagram is a social networking platform that allows users to connect and share photographs and short videos, either publicly or privately and, like Twitter, uses hashtags to identify subject material and specific topics. With more than one billion active daily users, Instagram continues to be one of the fastest growing social media platforms (Tankovska, 2021). Within the health realm, Instagram has been used to document patient experiences, engage in disease advocacy, advertise fundraising events, and connect users who may be impacted by the same disease (Braunberger et al., 2017; Demiris, 2016).

Video Streaming

YouTube and Vimeo are websites that host user-generated videos that can be either publicly or privately accessed on the web or through mobile applications. Video streaming has emerged as an embedded modality within Facebook and Twitter that users can experience in their home feeds and easily share through sharing video (Facebook) and retweeting (Twitter). The use of video streaming in nursing has emerged in the context of education as to learning, disseminating nurse-led interventions, and understanding of the illness experience through the study of patient-created videos (Harrison et al., 2017; Keim-Malpass et al., 2013).

Blogs

Blogs may have a broad or narrow topic focus or may be issue-specific. Blogs mirror the historic model of one voice, one view on an issue. One can either pitch a blogger to cover content or create one's own blog. The author/writer, or blogger, can do a deeper dive on issues and needs to be ready as the content expert to answer tough questions. Although most bloggers usually have expertise on a subject, nothing requires a blogger to be an expert; the follower needs to differentiate the credible expert from an individual who proliferates a dialogue with only opinion and not verified facts.

The number of blogs is growing exponentially. Bloggers want to attract interest to their topics and opinions on a regular basis, bringing loyal followers to a website. They also repurpose content, adding their own perspectives. Frequent updating is expected to attract new visitors and maintain repeat visitors to a blog website. Bloggers must heed the caution not to rant or face a loss of credibility and interest among readers. Blogs offer a unique opportunity to understand various illness perspectives and treatment experiences beyond the traditional clinic walls and can be used to drive nursing science (Keim-Malpass et al., 2014).

QR Codes

A QR code is a type of two-dimensional barcode read with a special application on smartphones and some tablets. Originally developed for marketing, QR codes can connect people in ways that have not been fully explored. They can provide access to prewritten text, connect to a website, send an email or a text message, and receive a telephone number or make a call. Codes can appear anywhere a user might want to seek more information such as magazines, signs, giveaways at meetings, flyers, and any print material.

Providing QR codes on organizational materials linking to information important to policymakers takes advantage of this technology. As they prepare briefs, backgrounders, and policy briefs, organizations can create their own QR codes to link back to more issue-specific information on their websites. In addition, a QR code linking to information about the organization can be provided on the back of a business card.

Uses of Social Media

Beyond its usefulness in influencing policymakers, social media can be a powerful tool for detecting emerging public health issues, crowdsourcing solutions to problems, and catalyzing social change.

Disaster and Disease Response

Social media monitoring has been used to track and/or predict the spread of infectious disease (Alessa & Faezipour, 2019; Ayyoubzadeh et al., 2020; Sinnenberg et al., 2017; Tang et al., 2018; van Lent et al., 2017). In addition, social media has been used to analyze public responses and fear related to certain diseases, such as COVID-19 (Chen et al., 2020; Lwin et al., 2020), Ebola (van Lent et al, 2017), and Zika virus (Ahmed et al., 2020; van Lent et al., 2017). Researchers have indicated that the upswing in the use of social media has decreased our perceptions of social distance, making it easier to give public attention to worldwide crises such as epidemics (van Lent et al., 2017). In addition, many believe that social media responses to certain tragic events and disasters, such as the Boston Marathon bombing in April 2013, have strengthened the disaster preparedness infrastructure and allowed public health professionals to more easily communicate needs and response strategies in real time (Côté & Hearn, 2016).

Crowdsourcing

Crowdsourcing originated in the business realm but has increasingly been recognized as an essential activity within the realm of participatory networking (McCartney, 2013). Within healthcare, crowdsourcing has generally been described as a social media model for enabling public involvement and can be viewed through the lens of patient- or clinician-initiated crowdsourcing. Generally, crowdsourcing can be used to engage large, diverse groups of people to participate in research, study digital strategies, respond to emergencies, and even gather opinions regarding difficult diagnoses or treatment-related questions (Rumsfeld et al., 2016; Schemmann et al., 2016). A project crowdsourced through Twitter resulted in 40 scholars developing a new model for documenting social media contributions on curriculum vitae in the health professions (Acquaviva et al., 2020). Increasingly, there is momentum to involve patients through every phase in the research process through the advent of crowdsourced research protocols and participatory design (Franzoni & Sauermann, 2014; Schemmann et al., 2016). Digital media sources have also become an increasingly popular platform for public health interventions and clinician crowdsourcing (McCartney, 2013). Nearly any social media platform can be used to pose a crowdsourced question and elicit targeted responses. Although crowdsourcing has numerous benefits, digital engagement strategies can have unintended consequences including a lack of quality control of information delivery (Rumsfeld et al., 2016).

Political Activism

The Future of Nursing: Leading Change, Advancing Health report (IOM, 2011) calls for nurses to directly engage in health policy and lead the transformation of the U.S. healthcare system. Nursing has consistently been ranked among the most honest professions and represents a significant percentage of the U.S. workforce; however, this does not always translate into direct policy influence (Waddell et al., 2016). Nurses have a unique on-the-ground perspective, should be viewed as a critical policy-promotion resource, and should have the opportunity to engage in civic discourse and advocacy (Waddell et al., 2016). Nurses are actively finding better ways to convey civic engagement and political messages in a turbulent political environment, and often their engagement is enhanced through social media platforms (Matthews et al., 2017). Mobilizing nurses to engage in policy advocacy was a critical approach to influencing action on a VA rule to secure full practice authority for three categories of APRNs. In 2017, nurses were engaged in advocating for patients through the uncertainty of the repeal of the ACA. They mobilized through professional organizations (e.g., ANA) or used social media sites such as Facebook and Twitter to engage in political messages and urge others to contact their local representatives.

Using Social Media in the Workplace

Many organizations have adopted policies to direct the appropriate use of social media to protect the patients, staff, and institution. Protecting patient confidentiality, adhering to laws governing privacy, and maintaining appropriate patient–professional boundaries are typical areas addressed in policy. Numerous organizations around the world have issued guidelines about the use of social media, stressing how to avoid problems (ANA, n.d.-a; Barry & Hardiker, 2012; National Council of State Boards of Nursing [NCSBN®], 2011).

The ANA's "Social Networking Principles" provide a solid foundation for nurses seeking basic guidance on social media engagement:

- Nurses must not transmit or place online individually identifiable patient information.
- Nurses must observe ethically prescribed professional patient–nurse boundaries.
- Nurses should understand that patients, colleagues, organizations, and employers may view postings.
- Nurses should take advantage of privacy settings and seek to separate personal and professional information online.
- Nurses should bring content that could harm a patient's privacy, rights, or welfare to the attention of appropriate authorities.
- Nurses should participate in developing organizational policies governing online conduct (ANA, n.d-b)

Organizations have invoked policies to protect patients, staff, and their reputations. As with any new medium, a few individuals abuse it, and some have used social media without understanding its implications. As a result, some policies have been overly restrictive and have not allowed people to explore potential positive uses. Following accepted guidelines and etiquette for proper communication, as well as being tech-savvy, will lead to effective use of social media, such as Facebook and Twitter.

POLICY SOLUTION — The American Nurses Association and the 2020 Presidential Election

In response to the ANA nonpresidential endorsement, nurses expressed their views to the ANA and through the media regarding the two candidates using numerous media strategies, for example, Twitter, Facebook, and op-eds. Nurses individually realized their responsibilities to get involved by speaking up and out and taking action. One outcome, as noted earlier in this chapter was the *Newsweek* opinion column, "We Are Nurses, America's Most Trusted Profession. And We Support Biden." Anecdotally nurses shared their advocacy efforts in memorable social media posts. More specifically, the ANA reported that through the ANA RN Action Program in 2020, the number of grassroots advocates increased by 145% to almost 200,000 nurses; more than 437,000 messages were sent to Congress, and the text message subscribers increased by 116% (I. Lusis, personal communication, April 19, 2021).

In moving away from the ANA's policy to endorse a presidential candidate and after robust discussion, the ANA board voted to amplify its work with member engagement processes. One example is a development effort found on NursesVote.org website. The ANA reached out to "inside government" groups (see Chapter 4) in both the Trump and Biden administrations, thus building stronger relationships not only built on an election process and its outcome. To ensure that ANA's work continues at all levels of advocacy, administration, legislative, regulatory, grassroots, and political, the association developed a strategic comprehensive "100 Day Advocacy Plan" (Lusis, 2020).

IMPLICATIONS FOR THE FUTURE

Without question, the use of media has changed how people behave, how we communicate about health, and how we can advocate on the behalf of the patients we serve and our own profession. A large component of the nursing profession involves improving environmental, societal, and physical conditions that inhibit patients from maintaining optimal health status. Improving these conditions is an inherently political process because there is a finite amount of resources. Messages need to be crafted that resonate with not only their audience but also stakeholders involved in political and decision-making processes. In addition, more opportunities are needed for nurses to be the stakeholders contributing to this process. Media advocacy is one modality that can help accomplish these diverse tasks.

What is critical for the future is taking advantage of media advocacy to influence not only individual behaviors and beliefs but also public policy that creates change. Studies about social media have focused primarily on increased use and less on effect. Nurses and others can study the implications of using media to influence public opinion, health policy, and legislation. It is essential that nurses acquire basic skills and move to mastery of social media and traditional methods of media engagement so that they can be players in the world of converged media.

In perusing the internet for illustrations of nurses in the media, there is an abundance of feel-good stories but little coverage of public policy issues or nurses involved in political advocacy movements. Nurses have a responsibility to use media to convey the expertise and efforts of nurses to advance health policy issues. Every letter, background paper, policy brief, and presentation that addresses a current issue should be converted into media that are shared, archived, and repurposed. Social media interests, on the other hand, are almost without limits and reflect a consistent presence of engagement by nurses and nursing organizations. Taking advantage of all forms of media means greater exposure of nursing's views and builds support for nursing's role in advancing healthcare policy. Understanding how to advocate for individual patients and populations of interest, how to communicate about health policy, and how to apply advocacy to the role of the nurse must be a sustained component of our professional development.

KEY CONCEPTS

1. Nurses can use print, broadcast, and social media to reach a broader audience and establish a presence in the community.

2. Nurses have a responsibility to convey their vision, current thinking, and opinions to stimulate actions to effect better policies that serve our communities and nation.

3. Media advocacy combines mass communication with community advocacy.

4. Media advocacy includes working with media tools as well as with members of the media to have your message heard, advance opinions about issues, and influence policy decision-makers.

5. The effective use of social media has the potential to maximize influence on policymakers.

6. Using multiple media modalities can maximize the impact of media advocacy efforts.

7. Working with the media includes cultivating long-term relationships.

8. The Media Strategy Planner (Exhibit 10.1) can be used to guide media advocacy.

9. Message content needs to be short and concise, provide key details, and define the main issue by using no more than three themes of underlying support.

10. Responding to media representatives includes preparing the who, what, when, where, why, and how of the story and preparing key facts and background using a format known as the *journalism inverted pyramid*.

11. Messages should be specifically crafted for a target audience, which may include policymakers, the public, and journalists.

12. Letters to the editors, op-eds, organizational policy-oriented newsletters, policy briefs, backgrounders, tip sheets, letters to policymakers, and announcements can all be used to garner support for an issue.

13. Careful orchestration of events such as press conferences can maximize their impact.

14. A crisis communication plan can help mitigate the impact of a negative event.

SUMMARY

Media advocacy is a vital tool that nurses can use to transform health in communities and across the national landscape. A comprehensive media strategy is essential for bringing an issue to the attention of policymakers and the public. In order to achieve the desired policy outcomes, nurses need to think strategically, speak concisely, and communicate persuasively.

Nurse leaders, together with their employers, professional associations, academic partners, and community organizations, can advance their views and positions through organized efforts to reach out to the media on a consistent basis. It is important to cultivate relationships with media representatives, make periodic contact to raise issues, provide background information, stand ready to address emerging issues, and give advance notice of developments related to nursing and healthcare and important to the community. The same strategies for cultivating relationships with media representatives can be used to develop relationships with PR staff within one's organization.

Responsible use of social media by individuals as thought leaders and organizations is an essential component of media advocacy. A planned strategy for integrating social media enables an organization to initiate or reinforce messaging and capture interests quickly on dynamic issues. Nurse leaders have a responsibility to learn the skill set needed for working with the media. Combining knowledge of media advocacy, the ability to express ideas in writing and oral presentations, and the use of current and emerging internet and other social networking resources can have a profound impact on influencing local policies, as well as more comprehensive national policy and politics.

END-OF-CHAPTER RESOURCES

LEARNING ACTIVITIES

1. Analyze a current issue for different media coverage (e.g., op-ed, press release, social media, press event, letters). What venue produced the most uptake? What organization or individual was cited most frequently?

2. Retrieve a set of talking points, or fact sheets, on a current policy issue from a nursing organization. Assess the ways the media has covered the topic and critique the impact of the information on the current state of the issue.

3. Identify nursing leaders you admire and analyze their use of social media. Do they have a following? Are their entries timely? Do they capture your attention? Are they amplified by others? What changes to their use of social media do you believe would enhance their messaging?

4. Retrieve an electronic health policy–oriented newsletter or a single story. Critique the contents to assess: Is the story newsworthy? Do the authors use the inverted pyramid or another writing style?

5. Using Exhibit 10.8, critique a recent policy brief. What are its strengths? How could it have been improved?

6. Select a previously published issue or current healthcare concern and submit a letter to the editor to a newspaper of your choice. Indicate the rationale for your selected paper.

7. Write an elevator speech about why you believe nurses should engage in policy advocacy for a general or specific issue.

8. Select a health issue and review the social media coverage to determine whether there is any bad or fake news related to the issue by establishing the following:

    a. Accuracy of claim(s) made by the author(s)

    b. Corroboration by other sources

    c. Reliability and legitimacy of the source

E-RESOURCES

Policy/Advocacy Websites for National Nurses Associations

- American Nurses Association https://www.nursingworld.org/practice-policy/advocacy/

- National Association of Hispanic Nurses https://www.nahnet.org/policy

- National Black Nurses Association https://www.nbna.org/pol

- National League for Nursing http://www.nln.org/advocacy-public-policy/government-affairs-action-center

Media Tips and Tools

- American Association of Colleges of Nursing. Media Relations Fact Sheets http://www2.smartbrief.com/getLast.action?mode=sample&b=ANA

- American Association of Nurse Practitioners. Media Tools for the NP https://www.aanp.org/press-room/media-tools-for-nps

- American Nurses Association. Media Backgrounders https://www.nursingworld.org/news/media-resources/media-backgrounders

- American Nurses Association. Media Resources https://www.nursingworld.org/news/media-resources

- Berkeley Media Studies Group Resources. Media Advocacy 101 http://www.bmsg.org/resources/media-advocacy-101

- Kaiser Family Foundation. Health Policy Communications http://www.kaiseredu.org/Tutorials-and-Presentations/Health-Policy-and-Communications.aspx

- Pew Research Center. Activism in the Social Media Age: https://www.pewresearch.org/internet/wp-content/uploads/sites/9/2018/07/PI_2018.07.11_social-activism_FINAL.pdf

Media Training

- Barbara Glickstein Strategies (training by Barbara Glickstein and Diana Mason) https://www.barbaraglickstein.com/media-training-1

- On the Spot Media Training and Coaching http://www.onthespotmediatraining.com

Health Policy Blogs

- American Nurses Association. Capitol Beat Blog http://anacapitolbeat.org

- American Nurses Association. NurseSpace http://www.ananursespace.org/ANANURSESPACE/BlogsMain/Blogs

- *Health Affairs.* Blog https://www.healthaffairs.org/blog

- Nurse.com https://www.nurse.com/blog

REFERENCES

Acquaviva, K. D., Mugele, J., Abadilla, N., Adamson, T., Bernstein, S. L., Bhayani, R. K., Büchi, A. E., Burbage, D., Carroll, C. L., Davis, S. P., Dhawan, N., Eaton, A., English, K., Grier, J. T., Gurney, M. K., Hahn, E. S., Haq, H., Huang, B., Jain, S., Jun, J., . . . Trudell, A. M. (2020). Documenting social media engagement as scholarship: A new model for assessing academic accomplishment for the health professions. *Journal of Medical Internet Research, 22*(12), e25070. https://doi.org/10.2196/25070

Ahmed, W., Bath, P. A., Sbaffi, L., & Demartini, G. (2020). Zika outbreak of 2016: Insights from Twitter. In G. Meiselwitz (Ed.), *Social computing and social media. Participation, user experience, consumer experience, and applications of social computing* (pp. 447–458). Springer. https://doi.org/10.1007/978-3-030-49576-3_32

Alessa, A., & Faezipour, M. (2019). Flu outbreak prediction using Twitter posts classification and linear regression with historical Centers for Disease Control and Prevention Reports: Prediction framework study. *JMIR Public Health and Surveillance, 5*(2), e12383. https://doi.org/10.2196/12383

American Academy of Nursing. (2017). *American Academy of Nursing announces neuroscience recommendations in Choosing Wisely® campaign.* [Press release]. https://www.aannet.org/news/press-releases/press-releases-2

American Association of Colleges of Nursing. (2017). *Nursing shortage.* http://www.aacn.nche.edu/media-relations/fact-sheets/nursing-shortage

American Association of Colleges of Nursing. (2018, October). *Policy brief: Title VII Nursing Workforce Reauthorization Act (S.1109/H.R. 959).* https://www.aacnnursing.org/Portals/42/Policy/Legislation/Workforce/HR959-S1109-Title-VIII-Reauthorization-Brief.pdf

American Nurses Association. (n.d.-a). *ANA social media principles.* https://www.nursingworld.org/social

American Nurses Association. (n.d.-b). *Board of directors.* https://www.nursingworld.org/ana/leadership-and-governance/board-of-directors/

American Nurses Association. (2015). *Code of Ethics for Nurses with interpretive statements.*

American Nurses Association. (2016). *American Nurses Association urges nurses to help stop gun violence.* [Press release]. http://www.nursingworld.org/functionalmenucategories/mediaresources/pressreleases/2016-News-Releases/ANAurgesnursestostopgunviolence-Pressrelease.html

American Nurses Association. (2017). *ANA community.* http://www.ananursespace.org/home

American Nurses Association. (2018, October 24). *ANA applauds nurses' MAT prescribing authority in support (H.R. 6).* [Press release]. https://www.nursingworld.org/news/news-releases/2018/opioid/

American Nurses Association. (2019, March 01). *ANA among first to partner with TIME's Up healthcare.* [Press release]. https://www.nursingworld.org/News/News-Releases/2019-News-Releases/ANA-Among-First-To-Partner-With-Times-Up-Healthcare/

American Nurses Association. (2020, June 01). *ANA condemns racism, brutality and senseless violence against Black communities.* [Press release]. https://www.nursingworld.org/News/News-Releases/2020/ANA-President-Condemns-Racism-Brutality-And-Senseless-Violence-Against-Black-Communities/

American Organization for Nursing Leadership. (2020). *Key issues for nurses.* https://www.aonl.org/advocacy/key-issues

American Printing History Association. (n.d.). *History of printing timeline.* https://printinghistory.org/timeline/

American Psychiatric Nurses Association. (2017, May 25). *Nurses expand access to needed treatment for opioid use disorder with complimentary MAT waiver training.* [Press release]. https://www.apna.org/i4a/pages/index.cfm?pageid=6260

Ayyoubzadeh, S. M., Ayyoubzadeh, S. M., Zahedi, H., Ahmadi, M., & R Niakan Kalhori, S. (2020). Predicting COVID-19 incidence through analysis of Google trends data in Iran: Data mining and deep learning pilot Study. *JMIR Public Health and Surveillance, 6*(2), e18828. https://doi.org/10.2196/18828

Barry, J., & Hardiker, N. (2012, September 30). Advancing nursing practice through social media: A global perspective. *Online Journal of Issues in Nursing, 17*(3), 5. https://doi.org/10.3912/OJIN.Vol17No03Man05

Betts, V. (2020, October 27). *ANA's presidential engagement policy and what YOU can DO!!* https://anacapitolbeat.org/2020/10/27/anas-presidential-engagement-policy-and-what-you-can-do/

Bird, S. E. (2011). Are we all producers now? *Cultural Studies, 25*(4–5), 502–516. https://doi.org/10.1080/09502386.2011.600532

Braunberger, T., Mounessa, J., Rudningen, K., Dunnick, C. A., & Dellavalle, R. P. (2017, May 15). Global skin diseases on Instagram hashtags. *Dermatology Online Journal, 23*(5), 13030/qt7sk410j3. https://escholarship.org/uc/doj

Carr, C. T., & Hayes, R. A. (2015). Social media: Defining, developing, and divining. *Atlantic Journal of Communication, 23*(1), 46 65. https://doi.org/10.1080/15456870.2015.972282

Chen, E., Lerman, K., & Ferrara, E. (2020). Tracking social media discourse about the COVID-19 pandemic: Development of a public coronavirus Twitter data set. *JMIR Public Health and Surveillance, 6*(2), e19273. https://doi.org/10.2196/19273

Cipriano, P. (2016, July 22). Proposed VA rule is about providing better care to veterans. *The Washington Post.* https://www.washingtonpost.com/opinions/Proposed-Va-Rule-Is-About-

Providing-Better Care-To-Veterans/2016/07/22/C5a50df4-4eb1-11e6-Bf27-405106836f96_Story. Html? Utm_Term=.87e7b8946669

Côté, E., & Hearn, R. (2016). The medical response to the Boston Marathon bombings: An analysis of social media commentary and professional opinion. *Perspectives in Public Health*, *136*(6), 339–344. https://doi.org/10.1177/1757913916644480

Demiris, G. (2016). Consumer health informatics: Past, present, and future of a rapidly evolving domain. *Yearbook of Medical Informatics*, (Suppl. 1), S42–S47. https://doi.org/10.15265/IYS-2016-s005

Diug, B., Kendal, E., & Ilic, D. (2016). Evaluating the use of Twitter as a tool to increase engagement in medical education. *Education for Health*, *29*(3), 223–230. https://www.educationforhealth.net

Dorfman, L., & Krasnow, I. D. (2014). Public health and media advocacy. *Annual Review of Public Health*, *35*(1), 293–306. https://doi.org/10.1146/annurev-publhealth-032013-182503

Dunne, S., Cummins, N. M., Hannigan, A., Shannon, B., Dunne, C., & Cullen, W. (2013). A method for the design and development of medical or health care information websites to optimize search engine results page rankings on Google. *Journal of Medical Internet Research*, *15*(8), e183. https://doi.org/10.2196/jmir.2632

Easley, J. (2017, May 24). *Poll: Majority says mainstream media publishes fake news*. http://thehill.com/homenews/campaign/334897-poll-majority-says-mainstream-media-publishes-fake-news

Everhart, K., Janssen, M., & Behrens, S. (n.d.). *Timeline: The history of public broadcasting in the U. S*. https://current.org/timeline-the-history-of-public-broadcasting-in-the-u-s/

Fact Checker. (2021, January). In four years, President Trump has made 30,573 false or misleading claims. *The Washington Post*. https://www.washingtonpost.com/graphics/politics/trump-claims-database/

Fitch, B., & Holt, C. J. (Eds.). (2012). *Media relations handbook for government, associations, nonprofits and elected officials* (2nd ed.). Thecapitol.net.

Franzoni, C., & Sauermann, H. (2014). Crowd science: The organization of scientific research in open collaborative projects. *Research Policy*, *43*(1), 1–20. https://doi.org/10.1016/j.respol.2013.07.005

Goldsmith, J. (2020, July 23). Twitter active daily users surge 34% to record 186m in q2, revenue dips, CEO Jack Dorsey apologizes for breach. *Deadline*. https://deadline.com/2020/07/twitter-active-daily-users-surge-34-to-186m-q2-revenue-dips-19-1202992835/

GW School of Nursing. (2018, May 8). *The Woodhull Study revisited press conference. (Minute marker 17:43)*. https://vimeo.com/269069064#t=1063s

Harrison, D., Reszel, J., Dagg, B., Aubertin, C., Bueno, M., Dunn, S., Fuller, A., Harrold, J., Larocque, C., Nicholls, S., & Sampson, M. (2017). Pain management during newborn screening: Using YouTube to disseminate effective pain management strategies. *The Journal of Perinatal and Neonatal Nursing*, *31*(2), 172–177. https://doi.org/10.1097/JPN.0000000000000255

Huang, E., Knittle, C., Wantuch, G., & Francis, T. (2020). How wired are U.S. hospitals? A study of patient-oriented interactive tools. *International Journal of Healthcare Management*, *13*(1), 72–78. https://doi.org/10.1080/20479700.2019.1640971

Institute of Medicine. (2011). *Future of nursing: Leading change, advancing health*. National Academies Press.

International Council of Nurses. (n.d.). Policy brief: The global nursing shortage and nurse retention. https://www.icn.ch/sites/default/files/inline-files/ICN%20Policy%20Brief_Nurse%20Shortage%20and%20Retention.pdf

Institute of Medicine. (2002). *Speaking of health: Assessing health communication strategies for diverse populations*. National Academies Press.

Jaspen, B. (2016). VA would join 21 states already lifting nurse practitioner hurdles. *Forbes*. https://www.forbes.com/sites/brucejapsen/2016/05/26/va-would-join-21-states-lifting-nurse-practitioner-hurdles/#43979bda348e

Keim-Malpass, J., Baernholdt, M., Erickson, J. M., Ropka, M. E., Schroen, A. T., & Steeves, R. H. (2013). Blogging through cancer: Young women's persistent problems shared online. *Cancer Nursing, 36*(2), 163–172. https://doi.org//10.1097/ncc.0b013e31824eb879

Keim-Malpass, J., Mitchell, E. M., Sun, E., & Kennedy, C. (2017). Using Twitter to understand public perceptions regarding the #hpv vaccine: Opportunities for public health nurses to engage in social marketing. *Public Health Nursing, 34*(4), 316–323. https://doi.org/10.1111/phn.12318

Keim-Malpass, J., Steeves, R. H., & Kennedy, C. (2014). Internet ethnography: A review of methodological considerations for studying online illness blogs. *International Journal of Nursing Studies, 51*(12), 1686–1692. https://doi.org/10.1016/j.ijnurstu.2014.06.003

Kiley, E., & Robertson, L. (2016, November 18). *How to spot fake news.* http://www.factcheck.org/2016/11/how-to-spot-fake-news/

Lusis, I. (2020, November 13). *ANA advocacy team prepares for a new administration and a new Congress.* Capitol Beat from the American Nurses Association. https://anacapitolbeat.org/page/3/

Lwin, M. O., Lu, J., Sheldenkar, A., Schulz, P. J., Shin, W., Gupta, R., & Yang, Y. (2020). Global sentiments surrounding the Covid-19 pandemic on Twitter: Analysis of Twitter trends. *JMIR Public Health Surveillance, 6*(2), e19447. https://doi.org/10.2196/19447

Mason, D. J., Nixon, L., Glickstein, B., Han, S., Westphaln, K., & Carter, L. (2018). The Woodhull Study revisited: Nurses' representation in health news media 20 Years later. *Journal of Nursing Scholarship, 50*(6), 695–704. https://doi.org/10.1111/jnu.12429

Matthews, G., Burris, S., Ledford, S. L., Gunderson, G., & Baker, E. L. (2017). Crafting richer public health messages for a turbulent political environment. *Journal of Public Health Management and Practice, 23*(4), 420–423. https://doi.org/10.1097/phh.0000000000000610

McCartney, P. (2013). Crowdsourcing in healthcare. *Maternal and Child Health Journal, 38*(1), 392. https://doi.org/10.1097/NMC.0b013e3182a41571

McGregor, S. C. (2019). Social media as public opinion: How journalists use social media to represent public opinion. *Journalism, 20*(8), 1070–1086. https://doi.org/10.1177/1464884919845458

Myers, C. R. (2019). ANA adopts new presidential election policy. *AJN: American Journal of Nursing, 119*(10), 19–20. https://doi.org/10.1097/01.naj.0000586136.65273.f8

National Council of State Boards of Nursing. (2011). *White paper: A nurse's guide to the use of social media.* https://www.ncsbn.org/social_media.pdf

Over 700 Signatories. (2020, October 02). We are nurses, America's most trusted profession. And we support Biden: Opinion. *Newsweek.* https://www.newsweek.com/we-are-nurses-americas-most-trusted-profession-we-support-biden-opinion-1535962

Oxford Lexico. (n.d.). Media. In *Oxford Dictionary.* https://www.lexico.com/en/definition/media

Robertson, L. (2020, November 05). *Trump tweets flagged by Twitter for misinformation.* https://www.factcheck.org/2020/11/trump-tweets-flagged-by-twitter-for-misinformation/

Roper ipoll. (n.d.). *Roper ipoll.* https://ropercenter.cornell.edu/ipoll/

Rumsfeld, J. S., Brooks, S. C., Aufderheide, T. P., Leary, M., Bradley, S. M., Nkonde-Price, C., Schwamm, L. H., Jessup, M., Ferrer, J. M., Merchant, R. M., & American Heart Association Emergency Cardiovascular Care Committee; Council on Cardiopulmonary, Critical Care, Perioperative and Resuscitation; Council on Quality of Care and Outcomes Research; Council on Cardiovascular and Stroke Nursing; and Council on Epidemiology and Prevention. (2016). Use of mobile devices, social media, and crowdsourcing as digital strategies to improve emergency cardiovascular dare: A scientific statement from the American Heart Association. *Circulation, 134*(8), e87–e108. https://doi.org/10.1161/CIR.0000000000000428

Salzmann-Erikson, M. (2018). Mental health nurses' use of Twitter for professional purposes during conference participation using #acmhn2016. *International Journal of Mental Health Nursing, 27*(2), 804–813. https://doi.org/10.1111/inm.12367

Schemmann, B., Herrmann, A. M., Chappin, M. M. H., & Heimeriks, G. J. (2016). Crowdsourcing ideas: Involving ordinary users in the ideation phase of new product development. *Research Policy, 45*(6), 1145–1154. https://doi.org/10.1016/j.respol.2016.02.003

Sigma Theta Tau International Honor Society of Nursing. (1997). *The Woodhull study on nursing and the media: Health care's invisible partner: Final report.* Center Nursing Press. http://hdl.handle.net/10755/624124

Sinnenberg, L., Buttenheim, A. M., Padrez, K., Mancheno, C., Ungar, L., & Merchant, R. M. (2017). Twitter as a tool for health research: A systematic review. *American Journal of Public Health, 107*(1), e1–e8. https://doi.org/10.2105/AJPH.2016.303512

Somaschini, A. (2019, June 29). *Memorandum to the American Nurses Association board of directors re: Presidential endorsements.* https://s3.amazonaws.com/nursing-network/production/files/84331/original/ANA_General_Counsel_Memorandum_to_BOD_6-28-2019_-_FINAL__281_29.pdf?1562164596

Tang, L., Bie, B., Park, S. E., & Zhi, D. (2018). Social media and outbreaks of emerging infectious diseases: A systematic review of literature. *American Journal of Infection Control, 46*(9), 962–972. https://doi.org/10.1016/j.ajic.2018.02.010

Tankovska, H. (2021, February 10). *Distribution of Instagram users worldwide as of January 202, by age group.* Statista. https://www.statista.com/statistics/325587/instagram-global-age-group/

U. S. Office of Special Counsel. (n.d.). Federal employee HATCH Act information. https://osc.gov/Services/Pages/HatchAct-Federal.aspx.

van Lent, L. G., Sungur, H., Kunneman, F. A., van de Velde, B., & Das, E. (2017). Too far to care? Measuring public attention and fear for Ebola using Twitter. *Journal of Medical Internet Research, 19*(6), e193. https://doi.org/10.2196/jmir.7219

Vogel, L. (2020, October 2). *Photo: A montage of some of the 700 nurses who are urging Americans to vote for former Vice President Joe Biden in the 2020 election.* https://www.newsweek.com/we-are-nurses-americas-most-trusted-profession-we-support-biden-opinion-1535962#slideshow/1645150

Waddell, A., Audette, K., DeLong, A., & Brostoff, M. (2016). A hospital-based interdisciplinary model for increasing nurses' engagement in legislative advocacy. *Policy, Politics, and Nursing Practice, 17*(1), 15–23. https://doi.org/10.1177/1527154416630638

Wakefield, M. (2017). Affordable Care Act needs mending not ending. *Grand Forks Herald.* http://www.grandforkshera ld.com/opinion/op-e d-columns/4240594-mary-wakefield-former-health-and-human-services-executive-affordable

The White House. (2020, May 6). *Remarks by President Trump at signing of a proclamation in honor of National Nurses Day.* https://trumpwhitehouse.archives.gov/briefings-statements/remarks-president-trump-signing-proclamation-honor-national-nurses-day/

CHAPTER 11

Applying a Nursing Lens to Shape Policy

GREER GLAZER AND ANGELA CLARK

The nursing lens . . ."is not simply a matter of parity. . . . It's a matter of perspective.
Without the nurses' voices and nursing lens, needed change cannot occur."
—Joanne Disch
Past President, AARP, American Academy of Nursing

OBJECTIVES

1. Understand the interconnectedness among policy, politics, health policy, and health reform.
2. Identify pathways for influencing policy at multiple levels (institutional, organizational, governmental: local, state, national, international).
3. Formulate strategies for expanding your influence and commitment to policy engagement.
4. Model your commitment to eliminating structural racism in the classroom, workplace, organization, and/or government.

THE POWER OF NURSES TO SHAPE POLICY

Nurses and midwives, 20.7 million strong, account for 50% of the global health workforce (World Health Organization [WHO], n.d.). Within the United States alone, the 4.3 million nurses are four times the size of the next largest group of providers. The weight of nursing's voice and the growing evidence on nursing's influence to shape policy are transforming care and health, including the definition of health. But how do we continue to reform healthcare and advance global population health? The immediate answer: individually and collectively. This chapter provides an overview of policy, politics, and the interconnected barriers, challenges, and opportunities that exist to assuage the geopolitical determinants of health. The power to shape policy is present in every role in nursing—from providers in the community and at the bedside, to advanced practice providers, researchers, academia, boards, political action committees (PACs), and professional organizations. This chapter's Policy Challenge describes the policy journey of an individual new to nursing.

Nursing's power to shape policy is essential to all facets of health. Policies exist at unit (microsystem), organizational, and societal levels. They are developed through processes that are individually driven or collectively based. They can address social issues, organizational effectiveness, or health. Up to this point, the role of nurses in policy development and implementation at all three of these levels has been

Marcus Henderson, MSN, RN,
Staff/Charge Nurse, Fairmount Behavioral Health System
Lecturer, University of Pennsylvania School of Nursing
Philadelphia, PA

In middle school, I cared for my great grandmother, who had Alzheimer's disease, and my great aunt, who had Down syndrome. I saw firsthand how home care, hospice, and acute care nurses helped maintain their dignity at the end of life. From this experience, I was able to find my voice at a young age. Now that I know that I have a voice, I try to use my voice as a force for change and to amplify the voices of others.

The strong women in my life, my mother, grandmother, aunts, great grandmother, and great aunts, served as important role models and provided me with resources of love and support, shaping me and my career as a nurse. One of my high school teachers, Jessica Way, a nurse, became my first nursing mentor. Mentorship has been important at every stage of my career. I believe that the mentor/mentee relationship gives each person perspective and can result in long-lasting relationships.

During high school, my activism began joining HOSA-Future Health Professionals, formerly Health Occupations Students of America the largest student organization preparing students to enter the healthcare field, and serving as president of the Pennsylvania Chapter from 2012 to 2013. The mission of HOSA is to empower future health professionals to become leaders in the global health community. The HOSA creed became my north star, "I believe through service to my community and to the world, I will make the best use of my knowledge and talents" (HOSA-Future Health Professionals, 2020).

As a high school student, I took the creed of service and leadership to heart, becoming an exemplar for the impact HOSA has had on my career, as it was a critical foundation for all that I have been able to accomplish in a very short time. I began my baccalaureate program at the University of Pennsylvania (Penn) in 2013. Upon enrolling in the undergraduate program, I immediately joined the local chapter of the SNAP and the NSNA. I attended the state convention that fall and was elected to the SNAP Board of Directors. I served on the SNAP board for four years, serving as president from 2015 to 2017, and served on the NSNA Board from 2016 to 2017. My SNAP/NSNA experience exposed me to the ANA and the use of evidence to inform policy and decision-making. Throughout my undergraduate career, the number of individuals I relied on for mentorship grew.

My professional involvement gave me the skills, leadership, and vision to compete for a $100,000 Penn President's Engagement Prize with my friend, Ian McCurry, for our project titled "Homeless Health and Nursing: Building Community Partnerships for a Healthier Future" in 2017. Up and Running Healthcare Solutions, a nurse-led case management organization, grew out of our passion for serving homeless individuals and was funded by Penn to provide individuals experiencing homelessness in Philadelphia with tools, partnerships, and support they need to achieve their health goals. Our organization sought to mitigate the effects that the SDOH can have on homeless individuals' health. We addressed these SDOH using community health workers, specially trained community members who understood homeless healthcare delivery on a personal level.

My nursing lens is evident in the organization we created as baccalaureate students at Penn. This equity lens focuses on SDOHs, their impact, individuals as members of a community, the social and professional responsibility to care for all, and advocacy for racial and social justice. My personal experience of having a White mother and Black father, growing up in a single-parent household, serving as a family caregiver, and being a first-generation college student is embedded in my nursing lens. For this, I had the honor and privilege to be elected to the ANA board of directors, nominated to the Committee on the Future of Nursing 2020–2030 at the National Academy of Medicine, and appointed to the National Commission to Address Racism in Nursing. At these tables, I provide the nursing lens of an early career nurse and millennial, grounded in equity, inclusion, social justice, and antiracism, toward advancing our profession.

ANA, American Nurses Association; NSNA, National Student Nurses' Association; SDOH, social determinants of health; SNAP, Student Nurses' Association of Pennsylvania.

inconsistent. There are increasing calls to use a broader lens to improve population health at a societal level. *Population health*, defined as the "health outcomes of a group of individuals, including distribution of such outcomes within the group," provides an opportunity for individuals, healthcare systems, agencies, and organizations to work together to improve health outcomes in the communities in which they serve (Kindig & Stoddart, 2003). Policy is a vehicle for making improvements in population health. Nursing has a long history of leaders who have worked to address population health. Lillian Wald, for example, is credited with founding public health in the late 1800s, created the Henry Street Settlement for marginalized populations focused on the social determinants of health (SDOHs). Public health nurses have followed her legacy by working to advance population health and achieve health equity within communities through health promotion, disease prevention and control, and advocacy.

Key healthcare organizations have definitions of *policy* that are helpful in understanding the scope of efforts to improve health. The Centers for Disease Control and Prevention (CDC, 2015) defines *policy* as "a law, regulation, procedure, administrative action, incentive, or voluntary practice of governments and other institutions". The WHO (2021) loosely defines *policy* as a complex dynamic process that requires the key elements of engaging stakeholders, situation analysis, and priority setting, bringing it all together, from vision to operational, costing plans, monitoring, and evaluation. Health policy in its broadest definition is *policy* aimed at individual and population health and health equity, where "everyone has a fair and just opportunity to reach their full health potential."

Equity and inclusion are important to improving population health. Policy groups and think tanks have identified essential goals for the improvement of health. The Institute of Medicine (IOM, now the National Academy of Medicine [NAM]) in *Crossing the Quality Chasm* (2001) identified six aims for healthcare improvement: safe, effective, patient-centered, timely, efficient, and equitable. The Institute of Healthcare Improvement (IHI) has called health equity the forgotten aim (Feeley, 2016).

Health in All Policies (HiAP) is one approach to policy development that incorporates the health of all communities and people to focus on and achieve health equity (CDC, 2016). HiAP advances broad definitions of health policy by appropriately emphasizing the impact of policy on the SDOH, which are the "conditions in the environments in which people live, learn, work, play, worship and age that affect a wide range of health, functioning and quality of life outcomes and risks" (Department of Health and Human Services [DHHS], n.d., para. 1). These conditions include economic stability, social and community context, health and healthcare, education and neighborhood, and built environment. HiAP provides a broader framework for nurses' policy activism to improve population health. Catherine Alicia Georges provides an excellent example of a nurse focusing on HiAP, stating, "nurses understand what people need and we advocate for their needs." She prepped Bronx, New York, community members for testimony on budget items about what communities needed and why they needed it from an HiAP perspective. She pointedly explained that an ambulance cannot get down the street in an emergency because of potholes; the elderly cannot walk on a sidewalk with a walker, exercise, or easily get groceries because of deteriorating sidewalks (see Section "Influencing Policy Through Organizations").

Improvements in the SDOHs cannot occur without changes in policy. The groundwork for addressing SDOHs is provided in Healthy People 2030 and the Sustainable Development Goals (SDGs) of the United Nations (UN). Healthy People 2030 provides a framework for addressing SDOHs (see Figure 11.1). It is clear that nurses must engage in organizational and local, state, and federal policy, applying a "health in all policies" strategy to achieve the goals of health equity, reduce, and, ultimately, close the health gaps (DHHS, n.d.). The UN SDGs, 17 in all, provide a road map for improving SDOHs from a global perspective (see Chapter 14). The SDGs, signed on to by all UN member nations in 2015, focuses on ending poverty and other deprivations must be included with efforts to "improve health and education, reduce inequality, and spur economic growth" while also addressing climate change and preserving oceans and forests (UN, n.d., para. 1). These two seminal documents focus on the achievement of their goals by 2030. Health reform through policy development and political implementation has a profound effect on bolstering health equity and population health. The CDC attributes the Ten Great Public Health Achievements of the last century to the interplay between policy, politics, and health. But addressing health reform requires political connectedness at all levels (CDC, 2011).

Nurses, given their various roles and placements across sectors, are uniquely positioned to lead and shape policy through advocacy supporting health reform. Nurses need to use their long-standing Gallup poll's first-place ranking of honesty and ethical standards across professions not for bragging but as an opportunity

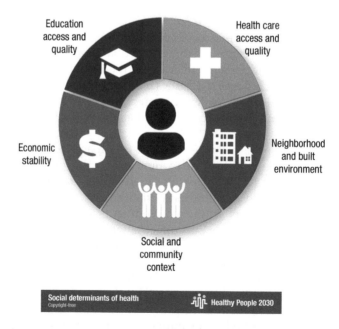

FIGURE 11.1 SDOHs and the Healthy People 2030 Framework

to leverage their influence on policy (Saad, 2020) In a recent survey regarding Americans' values and beliefs about national health insurance reform conducted by the Commonwealth Fund, *The New York Times*, & Harvard T.H. Chan School of Public Health (2019), Americans did not generally trust any major interest group other than nurses to improve the U.S. healthcare system. In fact, Americans trusted nurses (58%) to lead healthcare reform change, 28 percentage points higher than physicians, who were trusted to improve the healthcare system at 30%.

Nurses need to use their influence to get to policy tables. The future of health and healthcare is in the hands of nurses and the challenges are many. The fractured public healthcare system in the United States is buckling under the pressures of multiple epidemics, a global pandemic, and a system plagued with implicit bias and structural racism. Despite 16.9% of gross domestic product spent on healthcare in the United States, more than in any other country, the United States has the greatest income inequity, highest poverty rates, and some of the poorest health outcomes amongst the developed countries (Tikkanen, 2020). People of color and low socioeconomic status experience more disease burden and decreased life expectancy (Andrasfay & Goldman, 2021; Woolf & Schoomaker, 2019). Nurses have a front-row seat to the fractured public health system, but they need a seat at the policy table to bring forth their lens. Former Congresswoman Shirley Chisholm (n.d.) pointed out, "If they don't give you a seat at the table, bring a folding chair." It is necessary for nurses to be at the table in work settings, organizations, boards, and local, state, and national governments.

THE NURSING LENS

What differentiates nurses from others when engaging in the political process is the nursing lens, based on understanding nursing history, education, and practice experience. The nursing lens is a "viewpoint from which someone sees things holistically, considering the person, population or community in the larger context" (Disch, 2012, p. 170). The dominant view is that the history of nursing is grounded in social justice, health equity, public health, and community advocacy.

In nursing's history, this lens has also been grounded and limited by a Eurocentric, White viewpoint which negates the experiences of a growing number of nurses and patients. Regrettably, most nurses know little about other historic nurses who were persons of color (POCs) because this history is not part of textbooks, publications, or education. Most nurses know about Florence Nightingale. She is credited with establishing nursing as a profession, a holistic approach to health promotion, evidence-based practice, and recognizing the impact of the physical and social environment of health (as a precursor to the concept of SDOHs) in the second half of the 1800s. She has been studied, known, and beloved by almost all nurses. This status is exemplified by the WHO's recognition of 2020—the 200th anniversary of Nightingale's birth—as the International Year of the Nurse and Midwife.

However, "what is often unknown and rarely discussed in nursing history is Nightingale's racism and her political role in the genocide of indigenous people under British rule" (Stake-Doucet, 2020, "Nightengale and Colonialism"). In fact, the New Zealand Nurses Organization did not celebrate Nightingale in 2020 because of her role in advising Governor George Grey during the cruel era of repression against Maori anti-colonial uprisings. Nightingale's contemporary, Mary Grant Seacole, a Black Jamaican nurse, also served in the Crimean War and was known for her selfless treatment of wounded soldiers despite never being given an official position by Florence Nightingale. It is beyond the scope of this chapter to provide a more comprehensive picture of the many contributions of nurse leaders who were POCs; however, we recommend Darlene Clark Hine's *Black Women in White: Racial Conflict and Cooperation in the Nursing Profession 1890–1950*.

Despite nursing's complicated history, the American Nurses Association Code of Ethics for Nurses mandates the ongoing commitment to addressing SDOH, individual and population health, and healthcare equity. The code, containing ethical obligations for all nurses has nine provisions (www.nursingworld.org/practice-policy/nursing-excellence/ethics/code-of-ethics-for-nurses/coe-view-only/; see also Chapter 2). The code's interpretative statements expand on the principle of health as a human right, SDOHs, and nurses' roles in reducing disparities and generating health policy (ANA, 2015). In particular, Provision 8 states: "The nurse collaborates with other health professionals and the public to protect human rights, promote health diplomacy and reduce disparities." Provision 2 states: "The nurse's primary commitment is to the patient, whether an individual, family, group, community, or population." Provision 7 obligates each nurse, regardless of role or setting, to generate nursing and health policy (ANA, 2015). Provision 9 obligates our professional organizations to integrate principles of social justice into nursing and health policy (ANA, 2015).

The nursing lens is based on what we learn in our educational programs, which educate students to look at people holistically in the context of their families and communities. Nursing educational programs, when compared to physician education, for example, have traditionally included more content and coursework in community health, gerontology, health promotion and wellness, vulnerable populations, ethics, communication, evidence-based practice, and policy. Nursing is more than the treatment of illness and disease; it also focuses on health promotion and wellness. Students are taught to help people across the continuum and communities to reach their maximum health potential regardless of illness, disease, or conditions. Our educational system emphasizes the patient perspective, their assets, person-centered care, caring, and health equity.

Nursing practice occurs in many settings: in homes, hospitals, community health centers, schools, workplaces, retail clinics, churches, mosques, and synagogues, virtually anywhere. Nurses bring their well-developed skills in listening, assessment, interpersonal communication, ethical decision-making, critical thinking, ability to see the clinical and pragmatic side, and caring to each encounter. These perspectives facilitate nurses' abilities to seek personalized solutions that are pragmatic and realistic.

When nursing's history, educational preparation, and clinical practice are put together, the nursing lens provides a multifaceted understanding of care recipients from a holistic, broad perspective that reflects an understanding of the intersectionality of factors that determine health. The nursing lens reflects an understanding, articulation, and advocacy of the individual and community's perspective with the goal of attaining maximum health potential for all. Nurses are particularly effective in establishing effective interpersonal relationships that help people achieve their goals and do their very best work. Nurses can also readily size up situations and people. With this lens, nurses understand the human condition with all its intricacies and complexities. Thus, nurses can devise solutions or access resources where none seem to exist. The nursing lens is focused on the guiding question, "What is in the best interest of the patient?" as the north star. Our lens is not primarily focused on "What is in the best interest of the nurse?" Health and healthcare equity are our goals. Distinguished nurses who have used their lens to advance policy are listed in Exhibit 11.1. These exemplars illustrate the diversity of nurse leaders, and an in-depth discussion of additional nurse leaders and their approaches for using the nursing lens for policy leadership follows.

EXHIBIT 11.1 NURSE LEADERS IN PROMINENT POSITIONS

- Robyn Begley, DNP, RN, NEA-BC, CEO of the American Organization for Nursing Leadership, Senior Vice President and Chief Nursing Officer of the American Hospital Association, Chicago, IL
- Karen Cox, PhD, RN, FACHE, FAAN, President. Chamberlain University, Chicago, IL
- Regina S. Cunningham, PhD, RN, AOCN, FAAN, Chief Executive Officer, Hospital of the University of Pennsylvania, Philadelphia, PA
- Ernest Grant, PhD, RN, FAAN, President, American Nurses Association, Silver Spring, MD
- Susan Hassmiller, PhD, RN, FAAN, Senior Adviser for Nursing, Robert Wood Johnson Foundation, Director, Future of Nursing: Campaign for Action, Senior Scholar-in-Residence and Senior Adviser, National Academy of Medicine, Washington, D.C.
- Mary Jo Jerde, MBA, BSN, RN, FAAN, Senior Vice President UnitedHealth Group, Minneapolis, MN
- Brenda Marion Nevidjon, MSN, RN, FAAN, CEO of the Oncology Nursing Society, Pittsburgh, PA
- RADM Susan M. Orsega, MSN, FAAN, FNP-BC, FAANP, FAAN, Commissioned Corps Headquarters Director, U.S. Public Health Service, formerly Acting Surgeon General
- Betty Jo Rocchio, MS, RN, CRNA, CENP, Senior Vice President and Chief Nursing Officer, Mercy, St. Louis, MO
- RADM Sylvia Trent-Adams, PhD, RN, FAAN, FNAP, Principal Deputy Assistant Secretary for Health (retired)

Achieving the goals of health and health equity cannot be done by individuals alone. Associations have the capacity to amplify the voices of individuals. Most recently, the ANA along with every major nurses association has called for nurses to address structural racism. This is defined as racism that is embedded into laws, policies, and institutions, providing advantages to the dominant racial group while oppressing, disadvantaging or neglecting other racial groups (Williams et al., 2019). The COVID-19 pandemic has brought the issue of structural racism as an SDOH to the forefront as Blacks, Hispanics/Latinxs, and American Indians/Alaska Natives are more likely to be diagnosed and die from COVID-19 than others. The distinct disparities of COVID-19, nursing's historical focus on health, healthcare equity, and social justice, and adherence to the ANA Code of Ethics, necessitates that the nursing lens be used to address structural racism in all healthcare settings, educational institutions, workplaces, government, policies, laws, and regulations.

The following sections highlight selected examples of the diversity of roles that nurses hold that often are overlooked when advocacy and politics are discussed. These nontraditional roles are often overlooked because individuals mistakenly think that nurses in these roles have left the nursing lens behind. These nurses often hear from nurses in more traditional roles who state they could not consider such atypical roles because it would mean "giving up nursing" and the opportunities to advance nursing. Yet leaders like these who often started their careers providing direct patient care, indeed, found that they had many opportunities to have a positive impact on patients and nurses in their roles, even though their roles were less traditional. Although these leaders no longer function in direct care roles, their commitment to nursing and the patients they serve remains steadfast. Nurses must be involved and work to influence private and public policy through employment in their workplace, organizations, board membership, research, and government (local, state, national).

INFLUENCING POLICY THROUGH EMPLOYMENT

For many nurses, the road to policy starts at work and often by volunteering for a committee or responding "yes" when asked to serve on a committee. What better way to make a difference than policy work that impacts the lives of the public served by nurses or the work environment that impacts not only nurses, but the very people relied on every day to carry out work. Whether one is a new nurse or a seasoned nurse, a nurse in direct care, a leader on a unit or in the C-suite, an educator, or a researcher or holds an advanced degree, there is a role in policy for every nurse. There are multiple roles for active engagement in policy from its analysis, creation, implementation, evaluation, and/or modification, all of which need the nursing lens. Active engagement also includes role modeling and mentorship. It is an expectation that those with advanced degrees and named leadership positions have formal policy roles. However, many times, it is a nurse who does not hold a special title or credentials that can talk a colleague into starting a policy journey by demonstrating the importance of an issue, attending meetings, or getting involved in a policy project.

Often the best place to start down the road to policy is through committee work. Committee work not only provides opportunities to build political skills but also helps develop necessary networking skills, strengthen existing networks, and offer opportunities for mentorship. Organizations are often looking for members and chairpersons to lead committees or task forces, both in the work environment and in local communities. Often committee work can seem daunting; finding a mentor and getting familiar with fulfilling expectations is critical. Without guidance, committee members can lose sight of the work of the committee, or valuable time can be lost while members try to gather a sense of the committee. Both veterans and new members can benefit from formalizing the committee orientation process and bringing clarity to the policymaking and review process. The first step is expressing interest—and often just showing up. Highlighted here are two nurses Kevin Sowers and Antoinette Hays, both with impressive titles, who tell their story of how they became involved in policy work and now on a daily basis work to impact policy beyond nursing.

Kevin W. Sowers, MSN, RN, FAAN, president of the Johns Hopkins Health System and executive vice president of Johns Hopkins Medicine, is first, a nurse. Sowers's nursing lens is the commitment that the patient and their loved ones are central to everything done in healthcare, despite frequent changes in technology, care models, and disruptions across organizations. He remains committed to thinking through policy at all levels to support and balance this tenet. Sowers understood the need for and importance of hard work. He spent his formative years growing up in poverty and focusing on voice and piano and spent his summers days working at the county nursing home providing music therapy and his evenings at his second job as an orderly, feeding people, bathing them, and assisting with nightly routines. He fell in love with making a difference in people's lives and was inspired to make a career change to nursing, a decision that did not reflect the workforce at the time when men were not as prominent in the field. Sowers's supportive mother instilled in him the belief in something bigger and was very influential in his decision. She was right in recognizing that he had the passion and compassion to create change and make a real difference for patients and nurses alike.

Sowers started his professional nursing career as an oncology staff nurse at Duke in 1985, where he was promoted to assistant nurse manager and nurse manager before accepting a vice president role and senior vice president role at Duke Hospital. Sowers credits the development of a succession plan by the hospital's CEO and chief operations officer (COO) as a critical moment in his career. Senior leadership wanted two people to know everything about Duke Hospital, Sowers and his counterpart were each assigned half the hospital and instructed to learn every aspect of the healthcare organization over the year and, at the end of the year, they would swap portfolios. This experience, while challenging, allowed him to understand how to drive change at all levels within the organization.

Sowers's contributions include extensive publications and consultations on leadership, mentorship, and organizational change. He has been very active among professional organizations and boards, both current and past, including the American Hospital Association (AHA) Health Systems Council, Maryland Hospital Association Executive Board, the Vizient Board of Directors, the Association of American Medical Colleges' (AAMC) Council of Teaching Hospitals and Health Systems Administrative Board and previously chair of the AmSurg board, the North Carolina Hospital Association Board of Trustees, the American Heart Association, Susan G. Komen, and the Oncology Nursing Society (Johns Hopkins Medicine, n.d.; Rossbach, 2018).

Sowers attributes his success to relationships, collaboration, and being succinct in message delivery, intent, rationale, and outcome-oriented. "You have to be able to tell your story. When I go into any legislators' office, I always begin with 'as a nurse. . . .' I've found the power behind being a nurse and having people know I'm a nurse is immensely helpful. It begins a different dialogue and a different listening session because I'm coming from the place of a nurse versus an administrator."

> Sowers also exudes an expansive warmth during conversation, which evokes listening. He says, "Relationships, both internal and external to the organization, are important and it's important to build relationships with city, state, and federal officials outside of a crisis; the first time you sit down with someone, you don't have a relationship or credibility. Sitting down with them early on, before a crisis or conflict, allows you to establish a relationship and the trust needed to effectively navigate crisis."

Sowers has standing meetings with the legislators because

> "it's important that to have ongoing dialogue; every conversation can't come with an ask. Remain collaborative and partner using language that is about partnership and collaboration. When negotiating you will never get everything you want. Back off 80% and talk about the 20% that can be negotiated and prepare yourself to be informed for the 20% discussion. Look at the resources around you, most organizations have government affairs, they can help inform data points for discussions. Understand a politician or senior official's beliefs and agenda. Develop a strategy on how to manage the communication before you go into the room and negotiate."

An example of this strategy was seen while responding to healthcare delivery disruptions during the COVID-19 pandemic. Providers were able to consider seeing patients and providing care through telehealth, but practices were sustainable due to several legislative issues that needed to be addressed. Issues including licensure, liability, billing (Rothman & Sowers, 2020):

"We wanted to highlight how to change policy to allow us to continue using these innovations from a regulatory perspective. We strategically chose an evidence-backed opinion piece in the Washington Post because we know that is what Congress reads. It's important to understand the people who need to be brought to the table to inform policy development and change."

Antoinette Hays, PhD, RN, became the 10th President of Regis College in Weston, Massachusetts, a comprehensive liberal arts institution in 2011. It is abundantly clear to her how her experiences as a nurse were key motivators and set the groundwork for her current role as college president. What were these experiences? As a baccalaureate student at Boston College between 1970 and 1974, she was empowered to speak up for her patients, learned a patient-centered approach and the critical role of patients in care decisions. Upon graduation, she chose the field of geriatrics because she saw the incredible needs in long-term care, the challenge of managing multiple medical comorbidities, and the need to improve the quality of care for older adults. Very quickly, she experienced two profound realities in geriatric care: first, the essential skill of multitasking, as she was often the only professional nurse on a clinical unit, and, second, how ageism affected the social, economic, and policy injustices related to the care of older adults. Early on, she also recognized the social and economic injustices within the nursing profession. Antoinette's passion to influence change and policy was ignited and in 1976, she enrolled in the Geriatric Nurse Practitioner Program and master's Program in Gerontology and Community Health at Boston University (BU), graduating in 1978. In partnership with the medical team, she then launched the Geriatric Nurse Practitioner role at the Boston Visiting Nurses Association (VNA), creating a linkage between the new role of the APRN in the care of the geriatric client across the healthcare system, from home to hospital, to long-term care and, in many cases, back home.

Hays's academic career evolved significantly through this experience, and in 1979 she was recruited to be an assistant professor in the Graduate Geriatric Nurse Practitioner Program in the BU School of Nursing with a joint appointment in the Department of Geriatric Medicine at the medical school. In that position, she was charged with the development and launch of a new Multidisciplinary Acute Geriatric Consultation Program at BU Hospital (now known as the BU Medical Center). This role afforded her opportunities to build curriculum across disciplines (advanced nursing practice, medical students, medical residents, graduate students in social work), engage in clinical research, take part in national conferences, and author many peer-reviewed publications. In 1980, this program became a national model for acute geriatric care and was integral to an inaugural Geriatric Medical Fellowship Program, becoming a mandatory rotation for all medical residents at BU Hospital.

This opportunity in academia gave Hays the impetus to seek a doctoral degree, as she saw a pathway to improving healthcare delivery for the geriatric population through education and research. She chose the Heller School of Social Policy at Brandeis University in Waltham, Massachusetts, where she could focus her studies on the importance of nurses being at the policy tables to influence change in geriatric care. Too many times she saw healthcare providers feeling helpless as victims of the policy arena and it became clear to her that nurses needed to be at the table with data to advocate for change rather than remain frustrated onlookers.

During Hays's doctoral studies, she had the opportunity to help launch a new Nursing Leadership and Advanced-Practice program at Regis College, incorporating curriculum to prepare future nursing leaders and advanced nurse practitioners within a policy research and practice framework. In 1993, she was hired by Regis College as an assistant professor, then moved up the ranks as dean of the School of Nursing, Science and Health Professions (from 2006 to 2011) until being selected as the college's president in 2011. During this time, she was very active in the Massachusetts Association of Colleges of Nursing (MACN). While a board member and treasurer of MACN, the Nursing Deans and Directors began meeting with the Massachusetts Chief Nurse Executives (CNOs) through joint meetings of the MACN and the Massachusetts Organization of Nurse Executives. Hays's lens of looking at systems contributed to the group's understanding that academe could not move forward without practice and vice versa. Massachusetts became a leader in operationalizing academic practice partnership in the mid-2000s.

Throughout Antoinette's nursing career as a bedside nurse, nurse practitioner, faculty member, and dean, she was often presented with challenges to launch a new innovative role or program. Although the challenges posed were daunting at times, she loved the opportunity to "step out of the box" and challenge the norm, always with a nursing lens on how systems could be improved to enhance practice experiences and the quality of patient care outcomes. She learned the critical role of system analysis and research to convince others of the importance of innovation in practice, a principle that became integral to her work whether on clinical teams, with faculty partners, administrators, or with global partners in Haiti, working to improve outcomes in healthcare and in higher education.

Aware that change could only happen with the support and buy-in of others, the role of consensus builder became a priority for Hays. Excellence tempered by gentleness had always been Hays's style as a provider, teacher, or leader, which served her well as an innovator in the United States, in Haiti, and, now, as a university president. Her years in nursing practice and nursing education supplied the platform through which she learned to be a strategic partner, policy advocate, and change agent. She continues to use her system assessment skills every day, whether in the context of the interconnectedness of a healthcare organization, a community, or a related industry. Recognizing interdependence within any system has been essential to Hays's success as a leader, policy influencer, and educator focused on outcome improvements. Partnerships have always been central to her practice, whether in patient care, education, business, or globally; she appreciates the value of collective intelligence in improving outcomes in patient care, student success, or in a university's success.

Often quoted as saying, "No is not an option" (although she is open to discussion) and "Don't tell me why we can't . . . help me figure out how we can!" Hays has always led with great passion and compassion for what she believes to be the right thing to do and strives to instill inspiration in others to get the work done.

Influencing policy through the workplace does not require a leadership position, it is important for every nurse to be involved in policy development, implementation, and evaluation. Staff nurses can initiate and join committees on their units to develop policies for their patients that will improve outcomes. They can also initiate and join committees on their units that will address their own health and well-being. Similarly, nursing faculty can initiate and join committees in their schools/colleges that will improve student learning and success. They can also initiate and join committees at their schools/colleges that will address their own health and well-being. Getting your feet wet at the local level will give you the confidence and experience to increase your involvement in your workplace, whether it be at the hospital or school/college level.

INFLUENCING POLICY THROUGH ORGANIZATIONS

Organizations are just like people. They have values, mission or purpose, a vision, and can be influenced by those involved or associated with the organization. In fact, often leaders in organizations have a significant role in determining values, purposes, vision, and strategic actions. These elements will guide/determine organizational positions and establish recommendations on issues of importance to the organization. These organizational positions and recommendations provide the foundation on which issue or policy they will seek to influence.

Organizational values impact policies. Some values are central to the mission and vision of the organization, and therefore, they endure over time. For example, ANA collaborated with the nursing community in 1991 to develop Nursing's Agenda for Health Care Reform (Betts, 1996), which was then updated in 2008. Previous organizational positions and recommendations guided ANA's policy position that healthcare is a basic human right and that all people deserve access to essential healthcare services. Nursing's blueprint for healthcare reform, endorsed by an overwhelming majority of specialty nurses associations, served as a guide for the development of the Patient Protection and Affordable Care Act (ACA) that was passed in 2010.

Beverly Malone, PhD, RN, FAAN, is a strong example of an American nurse who has influenced health policy through her leadership of three major national and international organizations: the ANA, the Royal College of Nursing (RCN) of the United Kingdom, and the National League for Nursing (NLN). In 2020, she was ranked fifth by *Modern Healthcare's* "100 Most Influential People in Healthcare," the fourth time in the past decade she was included on this list. She was also named one of five "Inaugural Minority Healthcare Luminaries" by *Modern Healthcare* for her achievements that are reshaping healthcare. Her great grandmother, who was a healer in the community, served as her earliest role model: "She required everyone to eat before drinking and taught me how you work with the community." Malone's experience as a psychiatric–mental health nurse, clinical specialist, administrator, and faculty member influenced her nursing lens as she learned it was always about relationships. She believes that policy has so much to do with relationships that we do not always appreciate. Being a nurse meant that Malone had policy inside of her, as all nurses do. "How do you walk into a room and end up doing something personal with a patient and family if you don't have the ability to relate in an incredibly personal way?" Malone's nursing lens as an African American nurse is focused on equity and on always making sure people are taken care of, including those not able to care for themselves and those with mental health problems.

While Malone was working on her doctorate, her mentor, Dr. Hattie Bessent, wanted her to go to Washington, D.C., to work in the policy arena so she could really understand federal policy. In 1979, with children 4 and 6 years old, she worked during one summer as a legislative intern for Senator Inouye (D-HI), becoming the first African American nurse on the hill. She returned the next summer when she truly understood policy and how to work with government.

An example that highlights the importance of relationships and communication took place when Sen. Inouye asked Malone to find money to build a rehabilitation center in Hawaii. She asked the deputy assistant secretary for the money, but he replied he did not have any money available for this project. When she reported that back to her boss, he told her to check if it was true that the administrator did not have any money. When Malone found out that there was money, she was told to call the officer and tell him that he was lying. As a skilled psychiatric nurse,

Malone got on the phone and said, "It seems there was a misunderstanding: we need the $500,000 that you have for the center in Hawaii. The senator said that if you don't put the money in your proposed budget forward, then you won't have any money at all." The money was quickly found, and the rehabilitation center was built. Malone used her interpersonal communication skills as a nurse and did not call the appointed officer a liar, which would have likely ended their conversation. Malone had developed the relationship skills to get things done.

Malone has a favorite saying, "I can be delayed but not defeated." She shares an example of perceived failure when she was Interim Vice Chancellor, Academic Affairs at North Carolina Agriculture and State University in 1994, where she had been a dean and professor since 1986. During her tenure as interim vice chancellor, she had provided leadership for a successful Southern Association of Colleges and Schools (SACS) accreditation visit and a Family Science and Environment accreditation visit. The campus was healing, you could feel the mood changing, and positive and warm things were happening. She applied for the permanent position and, unexpectedly, did not get it. She immediately thought she was done; then she realized that was just a delay. "Sometimes you have to get to a place, turn around and look back to see the opportunities." Malone needed this twist in her plans and a closed door to get to her next big opportunity: She became the president of the ANA in 1996, serving until 2000. She served on ANA's board of directors, second vice president, chair of the Legislation Committee, vice chair of the Ethnic Minority Fellowship Program, and member of the Finance Committee. "You don't just become president of an organization one day without having provided prior significant service in the organization," and Malone had served previously at the state level in leadership positions.

As president of the ANA, she represented the association on issues affecting the nation's healthcare and the professional requirements of a diverse nursing workforce to provide safe quality care. She worked closely with the President of the United States' Office and Congress providing consultation, testimony, and serving on numerous federal commissions, committees, and taskforces. Significant ones during this time include President Clinton's Advisory Commission on Consumer Protection and Quality in the Healthcare Industry (1996–1998), where she helped develop The Patients' Bill of Rights, National Forum for Healthcare Quality Measurement and Reporting (1998–1999), and appointment by President Clinton to the World Health Assembly (1998, 1999). She represented nurses and nursing at various press conferences in support of the Patients' Bill of Rights and the Patient Safety Act.

At the end of Malone's ANA Presidency, she was appointed Deputy Assistant Secretary for Health (1999 to 2001), serving as the senior advisor to the Assistant Secretary of Health. She also provided advice and counsel to the secretary of the DHHS on public health and science issues. Her portfolio included mental health, international healthcare issues, food safety, disaster relief, and any issues related to the nation's public health that arose.

Opportunity came knocking in 2001 when Malone became the general secretary for the RCN of the United Kindgom—the largest professional union of nursing staff in the world—until 2007. With well over 400,000 members practicing across all settings in the National Health Service (NHS), as well as the independent and not-for-profit sector in all four U.K. countries (England, Scotland, Wales, and Northern Ireland), the RCN's mission is to represent nurses and nursing, promote excellence in practice and shape health policies. As the chief executive, reporting to the U.K.-wide elected RCN Council, Malone provided leadership to more than 1,000 staff in transforming the organization to better meet the needs and desires of members. Intensive influencing and legislative activities included regular meetings with the government (the prime minister, the Chancellor of the Exchequer, the secretary of state for health) and politicians of all mainstream U.K. political parties, as well as senior government officials and representatives of major organizations in U.K. public life. During Malone's tenure as general secretary, she was appointed by Prime Minister Tony Blair to the World Health Assembly between 2002 and 2003, which landed her an invitation to a state dinner seated next to Prince Charles.

Malone returned to the United States in 2007 as chief executive officer of the NLN, a position she still holds today. Dedicated to excellence in nursing education, the NLN is a membership organization for nurse faculty and leaders in nursing education. Its 40,000 individual and 1,200 institutional members include nurse educators, education agencies, healthcare agencies, and interested members of the public who can access faculty development programs, networking opportunities, testing and assessment, nursing research grants, and public policy initiatives. Malone has served on the DHHS National Alliance for Suicide Prevention and DHHS Advisory Committee on Minority Health. She has testified before Congress, subcommittees, and federal agencies on Title VIII appropriations (funding for nursing education) and funding for the Nurse Education Act.

Malone's prolific policy contributions via leadership in national and international organizations have always been through her nursing lens of equity, service, putting patients at the center of whatever she is doing, taking care of others, and based on excellent relationships and communication. "Nurses are committed to taking care of patients and creating a better place for them." She believes that any nurse can do policy work. "It is a cinch by an inch, it's hard by the yard. Understand we are the healers; even doing policy, we are in the business of healing." Malone reminds us that we do not exist as nurses without patients. "We are who we are because of our patients."

Catherine Alicia Georges, EdD, RN, FAAN, professor and chairperson of the Department of Nursing at Lehman College, is an exemplar of service leadership, shaping policy through boards and organizations, and a conduit for community and population health. Georges grew up in the U.S. Virgin Islands, where her godmother delivered many of the children on St. Thomas and her family was well connected with the nurses. Inspired by these relationships, she graduated from Seton Hall School of Nursing and then crossed the bridge to work in one of the most deprived areas in the Bronx and became involved with health promotion, restoration, and prevention for vulnerable populations. Georges began networking and established relationships with community stakeholders and politicians in the borough of the Bronx. Later on, she received her Master of Arts with an emphasis in community health nursing administration from New York University and a Doctor of Education from the University of Vermont. She remembers one of her nursing educational experiences with systemic racism included being required to include a picture with the school application (she decided not to apply to that school).

Georges's nursing lens is one of a holistic view with a clear understanding of the intersectionality of the SDOHs. Her pragmatic approach to problem-solving complimented her public health nursing background, allowing her to advocate for the needs of community members. An example of her early work includes prepping community members to testify for budget line items needed in their community as exemplified by the story at the beginning of the chapter in the discussion on HiAP. She magnified her influence and the voice of the community by serving on the Bronx Community Board #12, where she gained insights into news and the inner workings of the city that shaped policy. "Many elected officials don't know or have a sense of the health issues and social determinants. Nurses know the impact. Talk about it and bring forward the hard data. Nurses need to speak out."

As an active at-large member of the board of directors, for the New York Black Nurses Association, Georges communicated the needs of the lower middle-class areas in the Bronx. She expanded her role on the New York Black Nurses Association by serving as the treasurer, served on Governor Cuomo's advisory board and later became the president and founder of the "National Black Nurses Day on the Hill." She served as vice president and president of the National Black Nurses Association (NBNA), the DHHS Advisory Council on Nursing Education and Practice, and served on the AARP board of directors from 2010 to 2020.

When Georges's career began in the 1960s in New York City, everyone in her office was White, except all the housekeeping staff were Black. Race and gender often were roadblocks for her, but she has remained ambitious and committed to advocating for health equity, addressing racism, supporting Black nurses, and promoting outcomes for vulnerable populations. Her ambitions were fueled by the tremendous Black nurses she met, such as Dr. Betty Smith Williams, Dr. Rhetaugh Dumas, Dr. Gloria Smith, and Dr. Mary Elizabeth Carnegie who would talk with her about the history of Black nurses and where she needed to be. It is really amazing that Georges had no idea that these women were "bigshots," because they were so nice. She feels obligated to mentor others because of the mentorship that she received. Her efforts have resulted in research and program funding, speaking engagements around the globe, and invited proceedings to empower a culture of health and policy change. During momentous advancement in leadership roles, Georges has remained constant in her efforts to partner and advocate for African Americans and aging communities, and address the structural and racial barriers to healthcare. Service and policy advancements have led to George's recognition include, but are not limited to, the American Academy of Nursing (AAN) Living Legend, Women Who Lead Vitas Black History Month, Outstanding Women by New York Senator Larry Seabrook, and the ANA Minority Fellowship Program Public Service Award. Georges's father used to say, "The best you can do is give service to mankind," by continuing to show up, volunteering, speaking out, giving suggestions and solutions, and remaining connected.

Deborah Trautman, PhD, RN, FAAN, is president and chief executive Officer of the American Association of Colleges of Nursing (AACN). At a young age, Trautman knew she wanted to make a difference and improve the lives of those in her community. In a conversation with her one is struck by her genuine kindness and humility. While working as an aide in a long-term care facility, she recognized the quality of the work done by one of the nurses and knew she wanted to be like her: "She was a leader, organizer, and fun." While her career didn't start in formal policy development and she doesn't recall taking policy courses during nursing school, her nursing lens is grounded in health reform and complemented by her innate ability to develop relationships and communicate evidence.

Trautman's experiences as an ED nurse, staff instructor, and manager gave her the expertise to lead policy conversations. She believes that much of what helped her be a good nurse prepared her well in the policy arena. Early in her career, she noticed that nurses were often brought in after policy development and implementation "to clean things up," yet she thought, "if you just had nurses at the table in the first place." While in the ED, her boss connected her to serve as a representative for a statewide trauma system initiative in Pennsylvania; then during her doctoral studies, she had the opportunity to advance her role in domestic initiatives by serving on an interprofessional, diverse committee to reduce domestic violence for the state of Maryland. She advocated for better protections for women and safeguards to protect individuals. Her mentor, Dr. Jackie Campbell, was phenomenal in helping her develop her dissertation study to domestic violence screening. Trautman compared an electronic computer-based screening with an in-person screening to determine which had better results. The computer screening resulted in better information for detecting violence, which contradicted the prevailing beliefs. Her mentor suggested she continue her efforts driving evidence-based health reform and apply for the Robert Wood Johnson Foundation Health Policy Fellowship. Trautman was awarded the fellowship and served as Assistant to the Honorable Nancy Pelosi, Speaker of the House. Her role as a senior health policy staffer included advising the Speaker and the House on healthcare issues, current and pending legislation, and strategic policy considerations to advance health and healthcare. She coordinated activities with the Congressional health policy committee staff and Congressional offices and engaged in public speaking and liaising with professional associations, trade organizations, and constituents. While working on the ACA, Trautman was struck by the absence of health professionals at the table and thought that those who were at the table were most often advocating for their profession. One member of Congress wanted penalties in place for individuals who didn't adhere to ACA policies, Trautman was effective in communicating that penalties would be discriminatory. Trautman's interactions with patients and families and conservations with members of Congress all came together to guide her in working with the team that crafted appropriate language for this component of the bill.

After the legislative language was released and right before the House was going to vote, Trautman got a call from a freshman member of Congress who was hosting a town hall. Five hundred people, both red and blue constituents, were expected, and he requested she sit behind the curtain to help answer questions. The first question was posed by an elderly woman, who reminded Trautman of her great-grandmother, she shared that she just lost her husband of 50 years and was concerned about navigating the health system. Trautman was relieved that she seemed to have a supportive audience. The next person launched into "how could he dare support legislation to take control away from doctors and nurses and place into policymaker's hands?" Trautman's thoughts turned to feeling that perhaps the audience might be more combative than she had thought. The then congressman informed his audience that "he just so happens to have a nurse here that can provide more information." Trautman was surprised to learn that she would now be answering questions. However, she rose to the occasion with her usual command of interpersonal communication and positivity. Trautman helped explain the problems they were trying to fix; she was ready to have these difficult conversations because her nursing experience afforded her both knowledge competencies and human competencies. "Nurses will do whatever it takes to get the job done, we're less worried about the lane we're in and see boundaries differently."

While working on the ACA, there was strong disagreement, people were on the defense and Trautman felt that not enough had been done to educate individuals, "policies fail because people are not ready for it." This realization led to Trautman's next role as the executive director of Johns Hopkins Medicine, Center for Health Policy and Healthcare Transformation. The center's mission is to generate and disseminate knowledge and promote effective health policy. When reflecting on her work in policy at the federal level, Trautman posits that her roles in nursing—staff nurse, clinical nurse manager, director of nursing, vice president of patient care services—and experience handling any uncertainty that comes through the door conditioned her to shape policy. Trautman advised that it's important for nurses to remember that "we are not the only profession that has humanism; it may be more in our DNA than others and a lot of it is in our education and preparation, but we don't have to stand alone. We need to have the wisdom and confidence in our abilities to bring people together."

Trautman continues to shape policy in her role as president and CEO of the AACN. Through speaking engagements, congressional testimony, research, and dissemination, she is an avid policy advocate for nurses. She is a member of many organizations and professional affiliations including the ANA, Sigma Theta Tau, the AAN, Academy Health (advisory board member), the Nursing Organization Alliance, chair of the Interprofessional Education Collaborative, secretary and treasurer of the Federation of Associations of Schools of the Health Professions, and the Nursing Advisory Council, Joint Commission. She believes involvement in professional organizations is critical to expanding one's influence and the voice of nursing. She laments that membership in the ANA includes fewer than 10% of RNs and advanced practices nurses in the United States and strongly advocates that every nurse should be a member of their professional association or organization.

All of the previously mentioned leaders in this section were selected for their key roles in organizations. Each believes that there is great strength in joining together through organizational membership and leadership. Beyond the accomplishments of members joining together, organizations provide other mechanisms to exert influence. See political action committees and coalitions later in this chapter.

INFLUENCING POLICY THROUGH BOARD SERVICE

It is well known that nurses are knowledgeable about the challenges and issues on the frontline of healthcare. Yet too often, their expertise is not heard or taken into account in redesigning healthcare to make it cost-effective, safe, quality-driven, and person-centered. To address the nurse leadership vacuum in the boardroom, and in response to the *Future of Nursing: Leading Change, Advancing Health* report's (IOM, 2011) recommendations, the Nurses on Boards Coalition (NOBC) was created in 2014. This national organization is laser-focused on recruiting and recommending nurses for board service. Its nationally coordinated approach was successful in moving a nursing perspective into America's boardrooms. The goal was to place over 10,000 nurses on local, state, and national boards by 2020, which was achieved (NOBC, 2021) (www.nursesonboardscoalition.org). The following individuals illustrate the importance of nurses being at the table where their voice and vote help determine critical decisions that impact patients and their communities.

Betty Smith Williams, DrPH, MN, MS, FAAN, is a public health nurse, dean, and formidable trailblazer. A nurse since 1954, her 34-page curriculum vitae shows her commitment to service organizations beginning in 1958, from the executive board of the Los Angeles Chapter of Delta Sigma Theta, Inc. to the board of Directors of Blue Cross of California. Throughout her impressive tenure, she holds many firsts: she was the first Black person to wear the cap from the Frances Payne Bolton (FPB) School of Nursing, the first Black person to be hired by California State College, the first Black person to teach nursing at a higher education institution in the state of California, and the first Black nursing dean in Colorado. Williams believes that being a Black person impacted her entire life and career. Her first experience with a Black teacher was as a freshman at Howard University. She didn't know many Black nurses, and no one looked like her in a lot of situations. She didn't have a Black professor at FPB.

Smith experienced systemic racism throughout her nursing career, starting with her application to a direct-entry nursing program after getting a bachelor's degree in zoology at Howard University. When one program declined her application, she questioned them about the reason for nonacceptance. They asked her to take an examination (which others had not been required to do) and when she received a high score, was subsequently admitted. When she was teaching, she was usually in situations with the White majority, and she had some experiences that were discriminatory. As a voice for Black communities and ethnic minorities, Williams understood from a young age the many motivations behind politics. Her mother held county political party offices and was a local founding member of the National Association for the Advancement of Colored People (NAACP). She remembers when she was little, people coming to their home and putting money on their table. Her parents told her that "something happened to some boys." She later learned her parents were providing support and money to defend the nine young Scottsboro Boys (www.history.com/topics/great-depression/scottsboro-boys). She learned very young that when you do things together with other people, you have a voice, and you can get something done. Williams's nursing lens is one of civil rights, affirmative action, and human rights. She says that "if something violates your values, you speak up for what you believe in."

During her formative years, she was active in Girl's Club; in college, she was active in her Delta Sigma Theta chapter. Through her sorority, she had a lot of experiences with dynamic professional women and was introduced to some "heavy hitters." Upon graduation, she began practicing, then teaching as a public health nurse, and joined the American Public Health Association. She has remained steadfast in her commitment to address health disparities in minority communities, advocating for equality in healthcare. With an upbringing in activism, Williams recognized early on that councils provided access to high achievers, and she knew she needed to unite Black nurses to address healthcare inequities. So, in 1968, she cofounded the Council of Black Nurses in Los Angeles (CBN-LA) and, in 1971, she cofounded the NBNA. Williams stated, "I thought black nurses needed a way to communicate with each other. We had no voice, but we understood our culture and our unique needs better than anyone else" (Robison, 2016, para. 4).

In 1997, she cofounded the National Coalition of Ethnic Minority Nurse Associations (NCEMNA) whose members are the Philippine Nurses Association of America, Inc., the NBNA, the National Alaska Native American Indian Nurses Association, the National Association of Hispanic Nurses, and the Asian American/ Pacific Islander Nurses Association. Williams served 14 years as NCEMNA's founding president and now is its president emerita.

While serving as assistant dean of nursing at the University of California Los Angeles, Williams was asked to serve on the board of directors for Blue Cross of Southern California during the 1970s, a time when female board leadership was rare. Board members met at a private club in downtown Los Angeles where women were not allowed on the second floor. She notified the chairman of the board that she would not serve on a board that did not allow all board members to fully participate. Asian, Hispanic, and Jewish board members followed her lead in advocating for inclusion and the meeting location was moved.

For 65 years, Williams has leveraged her public health background, extensive organizational network, and voice to address the inequities in Black and minority communities. She has continued to break the glass ceiling by cultivating power through shared voices and shaping policy through community-based research and political activism. Williams is a living legend of the AAN. Her extensive research, leadership, and service have resulted in many political advancements for aging health, ethnic and minority nurse pathways, collaborative models of healthcare, economic issues in nursing, and global issues in public health nursing.

Melanie Dreher, PhD, RN, FAAN, is dean emerita, Rush University, College of Nursing. From a family of nurses with Irish politics in her blood, Dreher is an influential nursing leader with expansive big-picture views of human experiences formed by years of diverse work. Dreher has made it her mission to make connections, be a decision-maker and advocate for policy change through board service. Her unique nursing lens was shaped by her training as an anthropologist, as a student of Margaret Mead: "For nurses to have [the] capacity to create policy, they have to stand back and look through a different lens, the skill of policy starts with an assessment of your own profession on the world stage—its strengths and its limitations (most of which are self-imposed)." Dreher's early work in anthropology took place in Jamaica, where she also examined the use of cannabis. Engaged in the study of norms and values, Dreher understood that nurses were missing an incredible opportunity: "Helping people live well is a huge undertaking." Armed with an understanding of the needs and standards (values and norms) of people and communities, she used her board positions to advocate for a focus on health and the patient experience. When board conversations included the need to cut expenses by reducing the nursing staff, she would use that opportunity to say that, as a nurse, her standards for patient care are extremely high. She was able to get agreement that high standards of care were a value most would expect and agree on. This helped her board colleagues to find a better solution once they understood that the "*real* business of hospitals is 24-hour vigilance by expert nurses."

Dreher's extensive experience in Jamaica helped shape her perspective on the importance of nurse confidence, "I observed a nurse intercept a physician while he was writing discharge notes on patient and quietly offered, 'Doctor, I need to make you aware that this patient is not ready to go home at this time.' The physician simply stopped writing, closed the chart, and said, 'Ms. Jones, you know more about this patient than I. Please keep me informed on his progress.' She didn't begin her sentence with 'I think' or 'I believe.' She was secure in her assessment to effectively advocate for the patient's welfare." "Nurses have to be visible. Make yourself heard beyond academia. Join the Rotary, the Chamber of Commerce, and identify yourself as a community resource, available to impart your wisdom to individuals and groups. Write letters to the editor of the newspaper. . . . People will see you and recommend you for all kinds of opportunities in policy leadership."

When serving as dean at the University of Iowa, a business colleague suggested to Dreher that the nursing profession could do itself a big favor by serving on powerful corporate boards. To her, that meant the health insurance industry. Keeping her eye on how to achieve this goal, she asked a banker new to Iowa City trying to establish himself to, if he had connections, help her get her on the Des Moines Board of Blue Cross Blue Shield. Within 2 months, she was interviewed and offered a position on its subsidiary board where she continued to serve even after relocation to Chicago. A few years later, she was "promoted" to the Wellmark Inc. board, on which she still serves. In the meantime, she was recruited for the board of directors for Trinity Health, which became the second-largest private hospital/healthcare system in the country. According to Dreher, "board success requires showing up and showing what you got, armed with data and the rich experience that nurses bring."

As a dean, Dreher's voice shaped policy on the boards of Sigma Theta Tau International, the AACN, and the National Institutes of Health (NIH). In her retirement, her policy work has continued with board service at a variety of organizations like Wellmark, Trinity Health, the Chicago Board of Health, AvaSure Inc, Patients Out of Time, the Loyola University Board of Trustees, and the University of Minnesota School of Nursing Visiting Committee. Her innovative programs at Rush University shaped the future of nursing education (Callahan, 2019; Clarke & Dreher, 2017).

While engaged in leadership roles and extensive board service, Dreher maintained an active research program related to the use of cannabis for more than 40 years. Her work in this arena has both promoted social justice and transformed public opinion. Although her research was not especially welcomed by the nursing academic community, she found an eager audience in social science, education, psychiatry, and medicine. Her work was cited in the *New York Times*, the *Wall Street Journal*, and even the *High Times* and *Rolling Stone*. These publication outlets created opportunities for public awareness, visibility for nursing, and policy change beyond what was usually available in traditional academic journals.

Bobbie Berkowitz, PhD, RN, NEA-BC, FAAN, dean and professor emerita, Columbia University School of Nursing. For anyone who knows Bobbie Berkowitz, it is hard to believe that she says she was once very shy and introverted as a child. She realized that it was not going to get her where she wanted to go, so she worked hard to get comfortable with stepping forward. Her story shows how she was able to overcome her introversion and become a Nursing giant. As a second grader, Berkowitz was hospitalized with rheumatic fever. Extended hospitalization resulted in isolation and the nurses caring for her became her world. This was when she realized her early excitement for nursing. Her parents were not college-educated, but they were supportive of her choice to go to college to be a nurse and continue onward for a PhD. They would say, "We don't understand it but we know you do. If this is what you want, we are there for you." Berkowitz persevered throughout school, first becoming a candy-striper and nurse's aide before attending the University of Washington for nursing. Despite a passion for public health, Berkowitz accepted a position in Seattle as an oncology nurse after graduation. Once she realized that was not a good choice for her, she jumped at the opportunity to work as a public health nurse and began visiting families, serving as a school nurse and at the public health clinic.

The nursing director and health officer of the health department had great confidence in Berkowitz's ability to interact with all types of people and saw in her a gift for managing complex situations and scenarios. They supported her return to school for her master's degree, and upon graduation, she returned to the local health department and became the nursing director. As Berkowitz continued her education, pursuing a PhD, she transitioned to a more senior leadership position as the nursing director at the Seattle King County Department of Public Health. At that time, the governor of Washington was interested in creating the possibility for a universal health plan for the state. He created a task force whose role was to develop the framework for a universal health plan that could be sent to the legislature for approval. Berkowitz was appointed to the task force and when the plan was completed it was passed by the legislature. Berkowitz's nursing lens was underpinned by public health nursing. "You see what the world looks like from the eyes of those you work with."

This experience led to her appointment as the deputy secretary for the Washington State Department of Health. Berkowitz had many meetings with legislators and learned what they cared about in terms of public health. "There is limited understanding of the role of public health and why it is so critical to people. This legislation helped raise the visibility and value of public health."

During her time at the Washington State Department of Health, she was approached by the Robert Wood Johnson Foundation about leading a program called "Turning Point." It would be a 10-year grant focused on modernizing states' public health statutes, improving health quality, enhancing the utilization of information technology, creating performance management systems, and nurturing public health leadership. To carry out the grant, she left the state health department and joined the faculty at the University of Washington School of Public Health. During those 10 years of the grant, she became the chair of the Department of Psychosocial and Community Health at the University of Washington School of Nursing. When the grant ended, she took a sabbatical to think about her next phase and was recruited by Columbia University to become the dean of the Columbia University School of Nursing. During that time, she also served as the president of the AAN (2015–2017).

At the end of 2018, she retired from Columbia University and moved back to Seattle. She believes strongly that serving on boards is essential for nurses. She currently serves on the board of advisors of the University of Washington School of Nursing, the board of trustees for the Swedish Health System, the National Advisory Board of the University of California Davis Health System, and the board of directors of the Nurse-Family Partnership. "Nurses need to lead through boards, that is where we can have significant impact shaping policies. And nursing needs to be part of corporate board work where board members have a major leadership role."

Drs. Williams, Dreher, and Berkowitz are exemplars of how board membership and leadership shape policy through the nursing lens. Board membership allows nurses to serve as advocates and ambassadors for healthcare agendas while providing opportunities to oversee the strategic direction for nonprofit or for-profit organizations. The NOBC is promoting the impact of the nursing profession and recording board service. As of January 2021, 10,061 nurses had reported current service on boards (NOBC, 2021b). Coalition members include 16,514 nurses who self-identified race and ethnicity. Nearly 72% identified as White, White non-Hispanic, followed by 12% identifying Black or African American. Asian, American Indian, or Alaska Native, Hispanic Latinx, and Native Hawaiian or Other Pacific Islander comprised 8% of members, and those identifying as Other were about 7%. While nurse presence on boards and committees has increased, there is a great need to expand the presence of nurses on boards at local, state, and national levels, and a continued need to grow minority board leadership. Our nursing lens on boards is needed to improve healthcare delivery systems and promote health outcomes and healthier communities.

INFLUENCING POLICY THROUGH RESEARCH

Health policies are often promoted and developed without the benefit of research to support or refute a stance. Likewise, many researchers have focused on designing, implementing, and analyzing their research without effectively considering policy. Nursing research provides a unique view of what it is like for our patients to experience healthcare and thus provides essential input into each step of the policy process. As discussed in Chapter 5, nursing has a long history, beginning with the research by Florence Nightingale in impacting public policy. The following highlighted leaders demonstrate how nurses can purposefully impact policy through research.

Peter Buerhaus, PhD, RN, FAAN, FAANP(h), says that it was his best decision ever to become a nurse. His father was a hospital administrator and ran a community hospital. His parents invited candidates for positions in the hospital to their house to share dinner with their family. Based on these discussions and the experiences of his older sister, who was a nurse, Buerhaus decided to choose nursing as a career. He worked as a staff nurse and head nurse at a small hospital in New

Hampshire and went to graduate school at the University of Michigan to focus on nursing health services administration. He then went to Wayne State University, where he pursued advanced education in healthcare economics and nursing. Stints at the University of Iowa, a fellowship at Johns Hopkins, a Robert Wood Johnson program in finance, and the Public Health School at Harvard followed. There he met colleagues whom he collaborated with on early studies that were enormously powerful in shaping private and public policy. Buerhaus believes his career success was based on his background as a nurse researcher, economist, and policy expert. As an RN, healthcare economist, and health services researcher, he describes his nursing lens as understanding the role of the nurse in addition to his background as an economist and health services researcher. He understands outcomes that nurses can achieve clinically and can explain nuances about what is going on to nonclinical team members. His nursing lens focuses on clinical outcomes, quality, and cost. Buerhaus says that it is important for nurses to understand that their job is about patient care and they should excel clinically, but their role is also to improve outcomes and keep the cost the same or lower. From their first care plan, nurses should be thinking about clinical conditions, quality, and cost for every person.

Buerhaus is best known for his research on the nursing and physician workforces in the United States. Five (of his 150 plus publications) are designated as "classics" by the Agency for Healthcare Research and Quality (AHRQ) Patient Safety Network. Based on Buerhaus's research expertise, he was appointed chair of the National Health Workforce Commission that was established under the ACA in 2010. This commission was established to advise Congress and the administration on health workforce policy, provide data and analysis on problems facing health care, and align federal healthcare workforce resources with national needs. It was created to

> "serve as a national resource for Congress, the President and states and localities; communicate and coordinate with federal departments; develop and commission evaluations of education and training activities; identify barriers to improved coordination at the federal, state and local levels and recommend ways to address them; and encourage innovations that address population needs, changing technology and other environmental factors"

(Merrill, 2010, para. 2).

Two things about the workforce commission are important to know. First, Buerhaus, the only nurse appointed to the commission, was selected to be chair of a 15-person group including physicians and experts in health systems, health plans, public health, workforce, and health equity. His research expertise landed him a seat on the commission, and his appointment as chair likely resulted from the perception that he is considerate, fair, and guided to do the right thing. Second, although this commission was established and members were appointed to serve, it was never appropriated by Congress and never was operational because the federal spending process consists of authorization followed by appropriations. This example illustrates what happens all too frequently: A major piece of legislation establishing a program, activity, or agency is authorized, passes in Congress; however, the second step in the process—appropriation of funding—never occurs. We need to be cognizant of this and continue our advocacy through the appropriations process.

There are many outstanding examples of the influence of Buerhaus's research on policy. We highlight his team's publication, *Nurse Staffing and Quality of Care in Hospitals in the United States* (Needleman et al., 2002) because of the impact it had in multiple areas. It contributed to (a) Medicare's adoption of recommendations for changing the way inpatient complications are coded that made it possible to distinguish community-acquired versus hospital-acquired complications and (b) language used in The Nurse Reinvestment Act (DL 107-205) sponsored by Representative Lois Capps (D-CA) and signed into law in August 2002. Unfortunately, the 107th Congress adjourned in November of 2002 without appropriate funding. The following year, Congress authorized appropriations for all programs, which has continued to this time.

Loretta Sweet-Jemmott, PhD, MSN, RN, FAAN, was hit by a car when she was 7 years old and realized during her long-term hospitalization that the ladies with white uniforms were supportive and made her feel good. That was the beginning of Jemmott's quest to become a nurse. When she enrolled in a local public university to pursue her degree in nursing, she experienced discrimination and racism, including being chastised by the professor in front of a large class. She, along with other Black nursing students, suffered from many painful racial experiences preventing them from obtaining their nursing degrees at that institution. Determined to be a nurse, she transferred to Hampton University, a historically Black college and university, which she loved. While there she was inducted into the Student Leadership Program and became Ms. Hampton University.

After graduation, Jemmott volunteered at a local adolescent community sexual health clinic and was asked to teach classes to teens in an effort to reduce teen pregnancy. One year later, she became the clinic's executive director. She did not understand why teens knew what to do to reduce their risk for pregnancy and sexually transmitted infections but didn't do it. Therefore, she enrolled in the adolescent psychiatric and mental health nursing master's program at the University of Pennsylvania, followed by a PhD program in education, focusing on sex education. Although she worked in a private office in psychiatric–mental health in downtown Philadelphia and wanted to be the "Black Dr. Ruth," she moved to New Jersey for her first faculty position at Rutgers University, making her the only Black professor in the nursing school and the first to get tenure. From there she went to Columbia University, and shortly thereafter went to the University of Pennsylvania School of Nursing, where she stayed for 20 years and was the first and only Black faculty member promoted to the rank of full professor and the first to have an endowed chair.

Jemmott is best known for her theory-driven, culturally competent, translational, and community-engaged research on HIV/AIDS prevention with "perhaps the most consistent track record of evidence-based, HIV risk-reduction interventions" (Drexel University: College of Nursing and Health Professionals, n.d.). As an expert in health promotion research, she has led the nation in understanding the psychological determinants for reducing sexual risk-related behaviors. Her premier contribution is the development of knowledge on how best to facilitate and promote positive changes in health behaviors.

Jemmott describes her nursing lens as caring, sincere listening, and being there. "If you design an HIV/sexually-transmitted infection (STI) risk reduction intervention and the teens get a sense that you genuinely care about them, all the theories and concept of caring are taken to the next level. The adolescents want to know that you see them, that you hear them, that you understand them, that you really care about them, and would advocate for them. They need to know that you are just not giving them the knowledge to be safe sexually. You are also building up the confidence (self-efficacy) to be safe sexually while preparing them with the skills and the positive attitudes and beliefs needed to do it."

Jemmott and her husband, John Jemmott III, have received more than $150 million in National Institutes of Health (NIH) funding to design and test interventions to reduce the risk of HIV and other STIs among diverse populations worldwide. As a translational researcher with global impact, she has transformed her NIH-funded evidenced-based research outcomes for use in real-world settings. To date, eight of her evidence-based interventions have been designated by the CDC and the DHHS Office of Adolescent Health for national and international dissemination. Three of her evidence-based interventions have been developed into programs by community-based organizations and clinics in high-risk urban areas. Her research has changed public policy as it relates to theory-driven, culturally appropriate, evidence-based HIV risk reduction interventions in community and clinical settings. As a way to impact policy she was invited to present her research to the U.S. Congress and at an HIV Prevention Briefing and at the NIH's Consensus Development Conference on Interventions to Reduce HIV Risk Behaviors. Jemmott's research expertise contributed to her receiving the U.S. Congressional Merit Award and election to membership in the IOM, an honor afforded to very few nurses.

The Jemmotts' work with abstinence-based education showed more delayed initiation of sexual activity in middle school children than other kinds of sex education and was subsequently used to support policy for school-based abstinence-only sex education programs implemented by President George Bush. However, it is important to note that the Jemmotts' research differed from other abstinence-only programs in that they did not tell adolescents to abstain from sex until marriage. The curriculum, in fact, does not mention marriage or morality. Upon this realization, the White House team stopped using this evidenced-based program because they wanted pure abstinence-only-until-marriage programs, not abstinence-based programs. This example highlights how research results may be politicized and used by others for purposes never intended by the researchers.

Jemmott's nursing lens has been influenced by being a Black woman in the United States and having experienced racism and exclusion throughout her life, including many experiences in her nursing career. Her advice to others is to be strong and keep pressing on. "You can't let oppression and institutional racism block your success. You must have faith, determination, and resilience to push on and succeed despite whatever comes your way. You have to speak up, stand up, and advocate for yourself when others do not want you in the room or at the table." She believes she has been successful in shaping policy at the federal level because of what her mother calls *gumption*—the fire in her belly that pushes her through the door when people try to close the door. It is this spirit that keeps her going. "This is a lifelong journey and God sending His angels." Her nurse mentors, including Angela McBride, Rhetaugh Dumas, Nancy Bergstrom, Ada Sue Hinshaw, Beverly Malone, Neville Strumpf, and Linda Burns Bolton, were always there for her, took her out of her comfort zone, encouraged her, and introduced her to other successful scholars. Early on, they told her that she would be an "up-and-coming star," and she certainly has accomplished that.

The impact of Drs. Buerhaus and Jemmott's research on health policy has been extensive. All nurse-researchers should identify policy implications for their work, effectively communicate their findings to policymakers (which is different from a scientific presentation), and advocate for policy implementation and change where warranted.

INFLUENCING POLICY THROUGH GOVERNMENT SERVICE

Many roads lead to advocacy and politics. However, many visualize one road when they think of politics, and they assume that road is a straight path for running for and getting elected to a public office. Often, the offices that come to mind are high profile at the state and or national level. In reality, elected positions reflect only a small number of political opportunities. Many political roles are less visible but are vital to nursing and to healthcare policy development. Nurses do, and many more can, hold appointed positions or volunteer for positions. One can be appointed to an office or a committee or be elected. The following exemplars show the range of government opportunities available and the power that nurses can and do hold.

Local Government

Carol Roe, JD, MSN, RN, always knew she wanted to help people and was influenced to become a nurse by reading Cherry Ames and Sue Barton novels as a child. She went to law school so she could be a more effective advocate for nursing and patients in the public policy arena. She began her career as a diploma-prepared nurse, and each time she returned for more education, it was partially because she was unhappy with the leadership and the often-heard adage "if you can't beat them, join them." In her illustrious career, Roe served as a nurse administrator, clinical nurse specialist, faculty member, lobbyist, nursing regulator, compliance officer, risk manager, and mayor.

Several experiences are important to highlight: Roe was assistant director of medical–surgical nursing at University Hospitals of Cleveland from 1979 to 1989 and greatly enjoyed her job, especially the positive working relationships. While trying to revamp the nursing documentation system to not just make it medically directed but also include nursing diagnosis, Roe worked with lawyers who objected to her intentions. At that same time, Roe went to the state capitol to testify on behalf of changing the Ohio Nurse Practice Act, which, for the first time, would update the definition of nursing practice. The major opposition to the amended definition, which would allow for recognition of nurse practitioners was from hospitals. These two experiences were the tipping point leading to Roe's pursuit of a law degree. Roe's nursing lens has always been "What is in the best interest of the patient?" Her own passion for healthcare policy and politics grew out of her student public health experiences. When she made home visits with chronically ill children, she realized that some families were unable to pay for needed care. Roe learned about the role of insurance in the healthcare delivery system and came to believe that access to appropriate healthcare was a right, not a privilege.

While working, Roe was heavily involved in the Ohio Nurses Association (ONA), as well as in party politics. She believes the best place in the world for nurses to learn about expanding their influence is within professional organizations. Marta Reeder, president of ONA, served as a valued mentor, demonstrating that one can be a nursing administrator, genuinely understand and appreciate staff nurses, and still articulate the positions of staff nurses in the workplace. Roe was also very active in Democratic Party politics, political campaigns for city and state legislators, as well as presidential elections.

Roe's commitment to having more women serve in office led to working on women's campaigns, women's issues, and active membership in the National Organization of Women. It is important to note that she also supported candidates monetarily, critical to a candidate's ability to win an election. Despite Roe's heavy involvement in political campaigns, she never considered running for office, as she knew how much money it took to run a successful campaign. This changed in 2015 when Roe believed the neighborhood in which she lived was not being adequately represented on her city council, and she was approached by those she had forged relationships with through her prior political involvement. She successfully ran for the city council, serving from 2016 to 2019. She was selected by her fellow councilmen to be mayor of Cleveland Heights in 2018 to 2019 because of her expert listening skills gained through nursing education and experience.

Roe's success as a mayor resulted from the view and embodiment of leadership as not just telling others what to do. The most successful leaders inspire others and take joy in watching people they have mentored succeed. Successful leaders look for failures in systems rather than failures of people when something does not turn out as expected or something goes wrong. As city councilwoman and mayor, she provided oversight of the city manager in governing Cleveland Heights, a city of 46,000 residents with an annual budget of $78 million. Other duties included recommending legislation, responding to constituent concerns, representing the city at community events and meetings chairing the Administrative Services Committee, serving as president of the city council, and representing the city in the Ohio Mayors Alliance and Northeast Ohio Mayors Association.

State Government

Sue Birch, MBA, BSN, RN, has more than 35 years of progressive healthcare administrative experience in the public and private sectors. She has extensive community, regional and national involvement with healthcare transformation, including service delivery, program reform, and population health. Upon graduation from her baccalaureate program in nursing at the University of Colorado in 1982, she worked as a staff and charge nurse on an inpatient medical–surgical unit. She never returned to inpatient care and has focused on primary care and prevention, assisting in the development and implementation of ambulatory services at Kaiser Permanente, St. Joseph Hospital between 1984 and 1989. In 1988, she completed her MBA and from 1990 to 1992, Birch founded and ran a nurse consultant firm that provided consultation services for community agencies that included childcare centers, schools, and camps.

After moving to rural Colorado, Birch was the executive director and CEO of Northwest Colorado VNA from 1992 to 2010. In that position, she was responsible for a $9 million operating budget, leading and supervising a multidisciplinary management team and staff of 150. During this time, the agency purchased the Haren Assisted Living Center, built a co-located community center, and was recognized nationally for extensive aging well services.

Governor John Hickenlooper (D-CO) became familiar with Birch's track record and knew of her work on the ACA. He was in need of some political balance on his team and thus, appointed her to a cabinet post as Executive Director Colorado Department of Healthcare Policy and Financing, which had oversight of public insurance, health delivery and health policy development, and the implementation of the ACA for the state from 2011 to 2017. Leading a department with a $9 billion budget and responsible for the administration of healthcare coverage for 1.4 million Colorado residents, her experience as a Robert Wood Johnson Executive Nurse Fellow (RWJENF) and postwork with "social justice warriors" enabled her to exquisitely balance mission and margin. These experiences enabled her to see both clinical and programmatic sides of an issue.

A critical learning experience embedded in Birch's 3-year RWJENF program was spending time with economists at the Brookings Institution, looking at quantifying costs of care and how investments matter. She then realized that in policy work, you need to follow the money and make your case. Under Birch's leadership, the department successfully expanded coverage to more than 400,000 low-income, previously uninsured Coloradoans while focusing on containing costs and improving service delivery. She is very proud of having convinced the governor to expand Medicaid coverage. In 2012 and 2013, the department received the highest bonus of any state for its innovation and modernization of eligibility and enrollment systems by the Centers for Medicare and Medicaid Services (CMS). In 2017, Colorado ranked sixth in the Commonwealth Fund's scorecard on State Health System Performance.

History repeated itself in 2018, when Governor Jay Inslee, impressed by her work in Colorado, convinced Birch to move and serve as a cabinet member directing the Washington State Health Care Authority, which she still directs today. Birch oversees efforts to transform the healthcare system, helping ensure that Washington residents have better access, improved care, and at lower costs. With a budget of $14 billion, Birch leads the agency, which is the state's largest healthcare purchaser, serving nearly 2.7 million residents through Medicaid, the Public Employees Benefits Board Program, School Employees Benefits Board Program, and COFA Islander Health Care Program. Under her leadership, there have been a number of firsts: launched the first state-based public option in the United States in collaboration with the Washington Health Benefit Exchange and the Office of Insurance Commissioner and implemented the first Hepatitis C Elimination Program partnering with AbbVie on a population-health and modified-subscription financing model. In 2019, Washington ranked fourth in the Commonwealth Fund's scorecard on state health system performance achieved through alignment of achieving better population health, rewarding high-quality care, and curbing health costs.

Other unique transformation features include movement toward more integration of behavioral and physical health, empowering the members, using data to improve care, focusing on communities, and reshaping the workforce. Birch is passionate about cross-agency collaboration. For example, her team works closely with the state's long-term services and support system at a sister agency. The system is ranked number one in the United States by the AARP.

Birch's primary care/prevention focus, acquired from her earliest clinical nursing experiences, from her public health experience at the VNA and state government agencies and from her MBA contributed to her nursing lens of social justice and equity and population health, focus on communities, and goal of high-quality care while curbing costs and generating revenue. In fact, the Washington Department's Health Home model and Medicaid Program saved almost a quarter billion dollars in shared savings that were returned to the state. Birch is a towering example of a nurse with big systems skills and thinking being able to impact people at an individual and population level. At the individual level, Birch's early experience with her diabetic grandmother imprinted her with the caring compassion and an understanding of medical complexity that was needed to provide quality care. At the population level, she strives to operationalize health that is so far beyond medical complexity and place matters. She has been responsible for transforming two state departments of health to their fourth and sixth rankings for system performance.

Birch believes her success is related to having developed open, transparent teams that engage in "productive conflict." "We cannot shy away from healthy tension. It does not have to be an ugly process, although sometimes it is. It is important to align energies." A supportive environment and family that was able to flex enabled her to move into jobs in other states. Patience, tenacity, persistence, and her ability to gauge the systems' capacity for change enabled her to do transformative policy work. Last, Birch is passionate about having healthy people everywhere. "I think that when we can find passion in someone and marry passion with the profession, then that is when the magic happens. Nurses' perspectives are important."

Federal Government

Patricia Brennan, RN, PhD, FAAN, FACMI, is an RN and industrial engineer, with a Bachelor of Science in Nursing and Master of Science in Nursing, and a Master of Science and PhD in Industrial Engineering. She was introduced to computer technology in her baccalaureate program at the University of Delaware, worked as a staff and clinical nurse manager in an ICU and psychiatric unit, learned about professional nursing knowledge in her master's program at the University of Pennsylvania, and realized that engineering would give her more tools and training to do what she wanted to do for nursing. Upon graduation from her PhD at the University of Wisconsin–Madison in 1986, she held a faculty appointment in Nursing, Systems and Control Engineering, and Sociology at Case Western Reserve University and rose from assistant professor to professor in 10 years. She returned to the University of Wisconsin–Madison in 1996 as a professor of nursing and industrial engineering, serving as a department chair of Industrial Systems Engineering, a faculty member in both schools, and theme leader of the Living Environments Laboratory of the Wisconsin Institutes for Discovery. Since 2016, Brennan has served as the director of the National Library of Medicine (NLM), one of the 27 institutes and centers at the NIH.

What is so important about Brennan, a nurse being appointed as NLM director? The NLM is the world's largest biomedical library, which supports and conducts research, development, and training in health information and technology and biomedical informatics, coordinates an 8,500-member network of the NLM to promote and provide access to health information in communities across the United States, and makes a portion of their print and electronic collection public. Specifically, the functions of the NLM include (a) assist the advancement of medical and related sciences through the collection, dissemination, and exchange of information important to the progress of medicine and health; (b) serves as a national information resource for medical education, research, and service activities of Federal and private agencies, organizations, and institutions; (c) serves as a national information resource for the public, patients, and families by providing electronic access to reliable health information issued by the NIH and other trusted sources; (d) publishes in print and electronically guides to health sciences information in the form of catalogs, bibliographies, indexes, and online databases; (e) provides support for medical library development and for training of biomedical librarians and other health information specialists; (f) conducts and supports research in methods for recording, storing, retrieving, preserving, and communicating health information; (g) creates information resources and access tools for molecular biology, biotechnology, toxicology, environmental health, and health services research; and (h) provides technical consultation services and research assistance (NLM, 2014).

The NLM plays a critical role in translating biomedical research into practice. The NLM's research and information services support scientific discovery, healthcare, and public health. The NLM pioneers new ways to make biomedical data and information more accessible, which enables researchers, clinicians, and the public to use its vast collection of biomedical data to improve health. Brennan's nursing lens originates from being trained in the community health mental health model in her master's program in nursing. Her faculty helped her realize that nursing research, which contributes to nursing science, had important policy implications. At the same time, she is mindful of how policy impacts her work. Her nursing lens is based on the ANA's definition of *nursing*, Brennan believes in a patient-centered approach to healthcare, ensuring that patients' perspectives and values guide decisions.

Brennan's view of health is based on ANA's definition, "the protection, promotion, and optimization of health and abilities, prevention of illness and injury, alleviation of suffering through the diagnosis and treatment of human response, and advocacy in the care of individuals, families and communities and populations" (ANA, 2010). Brennan believes that public communication is vital to bridge the gap between research and policy. Her PhD advisor taught her that "if you are trying to do something innovative, you have to educate people along the way that it is safe, effective and essential. You always need to educate both patients and professionals." Brennan has taken communication very seriously in her role as NLM director by publishing a weekly blog since 2016 in which she shares her insights as director and fosters a two-way dialogue, as well as engaging with stakeholders through Twitter @NLMdirector.

Brennan's prolific funding from federal, state, foundation, and institutional sources for her research has been at the intersection of computers and nursing in practice and education. She does not believe that we would be as close to where we are today with self-monitoring if it weren't for her work in the 1980s. Her research expertise led to her appointment to an astounding number of federal advisory boards from the following agencies prior to becoming NLM director: the AHRQ, the Department of Commerce, the DHHS, the NIH, the National Institute of Nursing Research, the National Academies of Science, the National Academy of Engineering, the National Research Council, and the IOM. Despite Brennan's highly successful career, she is humble about her numerous contributions and has a wicked sense of humor.

Mary Wakefield, PhD, RN, FAAN, currently visiting professor and distinguished fellow of the Joseph H. Blades Centennial Memorial Professorship in Nursing, the University of Texas at Austin, is a trailblazing role model for nurse's involvement in health policy, becoming the administrator for the Health Resources and Services Administration of the DHHS from 2009 to 2015 and DHHS Acting Deputy from 2015 to 2017. As acting deputy secretary, she served in the second-most senior position at DHHS providing leadership and direction to an agency with a $1 trillion budget (almost one fourth of federal spending), with approximately 80,000 employees and contractors globally. The DHHS administers more grant money than all other federal agencies combined. It is responsible for regulating new pharmaceutical drugs and food products, administering the biggest government healthcare programs, and preventing the outbreak and spread of diseases. Its mission is "to enhance the health and well-being of all Americans, by providing for effective health and human services and by posturing sound, sustained advances in the sciences underlying medicine, public health and social services" (DHHS, 2018, "Mission Statement"). The DHHS has 11 operating divisions, including eight agencies, including, but not limited to, the AHRQ, the Agency for Toxic Substances and Disease Registry, the Food and Drug Administration, the CDC, the Health Resources & Services Administration (HRSA), the Indian Health Service, the NIH, and the CMS. The CMS administers Medicare, Medicaid, the marketplace, and the Children's Health Insurance Program (CHIP).

The mission of the HRSA is "to improve health outcomes and address health disparities through access to quality services, a skilled workforce, and innovative, high-value programs" (HRSA, 2019, para. 1). HRSA "provides healthcare to people who are geographically isolated and/or economically or medically vulnerable" which includes people living with HIV/AIDS, pregnant women, mothers and their families, and those unable to access high-quality healthcare. The HRSA supports the training of health professionals; distribution of providers to areas where they are needed most (medically underserved areas); improvements in healthcare delivery; oversees organ, bone marrow, and cord blood donation; compensates people harmed by vaccination; and maintains databases that flag providers with a record of malpractice, waste, fraud, and abuse (HRSA, 2021). The agency consists of five bureaus—the Bureau of Health Workforce, the Bureau of Primary Health Care, the Healthcare Systems Bureau, the HIV/AIDS Bureau, and the Maternal and Child Health Bureau—and includes the Federal Office of Rural Health Policy, the Office of Global Health, and the Office of Health Equity. As administrator of HRSA, Mary led and directed the agency with a $10.3 billion budget with more than 1,850 civil service and commissioned officer employees, with overall management of all HRSA programs and activities.

Wakefield led these federal agencies with her nursing lens. She said that when she graduated from her baccalaureate and even her master's program, she did not fully understand the impact of health policy on the patient, family, and community. She did not realize how policy directly impacted what she could or couldn't do as a nurse. As she gained clinical practice, she realized how much policy affected virtually everything in healthcare—from details such as the width of hospital room doorways to issues such as the mismatch between Medicaid eligibility and needed coverage of large segments of the uninsured population. As a nurse, she recognized the influence of the profession on health, but she learned rapidly that at times, state and federal health policy can be even more influential. An example that Wakefield recalls vividly, clearly makes this point. A woman, clearly distressed, explained that she had a job, had a couple of kids, was a single parent, had chronic conditions, and had no health insurance. The patient asked Mary, "What can you do to help me?" and Mary remembers to this day a feeling that was antithetical to her professional education; she could do nothing. This experience showed Mary that there is a larger context to caring for patients. Nurses know how and what patients and their families face. She knew from firsthand experience what is in the best interest of the patient. She said that in every single leadership position she has had since the crucible experience, she looks at decisions from the lens of how well we are serving those with needs. Her "north star" is always "What is in the best interest of the patient?" Mary's nursing lens also includes looking at people holistically, seeing individuals in their environments, and thinking about how an injury or illness will impact patients after they leave our healthcare settings and return to their family and community. She also is focused on prevention; how can we keep patients from needing to return to the healthcare system? She cites her experience as an ICU nurse in a small hospital in North Dakota as shaping her thinking. Some of her patients were admitted with diagnoses like preeclampsia and strokes. Many she saw were clearly patients who would have never been in the ICU if only upstream the problems could have been solved. She saw the ICU as a Band-Aid that reflected a broken primary care and public health system.

Wakefield has many examples of how she shaped policy and says that it is important for nurses to be in positions like she has occupied so that developing and implementing has the benefit of nursing expertise. She is particularly proud of her role in reconfiguring nursing programs at the HRSA to be veteran-friendly, enabling retired military personnel to move into nursing programs more easily, which is still being funded today.

Wakefield's trajectory into policy work is fascinating and one that nurses should emulate. This started with having a strong faculty member in her undergraduate program who facilitated nursing student engagement in the state nurses association. Students were encouraged to attend state nurses' meetings and annual conferences. It was a safe incubator for her to observe and learn from nurse leaders working to influence healthcare outside of healthcare delivery settings. She believes that involvement in professional nursing associations with a strong policy focus (e.g., the ANA, the AAN, the Emergency Nurses Association) helps nurses develop leadership skills and policy-related expertise. Active professional association engagement facilitates building important connections/relationships with others, developing broader and deeper understanding of health and healthcare, and being involved in political and policy processes.

At 31 years old, Mary was teaching health policy content derived from state-level experience and published literature. Without having had federal experience, she was not entirely comfortable teaching material she didn't know personally. Consequently, she volunteered to work in the Washington, D.C. office of one of her state's U.S. Senators during her summer break. She was told that they would be happy to have her volunteer but that they had a permanent health legislative assistant position available. Wakefield got the position as a legislative assistant and later chief of staff to Senator Quentin Burdick (D-ND) in 1987, followed by chief of staff for Senator Kent Conrad (D-ND) from 1993 to 1996. She served as the director of the Center for Health Policy, Research and Ethics at George Mason University from 1996 to 2001, and returned to where her first faculty position was at, the University of North Dakota, in 2001 to 2009 to lead the expansion of the Center for Rural Health. The center became a nationally recognized rural health resource. The totality of Wakefield's prior experiences in the health policy arena in academe, professional organizations, and government, excellent relationships in each sector, as well as her initiative in pursuing Capitol Hill experience, led to her appointments to top-level administrative posts in the federal government.

While working in the U.S. Senate, Wakefield, routinely introduced herself as a nurse and would often hear responses like "Well then what are you doing here?" to which she responded, "It's because I am a nurse that I'm here working in health policy. This is why I'm here." While Wakefield is clearly an extraordinary nurse policy expert, wouldn't it be wonderful if more nurses followed their own paths to leadership at the national level?

The nursing lens is critically needed in government service at the local, state, and federal levels. It provides opportunities for the advancement of nursing's values and agenda to improve health for more people. These nurse leaders, Carol Roe, Susan Birch, Patricia Brennan, and Mary Wakefield, used the values instilled in their early formative nursing experiences to shape their actions to influence policy. Their representation at each of these levels of government benefited the constituencies they served. Nurses have also taken on the challenge to influence policy through elected office at the federal level. See Policy on the Scene 11.1 for nurses serving in the 117th Congress.

EXPANDING YOUR INFLUENCE

Influence is the innate, cultivated, or capacity to invoke movement. Expanding and accelerating your personal influence can be accomplished by knowing one's worth and one's work, gaining visibility, building relationships and partnerships, and being prepared. As Alicia Georges said, "show up, volunteer, speak out. Many elected officials don't know or have a sense of the health issues and social determinants; nurses know the impact."

POLICY ON THE SCENE 11.1: Nurses Elected to the 117th Congress

Nurses in the 117th Congress not only represent the constituencies of their districts, but they also give voice to important healthcare issues that need to be addressed at the federal level. As nurses and healthcare professionals, they bring a unique lens to the policy discussions that have the potential to impact the health of millions.

Rep. Eddie Bernice Johnson (D-TX-30) is the longest serving nurse in the House of Representatives, representing Texas for her 14th term. As the first nurse to be elected to the U.S. Congress in 1993, she was also the first African American and the first woman to chair the House Committee on Science, Space, and Technology (Johnson, n.d.). With previous experience as a psychiatric nurse, she advocates for healthcare reform and works to decrease the stigma surrounding mental illnesses. Congresswoman Johnson works to create public health policy changes and has helped pass the National Suicide Hotline Improvement Act (H.R. 2345) and has cosponsored the Helping Families in Mental Health Crisis Act (H.R. 2646). Her amendment to the Violence Against Women Act was reauthorized to further protect victims' housing security. She received the Texas Hospital Advocacy Tribute for her efforts in improving public policy by expanding access to healthcare and lowering health insurance premiums. Her contributions to healthcare led to her induction as a fellow in the AAN.

Rep. Lauren Underwood (D-IL-14) is the youngest African American woman to serve in the House of Representatives. In efforts to decrease maternal healthcare disparities and improve maternal health outcomes, she cofounded and currently co-chairs the Black Maternal Health Caucus. Her proposed Black Maternal Health MOMNIBUS Act is a multifaceted approach designed to address all aspects of the maternal health crisis in American that disproportionately women of color. She taught future nurse practitioners at Georgetown University's online master's program and has helped to implement the ACA while working for the DHHS (Underwood, n.d.). Congresswoman Underwood prioritizes accessible and affordable healthcare for all people and has introduced the H.R. 1010 bill to better protect those with preexisting conditions by giving them continued insurance coverage.

Rep. Cori Bush (D-MO-01) is serving her first term in the House of Representatives as the first African American woman to represent Missouri (Handy, 2020). Her roles as nurse, pastor, community organizer, and childcare worker influence her lens. She hopes to decrease discrimination, poverty, inequality, and insecurity to better protect vulnerable populations. In her efforts to create improved and safer communities, she supports Medicare for all, housing for all, and education for all (Bush, n.d.). Congresswoman Bush has promised to promote prison, criminal justice, and immigration reforms along with gender equality.

Rep. Karen Bass (D-CA-37) represents California in her sixth term in Congress. Congresswoman Bass was a vocational nurse and then worked as a physician's assistant before being elected to Congress. This occupational shift transferred her bedside manner skills into diplomacy and allowed her to continue her passion to address human service issues (Daniels, 2015). One interest area involves advocating for the health of children, as she founded the bipartisan Congressional Caucus on Foster Youth (Bass, n.d.). With a focus on expanding healthcare access, she also chairs the Subcommittee on Africa, Global Health, Global Human Rights and International Organizations, under the House Committee on Foreign Affairs.

Having a background in nursing and health provides an important lens for members of Congress regarding the development and passage of legislation impacting health. Not only can these legislators propose health-focused legislation, but they can also identify the health implications of legislation designed for other purposes.

Being strategic is setting a vision, and balancing it with realism. Key elements of being strategic include knowing your worth, gaining visibility, building relationships and partnerships, and being prepared. Our policy exemplars provide advice and specific actions that can be taken to expand one's influence. See Exhibit 11.2.

While it is important to expand one's influence on an individual level, influencing policy is very often a group effort. Many of the leaders highlighted thus far expanded their influence through active engagement in the ANA, state nurses associations, and specialty associations, as well as interdisciplinary and community groups. Often, the participation of these leaders has not been limited to a single association or interest group. Participation in multiple groups expands

EXHIBIT 11.2   ACTIONS TO EXPAND YOUR INFLUENCE

STRATEGY	ACTIONS
Knowing Your Worth Nurses are moving into major leadership roles. Don't defer because of a fear of not understanding the landscape of corporate and political systems. Nurses have this capacity. Bobbie Berkowitz	▪ Be able to tell your story. ▪ Learn from failures; there is power in humility. ▪ Despite challenges, hold to your values. ▪ Understand the skills and attributes unique to nursing. ▪ Communicate others' stories through the nursing lens. ▪ There is not one pathway for nurses; follow your passion and aim to develop progressive skills and experiences. ▪ Commit to lifelong learning. ▪ Build your intellectual, social, political, and financial capital (see Chapter 7).
Being Prepared Be tenacious, armed with data, listen to your heart, and believe in what you know is the right thing to do. Antoinette Hays	▪ Don't just present problems, provide suggestions and solutions. ▪ Bring hard evidence and data. Many elected officials don't know or have a sense of health issues and social determinants. ▪ Respond to those who think differently with well-thought-out strategy, not emotion. ▪ No is not the only option. ▪ Know your audience, know the opposing argument; there is a way to engage all. ▪ Always have a short list of take-home points that you want to convey.

(continued)

EXHIBIT 11.2 ACTIONS TO EXPAND YOUR INFLUENCE (*CONTINUED*)

Gaining Visibility While the skill of policy starts with self-assessment and belief, you have to make yourself visible; people will see you and recommend you. Show them what you've got! Melanie Dreher	▪ Volunteer: in your organization/workplace, in your community, in your profession, for the cause you are passionate about. ▪ Show up: in your organization/workplace, in your community, in your profession, for the cause you are passionate about. ▪ Share information and generate knowledge through the use of social media. Make digital connections with community leaders, experts across professions, stakeholders, and lawmakers. ▪ Disseminate original research, evidence-based best practices, informed opinions, and thoughts through strategically appropriate media.
Building Relationships and Partnerships Find people that you can learn from, ask people for their help, and watch people, so you can learn how to master situations. Carol Roe	▪ Relationships are important, and partnerships are central to influencing policy. Understand and appreciate the value of collective intelligence to shape policy, drive change, and improve outcomes. ▪ Build effective interprofessional teams and partnerships. ▪ Find a mentor, know who your mentors are, and be a mentor. ▪ Remember that partnerships go two ways. ▪ Align your allies and understand your opponent's viewpoints. ▪ Establish trust. ▪ Don't always come with an ask. ▪ Be balanced and fair. ▪ Manage up—every CNO should make the CFO their best friend.

CFO, chief financial officer; CNO, chief nurse executives.

one's network and influence. It also creates opportunities for synergy in working toward common goals.

Partnerships are powerful mechanisms for expanding one's influence. Two particularly important partnerships are PACs (see Chapter 7) and coalitions (see Chapter 6). Within organizations, PACs allow the voices of organizational members to influence politics by providing opportunities to both educate candidates and hold candidates accountable. With hard money raised by their members, PACs can leverage funds to work for or against a candidate, and nurses within PACs can work together on issues affecting nursing and health (Groenwald & Eldridge, 2020). Of important consideration is that PACs require association membership. For example, the ANA–PAC cannot accept donations from nonmembers because of federal regulations. The ANA–PAC contributed $264,750 to federal candidates during 2019–2020 (The Center for Responsive Politics, 2021). If ANA membership rose to 50% of practicing nurses, and each nurse committed to giving $100 per year, an estimated $200 million dollars, nearly a 1,000-fold increase, would be available to expand the influence of nursing's lens.

Coalitions play an important role in influencing changemakers in policy and can increase effectiveness and the likelihood of seeing the desired changes be implemented (McGetrick et al., 2019; Wendl & Cramer, 2018). More participation from individuals in coalitions also supports higher acceptance rates of proposed solutions to problems (El-Ansari et al., 2004). The Nursing Community Coalition, specifically, is made up more than 60 national nursing organizations to include viewpoints from RNs in policy advocacy. This group focuses on addressing healthcare issues and influencing practice, education, research, and regulation through promoting policy changes (Nursing Community Coalition, 2020). Other notable nursing coalitions are illustrated in Exhibit 11.3.

EXHIBIT 11.3 SELECTED NURSING COALITION EXEMPLARS

COALITION	PURPOSE AND SCOPE OF WORK
Camden Coalition camdenhealth.org	Focus is on individuals and families with complex needs. Partners with local stakeholders to improve behavioral health services, such as the SJBHIC. Initiatives include testing new models of care.
Future of Nursing: Campaign for Action campaignforaction.org	Outgrowth of the *Future of Nursing* report (IOM, 2011). Sees nurses as stakeholders in providing accessible and equitable care while promoting the well-being of all patients. They encourage nurses and nursing organizations to get involved with community leaders to initiate changes that advance health.
Health Professions and Nursing Education https://www.aamc.org/advocacy/hpnec/	Includes 80 different organizations representing schools, students, and healthcare. They advocate for support regarding the development of programs to enhance the training of the nurses of tomorrow.

SJBHIC, South Jersey Behavioral Health Innovation Collaborative.

LESSONS LEARNED

When discussing failures with the policy shapers in this chapter, it was evident that losing (at some point) is inevitable, but failure isn't an option. The term *failure* was viewed more as an opportunity to demonstrate resilience. Dr. Birch reflects that "patience, tenacity, and persistence are needed to pull off transformations." Dr. Jemmott's lessons have culminated that when things don't go your way, "it hurts for a minute." Her pains come from experiences with structural racism: White students didn't want her to be their teacher, her published research received critiques—and she was not allowed the opportunity to respond with a published rebuttal. "The challenges continue, and you have to be strong and keep pressing on, we are not any better than we were before; now people are not hiding what they think. You can't let oppression and structural racism block success."

This candid and vulnerable look into the personal journey of nurses who are shaping policy by addressing health reform is framed in the nursing lens, shaped by personal experiences and the experiences of our patients. Health reform is an excruciatingly difficult process; people want an easy answer, and there's not one, even when you're in the highest office (Blumenthal & Morone, 2010). Lessons learned from nurse leaders illuminated throughout this chapter are echoed by Trautman's account of *The Heart of Power: Health and Politics in the Oval Office* (Blumenthal & Morone, 2010): be passionate, have a plan, be part of and deploy a talented team, go public to create momentum, speed is important, be willing to overrule advisors, and be willing to lose.

OUTCOMES

Nurses are influencing policy at the highest levels in partnership with some of the most senior legislators. For example, Dr. Trautman's leadership during the rollout of the ACA, and Dr. Buerhaus's research and evidence generating funding from the federal government, support the nursing workforce and full practice authority for APRNs. Dr. Dreher's work addresses policy with health insurance companies to promote patient outcomes. Dr. Birch's leadership expands coverage to low-income, previously uninsured patients. Dr. Jemmott's work develops evidence-based programming to reduce sexually transmitted diseases in underserved populations. Sower's work removes policy barriers that keep patients from getting the services they need across state lines. And there are the barrier breakers like Dr. Williams, who granted marginalized, underserved communities a voice by uniting Black nurses to form the NBNA, in response to the ANA not permitting membership to Black and minority nurses. The resounding denominator for policy change across nurse leaders, influencing policy at all levels and in all settings, is unity. Together we must address social injustices, health inequities, and advocate for our communities' public health; the power is in each of us.

| POLICY SOLUTION | The Nursing Lens of a Millennial Preparing for Policy Leadership |

Marcus Henderson MSN, RN

I believe that nurses can and should be a part of all health and policy conversations given the lens we provide. We have our own scope of practice and autonomy. I don't think this is stressed enough in school. Nurses need to understand their worth.

My clinical experience postgraduation in community health and psychiatric–mental health nursing since 2018 added this set of knowledge and skills to my nursing lens. My work with children and adolescents in mental health and homeless individuals in the community has allowed me to witness firsthand the failures of our healthcare and social services systems, which fuels my continued service to my community and the profession. My nursing lens informs my practice, teaching, and leadership.

My mentors saw my potential when I did not see it myself. This has been a key lesson for me about the importance of mentorship. Mentorship is a reciprocal process in which the mentor and mentee grow together. My mentors helped me to strengthen my voice. They have always brought me alongside them and kept me grounded so that I could be an agent for change and a role model to others. They taught me that in order to move our profession and nation forward we must ensure that all voices have a seat at the table. I carry these lessons with me every day. I want students and nurses to understand the complexity of SDOHs and health equity and that we have lots of work to do to impact policy in our communities. Our profession is 4.3 million nurses strong, and we practice in communities across the country. If we collectively come together, I don't see how we can't move the needle toward a more fair and just future for all.

SDOHs, social determinants of health.

IMPLICATIONS FOR FUTURE

Nursing's long history is filled with seminal documents identifying the nursing profession's preferred future. The latest in this long line is the recently released *Future of Nursing 2020–2030: Charting a Path to Achieve Health Equity* (National Academies of Science, Engineering, and Medicine, 2021). This future cannot happen without all nurses using their lens to take part in policy to create that future. We propose here that the actions that individual nurses take are as important as the collective policy decisions that impact the profession of nursing and the health of the people we serve. We cogitate for a number of actions for reform we deem to be essential to moving the profession forward: understanding of the full history of nursing, the potential of HOSA as a pipeline for nursing, increasing membership in the NSNA and the ANA; embedding policy throughout nursing curricula; and continuing work to include nurses on boards.

Nurses' knowledge and understanding of the *true* history of nursing is incomplete. Nursing's history needs to be rewritten to include marginalized and underrepresented nurse leaders. This true history needs to be integrated into all nursing curricula.

Numerous potential pipelines to nursing have been untapped. HOSA as exemplified in this chapter, with a membership of more than 165,000 distributed across 3,000 chapters. Most nurses are not aware of HOSA, nor that approximately 45% of its membership is composed of individuals from minority groups. If every college or school of nursing partnered with a local HOSA chapter or another pipeline group, this would surely facilitate to increase nursing workforce diversity.

Many of the leaders identified in this chapter harken back to their early involvement in professional nurses associations such as the ANA and others. Minimally, all faculty members should be role models of policy activism and be members of professional nurses associations, minimally the ANA and the state nurses association. Likewise, should it not be an expectation for all prelicensure students to be a member of the student nurses association and that all graduate students be members of the professional nurses association. Some programs cover memberships through student fees.

Policy content and conversations need to be integrated across all nursing curricula rather than only being included in a policy course. The impact of policy on patients, their families, and the community should be included in each clinical course, and each daily clinical conference. The potential political and economic impact of infusing our teaching with conversations about policy implications would enhance nurses' policy readiness. This would prepare nurses to achieve clinical competencies that include the new nurse advocacy standard outlined in the ANA's (2021) *Nursing: Scope and Standards.*

As noted, the largest group of healthcare providers are nurses. The first *Future of Nursing* report (IOM, 2011) was a call to action for nurses to have an increased role in reforming the healthcare system. As noted, this led to the formation of the NOBC, with its achievement of 10,000 nurses on boards. These efforts need to be continued. What is important now is to be strategic in ensuring that nurses are on the boards of each of the very large multisite health systems that are the players in partnerships and strategic alliances. Similar efforts need to be made for nurse representation on collegiate and university boards.

The leaders highlighted in this chapter had visions molded by their nursing lens. Without a vision, without a road map, without big audacious goals, strategies are not developed, change cannot be measured, and the profession of nursing will not march (see Chapter 1). We propose this set of goals as a beginning in Exhibit 11.4.

EXHIBIT 11.4 **ROAD MAP FOR NURSING'S VISION**

TARGET DATE	GOALS
2040	✓ Fifty percent of RNs will be members of the American Nurses Association. ✓ Each healthcare facility will have an RN on its board. ✓ Each university/college with a school/college of nursing will have an RN on its board. ✓ The CEO of 10% of healthcare facilities will be an RN. ✓ Ten percent of universities/colleges will have an RN as the president.
2050	✓ There will be an RN on the cabinet of every state legislature. ✓ Ten percent of Congress will be RNs. ✓ The president of the United States will be an RN. ✓ All APRNs will have full practice authority. ✓ Our nursing workforce will look like the U.S. population. ✓ Systemic racism will be eradicated.

KEY CONCEPTS

1. The power to shape policy is present in every role in nursing—from providers in the community and at the bedside, to advanced practice providers, researchers, academia, boards, PACs, and professional organizations.

2. In nursing's history, the nursing lens has also been grounded and limited by a Eurocentric, White viewpoint that negates the experiences of a growing number of nurses and patients.

3. The distinct disparities of COVID-19, nursing's historical focus on health, healthcare equity, and social justice, and adherence to the ANA Code of Ethics, necessitates that the nursing lens be used to address structural racism in all healthcare settings, educational institutions, workplaces, government, policies, laws, and regulations.

4. What differentiates nurses from others when engaging in the political process is the nursing lens, based on understanding nursing history, education, and practice experience.

5. Nurse leaders have made extraordinary contributions to health policy in a variety of roles in the public and private sectors.

6. The stories of nurse exemplars provide valuable guidance and inspiration to nurses who may be hesitant to embark on the path of policy leadership.

7. It is possible to blend one's passion for nursing with serving the public through policy advocacy.

8. Advanced education and professional association involvement are some of the commonalities among nurse policy leaders that led to long-term policy advocacy.

9. Having mentors and serving as mentors are important aspects of policy leadership development.

10. Involvement in policymaking leads to additional networking opportunities that may make an impact on policy.

11. Leadership and advocacy are important in creating the preferred future for nursing and a healthcare system responsive to the needs of the public.

12. Nurses need to assume their rightful place in policy leadership and in partnership with others in shaping our healthcare system.

SUMMARY

Our responsibility as nurses and the goal of governments around the world is achieving better health by addressing the SDOHs and barriers at all levels. Nurse leaders, when asked to describe their "nursing lens," have highlighted several important attributes and characteristics that nurses bring to policy development and reform. While answers were uniquely based on lived experience, interprofessional engagement, and social context, similarities included a clear assessment of needs, remaining committed to the health and wellness of patients/persons/ populations, and the critical importance of communicating these needs to policymakers. Nurses must be at the table before policies are created.

In a 12-month period in the United States beginning in 2020, we witnessed a crippling national response to a global pandemic while drug-related overdoses surged in response to pandemic-related stressors, both the pandemic and epidemic disproportionately affecting minorities, and then watched as racially fueled, violent protestors stormed the U.S. Capitol. As Villarruel and Broome (2020) highlight these "injustices in law enforcement and health inequities are not new occurrences—nor are they rare" (p. 375) this is the fabric of structural racism, woven throughout our policies, practices, and cultural norms. The nursing lens is firmly grounded within the context of social justice and is essential to naming and dismantling structural racism and addressing these atrocities (Villarruel & Broome, 2020). Shaping policy is the responsibility of every nurse, at all levels, and is the salvation of our democracy. The prominent nurse leaders in this chapter have paved the way, but our work is clearly just getting started.

At times, situations and violations of personal and professional values may be challenged and require individuals to be courageous and act. There is no single pathway to policy, so be guided by your nursing lens, be courageous and act to address the situation, and hold true to your and the professional values.

END-OF-CHAPTER RESOURCES

LEARNING ACTIVITIES

1. Select one of the nurses profiled in this chapter who impressed you the most. How would you approach a conversation with the person? What questions would you ask? What type of advice would you seek to enhance your policy journey?

2. Think about an issue that affects you? How could a policy change address the issue? Explain how your nursing lens would be beneficial in preparing for your advocacy.

3. What community organizations have missions that align with your ideals? Who serves on the community board? What is the process for an appointment/selection? How would you prepare for the selection process?

4. Consider the healthcare policies (national, state, local, facility) that have been changed or enacted in response to the COVID-19 pandemic. Choose one that you think was developed through a nursing lens and provide the rationale.

5. Select someone who is an effective leader in any field. What do they do that makes them effective? How can you apply similar strategies to being a nurse leader?

6. How many people from diverse backgrounds hold leadership positions in your organization or community? How about your representatives to the state and federal government? Does this reflect the community in which you live and work? Why is this important?

7. Examine your organization's recruitment, admission/hiring, or promotion practices or policies. How would a policy implementation or change affect representation? Why would this beneficial?

8. Choose one topic from Exhibit 11.4, to identify stakeholders and discuss specific strategies for its achievement.

E-RESOURCES

- American Association of Colleges of Nursing. Policy and Advocacy https://www.aacnnursing.org/Policy-Advocacy

- American Nurses Association. Health Policy Resources https://www.nursingworld.org/practice-policy/health-policy/

- Emerging RN Leader https://www.emergingrnleader.com/nurse-leader-development/

- Kaiser Health News www.khn.org

- Nurses on Boards Coalition https://www.nursesonboardscoalition.org

- Scottsboro Boys https://www.history.com/topics/great-depression/scottsboro-boys

REFERENCES

American Nurses Association. (2015). *Code of ethics for nurses with interpretive statements*. Author. https://www.nursingworld.org/practice-policy/nursing-excellence/ethics/code-of-ethics-for-nurses/

American Nurses Association. (2021). *Nursing: Scope and standards for practice* (4th ed.).

American Nurses Association. (2010). Nursing's social policy statement: The essence of the profession. (2010 edition).

Andrasfay, T., & Goldman, N. (2021). Reductions in 2020 US life expectancy due to COVID-19 and the disproportionate impact on the Black and Latino populations. *Proceedings of the National Academy of Sciences, 118*(5), e2014746118. https://doi.org/10.1073/pnas.2014746118

Bass, K. (n.d.). *Biography*. Representative Karen Bass. https://bass.house.gov/about/biography

Betts, V. T. (1996). Nursing's agenda for healthcare reform: Policy, politics, and power through professional leadership. *Nursing Administration Quarterly, 20*(3), 1–8. https://doi.org/10.1097/00006216-199602030-00003

Blumenthal, D., & Morone, J. (2010). *The heart of power: Health and politics in the Oval Office.* University of California Press.

Bush, C. (n.d.). Cori Bush: Congresswoman for Missouri's 1st. *Biography*. https://bush.house.gov/about

Callahan, A. (2019, September 2). *To justify using weed, some pregnant women cling to an old and dubious study.* Scientific American. https://www.scientificamerican.com/article/to-justify-using-weed-some-pregnant-women-cling-to-an-old-and-dubious-study/

Camden Coalition of Healthcare Providers. (2020). *Mission.* https://camdenhealth.org/

Centers for Disease Control and Prevention. (2015). *Definition of policy.* https://www.cdc.gov/policy/analysis/process/definition.html

Centers for Disease Control and Prevention. (2016). *Health in all policies.* https://www.cdc.gov/policy/hiap/index.html

Centers for Disease Control and Prevention. (2011). Ten great public health achievements – worldwide 2001–2010. *Morbidity and Mortality Weekly Report, 60*(24), 814–818.

The Center for Responsive Politics. (2021). *American medical assn.* Open Secrets.org. https://www.opensecrets.org/political-action-committees-pacs/american-medical-assn/C00000422/candidate-recipients/2020

Chisholm, S. (n.d.). *A seat at the table.* https://www.bringyourownchair.org/

Clarke, P. N., & Dreher, M. (2017). Transitions and transformations in nursing leadership. *Nursing Science Quarterly, 30*(1), 34–37. https://doi.org/10.1177/0894318416680532

The Commonwealth Fund, The New York Times, & Harvard T.H. Chan School of Public Health. (2019). *American's values and beliefs about traditional health insurance reform.* https://cdn1.sph.harvard.edu/wp-content/uploads/sites/94/2019/10/CMWF-NYT-Harvard_Final-Report_Oct2019.pdf

Daniels, J. Z. (2015, July 1). *From the bedside to the halls of Congress: Our national nurses.* Minority Nurse. https://minoritynurse.com/from-the-bedside-to-the-halls-of-congress-our-national-nurses/

Department of Health & Human Services. (2018). *Introduction: About HHS.* https://www.hhs.gov/about/strategic-plan/introduction/index.html

Department of Health and Human Services. (n.d.). *Healthy People 2030: Social determinants of health.* https://health.gov/healthypeople/objectives-and-data/social-determinants-health

Disch, J. (2012). The nursing lens. *Nursing Outlook, 60*(4), 170–171. https://doi.org/10.1016/j.outlook.2012.05.004

Drexel University: College of Nursing and Health Professionals. (n.d.). *Loretta Sweet Jemmott.* https://drexel.edu/cnhp/faculty/profiles/JemmottLoretta/

El-Ansari, W., Phillips, C. J., & Zwi, A. B. (2004). Public health nurses' perspectives on collaborative partnerships in South Africa. *Public Health Nursing, 21*(3), 277–286. https://doi.org/10.1111/j.0737-1209.2004.021310.x

Feeley, D. (2016). *Equity: The forgotten aim?* Institute of Healthcare Improvement (IHI). http://www.ihi.org/communities/blogs/equity-the-forgotten-aim

Future of Nursing: Campaign for Action. (n.d.). *Our network.* https://campaignforaction.org/our-network/

Groenwald, S. L., & Eldridge, C. (2020). Politics, power, and predictability of nursing care. *Nursing Forum, 55*(1), 16–32. https://doi.org/10.1111/nuf.12377

Handy, B. (2020, November 16). *Cori Bush, a nurse and activist, becomes the first Black woman to represent Missouri in Congress.* The New Yorker. https://www.newyorker.com/magazine/2020/11/16/cori-bush-becomes-first-black-woman-and-first-nurse-to-represent-missouri-in-congress

Health Professions and Nursing Education Coalition. (2020). *HPNEC background.* https://www.aamc.org/advocacy/hpnec/

Health Resources & Services Administration. (2021). *Strategic Plan FY 2019-2022.* https://www.hrsa.gov/about/strategic-plan/index.html

Hine, D. C. (1989). *Black women in white: Racial conflict and cooperation in the nursing profession 1890–1950.* Indiana University Press.

HOSA = Future Health Professionals. (2020). *HOSA handbook: Section C. Guide to managing and organizing a HOSA chapter.* https://hosa.org/wp-content/uploads/2012/08/Section-C-2017-Final.pdf

Institute of Medicine. (2001). *Crossing the quality chasm: A new health system for the 21st century.* National Academies Press. https://doi.org/10.17226/10027

Institute of Medicine. (2011). *The future of nursing: Leading change, advancing health.* National Academies Press. https://doi.org/10.17226/12956

Johns Hopkins Medicine. (n.d.). *Kevin W. Sowers, M.S.N., R.N., F.A.A.N.* https://www.hopkinsmedicine.org/about/leadership/biography/kevin-sowers

Johnson, E. B. (n.d.). *Meet Eddie Bernice.* U.S. Representative Eddie Bernice Johnson representing the 30th district of Texas. https://ebjohnson.house.gov/about/meet-eddie-bernice

Kindig, D., & Stoddart, G. (2003). What is population health? *American Journal of Public Health, 93*(3), 380–383. https://doi.org/10.2105/ajph.93.3.380

McGetrick, J. A., Raine, K. D., Wild, T. C., & Nykiforuk, C. (2019). Advancing strategies for agenda setting by health policy coalitions: A network analysis of the Canadian Chronic Disease Prevention Survey. *Health Communication, 34*(11), 1303–1312. https://doi.org/10.1080/10410236.2018.1484267

Merrill, M. (2010). *GAO names 15 members to National Health Care Workforce Commission.* Healthcare Finance. https://www.healthcarefinancenews.com/news/gao-names-15-members-national-health-care-workforce-commission

National Academies of Science, Engineering, and Medicine. (2021). *The future of nursing 2020–2030: Charting a path to health equity.* National Academies Press. https://doi.org/10.17226.25982

National Library of Medicine. (2014). *Functional statement.* https://www.nlm.nih.gov/about/functstatement.html

Needleman, J., Buerhaus, P., Mattke, S., Stewart, M., & Zelevinsky, K. (2002). Nurse-staffing levels and the quality of care in hospitals. *New England Journal of Medicine, 346*(22), 1715–1722. https://doi.org/10.1056/NEJMsa012247

Nursing Community Coalition. (2020). *About.* https://www.thenursingcommunity.org/members

Nurses on Boards Coalition. (2021a). *About.* https://www.nursesonboardscoalition.org/about/

Nurses on Boards Coalition. (2021b). *To improve the health of communities and the nation through the service of nurses on boards and other bodies.* https://www.nursesonboardscoalition.org/

Robison, D. (2016, Fall). Uniting nurses of color a pioneer in the field. *THINK Fall 2016*. Case Western Reserve University. https://case.edu/think/fall2016/nurses-of-color.html#. YNss9ehKiUl

Rossbach, M. (2018, April 9). *Introducing Kevin Sowers*. Johns Hopkins Medicine. https://www. hopkinsmedicine.org/news/articles/introducing-kevin-sowers

Rothman, P. S., & Sowers, K. (2020, December 10). Opinion: Telemedicine is a godsend during a pandemic. But state licensing rules get in the way. *Washington Post*. https://www.washington-post.com/opinions/2020/12/10/telemedicine-is-godsend-during-pandemic-state-licensing-rules-get-way/

Saad, L. (2020, December 22). *U.S. ethics ratings rise for medical workers and teachers*. https://news. gallup.com/poll/328136/ethics-ratings-rise-medical-workers-teachers.aspx

Stake-Doucet, N. (2020, November 5). *The racist lady with the lamp*. https://nursingclio. org/2020/11/05/the-racist-lady-with-the-lamp/#footnoteref9

Tikkanen, R., & Abrams, M. K. (2020). *U.S. health care from a global perspective, 2019: Higher spending, worse outcomes?* Commonwealth Fund. https://www.commonwealthfund.org/publi-cations/issue-briefs/2020/jan/us-health-care-global-perspective-2019

Underwood, L. (n.d.). *Biography. Lauren Underwood: 14th District of Illinois* https://underwood. house.gov/about/biography

United Nations. (n.d.). *The 17 goals*. https://sdgs.un.org/goals

Villarruel, A. M., & Broome, M. E. (2020). Beyond the naming: Institutional racism in nursing. *Nursing Outlook, 68*(4), 375–376. https://doi.org/10.1016/j.outlook.2020.06.009

Wendl, M. J., & Cramer, M. E. (2018). Evaluating effective leadership and governance in a Midwestern agricultural safety and health coalition. *Workplace Health and Safety*, (66)2, 84–94. https://doi.org/10.1177/2165079917729172

Williams, D. R., Lawrence, J. A., & Davis, B. A. (2019). Racism and health: Evidence and needed research. *Annual Review of Public Health, 40*(1), 105–125. https://doi.org/10.1146/annurev-publhealth-040218-043750

Woolf, S. H., & Schoomaker H. (2019). Life expectancy and mortality rates in the United States, 1959–2017. *JAMA, 322*(20), 1996–2016. https://doi.org/10.1001/jama.2019.16932

World Health Organization. (2021). *National health policies, strategies, and plans*. https://www. who.int/nationalpolicies/processes/en/

World Health Organization. (n.d.). *Nursing and midwifery*. https://www.who.int/hrh/nurs-ing_midwifery/en/

UNIT IV

Judging Worth and Advancing the Cause

CHAPTER 12

Evaluating Policy: Structures, Processes, and Outcomes

SEAN P. CLARKE AND PAUL LOGAN

> *One of the great mistakes is to judge policies and programs by their intentions*
> *rather than their results.*
> —Milton Friedman

OBJECTIVES

1. Identify the place of research and evaluation in the policy cycle.
2. Explain the process of evaluating policy using a structure, process, and outcome framework.
3. Describe the use of outcomes research as an influence on policy.
4. Compare and contrast program evaluation and outcome evaluation.
5. Analyze proposed policies for intended and unintended consequences.

This chapter focuses on tracking outcomes for ongoing monitoring and evaluation of policies and expands on the centrality of the use of evidence highlighted in Chapters 4 and 5. Assessing anticipated and unanticipated outcomes of enacted policies is examined using a structure, process, and outcome framework. Evaluation data can form the basis for discontinuing, amending, or expanding policy or assist in advocating for greater investments for a strategy or wider uptake of a specific initiative. The evaluation process is fundamental in the policymaking cycle, no matter whether one is involved in high-level (big-P, national and state) or local (little-p, local or organizational) service delivery policy.

Evaluation is the process of examining the end results or consequences of an intervention. An intervention can be a clinical treatment, which is the classic application of the term. A policy intervention can be a project, a program, or a package of services aimed at one or more stakeholder groups.

Evaluators ask a common set of questions and take similar steps when gathering and interpreting data to determine the effectiveness of policy. The heart of evaluation is collecting and reviewing evidence regarding inputs and outputs of a program or policy to determine whether a policy or program meets its intended goals. It involves taking stock of the structures, processes, and outcomes of an activity. These questions and steps apply across all levels of policymaking (i.e., at both the big-P or little-p levels) and, importantly, incorporate the perspectives of both the recipients of a program and its providers. Evaluation may look at interventions or programs as a whole or examine the impacts of a policy on various groups or on society at large.

357

An important example of how evaluation has informed advocacy relates to occupational injuries. The early focus of efforts to address occupational injuries was often on jobs that were traditionally viewed as highly dangerous such as mining and manufacturing. But since the establishment of the Occupational Safety and Health Administration (OSHA) in 1971, safety efforts have been applied across all work arenas. Occupational injuries across the nursing workforce are common even for the most routine tasks like injecting medications. The COVID-19 pandemic has again brought workplace safety for nurses to the forefront the focus on the supply of personal protective equipment (PPE) and, tragically, even the deaths of nurses and other healthcare workers. The following Policy Challenge illustrates the broad arenas of workplace safety for nurses, some successes realized to date regarding sharps injuries, and highlights the ongoing evolution of policy.

| POLICY CHALLENGE | Charting a Wider Path for Workplace Safety and Advocacy |

OSHA and numerous partners have raised the profile of workplace injuries and heightened awareness of preventive measures. The American Nurses Association (ANA) and specialty nurses organizations such as the Association of periOperative Registered Nurses (AORN) are examples of organizations that have been influential in policymaking so that nurses can be safe.

The nature of nurses' frontline work with the public creates a need for self-advocacy. Issues such as exposure to infection, chemicals, the potential for violence, and workplace injury are just some of the safety issues nurses face. A false assumption that injuries are inevitable despite the known risks or that society expects that injury risks be accepted without complaint undermines advocacy. The addition of a fourth aim to healthcare's Triple Aim of improving the experience of care, improving health, and reducing costs—that of improving the work life of providers (Bodenheimer & Sinsky, 2014)—makes it increasingly important to prevent workplace injuries. One of the recommendations of the *Future of Nursing Report 2020–2030: Charting a Path to Achieve Health Equity* (National Academies, 2021) is that action be taken to promote the well-being and health of nurses.

Sharps injuries also provide a good example of where much remains to be done in workplace safety. These injuries declined after the passage of the needlestick safety legislation, but that decline has leveled. A variety of policies, such as discouraging recapping of needles, ensuring widespread access to disposal containers, and using hands-free techniques (HFT) in the operating room, have done much to contribute to improved safety. Complacency may erode improvements in sharps safety (Daley et al., 2017). Needlestick and other sharps injuries and the potential for becoming ill with blood-borne diseases are still a concern with almost 400,000 injuries occurring among hospital-based healthcare personnel annually (Centers for Disease Control and Prevention [CDC], 2015). Considerable underreporting of injuries and a lack of information from other types of settings indicates that this number is likely to be much higher.

Evaluation is at the cornerstone of providing information for decision-making. However, this is a challenge because systems may not be in place for reporting needlestick injuries that may be occurring during the COVID-19 mass vaccination. Factors potentially contributing to problems in evaluation of needlestick injuries may include but are not limited to administration in multiple nontraditional sites, numerous providers, and the use nonstandard or unfamiliar equipment. Are policies related to sharps injuries where you work or volunteer adequate and up-to-date, and are safe practices embedded in workflows?

See *Policy Solution.*

LANGUAGE OF POLICY EVALUATION

The evaluation of policy touches on similar and/or overlapping concepts such as evaluation, research, policy analysis, quality improvement, and benchmarking.

Evidence is key to the policy-making process; all types of evidence are marshaled at each phase.

Evaluation

The purpose of evaluation in the policymaking cycle is to understand systems of services or policies assembled to address various issues or problems. Evaluation is necessary to make judgments about a policy's effectiveness and decide whether it is sufficient, needs modification, or should be discarded. The primary audiences for evaluation findings are those responsible for planning, implementing, and making decisions about services. In direct care nursing, policies often relate to promoting or restoring health, the safety and quality of patient care, and/or provider effectiveness.

Evaluators are most concerned with the practicalities of assembling sound data at a reasonable cost and in the timeliest manner because they need to know, often quickly, how well a policy or program is achieving its intended outcomes. Some features researchers might consider important in a research design are not always seen as critical by managers and policymakers in the evaluation process.

Research

Research, simply put, is the discovery of new knowledge. Researchers have a toolkit of techniques to uncover patterns that offer answers to larger questions in a scientific field by using different strategies depending on the methods tradition of which they are a part (i.e., qualitative, quantitative, mixed). In the end, there are many similarities between research and evaluation, even if the end goals are different. Nurses engaged in evaluation use many of the same data-collection sources as conventional researchers, including interviews, observations, and surveys.

Evidence is important in the policymaking process, and all types of qualitative and quantitative evidence from both highly formalized and informal data collection are used, as indicated in Chapter 5. Many researchers engage in evaluation projects as part of their portfolio of activities. Sometimes, carefully designed evaluation projects using the approaches discussed in this chapter are considered to have broader applicability and scientific value and are disseminated in the same venues as more conventional and less practically oriented research.

Policy Analysis

Policy analysis and its close cousin policy analysis research examine the context in which a policy is or could be introduced. They provide information about the likelihood of a policy's successful implementation. After implementation, they are used to examine how well a policy has achieved its intended outcomes and whether there have been unintended consequences. An analysis of government-level policies is often seen as the domain of social scientists, more specifically of political scientists and economists, but some nurse scholars also engage in this type of work.

However, policy is not only made at the state or country levels. Policies at the local (or little-p) level have extensive impacts on most nurses' work and work environments. Therefore, nurses and nurse leaders in practice settings must also be able to carry out policy analyses (Hewison, 2007). The initiation of new local policies or modification of existing ones often results when problems arise in practice settings or when circumstances emerge that are thought to require an accompanying policy. From an organizational standpoint, policies are best examined from a multidisciplinary approach. Often, this process involves contacting colleagues at other organizations or searching the literature and the internet for current best practices and guidelines, as well as information about their effectiveness. Nurses, as well as members of other disciplines, can be informed by these internal practices and can seek out and apply guidance offered by experts and professional groups.

Policy analysis examines specific criteria to evaluate a policy and includes developing policy alternatives, assessing the possible outcomes of each alternative, and selecting an alternative from the projected choices. An often-cited practical process for policy analysis can be found in the work of Bardach and Patashnik (2016), who developed a method for policy analysis with the following steps: (a) defining the problem, (b) assembling evidence, (c) constructing alternatives, (d) selecting criteria, (e) projecting outcomes, (f) confronting trade-offs, (g) deciding, and (h) telling the story. Some of these steps involve gathering data from the literature and other expert sources regarding a problem or issue, using best practices in addressing the challenge elsewhere and information specific to the location or site where one hopes to initiate the policy, whereas others involve analyzing this information and framing for communicating it to various decision-makers or stakeholders (see Chapter 4). Policy evaluation is often not as formal as research, and the sequencing of its steps is more flexible. It is often iterative with attention to both upstream and downstream processes and outcomes mixed together. These overall steps may seem familiar to nurses because the nursing process, the research process, and the policy analysis process are similar.

Quality Improvement and Benchmarking

Two other important ideas are *quality improvement* and *benchmarking*. Batalden and Davidoff (2007) define *quality improvement* as concerted efforts over time by all the stakeholders in healthcare to improve the health status of the population, care system functioning, and professional development or learning. We usually think of quality improvement as the work of managers or specifically designated work units within healthcare organizations charged with measuring and improving care system functioning, but Batalden and Davidoff's definition is broader and could even encompass the policy realm. Quality improvement draws on ideas from research methodology and evaluation but is yet another data-driven pursuit demanding high-quality outcomes data—it is another practical activity that many different disciplines can participate in.

Benchmarking is an activity comparing an object, an organization, or even a society against some sort of standard on a measure or measures. In healthcare contexts, benchmarks are used to describe a healthcare system (or a subset of the system, such as a clinic or nursing unit) in relation to others like it. The standard can be a national or international norm for staffing or patient outcomes or a "best in class" performance level. Organizations can even benchmark their performance against themselves over time. Benchmarks are obviously a major part of quality improvement, highlighting the areas calling for managerial action. They also provide a stimulus for higher level policymakers to confront and address reasons for suboptimal organizational performance and spur leaders to match or better the performance of peer organizations or even healthcare systems internationally. A good international-level example is work comparing the Organisation for Economic Co-operation and Development health system performance across countries. For example, Squires (2013) compares a range of countries on measures touching on healthcare expenditures, mortality, and quality. Numerous databases allow benchmarking of healthcare facilities and subunits (such as clinics or units). Some common examples that nurses in hospital and home care encounter on a regular basis include the National Database of Nursing Quality Indicators (NDNQI) and the Outcome and Assessment Information Set (OASIS). Efforts to integrate quality and benchmarking also include disease-specific initiatives, such as the Australian National Association of Diabetes Centres. This program integrates standards, accreditation, auditing, and benchmarking with quality improvement (Andrikopoulos et al., 2021).

Indicators are the specific measurements that are compared in a benchmarking process. Nurses in all settings and across all roles use and are often judged on some indicators (e.g., examination scores, numbers of publications, clinical practice benchmarks). Indicators related to quality and safety in clinical areas are familiar to nurses working in hospitals, clinics, and home healthcare. Patient fall rates, for example, are often measured and then benchmarked against those of similar units or institutions. The NDNQI specifically measures nursing quality and provides nurses with unit- and hospital-level measurement for benchmarking across state, regional, and national data. It should be noted, however, that finding indicators and benchmarks capturing nursing safety-related factors, such as occupational injuries, can be challenging.

Establishing and comparing an institution's data to local, state, and national benchmarks is one way to document progress and setbacks within an organization. After several years of mandatory reporting requirements for acute care hospitals to obtain full Centers for Medicare and Medicaid Services (CMS) reimbursement, benchmarks for patient safety outcomes, such as surgical site infections and hospital-associated infections, are readily available for those wanting to compare their own facility against other like facilities (e.g., number of beds, geographic location, teaching status). However, benchmarking data of healthcare worker occupational harm and injury rates are not readily available. Therefore, it is often difficult for organizations to assess progress in performance-improvement initiatives in this area.

With the increased emphasis on healthcare worker safety, including the update of the Triple Aim to the Quadruple Aim (Bodenheimer & Sinsky, 2014), the ANA Enterprise Healthy Nurse Healthy Nation initiative (ANA, 2021) and the *Future of Nursing 2020–2030* report (National Academies, 2021), there is an increased need and demand for benchmarking data of healthcare worker harm. Healthcare workers are faced with unique risks given the unpredictability and rapid pace of change. These injuries include bloodborne pathogen exposures, workplace violence incidents, and musculoskeletal disease related to patient handling. Performance improvement leaders are faced with challenges to compare their healthcare worker injury rates against other like facilities. OSHA (2016) regulation requiring annual electronic submission of injury and illness logs may enable researchers to examine and create benchmarking for comparison and improvement. In January 2021, OSHA issued guidance on protecting workers from COVID-19, which may eventually provide additional opportunities for benchmark development.

EVALUATING STRUCTURE, PROCESS, AND OUTCOME

A variety of program and policy evaluation models have emerged over the years. A structure, process, and outcome approach was first described by Avedis Donabedian, a health services research scholar who wrote highly influential papers and books on health service quality. This model has been popular in healthcare circles for decades. Donabedian's (1980, 1988) framework pushes clinicians, managers, and researchers to think about the services provided by professionals or the interactions with them that affect patients and communities and figure out raw materials use in terms of people, time, facilities, and equipment needed to deliver the services and the impacts they have on patients, providers, or society. His structure–process–outcome evaluation model is a classic, and many feel it remains applicable today.

Although by no means the only evaluation framework available, Donabedian's structure, process, and outcomes framework make intuitive sense to healthcare managers, clinicians, and program designers and are also useful for thinking about health policy. The framework can be used to study outcomes in healthcare settings and to examine the environment, as well as the personnel and work processes in those environments. For instance, we can easily apply the framework to a public health nursing team providing community outreach visits (structure) to connect at-risk families with resources (process) to facilitate coping, and teach healthy behaviors and parenting skills to at-risk families (outcome), with the end goal of enhancing child development and long-term family functioning (higher level, long-range outcomes). Another example would be a population health nursing team working with legislators to introduce regulation (structure) to reduce secondhand smoke exposure (process) with the intent of preventing downstream illness (outcome).

Donabedian's framework breaks down the components of a service or program into observable and measurable: structures, processes, and outcomes. Exhibit 12.1 illustrates how these may be applied in terms of high-level policy (big-P), as well as local service delivery (little-p).

EXHIBIT 12.1 EXAMPLES OF STRUCTURE, PROCESS, AND OUTCOME IN POLICY

COMPONENT	DEFINITION	LITTLE-P EXAMPLE	BIG-P EXAMPLE
Structure	Attributes of settings where healthcare is delivered: material and human resources, organizational structure	Hospital unit staffing, policies, procedures	Financial, space, and structural resources to establish state-wide emergency response systems
Process	Processes and actions of care delivery	Methods of fall screening implementation; falls prevention methods	Method of recording and transmitting patient falls with injury data to the NDNQI
Outcome	Effects of care on health status of patients and communities	Healthcare-associated pressure injury prevalence per 1,000 patient-days for a specific unit	Community mortality and morbidity measures

NDNQI, National Database of Nursing Quality Indicators.

Structure

The "structure" in Donabedian's framework is the "raw material" of healthcare (i.e., people and supplies), as well as the conditions or contexts of care provision. Structure encompasses human resources (the individuals who work to provide care and those who support this work), as well as processes for healthcare worker selection, training, assignments, and management. Structures can also include physical resources (e.g., equipment, supplies, physical space where care is provided). Finally, structure includes management supports for care: the organizational structure and decision-making mechanisms in a setting, the selection and support of managers, and management practices.

Several examples of structure cutting across both big-P and little-p policy were highlighted in the initial *The Future of Nursing: Leading Change, Advancing Health* report (Institute of Medicine, 2011). At a broad level, the report recommended that the proportion of nurses with baccalaureate degrees be increased to 80% by 2020 and that at a local level, residency programs be implemented for new nurses, new advanced practice nurses, and nurses transitioning to new practice areas.

Process

Processes are the elements of the care or services provided to a patient population—the services intended to improve health and quality measures. The activities of healthcare workers, the order in which they are carried out, and their quality or content are normally included. At the simplest level, processes might include whether a sterile technique was followed for a dressing change. Over the years, there have been some departures and popular reframing of structure, process, and outcomes from Donabedian's original writings. Some also would include management practices under the banner of "processes," but in Donabedian's original formulation, management approaches normally fall under "structures." In a management/policy context, using the example of local and national approaches to attain the 80% baccalaureate preparation of nursing staff mentioned earlier, a process evaluation might include an evaluation of the routes to the bachelor's degree among RN staff and the barriers and facilitators of achieving a bachelor's degree. Examining the details surrounding the initiation of a rapid response team in a hospital setting would be another example of process evaluation.

Outcome

Outcomes are downstream results or endpoints of care. Donabedian's work considers these primarily from a clinical point of view. Outcomes include "objective" health outcomes, such as the incidence of illness, illness severity, complications, and mortality. However, it is also important to consider "subjective" patients' and families' perspectives on health situations. The notion of quality of life is an important subjective measure. It allows for individually interpreted ratings of health states and their impacts, as well as the patient's perceptions of the quality of the care they have received and their satisfaction with their experiences.

Outcomes can be considered proximal or distal. Proximal outcomes are direct indicators of the impacts of treatment on visible manifestations of the phenomena (e.g., symptom levels, tumor size, blood pressure, scores on knowledge tests). Distal outcomes are reflections of the way a treatment or program affects a higher level of or more abstract functioning of individuals or systems (e.g., life satisfaction, job performance; Brenner et al., 1995). It is often easier to demonstrate an impact of a program on a proximal outcome and more difficult to show its impact on a distal outcome, even though the public (and decision-makers at higher levels of systems) are often more concerned about distal outcomes that have clearer impacts on patients and society.

Quality can be considered the degree to which the services are aligned with best practices (frequently the clinical point of view); this is more in line with Donabedian's notion of process, but it may also be considered the desirable end points that are achieved (e.g., recovery of function, return home, enhanced long-term survival) or undesirable end points (e.g., complications) that are avoided in the delivery of a service.

A number of important health system outcomes can also be considered from the perspectives of various stakeholders. These take on different forms for the consumer, for the organization, and for a health system or a wider society. Access and cost-effectiveness are outcomes of healthcare that can be examined from various positions in the healthcare system. Consumers tend to be more concerned with their personal experiences of care, while managers and policymakers tend to view the aggregate experiences across a service line or community. *Access* ("theoretical") can refer to the availability of personnel and facilities in the community, with or without examining whether there are enough "spaces" to meet demand. Or, in a practical sense, access can refer to the availability of affordable services within reasonable travel distances (Roberts et al., 2008).

A service can also be analyzed in terms of the resources consumed for a patient to achieve a certain health state. Financial outcomes, seen from the perspective of a healthcare consumer (patients and families), usually relate to costs of their insurance coverage (through taxes, insurance premiums, or both) and any out-of-pocket costs not covered by insurance, such as additional copayments, travel expenses, or other unreimbursed costs. Through the eyes of a healthcare provider and organization, outcomes relate to the expenses sustained in delivering services relative to the reimbursements they receive and whether there are deficits that must be compensated for by other revenue-generating activities (e.g., other healthcare services). For a government or insurance payer, financial outcomes are a balance between the outlays and the end points they are responsible for producing for their patients or citizens.

Interconnectedness

The connections between *structures, processes,* and *outcomes* are very important. Altering processes of care that have limited or highly indirect connections to desired outcomes is highly unlikely to produce improvements. Likewise, hoping to improve processes of care without ensuring that a critical mass of structures is in place to allow consistent implementation of sound practices is equally misguided. Some experts believe the first step in planning and evaluating a service or an initiative is to construct a diagram (one such type of diagram is called a *logic model*) that lays out the various components of an intervention or a policy and the preconditions for the outputs in terms of actions of the participants and then to identify the basic resources needed to make these actions possible. See Figure 12.1 for a comparison of the language used in Donabedian's framework and a simple logic model for a hypothetical diabetes self-care teaching program. A logic model (also known as a program theory) not only is a convenient tool for explaining the reasoning behind an intervention or policy but also provides a road map for evaluating interventions and policies.

Health is a complicated phenomenon with many facets that can be studied at many different levels from an individual level through the community and societal levels. It is influenced by a multitude of factors such as genetics, developmental

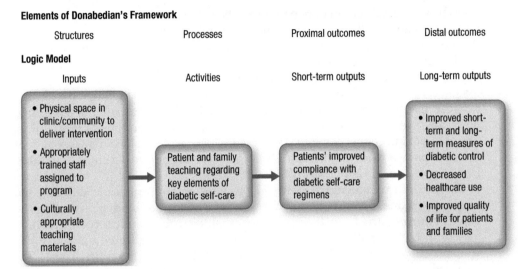

FIGURE 12.1 Comparison of Donabedian's framework and a logic model in a scenario of teaching self-care to individuals with diabetes.

and life history, the social and physical environment, and, of course, healthcare. In health policy, the aim is often to use government powers to improve population health usually, but not always, by influencing what happens in health service delivery.

The Patient Protection and Affordable Care Act (ACA), a legislative intervention signed into law in 2010, was intended to influence financing (structure), increase the use of appropriate services (process), and improve health (outcome) in the U.S. system. This complex law, from its inception, stimulated a great deal of controversy and, after its enactment, received much attention from researchers and policy analysts. Opinions regarding the legislation were very strong and varied markedly. But many in organized nursing have advocated for these reforms, especially the elements of the law that expanded access to health insurance and the lesser discussed, but still important, provisions touching on quality and cost of care, and the nurse workforce. From their initial casting through their modifications through the legislative process, structures to make purchasing health insurance coverage simpler and more affordable were intended to promote processes for the public and insurers to increase the health insurance coverage of individuals across age groups, with the goal of improving quality of care and health outcomes. The proponents and detractors of the ACA either embraced or dismissed various arguments for the legislation through the lens of their assumptions and political contexts/constraints.

The impact and future of the ACA are still debated more than a decade later. Interestingly, few results from evaluation research (and indeed little economic theory) have informed the public debate or the legislative activity over the act. However, many analyses have evaluated the ACA as a policy. There have also been many studies of public opinion about the impacts of the legislation, consumer experiences, and insurance carrier and healthcare provider responses to it. Changing political winds from many different directions have clearly influenced legislators' plans to repeal and replace the ACA with an alternative plan aimed at reducing expenses and improving access.

The interconnectedness of structures, processes, and outcomes is also reflected in research on nurse staffing and patient falls. In some studies, higher nurse-staffing ratios in acute care settings have been linked to decreased patient falls. In a study by

Kalisch et al. (2012) certain nursing interventions left unperformed were connected with more patient falls. *Staffing* was the structural variable, *missed nursing care* was the process variable, and *falls* was the outcome measure. The team found that lower levels of nurse staffing and missed care were linked to inpatient falls. Missed nursing care (classified as an error of omission) is increasingly associated with unintended consequences and poor outcomes. Systematic reviews highlight the linkage between the omission of care to structure, specifically inadequate nurse staffing; outcomes, specifically safety in community/primary care; and medication errors, urinary tract infections, patient falls, pressure injuries, critical incidents, quality of care, and patient readmissions in hospitals and nursing homes (Griffiths et al., 2018; Recio-Saucedo et al., 2018; Sworn & Booth, 2020).

The use of a unique nurse identifier provides an opportunity to illustrate the interconnectedness of structures, processes, and outcomes by demonstrating the value of nurses (structure), the visibility of their contributions (process), and how they contribute to patient outcomes. Advanced practice registered nurse (APRN) students should obtain a National Provider Identifier (NPI) number. The NPI is included on claims submitted to healthcare payors defined as covered entities under the Health Insurance Portability and Accountability Act (HIPAA). The importance of a unique nursing identifier across all practice settings is described in Policy on the Scene 12.1.

POLICY ON THE SCENE 12.1: UNIQUE NURSE IDENTIFIERS: MAKING NURSING VISIBLE AND DEMONSTRATING NURSES' VALUE

Isis Montalvo, MBA, MS, RN, CPHQ, Senior Consultant
Health Management Associates
Costa Mesa, CA

Employing unique nurse identifiers is a strategy highlighted by the *Future of Nursing 2020–2030* report (National Academies, 2021) that can enhance the visibility of nursing and demonstrate its value as payment as the healthcare system moves toward a value-based reimbursement model. It is an opportunity to capture the role of nurses in improving the social determinants of health, patient outcomes, patient safety, and the effectiveness of clinical care (Sensmeier et al., 2021). Using unique nurse identifiers places the focus, on being paid for the quality of care, not the quantity of care. Measuring nursing's quality of care through a unique nurse identifier enables evaluation of the impact of nursing care, since it would be directly linked within the electronic health record to the care provider. The identifier can provide a direct connection to the care rendered and an evaluation of resources at the time of care. It also can provide the means for educators and nurse researchers to aggregate and evaluate the outcomes of that care to improve nursing practice and educate staff on improvements needed.

In the United States, nurse-identifiers exist with the National Provider Identifier (NPI) used by the Centers for Medicare and Medicaid Services (CMS), and the National Council State Boards of Nursing ID (NCSBN ID) for reimbursement and to track licensures, respectively. The latter provides a unique opportunity in that it is available in the Nursys database and allows the tracking of nurses across multiple state licenses (NCSBN, n.d.). The Alliance for Nursing Informatics (ANI) joined forces with the Nursing Knowledge: Big Data Science Initiative Policy and Advocacy work group to recommend the use of the NCSBN ID as a nurse-identifier. The ANI (2020) issued a policy statement to this effect.

Nursys grants free access. This could facilitate researchers, and quality experts, access to demographic characteristics and nurse specialties to determine their relationships to patient outcomes. This is an important consideration, given Avedis Donabedian's quality framework on structure and process measures having an impact on outcome measures. Nurse-sensitive measures have been used for several decades to identify their respective impact on patient outcomes at an aggregate level and even by type of nursing unit.

The unique nurse identifier would provide a more direct connection to the nurse provider and the impact on patient outcome, and more information on the provider who may have contributed to the outcome. Staffing measures that speak to the structure of nursing care have been demonstrated to have an impact on patient outcomes. Having further demographic details on the providers, and the respective work environment where the care was provided, could expand the evaluation of the outcome on other factors. Similarly, processes of care connected to the provider could also be evaluated for their impact on the outcome of care. Moving into this space is in alignment with expanding nursing knowledge and contributes to addressing broader care needs across the continuum and care settings.

With a unique nurse identified, health systems, whether acute- or community-based, would have additional information that could assist with not just evaluating the outcomes of care but the cost of care as well. Social determinants of health, care coordination, and health inequity could further be evaluated by having a direct link to the provider's care and provide greater insight into population health measures. Population health measures benefit multiple stakeholders, such as public and private payers, community-based organizations, social services providers, and healthcare organizations. More important, these organizations could then improve the outcomes of the populations they serve, impacting care broadly.

Using a unique nurse identifier would be a useful means to serve many, across many segments in the evaluation of care and the populations served while, at the same time, increasing the visibility of nursing's impact. Wouldn't we want the opportunity to impact many populations served, advance the practice of nursing, and demonstrate the value of nursing?

In cases in which care delivery is not the direct focus of attention, government-level health policy may be aimed at improving one of the other social determinants of health (i.e., income, social and physical environments, health-related behaviors). Most public health and social policy interventions fall into this category (see Chapter 13). In either case, staff time, basic resources, or raw materials (structures) are transformed into services or contacts with a clientele that is expected to impact changes in their circumstances and then ultimately influence health-related outcomes. Policies of local agencies (processes) usually target narrower aspects of office, unit, or service functioning but relate to the way structures are used to accomplish the day-to-day work of an organization; the outcomes often relate to smooth organizational function or movement toward an organizational goal. In this case of local policies, the health status of the population is a tacit, or implied, downstream goal.

MEASURING CHANGE

Evaluation is investigating whether there has been a change in outcomes as a result of a program or policy. Specifically, it is the search for differences in a phenomenon of interest during the course of a change in contexts or activities in a system. The evaluation of a policy involves assessing changes in structures or processes (or both) that are related to policy implementation, along with possible changes in outcomes in the individuals targeted by a program or policy.

Evaluation approaches can be formative, summative, or a combination. Formative evaluations collect data *while* a policy or program is implemented, sometimes with the explicit purpose of providing feedback that can be used to tweak the program along the way. Other times, it is undertaken to understand how systems change over time. Summative evaluation involves collecting data *after* policies have been implemented or at the end of a program. Structure, process, and outcome data are being used to measure change at the local and national levels.

Another element of evaluation methods relates to prospective data (subjects are identified prior to implementation and followed forward in time) versus retrospective data (subjects are identified and information is gathered after the fact). When resources are scarce and policies are rapidly implemented, especially at the little-p level, it is common for policies, to be examined cumulatively and retrospectively and without a formal baseline data collection. Small-scale local "posttest only" evaluations may be quite informal.

In the years since value-based purchasing initiatives were instituted, hospitals have made significant changes to structures and processes, such as care bundles, in efforts to reduce these harm events to patients. Care bundles are groupings of evidence-based structures and processes that, when implemented together, result in significant reductions in certain negative events. Evaluating the impact of policies incentivizing these bundles is integral to modifying these policies appropriately and developing future initiatives.

In response to Medicare policy to deny payment for certain hospital-acquired conditions (HACs), Waters et al. (2015) examined whether this denial of payment improved outcomes in four of the eight HACs: hospital-associated pressure injuries (HAPIs), injurious falls, central line–associated bloodstream infections (CLABSIs), and catheter-associated urinary tract infections (CAUTIs). Combining data from the American Hospital Association, the Medicare Cost Report, and the NDNQI, the HAC initiative was associated with decreased rates of CAUTIs and CLABSIs. However, the HAC initiative was not found to be associated with a reduction in HAPIs and injurious falls. It was hypothesized that these two harm outcomes (HAPIs and falls) may not have had the same evidence-based care bundles of structures and processes that had been developed for CLABSIs and CAUTIs (Waters et al., 2015). Ideally, data can be used to continue to evaluate policies aimed at improving structures, processes, and outcomes at both the local and national levels.

Understanding Change Over Time

The heart of all research design is assessing differences over time or across settings or conditions; that is an element that research and evaluation share. For instance, a research study could ask whether mortality changes when a specific drug or treatment protocol is given to patients. Other variables (sometimes called *secondary outcomes*), such as blood pressure measurements, may also change alongside differences in the main variable of interest, the primary outcome. Perhaps the impact of the treatment on mortality moves in different ways after treatment, depending on the gender or age of the patient. In such a case, it would be wise to incorporate gender and age measures as biological variables. We also might be interested in how hospital length of stay or inpatient mortality varies across patients, hospitals, regions, or time. The Agency for Healthcare Research and Quality's (AHRQ)

Healthcare Cost and Utilization Project (HCUP; www.ahrq.gov/research/data/hcup/index.html) is a nationwide longitudinal U.S. database containing a range of hospital care indicators that can be used to track changes over several years. In addition, national patient registries can provide population-specific data for use in tracking outcomes over time (Taha et al., 2014).

The aim of a specific policy initiative involving the implementation of home visits by community nurses after the arrival of new babies in socially and economically vulnerable families (Olds et al., 2010) might be to improve short- and long-term child development. In this case, child development in targeted families would be measured before and after their participation in the program. When outcomes change after implementation, the policy or program appears to have also affected the structures or processes in a system, and evaluators have used various strategies to exclude competing explanations for outcomes improvements (e.g., the mere passage of time, other changes in the environment that were independent from the interventions); evaluators can be relatively confident making statements that the initiative was responsible for the change.

Data over time (longitudinal data) are very important for determining whether a policy or program is effective. In the home visit example, if the families receiving the intervention had considerable contact with nurses and the content of those interactions was closely aligned with providing information about optimal parenting techniques, anticipatory guidance, and timely referrals, this would strengthen confidence that any improvements seen were due to the policy. So would seeing persistent improvements for many years after the intervention. To take the example further, showing that the improved outcomes were seen only when nurses and not lay community workers conducted the intervention would suggest that it was relationship building with nurses that led to the improved outcomes for families and children (Bornstein, 2012).

Using Quantitative and Qualitative Approaches to Evaluation

In many cases, evaluators and policymakers want to understand what would happen without an intervention or initiative but are unwilling or unable to conduct a formal experiment. In situations in which randomized trials and other forms of experimentation are not possible, researchers in the social and health sciences have developed approaches to quantify what would have happened without a specific initiative in place. This has sometimes included finding groups or situations that provide a possible "control" or "comparison" group outside the research or evaluation initiative to gauge the outcomes of those targeted by a policy or an initiative. It could involve examining outcomes for a comparable group of vulnerable families in other areas of the same region who did not participate in the home visit program or examining outcomes for families in the same area but in the years before the program was implemented. To the greatest extent possible, the comparison group is constructed to be similar in all important respects to the intervention group.

In addition to having a control or comparison group, preferably one that individuals are assigned to randomly, the ideal quantitative evaluation approach involves a pretest before policy implementation, followed by a posttest after policy implementation. Posttest evaluation designs that involve measurements only *after* the enactment of a policy or program are extremely common. The likelihood of many competing explanations for any patterns seen complicates the drawing of conclusions from the data obtained from such designs. As discussed previously, a lack of planning and resources, both human and financial, contributes to the common use of post-test-only designs for evaluating policy.

It is important to realize that in most evaluations, the main outcome of interest fails to change. There are several likely explanations for this. First, most outcomes are the product of complex and often interrelated factors. Second, interventions or initiatives can only hope to address a small handful of the factors involved, and we may not understand the mechanisms as well as we think. Third, available outcome measures may simply not be as reliable as we might like. This latter situation is sometimes found in large, preexisting data sets or when data can be accessed only after a policy has been implemented. Examples of proxy data ("stand-in" variables) include using educational level for health literacy or self-rated health status for disease state. Fourth, sometimes data are collected and theoretically available for use in evaluation, but access to them is greatly restricted due to privacy concerns. This often leads to policy evaluators being unable to access and analyze the data. Many compromises have been made, including using proxy data to evaluate programs, but with compromises come debates about data quality that can render evaluations open to critique.

These approaches to evaluation are based on the measurement and the quantitative paradigm. A growing contingent of researchers and evaluators, as well as policymakers, recognize that quantitative approaches are not always the best or only methods for understanding the impacts of programs. Instead, they apply methods from qualitative research, including content analysis of various types of documents, interviews, focus groups, and field observation, to gain insights into the experiences of participants and stakeholders. Donabedian's framework and the elements of structures, processes, and outcomes are equally relevant, addressing the quality of the structures, evaluating changes in processes (or behavior changes of providers or patients), and understanding the outcomes perceived and lived by all involved. Although some view quantitative evaluations using well-structured quasi-experimental designs as providing more robust evidence for policy analysis, most agree that multiple types of data are needed to guide policy.

In addition to outcome data collected by the evaluator explicitly for the purpose of assessing program function, existing data sources can also be identified and accessed during the evaluation process. Both data sources result in two interconnected sets of issues: logistical and methodological. Logistical issues involve energy and the human and financial resources that must be invested, as well as access barriers that must be overcome. Methodological issues include ensuring that the data collected are of consistent quality, reliable and valid. For data to be collected, stakeholder interests must outweigh the costs and potential risks involved. These issues were referenced in the previous section, but they hold particular meaning for nursing because in many cases the impacts of policies involving nursing and nursing care are difficult to track. Commonly, not all the data needed to evaluate a program or a policy initiative are known or can even be collected. Often, there is a lack of measures, or assessments of key variables (structures, processes, outcomes) from the time *before* a policy is implemented. Regardless of the design, data necessary for policy evaluation require money, energy, and time. This is a basic reality of all research and makes using existing data sources in policy evaluation particularly attractive.

EXISTING DATA SOURCES

Analyzing existing data sources, as opposed to gathering new data, helps alleviate many of the resource constraints evaluators face related to original data collection. State and federal public policies have for some time attempted to ensure that the numbers and types of nursing personnel are sufficient to meet regions' and the nation's needs. For over two decades, the National Sample Survey of Registered Nurses, a federally sponsored, carefully planned representative survey of licensed RNs across the United States, was conducted every 4 years. It had a strikingly high response rate and was considered the authoritative source for understanding trends in entry to and exit from the profession, as well as educational and career paths of nurses. Thus, it was a key tool in planning state and national workforce policy (Spetz, 2010). The survey was defunded by the Health Resources & Services Administration after the 2008 data collection cycle, and for some time there were no plans to restart it (Spetz, 2013). (A modified version of the survey was conducted in 2018; see bhw.hrsa.gov/data-research/access-data-tools/national-sample-survey-registered-nurses.) Other researchers use U.S. Census datasets on employment across communities to get a sense of workforce trends (Auerbach et al., 2015; Buerhaus et al., 2017). Although the career paths of nurses are still difficult to track, researchers are still finding ways to justify and evaluate investments in the nurse workforce.

The evaluation of policies affecting the quality of nursing care has been impeded by a lack of systematic data collection about the trajectories of patients through the healthcare system and patients' experiences of health. To complicate matters, nursing is often "invisible" in data sets because variables that represent nursing's contributions have not been routinely collected. As a partial answer to that issue, nurse-sensitive indicators that are distinct from medical indicators have been developed and reflect the outcomes that nursing care can prevent or change. These measures are found in the NDNQI, established by the ANA in 1998 and now owned by Press Ganey. It is the largest global quality nursing database available to assist nurses and hospitals improve the quality of care and evaluate outcomes, and it helps make nursing's impact much more visible. Over 2,000 hospitals participate domestically and internationally.

Donabedian's structure, process, and outcome quality framework underpin the database. See Exhibit 12.2 for a list of commonly used measures and their relationship to the Donabedian framework. Using existing data sources, if they can be identified and accessed, saves time and resources. These data sources provide for a robust comparison for policy evaluation.

EXHIBIT 12.2 EXAMPLES OF STRUCTURES, PROCESSES, AND OUTCOMES MEASURES

STRUCTURES
Certified lactation consultant hours per 1,000 live births
Nurse turnover
Nursing care hour per patient day
Nursing care hours per patient visit
Nursing care minutes per surgical minute
Patient volume and flow
RN education
Skill mix
PROCESSES
Care coordination

(continued)

EXHIBIT 12.2   EXAMPLES OF STRUCTURES, PROCESSES, AND OUTCOMES MEASURES (*CONTINUED*)

Strategies to prevent HAIs
Pediatric pain management
Physical restraint prevention
Pressure injury prevention
OUTCOMES
Assaults on nursing personnel
CAUTIs
CLABSIs
Patient falls
Pediatric peripheral intravenous infiltrations
Physical/sexual assaults
Pressure injuries
VAE (including pneumonias)

CAUTIs, catheter-associated urinary tract infections; CLABSIs, central line–associated bloodstream infections; HAIs, healthcare-associated infections; VAE, ventilator-associated events.

ACCOUNTABILITY AND TRANSPARENCY IN EVALUATION

Healthcare systems are stunningly complex webs of providers, organizations, and programs. The resources invested are huge, and the stakes are high for all involved. However, consumers/citizens often feel that they have limited choices about how and where they receive care and have limited inputs into the decisions around the design and payment of services. In addition to incorporating the voices of consumers at the local level, such as having patient and family councils and inviting community members to serve on boards, a number of approaches have emerged to address such concerns. An accountability and transparency movement has emerged that emphasizes the freer exchange of information about operational details and outcomes of policies in the hands of consumers. This movement is not unique to healthcare by any means; it has well-known forms in elementary and secondary education (i.e., standardized testing to evaluate schools and teachers) and is coming of age in many other areas of public and social services, including policing and the justice system (i.e., police body cameras to document whether the use of force by officers is consistent with regulations in jurisdictions). The accountability movement is intended to hold local managers and system policymakers responsible for outcomes.

Accountability for outcomes of policymakers and executives/managers is part of a broader move toward "transparency"—a willingness to share information openly to permit outside examination of the operations of complicated organizations. Public reporting of healthcare structures, processes, and outcomes is increasingly common. Review or reporting of staffing levels in healthcare facilities; accreditation processes that focus on the verifiable presence of various types of equipment, supplies, and operating procedures; training and management practices; review of patient records and inspection of care practice; and public reporting of outcomes are all examples of measurement of structures, processes, and outcomes and their publication or diffusion to various audiences either in the form of individual measures or in summarized form. Data that compare the charges for specific surgical procedures (e.g., coronary artery bypass graft surgery) across a state, a region, a country, or even the world, for example, are routinely made public.

Government Accountability Programs

Data are available from a large number of hospitals regarding the deadliest hospital-acquired complications. The CMS (n.d.-a) routinely publishes results that compare data on each of the following settings: nursing homes, Medicare-certified hospitals, and home care (www.medicare.gov/hospitalcompare/search.html). There is a move to provide managers and clinicians with additional incentives for attaining certain outcomes by tying performance to some portion of remuneration. This movement, known as "pay for performance," exists in various forms in healthcare. In October 2012, reimbursement based on performance under the Medicare Hospital Value-Based Purchasing (HVBP) program began for acute care hospitals throughout the United States (Ryan et al., 2017). The HVBP can be traced to the Medicare Prescription Drug, Improvement, and Modernization Act of 2003 and the Deficit Reduction Act of 2005 that started with the voluntary public reporting of measures. With the passage of the ACA in 2010, the HVBP was mandated, providing rewards for how well hospitals meet selected quality measures. The program incentives have increased from 1% of diagnosis-related group revenue to 2% starting in October 2016 (Ryan et al., 2017). Since its inception, incentives have been expanded from clinical process and patient experience measures to spending measure outcomes, such as 30-day mortality rates for specific diagnoses (Ryan et al., 2017).

POLICY ON THE SCENE 12.2: VALUE-BASED PURCHASING AND APRNs

Anne Pohnert, MSN, BSN, RN, FNP-BC, Director of Clinical Quality, MinuteClinic

Tammy Todd, MSN, BSN, RN, CRNP, CPHQ, Senior Manager, Clinical Quality MinuteClinic

With the Medicare Access and CHIP Reauthorization Act of 2015 (MACRA), the CMS began working toward a value-based payment approach. The Quality Payment Program (QPP), which started on January 1, 2017, aims to reward high-value, high-quality Medicare clinicians with payment increases while, at the same time, reducing payments to those clinicians who aren't meeting performance standards. The QPP has two tracks to choose from, based on practice size, specialty, location, or patient population. Based on these criteria, clinicians can choose one track. In the Merit Incentive Payment System (MIPS), a practice may earn performance-based payment adjustments for the services provided to Medicare patients. The Alternative Payment Model (APM) is a customized payment approach developed by CMS, designed to provide incentives to clinicians who are providing high-quality, high-value care with a focus on particular clinical conditions, care episodes, or a population (CMS, n.d.-a).

The MinuteClinic is a large national group practice of approximately 1,100 retail medical clinics located in select CVS and Target retail pharmacies in 35 states and the District of Columbia. MinuteClinics are staffed by APRNs, primarily family nurse practitioners, as well as physician assistants (PAs). Since its founding in 1999,

MinuteClinic has emphasized the quality of care provided by APRNs and PAs, along with accessibility and cost-effectiveness, as a key strategy to help patients on their path to better health. In April 2021, MinuteClinic successfully submitted 2020 calendar year quality metrics to the MIPS for the first time. The months-long process to prepare to participate in the MIPS was complex and dynamic, requiring hours of project planning and the alignment of key organizational stakeholders and external partners.

We led the project. Executive sponsors included the president of MinuteClinic, the chief nurse practitioner officer, the medical director for quality and patient safety, and the senior director for payor relations. Key program partners included the director of provider credentialing, payer enrollment and medical coding, a regional director for payor relations, the enterprise analytics and reporting team, an executive manager on the clinical practice team, and members of the internal MinuteClinic Epic Electronic Health Record Team. External partners included Technical Solutions Engineers for Epic and other Epic personnel who specialize in supporting clients with developing quality measure reporting for programs such as the MIPS.

The four category weights for the MIPS are Quality (45% in 2020), Improvement Activities (15%), Promoting Interoperability (25%), and Cost (15%). Per the CMS, the Nurse Practitioner (NP) and Physician Assistant (PA) facing practices are currently excluded from the Performing Interoperability reporting category; therefore, there is an enhanced quality weighting and shift toward MIPS quality-focused measure outcomes. MinuteClinic 2020 MIPS reporting included a Quality scoring reweight of 70% and 15% weighting for the cost and improvement activities categories, respectively.

Throughout 2020, the MinuteClinic project team focused on learning the MIPS reporting process, identifying the quality measures to report, building the quality reporting framework in Epic, and mapping the clinical documentation behind the quality measures. The successful application to the MIPS program and subsequent reporting of quality measures for the 2020 calendar year was an exciting opportunity to demonstrate the quality of Advanced Practice Provider (NP and PA) practice in a large multistate convenient care practice. The overall project experience helped to strengthen MinuteClinic's organizational commitment toward improving process workflows and has supported focused efforts to improve quality health record documentation approaches. Additionally, this process has helped strengthen both internal and external quality reporting with a focus on national quality standards.

As the organization builds on the learnings from the 2020 MIPS submissions and prepares to submit the 2021 MIPS required data in early 2022, the MinuteClinic quality team and organizational stakeholders are aligned on strategic quality initiatives to improve workflows and clinical documentation to meet national quality standards and more firmly establish a consistent approach to MIPS reporting in years to come.

Considerations for Transparency

Several issues surround high-stakes measurement used for public reporting or payment to providers or workers' compensation. The first relates to differences in the clientele served by various healthcare agencies that may make interpreting the variability in outcomes challenging. Should healthcare providers serving patients with more complex or challenging conditions be compared with those serving patients with less complicated conditions on their outcomes or financial performance? Performing statistical adjustments to outcomes that take patient or institutional characteristics into account and that soften the impact of treatment "failures" on the indicators is called *risk adjustment*. For instance, it is arguably important to consider the ages, backgrounds, and disability status of patients or their clinical stability before drawing conclusions about the possible significance of healthcare-associated pressure injury or infection data as an indicator of the quality of nursing care. The debates are not simple ones—arguably more challenging cases deserve tailored care, and patients and their communities often experience negative events as failures, whether some cases are inherently "harder" than others. Preliminary data after the first year of the HVBP show that the financial impact on hospitals caring for more disadvantaged patients was worse (Ryan, 2013). These results indicate that processes for reviewing the data and determining payments need further refinement. The second issue relates to understanding meaningful differences across healthcare providers or in the same healthcare providers over time. Much can be made of very small differences that may be trivial, the result of minor fluctuations, or the result of relatively small numbers of cases going into the calculation of event rates.

Practical details of ensuring accurate and consistent data across agencies must be confronted. Intraorganizational differences in personnel and data-collection procedures without extensive external validation raise concerns for the rigor and quality of data. Criteria for determining incidence and rates of HACs, especially when case definitions are constantly being revised, could lead to different interpretations by data collectors and analysts. This leads to discrepancies and problems with comparing intraorganizational differences, especially when there is organizational motivation to minimize adverse events.

Underlying all these issues is the tension among professional organizations, consumers, and healthcare agencies about the public availability of data. As healthcare reform pushes for data transparency, it is believed that consumers, if they can easily access and understand the outcome data, will choose providers with good track records on quality and who offer lower prices. In a study done of almost 1,500 employees, it was found that cost was a major factor in choosing providers (Hibbard et al., 2012). Many in the Hibbard et al. study avoided providers who were less expensive because there seemed to be a perception that high cost equated with high quality. However, when the employees were presented with cost data and easy-to-understand information about provider and service quality, more consumers indicated that they would choose quality rather than basing decisions on cost alone.

Implications for Nursing of the Accountability and Transparency Movement

Accountability and transparency work in favor of increased investments in nursing. However, in many organizations, nursing services are considered overhead, costs of doing business, and areas for possible cost cutting. Relying on financial accounting approaches without an understanding of what are truly equivalent care structures and processes or without considering care outcomes can lead to decisions that cut staffing and other nursing resources but ultimately increase service costs. Broadening the range of indicators tracked and reported/used to drive reimbursement to include more process and outcome measures influenced by nursing care could support investments or reinvestments in structures of care. What is needed is a paradigm shift such that the financial bottom line is not the only outcome that should determine action.

In the case of nursing, we need to analyze the ways that nursing offers value to the public to keep citizens healthier, including helping individuals enjoy a greater quality of life and health. This involves identifying how outcomes for the public can be made tangible through measurement, exploring how nurses produce these outputs and what types of structures and processes are needed to achieve the outcomes, and considering whether and how the measurement of structure and process should be undertaken. It may also involve encouraging the public to insist on having access to important information regarding outcomes and educating the public about how to interpret outcomes data.

Although structures, processes, and outcomes and their relationships to one another are all important, many stakeholders beyond clinicians and managers are almost exclusively interested in "hard" patient and financial outcomes. Structure and process data seem to be much more important to the architects of policy and the managers of services than to many other stakeholder groups. This is perhaps why transitional care interventions by advanced practice nurses that facilitate coordination of services between community and institutional settings were fully embraced only when their impacts on outcomes such as hospitalizations and overall service use were demonstrated. Another example highlighting the work of nurses beyond cost can be found in care coordination, the value of which has been well demonstrated (Camicia et al., 2013). The ANA (2013) has published a framework identifying the structural components and measurement context for nurses' contributions to care coordination. The latter includes system, institutional, and individual/population contributors, impacting the ability of nurses to deliver high-quality care.

Historically, because the types of data that are most easily extracted from secondary data have involved negative outcomes (e.g., falls, pressure injuries) assumed to be preventable with more nursing staff and investments in nursing care structures, such secondary measures have been emphasized in data collection schemes to date. However, many researchers and leaders are working to develop and refine measures that cover more areas and domains of nursing practice and assess what nurses do to facilitate positive outcomes, rather than only examining a narrow range of negative outcomes. Down the line, we must strategize for the use of more nursing-relevant measures that can inform resource allocation decisions by suggesting where investments in healthcare settings should be made to improve outcomes.

Despite the promise of the accountability movement to provide leverage for the nursing profession, special emphasis on indicators, especially outcome measures alone, can be a double-edged sword and can result in unintended consequences. Boiling down the outputs of systems for delivering care to single measures or a collection of indicators, even if only for the sake of making the quantities of information accessible, results in clear lines separating "important" from less important aspects of system performance. Such divisions can distract individuals from aspects of care activities that are "unpaid." These activities, if seen as expected by management but not affecting reimbursement, can create ambiguity for staff. Furthermore, emphasizing grades or scores can force healthcare workers and managers to reallocate efforts without improving patient outcomes. For instance, increasing the burden on healthcare providers to maintain certain types of records can increase costs and divert attention from important work. Chasing favorable outcomes can persuade individuals and organizations to pursue any number of strategies from gaming, or steering outcomes, up to and including fraud. The public may not realize that the upshot may be that attention and other resources are diverted away from aspects of care influencing their well-being and toward activities that are not beneficial.

Accountability programs have popular appeal, even if their implementation is complicated. It may be risky to criticize outcomes-related policies even if the intent of the critiques is to warn consumers and policymakers about the unintended consequences of using poor measures. Speaking out against accountability initiatives may be seen as a self-protection tactic and tantamount to dodging responsibility for results. Within healthcare, rating schemes developed by organizations such as the Leapfrog Group, which distills a great deal of data regarding patient safety down to a single, easily interpreted letter grade, generate similar anxiety in leaders and clinicians—and some of their criticisms seem warranted (Castillo, 2012). Arguably, nursing as a profession needs to take on a greater role in developing outcomes science. Developing meaningful measures, affordable means for tracking data, and an understanding of the complex factors influencing evaluation is necessary to ensure the public's safety.

DOCUMENTING THE IMPACT OF POLICIES RELATED TO NURSING

Documenting how various policies affect the nursing profession is important first and foremost because patient well-being is influenced by nurses' actions. Policies can influence the structures under which nurses practice and thereby alter what nurses are able to do for their patients. It has been argued for some time that what is "good for nurses" is also in patients' best interest; this includes work satisfaction and other aspects of their work lives that influence their mental or physical health. Research on the Magnet Recognition Program, which identifies institutions applying best practices in managing nursing workplaces, provides support for this idea. A growing body of literature shows more favorable outcomes for hospitals that have achieved Magnet status compared with those that have not (Barnes et al., 2016; Kelly et al., 2011; Stimpfel et al., 2016). Several researchers make a compelling business case for the Magnet program (Drenkard, 2010; Stimpfel et al., 2016). This work continues to be important at a time of profound change and cost awareness in the healthcare system when it is becoming increasingly common to hear questions and concerns about the return on investments in single professions such as nursing.

Economic Evaluation: Costs in Relation to Outcomes

As costs of healthcare have increased, consumer expectations have risen, and payers, government agencies, legislators, and advocacy groups are debating whether healthcare expenditures can continue to increase at current rates. Economic evaluation, or the assessment of options in healthcare in terms of their costs and consequences, has therefore become increasingly important. Care delivered by RNs and advanced practice nurses is often thought of as offering a particularly high value, but relatively few nurses are accustomed to demonstrating this using data.

The steps in an economic evaluation are relatively simple, but the resources required for accomplishing them and the technicalities can be extensive. First, an attempt is made to measure all relevant benefits or to assign values to health states, and then all relevant costs of delivering services in specific ways are measured. Next, how those costs vary across treatment options or situations in which a program exists is determined. Then the ratio between outcomes and costs is calculated. Finally, an attempt is made to see how much this ratio is affected by assumptions made about the way that services are delivered, the most important elements of the costs and benefits, and the items that could be ignored. The last step is quite important; good economic evaluations always provide a sense of how the conclusions might be affected by making different assumptions.

There are several types of economic evaluation. The two most common approaches are (a) cost-effectiveness analysis (CEA), in which ratios of the total costs to the same measurable health outcomes obtained—lives saved, infections prevented, unit drops in blood pressure, or quality-adjusted life years—are calculated and compared for different treatment/care options and (b) cost–benefit analysis (CBA), in which monetary values are assigned to the different health states resulting from various healthcare approaches and the costs of treatments are then considered alongside these treatments (Glick et al., 2010; Stone et al., 2002).

A few examples may help with understanding the distinction between these two strategies and the application of these methods to policy-relevant questions. A CEA of a community-based intervention run by nurse practitioners and community health workers for patients at high risk of cardiovascular disease that drew on a randomized controlled trial found that relative to usual care, the intervention was able to reduce blood pressures and lipid levels for approximately $40 to $200 per percentage point drop in these measures (Allen et al., 2014). In another CEA, it was determined through computer simulations that providing for anesthesia needs of a 12-bed/station operating room using only nurse anesthetists would yield revenues of $3.3 million, whereas using only physician anesthesiologists would yield revenues of $1.3 million, and 1:6 supervision would yield revenues of $1.5 million (Hogan et al., 2010). A CBA of school nurses in Massachusetts public schools by Wang et al. (2014) reported that every dollar spent on nursing services saved $2.20 in lost teacher productivity related to teachers dealing with health-related tasks, as well as on preventable healthcare costs and lost parental productivity. Another CBA found that by reducing nurse turnover and the need for contingent/temporary staff, new graduate nurse residency programs appeared to save between $10 and $50 per patient day relative to institutions that use more traditional onboarding programs (Trepanier et al., 2012).

Economic evaluation is complicated by a number of factors. Economic analysis always involves comparing different approaches to care or investments in services against each other. Selecting which conditions to put side by side can be both methodologically and politically challenging, particularly if there is no obvious comparison or the comparison involves treatment approaches using very different health professionals. Another issue is finding consistent and accurate means of tracking all relevant costs and outcomes rather than restricting attention to the costs and outcomes for which data are most readily available. For instance, even though the amounts hospitals bill for their services can be learned, charges by healthcare providers have only a weak connection to the real costs of providing the services, with charges being notoriously much higher than what providers actually collect. Because charges can adversely affect the impact of interventions, the amount ultimately paid for services is preferred over the amount charged by the organization or provider (Petitti, 2000). Given uncertainties surrounding health outcomes, as well as differences across individuals in what outcomes or health states are most desirable and to what extent, it is often also difficult to assign values to different health states. Deciding on the frame of reference for analysis in terms of whose costs and benefits and over what time frames, given both the plurality of stakeholders and the longtime horizons for many benefits of healthcare, is a further challenge.

Economic analyses demand considerable time and expertise, and incorrectly conducted analyses can reach unhelpful and even damaging conclusions. Economic analyses, with insufficient attention to time horizons and the positions of the stakeholders, can reach counterintuitive conclusions. For instance, in accounting for the added costs of hospitalization for individuals who experience adverse outcomes, it can appear more cost-effective to make choices that lead to death (and death early in patients' hospital stays) than create conditions that require prolonged hospital stays to treat.

Conclusions about costs and benefits are also often meaningfully different for different stakeholders. Cost savings or value added for a provider or payor may not be value added from the patient's perspective. One analysis concluded that the net benefits of improved nurse staffing on patient outcomes may really accrue to patients and society rather than to individual hospitals (Twigg et al., 2015). This suggests that policy strategies for improving nurse staffing may need to consider where motivations can be leveraged (e.g., at the societal level).

The literature linking nurse staffing with patient safety outcomes in acute care hospitals has been at the heart of more than 20 years of advocacy work on the part of many, including nurses' professional associations in a number of countries, trying to fend off cuts in staffing and increases in nurse–patient workloads. These efforts have led to a more explicit examination of the unintended consequence of changes in nurse staffing whether due to nurse shortages or hospital cost cutting. One such unintended consequence receiving increasing scrutiny is nurse rationing of care.

Understanding Failures to Observe Unanticipated Change and Analyzing Unintended Consequences

Policies may fail to achieve the outcomes targeted by their originators or have unintended consequences. Policy initiatives may be based on incomplete or misinformed ideas about the factors that influence the outcomes being targeted. Various political forces may lead to adoption of policies that are not the ones most likely to produce desired responses. Downstream, the implementation of measures may also be incomplete or inconsistent; that is, structures are not being instituted or are failing to influence processes in the manner expected. Furthermore, attempting to engineer complex social systems with multiple actors can produce any number of reactions as stakeholders attempt to maximize or maintain their benefits and minimize their costs. Obamacare was designed to increase coverage of working-age adults by requiring employers of 50 or more employees to offer health insurance coverage to all employees working 30 or more hours per week. Some observers claimed that this provision would create a disincentive for employers to create new jobs and give more weekly hours to employees scheduled at the 30-hour-per-week threshold. This of course could be seen as bad in a time of economic challenges when workers need jobs and job creation is a priority (McVeigh, 2013). Thus far, analyses have concluded that the feared loss of jobs did not materialize (Garrett et al., 2017). However, it is clear that this concept played a role in efforts to repeal and replace Obamacare. As a general principle, stakeholders can and do shift their energies or resources into alternative behaviors that can undermine the original intent of a policy or program. As a result, the consequences of implementing a policy may fall well short of the expected or intended ones and the possibility of new desirable and undesirable effects that were never foreseen must be kept in mind.

A central concept in policy analysis is the notion of unintended consequences: changes that were not foreseen or intended by the creators of an intervention or a policy. Unintended consequences are not always bad, however. One example of a positive unintended consequence is found in examining health information exchanges (HIEs). HIEs, electronic-based exchanges that allow organizations, systems, and providers to share health information, are a direct result of the American Recovery and Reinvestment Act (ARRA) of 2009. Although benefits were anticipated in terms of enhanced quality of patient care and cost savings, concerns were raised about privacy invasions. At least one positive unintended consequence emerged: new possibilities for detecting disease outbreaks. Clinicians, officials, and researchers using syndromic surveillance can identify patterns of conditions and diseases that might point to a developing public health problem sooner, providing the opportunity for earlier response and intervention (McGowan et al., 2012).

Full evaluation of a policy tracks both costs and benefits and attempts not only to identify whether expected changes are observed in targeted outcomes but also to track what other related factors may be affected by the intervention. Commonly intended consequences of policies and programs include improved service quality, cost efficiencies, and health outcomes; increased and expanded access to services; and enhanced quality of life. Unintended consequences can be found by recognizing their potential to emerge when developing policy and examining a policy once it is in place for both positive and negative outcomes. See Exhibit 12.3 for a list of unintended consequences based on the work of Smith (1995) and Rambur et al. (2013). This was originally framed as a list of caveats when examining performance metrics but has broader implications for understanding "traps" that may lead to a failure to recognize unintended consequences. Obviously, engaging stakeholders directly impacted by policies in the development and implementation phases helps in anticipating potential consequences.

Deep knowledge of the targeted health problem or care-delivery issue with an understanding of the community and critical unbiased eyes is needed to draw up a complete list of consequences and select variables to include in an evaluation.

EXHIBIT 12.3   MINDSETS THAT LEAD TO MISSING UNINTENDED CONSEQUENCES AND EXAMPLES

Tunnel vision: Evaluating effectiveness based primarily on financial benefits
Measure fixation: Focusing on a metric such as 30-day readmission without full consideration of the patient's illness experience
Acontextual actions: Choosing patients for an evaluation who will likely experience the best results
Misrepresentation: Presenting only a subset of measured results or measured outcomes, either positive or negative or either expected or unexpected that supports conclusions
Gaming: Inadvertently encouraging clinicians to work to influence the measures without affecting the targeted outcomes (e.g., patients are told how to respond on satisfaction surveys)
Myopia: Focusing only on short-term results
Suboptimization: Pursuing a limited number of outcomes and selecting only those that are likely to show the greatest improvements
Ossification: Deterring innovation by overemphasizing strengths of existing approaches

Evaluations that leave out important consequences may sell the successes of a policy short or overestimate its benefits. Equally critical, evaluations perceived as omitting important considerations are particularly vulnerable to claims of bias. By virtue of their roles, nurses are well positioned to anticipate unintended consequences and think about how to place unintended consequences in context (Rambur et al., 2013).

DETERMINING SUSTAINABILITY

Sustainability refers to the persistence of changes in conditions or outcomes beyond the initial investments of resources in implementing interventions. As noted earlier in this chapter, many, if not most, program or policy evaluations fail to identify hoped-for improvements in the main outcomes of interest. Even fewer evaluations demonstrate sustained improvements in outcomes over time. People tire of messages and fail to be motivated by inducements or penalties; overall, systems tend to revert to their original states over time (Swerissen & Crisp, 2004). At the little-p level in hospitals, increases in the incidence of falls, rises in restraint use, lax hand hygiene, and inattention to alarms are examples of poor processes and outcomes that tend to resurface over the long term even when initial improvements are noted after an intervention of some kind.

Whether the resources normally available in a system are sufficient to cover the ongoing costs or expenses of a policy initiative is a common and recurrent question. Can a regulation be enforced sufficiently over time? Will behavior become widespread enough, or will people in various roles have enough knowledge and intrinsic motivation over time to continue proceeding in a certain way? Could the benefits of an initiative balance the costs and eventually lead to it "paying for itself"? If regulation is used as a means of influencing patients, providers, payers, and systems, will resources for inspection and enforcement of these regulations be available in the long term? Will the benefits of the policy, whatever it is, be sufficiently clear to maintain a critical mass of support over time?

Obviously, careful evaluation of a policy initiative can provide important information for making a case that an intervention is sustainable. Thinking about sustainability is critical from the moment a policy is conceived. If the structures needed to implement a policy are not thought through or are incompletely measured, the long-term costs and benefits of the intervention will be underestimated. Because of this problem, evidence-based practice (EBP) models include a final step of ongoing monitoring and/or evaluation. Without ongoing monitoring and evaluation, initial improvements often fade away.

OUTCOMES DATA AS GUIDES TO NEXT STEPS IN POLICY

The policy process is a cycle from problem identification; through agenda setting, policy formulation, selection, and implementation; and back to agenda setting after policies are selected and implemented. Some type of evaluation often takes place, even if it is on an informal basis and involves stakeholders gathering impressions and drawing conclusions about whether their aims were met and beginning the cycle anew. In terms of strategizing next steps, a number of basic options are available: Do nothing (i.e., to cease interventions and to let "natural" conditions take or retake hold), maintain the current course, increase investments or expand the scope of a policy, change course by withdrawing financial support or repealing regulations, introduce new policies that proceed in a different direction, or let others do something that takes the policy in a different direction. All these options appear to remain on the table with respect to the ACA. The unfolding policy debates were notable for the extent to which evaluation and research data often were only tangentially related to the new options proposed.

People seeking to influence the policy process must decide which options they wish policymakers to address. Formal analysis of a policy, including indicating the extent to which a policy has achieved its intended ends and determining what its other consequences have been, can be useful tools in determining how to move forward and as supports for arguments.

Many argue that evaluation is a fundamentally political process and that data will nearly always be seen as the tool of one side or another in a policy debate. Perhaps this is true, but in the long run, using data in a principled way and avoiding intentionally overstating or misstating facts is the best strategy for ensuring that data are seen as a potentially credible means of informing policy.

DEVELOPING POLICY SCHOLARSHIP IN NURSING

The future of healthcare increasingly requires health professionals to confront dilemmas about how to offer high-quality services that are accessible to the public at a reasonable cost. The pace of change in terms of social and economic forces hitting healthcare shows no sign of abating. Nurses and others must understand and attempt to influence the direction of policy for it to have greater benefit for their work. Most health professionals and researchers still have an uncomfortable relationship with policy and politics. They consider it, at best, a distraction from "higher yield" direct service to patients and, at worst, a convoluted and often distasteful process of manipulation and strategizing. However, many are now realizing that maintaining remoteness from policy is no longer a viable option. Beyond becoming informed about the policy process in general, it is important to learn about specific policies at various levels and eventually to share our experiences in advocacy, implementation, and evaluation.

Relatively few academic policy evaluators specialize in healthcare issues, and even fewer nurse researchers are involved in this area. There are some notable examples, however, at a few major centers across the country. If we turn our attention briefly to local policy initiatives, many are never formally evaluated at all; among those where some data are collected and/or analyzed, few are ever formally reported in any consistent or retrievable manner. Given the understandable emphasis in the nursing literature on updating clinicians on clinical matters and publishing reports of research studies, it is understandable that policy-focused articles are less commonly written or read. As a result, there is mostly an informal method of passing along information about what has worked in local policies and programs and certainly around nursing involvement in policy and its results.

Contexts and history are important for anyone hoping to translate approaches used in other communities or around other policy issues to new settings, but evaluation data (especially health outcomes data) can be quite influential in encouraging uptake of approaches from elsewhere. Articles about political involvement, state and national policy issues affecting nursing, and policy advocacy efforts involving nursing appear in publications such as *American Journal of Nursing*, *American Nurse*, *OJIN: Online Journal of Issues in Nursing*, and *Politics, Policy, and*

Nursing Practice. Anecdotal experiences with implementing policies and programs are dotted throughout the management and clinical literature; however, it is vital that published reports be structured in a manner that permits readers to intelligently assess the potential for replicating experiences and the likelihood of improving outcomes if they do. A number of scholars and journal editors developed the Standards for Quality Improvement Reporting Excellence (www.squire-statement.org) to assist groups in reporting local experiences of implementing and evaluating programs in a complete and rigorous manner, keeping in mind that there is likely to be a fair degree of variation in the nature of programs and content of evaluations. Perhaps nurses, nurse scientists, and leaders need more encouragement to write their experiences and more recognition needs to be given to those who share their experiences in local and higher level policies with broad professional audiences.

POLICY SOLUTION | Charting a Wider Path for Workplace Safety and Advocacy

Ongoing monitoring and evaluation of injuries, research, and policies are basic to safety advocacy. Even though we have passed the 20-year anniversary of the Needlestick Prevention and Safety Act, more work is needed to reduce sharps injuries with compliance and its oversight and to fully integrate policies and best practices into the work setting and expand these initiatives to outpatient, home care, and nontraditional settings, as well as settings with fewer resources. Ongoing efforts at the big-P and little-p levels remain crucial.

Continuing active research and sharing research results and practice and policy changes at all levels are vital to preventing the complacency that often sets in once new policies are in place. An integrative review on hands-free techniques in traditional settings identified broad categories of factors related to compliance, each representing a different structure or process influencing sharps injury outcomes, such as education and manager support (Linzer & Clarke, 2017). These factors provide opportunities for the development of additional policies and/or interventions to impact structure and process. However, there are still data to be collected and lessons learned from mass vaccinations. Persaud and Mitchell (2021) emphasize the importance of the hierarchy of controls such as leader and staff engagement, assessment and identification of safety gaps, enhanced worker training, standardization of safety practices, administrative policies, procurement of safer devices, and use of sharps injury logs. Each of these arenas provides an opportunity to address structure, process, or outcomes in the implementation and evaluation of policy at the little-p and big-P levels to decrease the number sharps injuries and increase the likelihood that healthcare professionals will report sharps injuries.

Policy work needs to continue regardless of one's role or practice setting because roles evolve, practice moves to nontraditional settings, and the unexpected occurs, requiring new ways of addressing structure, process, and outcome to evaluate policy. Key to integrating policies is the sustained engagement of nurses who may be directly impacted.

IMPLICATIONS FOR THE FUTURE

Outcomes and evaluation research are important tools in policy development and advocacy. Increasing debates about the role of government and of regulation in ensuring healthcare quality will mean that arguments for new health policies (or that justify existing programs) will need supporting data. In addition, educating the public about outcomes and their role as empowered consumers will also be increasingly important. Of course, many have become cynical about the shaping of political messages and the selective reporting or overt misrepresentation of facts, including research and evaluation data, in the fight for public opinion. In the past decades, there have been massive investments in research projects, and the conclusions that can be drawn from such studies have often been somewhat softer or nuanced than many would like. In the upcoming years there will probably be many stakeholders with more realistic expectations of program evaluations. This realism will more effectively guide policy and provide guiding policy and more understanding that the synthesis or summarizing of evidence may need to proceed in a different direction rather than expecting a small handful of studies to provide "the" answers to complex and often very polarizing health policy debates and challenges.

KEY CONCEPTS

1. Evaluation of outcomes is an integral component of accountable policymaking at all levels.
2. Evaluation takes many forms from the examination of specific clinical interventions to the impact of a policy on society.
3. Evaluation uses many of the techniques of conventional research (e.g., quantitative and qualitative methods, prospective and retrospective approaches).
4. The purpose of evaluation is to understand systems and services or policies that address various issues or problems.
5. Policy analysis research assesses how well the implementation of a policy has achieved its intended outcomes.
6. Benchmarking is a comparison against a standard of performance or level of quality.
7. Indicators are specific measurements that are benchmarked.
8. Nurse-sensitive indicators are outcomes that are believed to be particularly influenced by nursing.
9. Structure, process, and outcome is a frequently used framework for evaluation that takes into consideration people, facilities, equipment, and the delivery of services.
10. Missed nursing care, an error of omission, is tied to adverse patient outcomes, but much work remains for nurses across roles and settings to fully understand the structure–process–outcome dynamics of this worldwide issue.
11. Evaluation may be summative (after a policy is implemented) or formative (while a policy is implemented).
12. Demonstrating differences in outcomes is difficult because of the complexity of influences on many outcome variables, incomplete understandings of involved factors, imprecise measurement, and data access restrictions.
13. Outcome measurement may have both positive and negative unintended consequences that impact the direction of policy.
14. Pay-for-performance schemes and public reporting are examples of high-stakes outcome measurement initiatives.
15. A unique nurse identifier can be used to demonstrate the value of nursing.
16. Economic evaluation focuses on the comparison of different approaches to investments in care or services and the way that the results vary based on different assumptions.

17. The sustainability of outcomes needs to be included in the initial development of policy.

18. The development of the science of measuring structures, processes, and outcomes and developing and maintaining data sources is critical to enhancing visibility in policy circles.

SUMMARY

Sound data have enormous potential to influence the creation of worthwhile policies and assist stakeholders in evaluating the impacts of policies on key outcomes. Frameworks that describe how outcomes influence structures and processes for providing services are critical for designing evaluations; verifying that the connections between various elements of a policy or program to each other and to the intended outcomes is important. Obtaining data that assist in policy or program planning is often costly and complicated, but it is almost always possible to assemble some data even with lean resources. Documenting the contribution of nursing services to the public's well-being is a challenging but a vital pursuit. Economic analyses of policies and programs are becoming more common, and an awareness of concepts such as sustainability and unintended consequences is certainly key to using evaluation data for policies. The challenge to nursing is fostering a tradition of nursing scholarship that employs meaningful data to inform successful policies.

END-OF-CHAPTER RESOURCES

LEARNING ACTIVITIES

1. Identify a little-p or a big-P health policy related to an issue of interest to you. List intended and potentially unintended consequences of this policy.

2. Obtain a policy evaluation report or a research study and compare and contrast the elements of the policy evaluation with the elements described in this chapter. Describe the stated conclusion about the effectiveness of the policy in the report and the recommendations for next steps proposed by the authors. Identify why you support or do not support the conclusions of the report based on the data presented.

3. Select a little-p policy at work or in your educational program and discuss how outcomes for the policy are being formally measured. Discuss how the measures are reported and what changes for maintaining or modifying the measures and their reporting you would make and why.

4. Engage a colleague in a discussion of an example of missed nursing care reflecting on its connection to structure, process, and/or outcome. Identify the patient's and nurse's perspectives and implications for policy.

5. Reexamine Exhibit 12.2. Select a policy you would like to change related to one of the issues. Make a list of four or five questions that you would ask to determine whether the unintended consequences have not been fully explored because of the potential traps identified in the table.

6. Create a logic model illustrating the interconnectedness of structure, process, and outcome using a current health policy.

7. Identify two research or EBP questions in your practice setting that would yield relevant data and information to evaluate and direct future policy work.

E-RESOURCES

■ Agency on Healthcare Research and Quality. Healthcare Cost and Utilization Project (HCUP) http://www.ahrq.gov/research/data/hcup/index.html

■ Agency on Healthcare Research and Quality. *Patient Safety and Quality: An Evidence-Based Handbook for Nurses* http://www.ahrq.gov/professionals/clinicians-providers/resources/nursing/resources/nurseshdbk/index.html

■ Centers for Disease Control and Prevention. Developing an Effective Evaluation Report http://www.cdc.gov/eval/materials/Developing-An-Effective-Evaluation-Report_TAG508.pdf

■ Centers for Medicare & Medicaid Services https://data.medicare.gov

■ Centers for Medicare & Medicaid Services. Hospital Value-Based Purchasing Program https://www.cms.gov/Medicare/Quality-Initiatives-Patient-Assessment-Instruments/HospitalQualityInits/Hospital-Value-Based-Purchasing-.html

■ Needlestick Safety and Prevention Act of 2000, Pub. L. 106-430 https://www.govtrack.us/congress/bills/106/hr5178

■ National Database of Nursing Quality Indicators. Quality Improvement Solutions from Press Ganey http://www.pressganey.com/solutions/clinical-quality/nursing-quality

- Outcome and Assessment Information Set. http://www.cms.gov/Medicare/Quality-Initiatives-Patient-Assessment-Instruments/OASIS/index.html

- PSNet Patient Safety Network https://psnet.ahrq.gov/primer/missed-nursing-care

- Standards for Quality Improvement Reporting Excellence http://squire-statement.org

REFERENCES

Allen, J. K., Dennison Himmelfarb, C. R., Szanton, S. L., & Frick, K. D. (2014). Cost-effectiveness of nurse practitioner/community health worker care to reduce cardiovascular health disparities. *Journal of Cardiovascular Nursing*, 29(4), 308–314. https://doi.org/10.1097/JCN.0b013e3182945243

Alliance for Nursing Informatics. (2020, July 16). *Demonstrating the value of nursing care through use of a unique nurse identifier policy statement*. https://www.allianceni.org/unique-nurse-identifier

American Nurses Association. (2013). *Framework for measuring nurses' contributions to care coordination*. https://www.nursingworld.org/~4afbd6/globalassets/practiceandpolicy/health-policy/framework-for-measuring-nurses-contributions-to-care-coordination.pdf

American Nurses Association. (2021). *Healthy Nurse Healthy Nation*. https://www.healthynursehealthynation.org/

American Recovery and Reinvestment Act of 2009. (2009). Pub. L. No. 111-5, 123 § 115.

Andrikopoulos, S., James, S., & Wischer, N. (2021). What gets measured gets improved-Setting standards and accreditation for quality improvement for diabetes services in Australia. *Journal of Diabetes Science and Technology*, 15(4), 748–754. https://doi.org/10.1177/19322968211009910

Auerbach, D. I., Buerhaus, P. I., & Staiger, D. O. (2015). Do associate degree registered nurses fare differently in the nurse labor market compared to baccalaureate-prepared RNs? *Nursing Economic$*, 33(1), 8–12, 35. www.nursingeconomics.net

Bardach, E., & Patashnik, E. M. (2016). *A practical guide for policy analysis: The eightfold path to more effective problem solving* (5th ed.). CQ Press.

Barnes, H., Rearden, J., & McHugh, M. D. (2016). Magnet® hospital recognition linked to lower central line–associated bloodstream infection rates. *Research in Nursing and Health*, 39(2), 96–104. https://doi.org/10.1002/nur.21709

Batalden, P. B., & Davidoff, K. (2007). What is "quality improvement" and how can it transform health care? *Quality and Safety in Health Care*, 16(1), 2–3. https://doi.org/10.1136/qshc.2006.022046

Bodenheimer, T., & Sinsky, C. (2014). From Triple to Quadruple Aim: Care of the patient requires care of the provider. *Annals of Family Medicine*, 12(6), 573–576. https://doi.org/10.1370/afm.1713

Bornstein, D. (2012, May 16). *The power of nursing. The New York Times*. http://opinionator.blogs.nytimes.com/2012/05/16/the-power-of-nursing/?_r=0

Brenner, M. H., Curbow, B., & Legro, M. W. (1995). The proximal–distal continuum of multiple health outcome measures: The case of cataract surgery. *Medical Care*, 33(Suppl. 4), AS236–AS244. https://journals.lww.com/lww-medicalcare

Buerhaus, P. I., Skinner, L. E., Auerbach, D. I., & Staiger, D. O. (2017). Four challenges facing the nursing workforce in the United States. *Journal of Nursing Regulation*, 8(2), 40–46. https://doi.org/10.1016/S2155-8256(17)30097-2

Camicia, M., Chamberlain, B., Finnie, R. R., Nalle, M., Lindeke, L. L., Lorenz, L., Hain, D., Haney, K. D., Campbell-Heider, N., Pecenka-Johnson, K., Jones, T., Parker-Guyton, N., Brydges, G., Briggs, W. T., Cisco, M. C., Haney, C., & McMemamin, P. (2013). The value of nursing care coordination: A white paper of the American Nurses Association. *Nursing Outlook, 61*(6), 490–501. https://doi.org/10.1016/j.outlook.2013.10.006

Castillo, M. (2012, November 28). *Study on safest hospitals shows some surprising results.* CBS News. http://www.cbsnews.com/8301-204_162-57556061

Centers for Disease Control and Prevention. (2015, February 11). Sharps safety for healthcare settings. https://www.cdc.gov/sharpssafety/index.html

Centers for Medicare & Medicaid Services. (n.d.-a). APMS overview. https://qpp.cms.gov/

Centers for Medicare & Medicaid. (n.d.-b). Find & compare nursing homes, hospitals & other providers near you. Medicare.gov https://www.medicare.gov/care-compare/

Centers for Medicare & Medicaid. (n.d.-c). *Quality Payment Program overview*. https://qpp.cms.gov/about/qpp-overview

Daley, K. A., Laramie, A. K., & Mitchell, A. H. (2017). Sharps injuries remain major occupational safety concern for healthcare personnel. *Infection Control Today, 21*(11), 26–30. https://www.infectioncontroltoday.com/sharps-safety/sharps-injuries-remain-major-occupational-safety-concern-healthcare-personnel

Deficit Reduction Act of 2005. (2006). Pub. L. No. 109-171, 120 § 4.

Donabedian, A. (1980). Methods for deriving criteria for assessing the quality of medical care. *Medical Care Review, 37*(7), 653–698. http://mcr.sagepub.com

Donabedian, A. (1988). The quality of care. How can it be assessed? *Journal of the American Medical Association, 260*(12), 1743–1748. https://doi.org/10.1001/jama.1988.03410120089033

Drenkard, K. (2010). The business case for Magnet. *Journal of Nursing Administration, 40*(6), 263–271. https://doi.org/10.1097/NNA.0b013e3181df0fd6

Garrett, A. B., Kaestner, R., & Gangopadhyaya, A. (2017). *Recent evidence on the ACA and employment: Has the ACA been a job killer? 2016 update.* The Urban Institute, ACA Implementation—Monitoring and Tracking.

Glick, H. A., Polsky, D. P., & Shulman, K. A. (2010). Trial-based economic evaluations: An overview of design and analysis. In M. Drummond & A. McGuire (Eds.), *Economic evaluation in health care: Merging theory with practice* (pp. 113–140). Oxford University Press.

Griffiths, P., Recio-Saucedo, A., Dall'Ora, C., Briggs, J., Maruotti, A., Meredith, P., Smith, G. B., Ball, J., & Missed Care Study Group. (2018). The association between nurse staffing and omissions in nursing care: A systematic review. *Journal of Advanced Nursing, 74*(7), 1474–1487. https://doi.org/10.1111/jan.13564

Hewison, A. (2007). Policy analysis: A framework for nurse managers. *Journal of Nursing Management, 15*(7), 693–699. https://doi.org/10.1111/j.1365-2934.2006.00731.x

Hibbard, J. H., Greene, J., Sofaer, S., Firminger, K., & Hirsch, J. (2012). An experiment shows that a well-designed report on costs and quality can help consumers choose high-value health care. *Health Affairs, 31*(3), 560–568. https://doi.org/10.1377/hlthaff.2011.1168

Hogan, P. F., Seifert, R. F., Moore, C. S., & Simonson, B. E. (2010). Cost effectiveness analysis of anesthesia providers. *Nursing Economic$, 28*(3), 159–169. www.nursingeconomics.net

Institute of Medicine. (2011). *The future of nursing: Leading change, advancing health.* The National Academies Press. https://doi.org/10.17226/12956

Kalisch, B. J., Tschannen, D., & Lee, K. H. (2012). Missed nursing care, staffing, and patient falls. *Journal of Nursing Care Quality, 27*(1), 6–12. https://doi.org/10.1097/NCQ.0b013e318225aa23

Kelly, L. A., McHugh, M. D., & Aiken, L. H. (2011). Nurse outcomes in Magnet® and non-Magnet hospitals. *Journal of Nursing Administration, 41*(10), 428–433. https://doi.org/10.1097/NNA.0b013e31822eddbc

Linzer, P. B., & Clarke, S. P. (2017). An integrative review of hands-free technique in the OR. *AORN Journal, 106*(3), 211–218.e6. https://doi.org/10.1016/j.aorn.2017.07.004

McGowan, J. J., Kuperman, G. J., Olinger, L., & Russell, C. (2012). *Strengthening health information exchange: Final report HIE Unintended Consequences Work Group*. http://www.healthit.gov/sites/default/files/hie_uc_workgroup_final_report.pdf

McVeigh, K. (2013, September 30). *US employers slashing worker hours to avoid Obamacare insurance mandate*. http://www.theguardian.com/world/2013/sep/30/us-employers-slash-hours-avoid-obamacare

Medicare Prescription Drug, Improvement, and Modernization Act of 2003. (2003). Pub. L. No. 108–173.

National Academies of Sciences, Engineering, and Medicine. (2021). *The future of nursing 2020–2030: Charting a path to achieve health equity*. The National Academies Press. https://doi.org/10.17226.25982

National Council of State Boards of Nursing. (n.d.). Nursys overview. https://www.ncsbn.org/nursys.htm

Occupational Safety and Health Administration. (2016, May 12). Improve tracking of workplace injuries and illnesses a rule by the Occupational Safety and Health Administration. *Federal Register, 81*(92), 29623. https://www.gpo.gov/fdsys/pkg/FR-2016-05-12/pdf/2016-10443.pdf

Occupational Safety and Health Administration. (2021, January 29). *Protecting workers: Guidance on mitigating and preventing the spread of COVID-19 in the workplace*. https://www.osha.gov/coronavirus/safework

Olds, D. L., Kitzman, H. J., Cole, R. E., Hanks, C. A., Arcoleo, K. J., Anson, E. A., Luckey, D. W., Knudtson, M. D., Henderson, C. R. & Stevenson, A. J. (2010). Enduring effects of prenatal and infancy home visiting by nurses on maternal life course and government spending: A follow-up of a randomized trial among children at age 12 years. *Archives of Pediatric and Adolescent Medicine, 164*(5), 419–424. https://doi.org/10.1001/archpediatrics.2010.49

Patient Protection and Affordable Care Act of 2010. (2010). Pub. L. No. 111-148. 124 § 119-1025.

Persaud, E., & Mitchell, A. (2021). Needlestick injuries among healthcare workers administering COVID-19 vaccinations in the United States. *New Solutions : a Journal of Environmental and Occupational Health Policy, 31*(1), 16–19. https://doi.org/10.1177/10482911211001483

Petitti, D. B. (2000). *Meta-analysis, decision analysis, and cost-effectiveness analysis: Methods for quantitative synthesis in medicine*. Oxford University Press.

Rambur, B., Vallett, C., Cohen, J. A., & Tarule, J. M. (2013). Metric-driven harm: An exploration of unintended consequences of performance measurement. *Applied Nursing Research, 26*(4), 269–272. https://doi.org/10.1016/j.apnr.2013.09.001

Recio-Saucedo, A., Dall'Ora, C., Maruotti, A., Ball, J., Briggs, J., Meredith, P., Redfern, O. C., Kovacs, C., Prytherch, D., Smith, G. B., & Griffiths, P. (2018). What impact does nursing care left undone have on patient outcomes? Review of the literature. *Journal of Clinical Nursing, 27*(11–12), 2248–2259. https://doi.org/10.1111/jocn.14058

Roberts, M. J., Hsiao, W., Berman, P., & Reich, M. R. (2008). *Getting health reform right: A guide to improving performance and equity*. Oxford University Press.

Ryan, A. M. (2013). Will valued-based purchasing increase disparities in care? *New England Journal of Medicine, 369*(26), 2472–2474. https://doi.org/10.1056/NEJMp1312654

Ryan, A. M., Krinsky, S., Maurer, K. A., & Dimick, J. B. (2017). Changes in hospital quality associated with hospital value-based purchasing. *New England Journal of Medicine, 376*(24), 2358–2366. https://doi.org/10.1056/NEJMsa1613412

Sensmeier, J., Carroll, W. M., & Carter-Templeton, H. (2021). Improving patient outcomes through sharable, comparable nursing data using a unique nurse identifier. *CIN: Computers, Informatics, Nursing, 39*(2), 61–62. https://doi.org/10.1097/CIN.0000000000000706

Smith, P. (1995). On the unintended consequences of publishing performance data in the public sector. *International Journal of Public Administration, 18*(23), 277–310. https://doi.org/10.1080/01900699508525011

Spetz, J. (2010). The importance of good data: How the National Sample Survey of Registered Nurses has been used to improve knowledge and policy. *Annual Review of Nursing Research*, *28*, 1–18. https://doi.org/10.1891/0739-6686.28.1

Spetz, J. (2013). The research and policy importance of nursing sample surveys and minimum data sets. *Policy, Politics and Nursing Practice*, *14*(1), 33–40. https://doi.org/10.1177/1527154413491149

Squires, D. A. (2013). *Multinational comparisons of health systems data, 2012*. The Commonwealth Fund. http://www.commonwealthfund.org/Publications/Chartbooks/2013/Mar/Multinational-Comparisons-of-Health-Data-2012.aspx

Stimpfel, A. W., Sloane, D. M., McHugh, M. D., & Aiken, L. H. (2016). Hospitals known for nursing excellence associated with better hospital experience for patients. *Health Services Research*, *51*(3), 1120–1134. https://doi.org/10.1111/1475-6773.12357

Stone, P. W., Bakken, S., Curran, C. R., & Walker, P. H. (2002). Evaluation of studies of health economics. *Evidence-Based Nursing*, *5*(4), 100–104. https://doi.org/10.1136/ebn.5.4.100

Swerissen, H., & Crisp, B. R. (2004). The sustainability of health promotion interventions for different levels of social organization. *Health Promotion International*, *19*(1), 123–130. https://doi.org/10.1093/heapro/dah113

Sworn, K., & Booth, A. (2020). A systematic review of the impact of "missed care" in primary, community and nursing home settings. *Journal of Nursing Management*, *28*(8), 1805–1829. https://doi.org/10.1111/jonm.12969

Taha, A., Ballou, M. M., & Lama, A. E. (2014). Utilization of national patient registries by clinical nurse specialist: Opportunities and implications. *Clinical Nurse Specialist*, *28*(10), 56–62. https://doi.org/10.1097/NUR.0000000000000018

Trepanier, S., Early, S., Ulrich, B., & Cherry, B. (2012). New graduate nurse residency program: A cost-benefit analysis based on turnover and contract labor usage. *Nursing Economic$*, *30*(4), 207–214. https://www.nursingeconomics.net

Twigg, D. E., Myers, H., Duffield, C., Giles, M., & Evans, G. (2015). Is there an economic case for investing in nursing care—what does the literature tell us? *Journal of Advanced Nursing*, *71*(5), 975–990. https://doi.org/10.1111/jan.12577

Wang, L. Y., Vernon-Smiley, M., Gapinski, M. A., Desisto, M., Maughan, E., & Sheetz, A. (2014). Cost-benefit study of school nursing services. *JAMA Pediatrics*, *168*(7), 642–648. https://doi.org/10.1001/jamapediatrics.2013.5441

Waters, T. M., Daniels, M. J., Bazzoli, G. J., Perencevich, E., Dunton, N., Staggs, V. S., Potter, C., Fareed, N., Liu, M. & Shorr, R. I. (2015). Effect of Medicare's nonpayment for hospital-acquired conditions: Lessons for future policy. *JAMA Internal Medicine*, *175*(3), 347–354. https://doi.org/10.1001/jamainternmed.2014.5486

CHAPTER 13

Eliminating Health Inequities Through National and Global Policy

SHANITA D. WILLIAMS AND JANICE M. PHILLIPS

Health inequities arise because of a toxic combination of poor social policies, unfair economic arrangements and bad politics. These, in turn, affect the circumstances in which people are born, grow, live, work and age.
—Sir Michael Marmot (2008)

OBJECTIVES

1. Explain the link between social and economic conditions, public policies, and population health inequity in the United States and globally.
2. Describe U.S. inequities and the global context in which health inequities exist.
3. Analyze the health impacts of the social determinants of health.
4. Evaluate the social, structural, economic, and health policy determinants of health inequities.
5. Identify evidence-based policy strategies to address social and economic conditions that shape health inequities.
6. Recommend potential policy solutions for health inequities in the United States and globally.

In early 2020, the conjunction of the spheres of public health and infectious disease epidemiology laid bare the insidious inequities that have plagued the United States and the world. The novel coronavirus disease (COVID-19) pandemic was a cataclysmic public health event that engulfed the entire world in a real-time dialogue about the true nature of systematic and enduring inequities. When COVID-19 struck, no one was immune, and everyone was at risk. Yet, COVID-19 quickly unmasked the underlying health risks borne disproportionately by the world's vulnerable populations. The advantaged—shielded by their material and social resource reserves, adequate and flexible employment, and access to food and healthcare services—quickly adjusted and rebounded from the initial threat of the coronavirus. While the poor, elderly, and socioeconomically, and culturally disadvantaged experienced mounting losses and enduring despair. Months into the pandemic, the disadvantaged were more likely to have lost a job (Couch et al., 2020; Crossley et al., 2021; Groeger, 2020), be at increased risk for housing instability (Cai & Fremstad, 2020; Chun, et al., 2020; Greene & McCargo, 2020), more likely to have experienced extreme financial hardship and food insecurity (Morales et al., 2020; U.S. Global Leadership Coalition, 2020), and two to four times more likely to experience severe illness and death (Centers for Disease Control and Prevention [CDC], 2020a;

Figueroa et al., 2021; Maness et al., 2021; Sanchez, 2020; Selden & Berdahl, 2020; U.S. Global Leadership Coalition, 2020). Furthermore, the patchwork of social and economic public policies or "safety net" that should have been activated to stabilize and support the vulnerable was overtaxed and quickly collapsed (Moffitt & Ziliak, 2020). The nation's safety net frayed and unraveled as a consequence of too much need, insufficient targeted resources, and poor social and economic policies (Moffitt & Ziliak, 2020).

As a result of the 2020 pandemic, we lost the sense that health is a human right and that government policies would provide timely relief to those most vulnerable. We gained new insights into how entrenched inequities and inadequate social and economic policies shape poor health outcomes. The global COVID-19 pandemic has revealed to us now, more than ever before, that inequities are indeed a consequence of global economic forces, the sociopolitical environment, and a society's level of commitment to social justice (Bhala et al., 2020; Yancy, 2020).

Throughout the world, health inequities are inextricably linked to the unequal distribution of social and economic resources. When an unplanned public health catastrophe such as COVID-19 strikes, it happens in the context where vulnerable populations are already less likely to be in good health, less likely to have access to quality healthcare and services, and more likely to die prematurely when compared with the socially and economically advantaged. In the United States, those who live in poverty, the uninsured, the disabled, and people of color bear the brunt of the health-inequities burden—these are the same populations that are experiencing extreme COVID-19 illness and dying at a rate two to four times that of advantaged populations (CDC, 2020a). It is the vulnerable populations in the United States and the world who lack the healthy reserve of material and social resources required to survive and rebound from mortal threats such as a global pandemic (Avram, 2020; Bhala et al., 2020; U.S. Global Leadership Coalition, 2020).

Registered nurses (RNs) comprise the largest segment of the U.S. professional healthcare workforce, with 3.1 million employed in 2019 (U.S. Department of Labor, Bureau of Labor Statistics [BLS], 2020). Nurses have always been at the center of the interface where health systems and patients, families, and communities intersect. Nurses are strategically positioned to serve as key actors to advocate for the health and well-being of the nation. It is no accident that nurses are on the front lines of the COVID-19 pandemic in 2020 where they willingly accept the responsibility and risks that come with being a frontline, essential professional workforce. However, in addition to their taking care of patients and families on the front lines, it is equally imperative that nurses champion the right social and economic policies that can interrupt the cycle of poverty, disadvantage, and poor health. Policy advocacy on behalf of society's disadvantaged should be a fundamental element of professional nursing practice.

When people learn about healthcare inequities, they may assume that inequity-related issues do not exist in their own communities. However, one need not travel very far to observe the adverse health and healthcare impacts of poor social policies that perpetuate the status quo. Addressing national and global health inequities requires upstream, long-range policy approaches at the big-P (e.g., congressional) level to address their underlying root causes. There are also numerous opportunities in which nurses advocating for better health and healthcare can address inequities in their local communities (e.g., little-p level) to make a more immediate impact on the health of people in need. To strengthen nurses' advocacy activities, it is imperative that nurses engage and partner across professions and sectors to support and codevelop effective policies to address systemic inequities in health and healthcare.

This chapter presents a broad overview of the link between social and economic policy and health inequities and highlights the health impacts of social determinants on populations in the United States and across the globe. The terms *inequalities* and *inequities* are frequently used interchangeably. It is worth clarifying the distinction between the two related terms. *Inequalities* is a more general term, has been in the use for a much longer time, and is used much more frequently around the world. *Health inequalities* refer to population health summary measures associated with group- or individual-level attributes or differences that can be compared such as income, education, or race and ethnicity (Braveman, 2014; Health Resources and Services Administration [HRSA], Office of Health Equity, 2018; U.S. Department of Health and Human Services [USDHHS] HHRSA, 2020). By contrast, the term *inequities* involves normative judgments about the nature of social-group differences. Inequities are basically inequalities that are unfair, unjust, avoidable, and unnecessary that can be reduced or remedied through effective policy actions (HRSA Office of Health Equity, 2018; USDHHS HRSA, 2020). The assumption that health differences are unjust or unfair and can be acted on is the fundamental distinction between an inequality and an inequity. We intentionally chose the term *inequities* to emphasize our fundamental belief that effective public policies can ensure social justice is achieved in society.

In the United States, the nature of health inequities has traditionally focused on racial, ethnic, and socioeconomic status (SES)/class inequities in health and healthcare. This focus has expanded in recent years to include sexual orientation and gender identity. This chapter aims to extend the health inequities discussion beyond U.S. borders to include a global context that presents poverty and disadvantage as the root cause of underlying health inequities both within the United States and across nations. We conclude with a discussion of globally-informed policy approaches that may mitigate the social, economic, and structural determinants that drive health inequities in the United States.

The Policy Challenge in the following section illustrates how harmful social policies targeting vulnerable populations fuel preexisting health conditions that place the nation's poor, elderly, rural, and racial/ethnic populations at increased risk for adverse outcomes for COVID-19 and other public health threats. We highlight the example of menthol-flavored tobacco use in African American communities targeted by tobacco companies.

In the United States, tobacco use is a major contributor to the three leading causes of death among African Americans—heart disease, cancer, and stroke (Heron, 2019). African American children and adults are more likely to be exposed to secondhand smoke than any other racial or ethnic group. Despite more quit attempts, African Americans are less successful at quitting than White and Latinx cigarette smokers, possibly because of lower utilization of cessation treatments such as counseling and medication and the disproportionately increased use of menthol tobacco products (Babb et al., 2017; CDC, 2020b). Researchers have shown that menthol cigarettes may be more addictive and dangerous when compared to nonmenthol cigarettes (CDC, 2020b; Food and Drug Administration [FDA], 2013). In cigarettes, menthol is thought to make harmful chemicals more easily absorbed in the body, likely because menthol makes it easier to inhale cigarette smoke (CDC, 2020b; FDA, 2013). The increased risk profile related to menthol cigarettes has forced tobacco companies to target their menthol products in resource-poor and disadvantaged communities—likely because more advantaged communities would not tolerate the additional risk burden of menthol products. As a consequence, the tobacco industry began targeting and marketing menthol products to young African Americans in urban communities as early as the 1950s (Kary, 2020).

The tobacco industry aggressively targeted African American communities using a classic marketing mix approach of "price, promotion, product, and place." Tobacco advertisers deployed multipronged efforts such as supporting cultural events, making contributions to minority higher education institutions, supporting elected officials, civic and community organizations, and scholarship programs (CDC, 2020b; FDA, 2013). In addition, tobacco companies promoted the use of menthol cigarettes through culturally tailored advertising images and messages (CDC, 2020b; Smokefree.gov, 2015). Larger amounts of targeted menthol cigarette advertising in African American publications have exposed African Americans to more cigarette ads than Whites and other racial and ethnic groups (CDC, 2020b). African American neighborhoods have more tobacco retailers per capita densely located within them, which contributes to greater tobacco advertising exposure (FDA, 2013). In addition, using a mix of price promotions, retail, and point-of-sale advertising, menthol products are given more shelf space in retail outlets within African American and other minority neighborhoods (CDC, 2020b; Center for Public Health Systems Science [CPHSS], 2014). Tobacco companies frequently use price promotions such as discounts and multipack coupons—which are most often used by African Americans and other minority groups, women, and young people—to increase sales (CDC, 2020b; CPHSS, 2014). As a consequence of these targeted efforts, African American adults have the highest percentage of menthol cigarette use when compared to other racial and ethnic groups (CDC, 2020b; Kary, 2020). In addition, approximately 70% of African American youth ages 12 to 17 years who smoke use menthol cigarettes (CDC, 2020b). Yet, the tobacco industry efforts have been enabled by societal-level tobacco policies harmful to African American and other similarly disadvantaged communities (CPHSS, 2014; Kary, 2020).

National and Global Health Inequities

Researchers are constantly uncovering the deleterious health effects and the social and economic costs that systemic and persistent inequities have on individuals,

POLICY CHALLENGE | **The Case of Marquis: An Illustration of How Failure to Ban the Sale of Mentholated Tobacco Products Perpetuates a Lifetime of Health Risk and Preventable Deaths**

Larger-than-life billboards depicting African American men smoking Marlboro cigarettes were a frequent occurrence in the impoverished neighborhood where 12-year-old Marquis lived when growing up. The depictions of stylish African American men dressed up in suits carrying a leather briefcase in one hand and a long cigarette in the other hand seemed cool to Marquis. While some of his family members were already smokers, nothing intrigued Marquis more than seeing seemingly successful Black men in tobacco marketing ads. As a pre-teen, Marquis was unable to purchase cigarettes legally; however, he had easy access to cigarettes through older friends who smoked, family members who smoked, and the local corner-store owner that sold loose, single, and cheap Marlboro cigarettes to whoever had the coins.

The cool and refreshing menthol sensation Marquis experienced when smoking was soothing and appealing. At age 12, smoking an occasional menthol cigarette was relaxing and seemed harmless. However, the addicting power of the menthol cigarette ignited his desire to smoke even more. Fast-forward 25 years—Marquis has been smoking two packs of cigarettes per day for 20 years, and his health risks and life trajectory have taken a totally predictable turn for the worst. Marquis, a 37-year-old African American male is living with a diagnosis of aggressive lung cancer and heart disease. In spite of his difficulty breathing due to his diagnoses, Marquis continues to smoke as he struggles to overcome his addiction to menthol-flavored cigarettes.

communities, and societies. Societies throughout the world with increased access to material and social resources—the educated, employed, socially connected—experience better health and longer life. Furthermore, this health advantage is patterned along a social and economic gradient whereby as one's status on the social and economic hierarchy increases, health progressively improves (Marmot & Allen, 2014; Singh et al., 2017; Singh & Jemal, 2017). Race/ethnicity, gender, sexual orientation, SES, and the natural and built environment are the social constructs on which inequities are built. Nurses who advocate for the elimination of national and global health inequities must be aware of how social constructs or determinants are used to shape the health and health outcomes of our patients, communities, and society.

With the global COVID-19 pandemic, public health and the environment are receiving much more attention in the United States and globally. Environmental exposures that fuel increased health risk and poor health outcomes are often overlooked in the discussion of health inequities. As in the case with COVID-19, there is often a fivefold increase in negative environmental exposures for the disadvantaged when compared with the advantaged populations (Gouveia, 2016; Landrigan et al., 2016; Sly et al., 2016). Negative environmental exposures include violent and unsafe neighborhoods, inadequate housing, injuries, noise pollution, poor sanitation, toxic waste, contaminated water supply, cigarette smoking, and exposure to secondhand smoke. Negative environmental exposures are not limited to other nations and can be found in many communities in the United States. See Policy Solution 13.1 later in this chapter for a discussion of how legislation, especially when enacted without applying a health equity lens, can perpetuate negative environmental impacts on the health and well-being of disadvantaged populations.

Race, Ethnicity, and U.S. Health Inequities

Social, economic, and class inequities that are pervasive and systemic across nations are frequently articulated in the United States as racial and ethnic disparities. Race and ethnicity have historically served as a proxy (or substitute) for SES and social class primarily because racial and ethnic minority groups in the United States are consistently overrepresented among the poor and disenfranchised. Racial/ethnic data collected in the United States have facilitated tracking disparities by racial and ethnic categories rather than by social class (National Research Council Panel on the DHHS Collection of Race and Ethnic Data et al., 2004). Yet race and ethnicity are complex social phenomena that have been shown to have real health impacts not fully explained by biological, genetic, or environmental determinants.

Take, for example, the case of Hispanic/Latino (or the gender- and LGBTQ-inclusive term *Latinx*) ethnicity and health outcomes in the United States. Researchers have shown that generally Whites experience improved health outcomes compared with racial and ethnic minorities. In a now-classic study, Jones et al. (2008) examined discordance between self-identified race and ethnicity (What race or ethnicity do you consider yourself?), socially assigned race and ethnicity (What race or ethnicity do others classify you?), and self-rated health outcomes (Do you rate your health as poor, fair, good, or excellent?). They found that Hispanics/Latinx who were socially assigned as "White," although they classified themselves as Hispanics/Latinx, experienced large and statistically significant advantages in health status relative to self-identified Hispanics/Latinx, who were also socially classified as Hispanics/Latinx (Jones et al., 2008). Furthermore, the socially assigned "White" Hispanics/Latinx experienced health outcomes that were statistically the same as U.S. Whites. The authors' major conclusion was that socially assigned categories of ethnicity had a significant and measurable impact on an individual's self-rating of health status.

The significant point about the findings of Jones et al. (2008) is that self-rated health is a proven proxy indicator of physical health outcomes, including morbidity and mortality (Harris et al., 2015; Lorem et al., 2020; Schnittker & Bacak, 2014). This example of self-identified versus socially assigned ethnicity is also important in that it reveals one mechanism by which socially assigned race and ethnicity in the United States can impact the physical health outcomes of members of a social group.

In the United States, it is the complex meaning of *race* and *ethnicity*, and the way they are used to assign value and life opportunities in society, that poses the greatest challenge to addressing health inequities, particularly those driven by race, ethnicity, and socioeconomic/class differences among populations. However, the global context allows us to understand more fully that even in the United States, health inequities are not simply about race and ethnicity. A global assessment of socioeconomic/class, gender, and sexual identity patterns of health inequities confirms the role of broader societal-level factors, such as human development, gender inequality, gross national product, income inequality, and healthcare system infrastructures, as the fundamental determinants of health inequities among populations and among nations (World Health Organization [WHO], 2017).

SOCIAL DETERMINANTS OF HEALTH INEQUITIES

> *The moral test of government is how that government treats those who are in the dawn of life—the children; those who are in the twilight of life—the elderly; those who are in the shadows of life—the sick, the [poor], and the [disabled].*
>
> —Hubert H. Humphrey (1977)

There is consensus among social and public health researchers that widespread health inequities experienced by social groups in the United States and throughout the world cannot be solely explained by individual-level determinants such as health-related behaviors. Consequently, there have been increased efforts to better understand factors that lie outside of an individual's control such as social-, economic-, and policy-related factors that contribute to persistent and inequitable health outcomes.

Social determinants of health (SDOHs) can be understood as the conditions in which people are born, grow, live, work, and age—including the health system—and are shaped by the distribution of money, power, and resources at global, national, and local levels, which are themselves influenced by policy choices. Research on SDOHs and their contribution to population health disparities emphasizes the complex role that social structures and economic systems play in the health of populations. WHO confirmed in its landmark 2008 Commission on the Social Determinants of Health report (WHO, CSDH, 2008) that SDOHs are indeed mostly responsible for health inequities—the unfair and avoidable factors in health status—within and among countries. By examining key economic and social conditions that collectively form the composite measure of SES—income and employment, education, and access to care and health insurance—we can illustrate the potential health impacts of social determinants on populations in the United States.

Income and Employment

Income and employment opportunities are critical to achieving and maintaining optimal health and accessing healthcare services (CDC, 2020a; HRSA Office of Health Equity, 2018; LEAD Center, 2015; Robert Wood Johnson Foundation [RWJF], 2013). Income and employment are directly related to morbidity and mortality outcomes in almost every health outcome. Health-related diabetes, cardiovascular disease (CVD), cancer, and infectious disease outcomes follow a consistent income and employment gradient: As income and employment increase, mortality and morbidity decrease. Subramanian and Kawachi (2004) state, "Income poverty is a risk factor for premature mortality and increased morbidity" (p. 78). Take, for example, the well-established association between income and CVD and its associated risk factors, such as hypertension, cholesterol, smoking, diabetes, and physical inactivity. Quarells et al. (2012) examined the impact of education, employment, income, and stress on CVD clinical risk factors in rural and urban men older than the age of 18. Quarells et al. reported that lower education, unemployment, lower income, and general stress were each significantly correlated with the presence of two or more CVD risk factors. In an earlier study of CVD risk and involuntary late-career unemployment, researchers found that displaced workers who lost their jobs late in their careers were more than twice as likely to have a myocardial infarction and stroke compared with employed persons (Gallo et al., 2006). The investigators recommended that healthcare providers consider involuntary unemployment a significant risk factor for CVD. In a recent 2020 Health Equity Report, government scientists found that unemployed adults had an 87% higher heart disease prevalence when compared to adults with full-time employment. Adults with lower education and income levels had a higher prevalence of heart disease compared to high-education, high-income adults (USDHHS HRSA, 2020).

One of the challenges with income and employment as a determinant of health is the lack of intergenerational income mobility or movement into the middle class. Disadvantaged groups are frequently not able to rise out of poverty and mitigate its attendant health risks. A 2013 study by Chetty et al. examined the degree to which children can rise out of poverty. Factors having a positive impact on increasing income mobility included (a) a greater geographical dispersion of the middle class, (b) better-than-average schools, (c) a higher proportion of two-parent households, and (d) an engagement with community and religious organizations (Chetty et al., 2013).

Education

Educational attainment is inextricably linked with income and employment and reliably influences future earning potential and employment opportunities (USDHHS HRSA, 2020). Poor, vulnerable, and disadvantaged children, youth, and young adults typically receive poor-quality education exposures and often fail to graduate from high school (Figure 13.1; de Brey et al., 2019; Musu-Gillette et al., 2017; U.S. Census Bureau, Current Population Survey, 2020). For example, nearly twice as many adults with disabilities did not complete high school and subsequently live below the poverty level compared with the U.S. adult population (Goodman et al., 2019).

A person's level of education is closely linked to global population health outcomes. There is a common expression applied to international education that states "when you educate a woman, you educate a nation. When girls are educated, their countries become stronger and more prosperous" (Wodon et al., 2018). Extensive

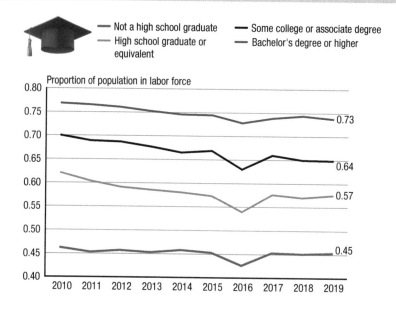

FIGURE 13.1 Labor force participation by level of education among population age 25 and older.

Source: U.S. Census Bureau, Current Population Survey. (2020). *Annual social and economic supplement (CPS ASEC) 2010-2019*. https://www.census.gov/library/visualizations/2020/comm/labor-force-by-education.html

national and international data show that women and girls who are educated and are gainfully employed in meaningful work are more likely to delay childbirth and to increase spacing between births and are less likely to deliver low-birth-weight infants. Hence, educated women are more likely to experience healthy maternal and childbirth outcomes (MacDorman et al., 2013, 2014; Matijasevich et al., 2012).

Infant mortality rate (IMR) is an important indicator of a nation's health (CDC, 2021; MacDorman et al., 2013; Mathews & Driscoll, 2017). The IMR is tracked and measured throughout the world, providing local and global comparative health-care outcome data for nations. In the United States, IMRs are highest among racial and ethnic minorities, the poor, and women living in southern states. As with maternal outcomes, infant mortality is also closely linked to education. Researchers have shown that education status and race and ethnicity interact and result in cumulative disadvantage, such that racial and ethnic minority women with low educational attainment experience the highest IMR among all women in the United States (Li & Keith, 2011; Singh & Kogan, 2007). In fact, there is a clear inverse association between educational attainment and IMR; as women's educational attainment increases, IMRs decrease. The IMR among mothers with less than a high school diploma is more than the IMR of mothers with a bachelor's or higher degree (Mathews et al., 2015). There is also mounting evidence that links lower education, poverty, and childhood obesity. Data from the CDC show that obese children miss more days of school compared with children with normal weights. More missed days at school are linked to poor academic performance, and poor academic performance is correlated with reduced employment opportunities and an increased likelihood of poverty in adulthood (CDC, 2017).

Access to Care and Health Insurance

Health insurance—private and, especially, employer-based insurance—is the gateway to accessing health and healthcare services in the United States. Higher status occupations and jobs are correlated with employer-based insurance, which is associated with increased access to healthcare services. Yet private, employer-based insurance, although considered the preferred method of payment by healthcare systems and its providers, can frequently lack key coverage provisions that require additional copays and deductible and other out-of-pocket costs. See Figure 13.2.

Often, persons in lower status occupations often lack employer-based health insurance and frequently do not have the resources available to pay for private insurance. Consequently, low-status occupations such as frontline and essential service-oriented, trade, and labor sectors populate the ranks of the uninsured in the United States. Hence, health insurance type (public, private, employer-based) is a key indicator of SES and social class status in the United States. The type of health insurance status is also strongly correlated with race, ethnicity, and SES. See Figure 13.3. Public insurance or Medicaid is a primary source of health insurance for racial and ethnic minorities and the poor, primarily because they are unemployed or hold part-time or full-time, lower sector occupations that frequently do not offer health insurance to their employees (Cha & Cohen, 2020). Several studies have shown that persons with public insurance or Medicaid experience decreased access to care and poor health outcomes comparable with outcomes for the uninsured population in the United States. In essence, having public health insurance or Medicaid offers no health advantages over having no insurance coverage (LaPar et al., 2010). Experts posit that as many as 2 million Black/African Americans and 3 million Hispanic/Latino/Latinx may lose their employee-sponsored insurance coverage by the end of 2020, further widening the equity gaps in healthcare coverage (Sloan et al., 2020; Waddill, 2020).

Healthcare workers are not immune to having inadequate health insurance. Approximately 11% of the healthcare workforce lack quality health insurance, with ambulatory care workers being 3.1 times more likely and residential workers

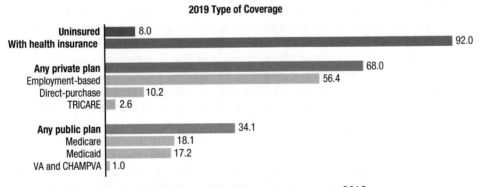

FIGURE 13.2 Percentage of people by type of health insurance coverage, 2019.

Source: U.S. Census Bureau, Current Population Survey. (2020). *Annual social and economic supplement (CPS ASEC).* https://www.census.gov/library/visualizations/2020/demo/p60-271.html

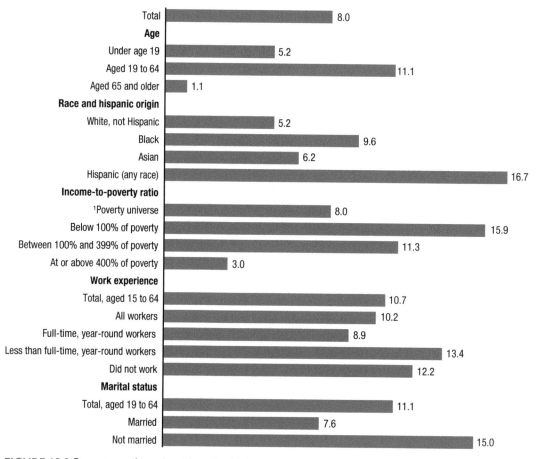

FIGURE 13.3 Percentage of people without health insurance coverage by selected characteristics: 2019.

Source: U.S. Census Bureau, Current Population Survey. (2020). *Annual social and economic supplement* (CPS ASEC). https://www.census.gov/content/dam/Census/library/visualizations/2020/demo/p60-271/figure2.pdf

4.3 times more likely to be uninsured; service workers are 50% more likely to lack insurance than are workers involved in diagnosing and treating illness (Chou et al., 2009). Similar results were found in an earlier study, with 23.8% of health aides, 14.5% of licensed practical nurses, and 5% of RNs uninsured; for employment setting, 20% of nursing home workers, 8.2% of medical office workers, and 8.7% of hospital workers were uninsured (Case et al., 2002). Very often, per diem nurses and adjunct nurse faculty have several part-time positions and thus do not have health insurance.

Cancer survival offers another example of the link between health insurance status and health inequities. Niu et al. (2013) found that uninsured and Medicaid-insured patients with breast, colorectal, lung, non-Hodgkin lymphoma, bladder, and prostate cancers had significantly higher risks of death than privately insured patients. Similarly, Robbins et al. (2010) reported in a study of patients with rectal cancer in which those with Medicaid insurance or no insurance were twice as likely to die in 5 years than were patients with private insurance.

The researchers found that the disparity in risk of death from cancer by insurance status was approximately 15.5 times larger than the disparity in risk of death from noncancerous causes (Robbins et al., 2010). Furthermore, insurance status is associated with not only inequities in cancer survival but also differences in cancer stage at diagnosis and treatment options. The American Cancer Society reported that a lack of health insurance, along with other barriers, prevents Americans from receiving optimal cancer care. Despite the passage of the Patient Protection and Affordable Care Act (ACA) in 2010, Latinx and Blacks remain most likely to be uninsured (16.7% and 9.6%, respectively). This compares to 5.2% of non-Hispanic Whites (U.S. Census Bureau, Current Population Survey, 2020). The uninsured and members of racial and ethnic minority groups are more likely to be diagnosed with a late-stage cancer, resulting in fewer, costlier, and less effective treatment and poorer cancer outcomes (American Cancer Society, 2020). Cancer is an example of the impact of health insurance status on health outcomes because it highlights the role of insurance as a gateway to healthcare services. A cancer diagnosis also exposes the cumulative effects of disadvantage over the life course, whereby the progression of cancer from initiation to detection can be a marker of cumulative social, economic, and political disadvantage (Halfon et al., 2020).

Illness accompanied by a lack of insurance can be a pathway to poverty. The COVID-19 pandemic of 2020 is a case example. According to the World Bank, the COVID-19 pandemic will fuel extreme poverty worldwide. Policy experts project that the global pandemic and economic crisis will push 1.4% of the global population into extreme poverty, with estimates of poverty rising from the current 88 million to 150 million people worldwide (World Bank, 2020). Racial ethnic minorities and other underserved populations who already lack employment or access to a livable wage and health insurance are at an increased risk for extreme poverty (World Bank, 2020).

In addition to racial and ethnic minorities and the poor, other vulnerable populations such as the nation's disabled populations and low-income seniors also depend on Medicaid as both a primary and a secondary source of health insurance. Persons with disabilities and low-income seniors are continually threatened by the potential of inequities in healthcare access and lower quality care services. Hence, quality, coordinated, and accessible care is a critical issue for all uninsured vulnerable populations, as well as those dependent on Medicaid. The Medicaid expansion resulting from the enactment of the ACA has had a significant impact on improving the health and well-being of our most vulnerable and underserved populations. Since the implementation of ACA exchanges and Medicaid expansion in October 2013, an additional 25.2% or 14.2 million people in 49 states enrolled in Medicaid and the Children's Health Insurance Program Payment and Access Commission (2020). Expanding access to care through Medicaid and ensuring that Medicaid users receive equitable healthcare is necessary for ensuring greater equity in health coverage and healthcare services. Nurses are in a key position to advocate for equitable, quality care for all persons, regardless of insurance status. For a detailed discussion of Medicaid-related issues and priorities for the expansion of Medicaid via the ACA as presented by the Kaiser Family Foundation, please visit www.kff.org/Medicaid.

HEALTH POLICY: NATIONAL AND GLOBAL

Health policy is a subcategory within social policy, and social policy is located within the larger framework of public policy. Public policies inform social policies, which in turn shape health policy at the local, state, national, and global levels. Policies frequently reflect unspoken values and are in turn shaped by the economic and political climates of countries. Policy efforts can be directed to act at the level of the individual within countries or can influence action on the SDOHs, which operate outside the level of the individual and across nations. Yet policy-making is insignificant unless policies are implemented more broadly in society.

What does it take to interrupt the cycle of social and economic disadvantage so closely linked with health inequities throughout the world and the United States? There is a general national and international consensus that addressing health inequities requires cross-sectoral policy solutions that span the life course. Put simply, eliminating health inequities requires equitable access to the material and social resources necessary for health. Therefore, effective U.S. and global policies to eliminate health inequities must contain, to some extent, elements of effective education, employment, and housing policies, among others. Policy solutions and committed resources are also necessary to achieve population health equity.

Despite the continued uncertainty regarding the future of the ACA in its current form, the need to reduce health inequities in the United States remains an ongoing and critical challenge. Social and economically disadvantaged populations continue to experience disproportionate adverse health impacts compared with their advantaged counterparts. Healthy People 2020 had broadened its focus on eliminating disparities to include a focus on achieving health equity, eliminating disparities, and improving the health of all groups (USDHHS, 2014), Healthy People 2030 has maintained focus on achieving health equity (USDHHS HRSA Office of Health Equity, 2020). The ACA's increased emphasis on improving community and population health, in addition to increasing individuals' access to care, has mandated that hospitals and health systems step up their efforts to contribute to the improvement of community and population health outcomes through its *Community Benefit Standards* (Carroll-Scott et al., 2017). However, despite the *Community Benefit Standards* that had been in effect for nearly a decade, when COVID-19 emerged as a worldwide pandemic and threat to the public's health, hospitals and community health systems were under-resourced and unprepared to take on the public health crisis. At the beginning of the pandemic, the U.S. House of Representatives passed the ambitious Health and Economic Recovery Omnibus Emergency Solutions Act (HEROES Act, 2020) to stimulate a failing economy precipitated by an economic shutdown and massive job losses. However, the legislation failed to pass the Senate. Nearly one year into the pandemic, through the Coronavirus Aid, Relief, and Economic Security Act (CARES Act; U.S. Department of Treasury, 2020), there remains only a patchwork of legislation to support a U.S. public health safety net under severe strain. The global hunger crisis is a sign of the fragile safety net in the United States and around the world. World hunger has intensified during the 2020 coronavirus pandemic. Nations throughout the world face the double threat of hunger and the coronavirus, and millions of children and families are facing food insecurity for the first time (Huizar et al., 2020; Wolfson & Lueng, 2020).

In the next section, we discuss in detail a policy-driven strategy, Health in All Policies, which holds promise for strengthening the nation's safety net, improving population health outcomes, and reducing health inequities.

Health in All Policies

Health in All Policies (HiAP) is a collaborative approach to improving population health by incorporating health considerations into the policymaking process. The HiAP: Framework for Country Action mandate originated with the WHO (2013) and has since gained momentum in the United States and around the world. The HiAP field resonates with the current emphasis on embracing upstream approaches to address health inequities by acknowledging the role of SDOH in influencing health outcomes. The HiAP approach to policymaking integrates the social determinants known to influence health (i.e., housing, education, food security, transportation), into public policies. In the United States, several state, federal, and local governments have adopted the HiAP approach in their policies and policy decision-making (Rudolph et al., 2013). Multiple sectors, such as housing, transportation, streets and sanitation, and public education, to name a few, are considering the health implications when designing their public policy agendas. Multisectoral collaboration across sectors and policy areas in government is necessary to ensure the success of a HiAP approach. Webb (2012) provides an excellent discussion on evidence-based policymaking and outlines the policies needed to modify factors influencing health, noting that to be optimally effective, policy work needs to be focused at the appropriate level. See Exhibit 13.1—a quick guide with local-, state-, and federal-level policy approaches for a variety of social determinants. Proponents of the HiAP approach believe that collaboration across various sectors can improve efficiencies, reduce redundancy, facilitate sharing of resources, and reduce cost and improve outcomes (Williams et al., 2018).

Multisectoral policies that have the greatest impact on health include early childhood care and youth development, child poverty, inclusive economic investment strategies, and programs to enhance job readiness and promote fair, equitable, and safe work opportunities and conditions. See Exhibit 13.2 for a select list of SDOHs, potentially impactful policies, and opportunities for nurses to advocate on behalf of poor, disadvantaged, and vulnerable populations within these four policy-sensitive areas.

EXHIBIT 13.1   LEVELS OF EVIDENCE-BASED ADVOCACY TO ADDRESS DISPARITIES IN THE SOCIAL DETERMINANTS OF HEALTH

In order to be most effective, advocacy for the various policy strategies described in this review must be directed to the proper policymaking entity. This table provides a guide as to which level of government advocates should approach regarding the respective evidence-based policy strategies.

Policy to Modify Factors Influencing Health	POINT(S) OF POLICY ADVOCACY		
	Local	**State**	**Federal**
Economic and Social Conditions			
Child and Youth Development/Education			
Home Visiting	•	•	•
Family Income Supplementation	•	•	•
Early Childhood Development Programs*	•	•	•
Economic Development			
Training Incentives		•	
Entrepreneurship Training	•	•	
Enterprise Zones		•	•
Empowerment Zones			•

(continued)

EXHIBIT 13.1   LEVELS OF EVIDENCE-BASED ADVOCACY TO ADDRESS DISPARITIES IN THE SOCIAL DETERMINANTS OF HEALTH (*CONTINUED*)

Policy to Modify Factors Influencing Health	POINT(S) OF POLICY ADVOCACY		
	Local	State	Federal
Poverty Reduction			
Transfer Programs		•	•
Living Wage Ordinances	•	•	•
Expanded Health Insurance		•	•
Living and Working Conditions			
Healthy Homes			
Integrated Post Management	•	•	
In-Home Tailored Asthma Interventions*	•	•	
Smoke-Free Policies*	•	•	
Lead Hazard Control*	•	•	•
Housing Choice Voucher Program*		•	•
Healthy Neighborhoods			
Urban Design and Land Use*	•		
Farmers' Markets	•		
Community Gardens	•		
Transportation-Related Improvements	•	•	
Zoning Ordinances	•		
Retail Food Stores	•	•	•
School-Based Violence Reduction*	•		

Source: Reprinted with permission from Webb, B. C. (2012). Moving upstream: Policy strategies to address social, economic, and environmental conditions that shape health inequities. Joint Center for Political and Economic Studies. https://jointcenter.org/wp-content/uploads/2014/06/Moving-UpStream.-Policy-Strategies.pdf

* *Sufficient evidence-base to support widespread implementation.*

Global Policies to Reduce and Eliminate Health Inequities

Globally, several countries have mobilized and formed regional alliances to develop frameworks that address the SDOH and health inequity within the context of a nation's political, social, and economic systems. In a call for public health advocates for public policy to address social inequities throughout the world, George Annas (2013) wrote:

> The health and human rights movement should be able to make a difference by focusing public health advocacy on promoting a universally accepted framework of government obligations. Evidence-based public health advocates should loudly and insistently make the case for governments to put population-based prevention programs, such as vaccination, clean water, decent sanitation, basic medical care, and a universally available safety net, as budgetary priority items—ones that should be protected and even expanded in times of economic recession and depression, when vulnerable populations are most at risk. (p. 967)

Many resource-poor and developing nations around the globe are working in concert with governmental and private-sector entities to develop public health infrastructures to deliver population-level healthcare to meet the needs of its citizens (Council on Foreign Relations, 2013). Private foundations are also taking a leading role. For example, the Clinton Foundation (n.d.) began an initiative in 2002 to address the HIV/AIDS crisis in developing nations. This has been expanded to include work on malaria, access to new vaccines, and efforts to lower infant mortality. The Bill and Melinda Gates Foundation (n.d.) is working to address hunger and poverty through investment in science and technology. In the United States, the public health infrastructure also needs increased funding and coordination of multiple sectors and resources to meet the public health needs of the population.

Maani and Galea (2020a, 2020b) argue that the decline in federal support for building public health infrastructure coupled with a lack of predictable funding for public health has hampered the nation's ability to render a robust preparedness and response effort to the current pandemic. These authors note that our preoccupation with the political discourse did not serve us well regarding containing the infectious disease outbreak. As our state public health departments continue to be underfunded, federal support is needed to build a more robust response to public health threats across the entire country. Maani and Galea (2020a, 2020b) call for a bipartisan commitment to funding public health infrastructure as a critical step toward ensuring economic security and better health for the U.S. population.

U.S. Healthcare System: Policy and Legislation

Health care systems are social and cultural institutions, that are built out of the existing social structure, and carry its inequities within them.
—Mackintosh (2001, p. 175)

Healthcare systems play a key role in generating and perpetuating social group health inequities. The U.S. healthcare system is a complex amalgamation of private, for-profit, and public entities (e.g., military, veterans) with various health service and delivery goals. The healthcare system is expected to deliver quality healthcare services to meet the health needs of the population, increase access to care for disadvantaged and underserved populations, and decrease health and healthcare inequities. Furthermore, the health system must interface and balance the interests of patients and consumers, businesses and purchasers, labor, health plans, clinicians and providers, communities and states, and suppliers. Too frequently, however, the U.S. health system enables exclusionary and inequitable practices that limit access based on health and healthcare by insurance status. Limiting care based on payment methods or inability to pay routinely results in inequitable healthcare experiences.

The ACA (2010) is one of the most comprehensive pieces of legislation enacted in the past 40 years and has direct implications for eliminating health inequities. The passage of the ACA presented new opportunities for implementing cross-cutting interventions and strategies that are driven by economic and educational policy framed in the context of the SDOH. The ACA intentionally created a paradigm shift from a focus on disease management to health promotion. This shift not only addressed healthcare reform but also created more opportunities to eliminate health inequities. Included among other provisions are specific efforts to address minority health within the federal government. Offices of Minority Health were created within six federal agencies: The Agency for Healthcare Research and

EXHIBIT 13.2 SELECT SOCIAL DETERMINANTS OF HEALTH, POTENTIAL IMPACTFUL SOCIAL POLICIES, AND NURSE ADVOCACY OPPORTUNITIES

SOCIAL DETERMINANT	DEFINITION	NEED/RATIONALE	EVIDENCE-BASED PROGRAMS/POLICIES	NURSE ADVOCACY OPPORTUNITIES
CHILD AND YOUTH EDUCATION AND DEVELOPMENT				
ECE (Aron et al., 2015; Webb, 2012)	Critical period in a child's development of personality, cognition, language, and behavior Establishes a solid and broad foundation for lifelong learning and well-being	Children with low SES backgrounds experience increased physical, social, emotional, language, cognitive, and behavioral delays Delayed ECE is linked to depression, attention deficits, and poor academic achievement in later school years	Maternal, Infant, and Child Home Visiting Programs Early Childhood Development Programs Early Childhood Education (pre-school/pre-K) Programs Childcare assistance programs Food/nutrition programs	Partner with ECE professionals to support ECE funding/programs Support universal access to quality and affordable childcare education/services Support high-quality free ECE for low- and middle-income families Support publicly funded center-based programs for children 3–5 years of age
Child Poverty (Kirkpatrick et al., 2010; Osypuk et al., 2014; Wicks-Lim & Arno, 2017)	Condition in which a child lacks basic resources such as food, clothing, and shelter that may inhibit social, emotional, language, cognitive, and behavioral development Children experience poverty as an environment damaging to their mental, physical, emotional, and spiritual development	The majority of poverty-stricken children are born to poor parent(s) The major cause of child poverty is adult poverty fueled by low education attainment, unemployment, housing instability and food insecurity, and single parent/caregiver households Childhood poverty produces negative impacts on education, nutrition/health, psychological, and behavioral/social outcomes that persist into adulthood and subsequent generations	Programs to increase parent/caregiver education attainment /employment opportunities Policies to supplement parental/caregiver household income (e.g., Federal Earned Income Tax Credits) Educational development opportunities for parent/caregivers Fair housing opportunities Universal child health benefits/insurance	Support policies/programs to address adult/child poverty Support programs that expand economic opportunities for disadvantaged/rural girls Influence policy dialogue on poverty reduction to include children's experience of poverty in addition to poverty's negative economic and social impacts

Youth Development (Aron et al., 2015; Gennetian et al., 2012; Webb, 2012)	Process that prepares a young person to meet the challenges of adolescence and adulthood and achieve their full potential Activities and experiences that help youth develop social, ethical, emotional, physical, and cognitive competencies	Programs demonstrate a positive effect on the youth's school achievement, motivation, and social behavior, especially for boys	Educational development opportunities for youth School–community partnerships School-based centers for disadvantaged young people Community-based mentoring programs (i.e., Big Brothers Big Sisters of America; 4-H Clubs) Rehabilitative and violence prevention programs	Support efforts of other youth, adults, communities, government agencies, and schools to provide opportunities for youth to enhance their interests, skills, and abilities Support policies and legislation that advance youth development Inject ideas and information about youth development into communications with lawmakers Become an expert on the dynamic challenges in the youth development policy field
FAIR EMPLOYMENT AND LIVING WAGE				
Living Wage (Aron et al., 2015; Osypuk et al., 2014)	Affords the wage earner and their family the most basic costs of living without the need for government support or poverty programs	Policies that provide additional income can be effective in improving health	Statutory minimum wages FLSA Program	Support federal, state, and local minimum wage campaigns

(continued)

EXHIBIT 13.2   SELECT SOCIAL DETERMINANTS OF HEALTH, POTENTIAL IMPACTFUL SOCIAL POLICIES, AND NURSE ADVOCACY OPPORTUNITIES (*CONTINUED*)

SOCIAL DETERMINANT	DEFINITION	NEED/RATIONALE	EVIDENCE-BASED PROGRAMS/POLICIES	NURSE ADVOCACY OPPORTUNITIES
Job Security (Bambra et al., 2010)	An assurance that an individual will keep their job without the risk of becoming unemployed Continuity in employment	Job security offers greater economic security and increased ability to accumulate wealth, enabling individuals to obtain healthcare when needed, to provide themselves and their families with more nutritious foods, and to live in safer and healthier homes and neighborhoods with supermarkets, parks, and places to exercise—all of which can promote good health by making it easier to adopt and maintain healthy behaviors	Job/skills development and training FMLA Paid parental leave	Support policies and programs that increase education and job training opportunities Support policies that maintain employment security after the birth or adoption of a child or other major life event
Safe Working Conditions (Burgard & Lin, 2013)	Workplace free of known health and safety hazards to reduce the risk of accidental injury, death, or disease	Lower paying jobs are associated with more occupational hazards, including environmental and chemical exposures (e.g., pesticides, asbestos) and poor working conditions (e.g., shift work with few breaks, potentially harmful tools) that put them at higher risk of injury and fatality	Workplace safety laws (e.g., OSHA) State worker's compensation programs	Support labor laws that ensure employers enforce safety standards for employees

Education Attainment (Aron et al., 2015; Webb, 2012)	Highest degree of education an individual has completed	Educational attainment is a powerful and valid predictor of SES, long-term health and well-being, and quality of life Plays a significant role in shaping employment opportunities and increasing social and personal resources Increased educational attainment leads to better employment opportunities and higher income, which are linked with better health	Supplemental funding for public education State Need Grant programs Higher Education Affordability programs such as (i.e., College Bound Scholarships) college and career readiness programs Recruit and retain adult students Work-based learning programs	Support educational attainment policies such as Student Achievement Councils Promote workforce training and employment services Support Title I of the Workforce Investment Act Support legislation addressing entrepreneurship education at the K–12 level

SOCIAL PROTECTION

Income Inequality (Aron et al., 2015; Marr et al., 2015; Osypuk et al., 2014; Webb, 2012; Wicks–Lim & Arno, 2017)	The unequal distribution of income and opportunity between advantaged and disadvantaged groups in society	Inequalities in income/wealth, education, nutrition, and healthcare access contribute to health inequities	Earned income tax credits Child tax credits Unemployment insurance Minimum wage laws Universal health benefits/ expanded health insurance	Support family income supplementation programs and policies

(continued)

SOCIAL DETERMINANT	DEFINITION	NEED/RATIONALE	EVIDENCE-BASED PROGRAMS/POLICIES	NURSE ADVOCACY OPPORTUNITIES
Social Status (Osypuk et al., 2014; Webb, 2012)	A person's standing or importance in relation to other people within a society. The relative rank that an individual holds, with attendant rights, duties, and lifestyle, in a social hierarchy based on honor or prestige	Social status is linked to health outcomes; as social status increases, health and health outcomes improve	Entrepreneurship training	Support maternal, child, and youth development policies and programs. Support education and job training policies and programs
LIVING ENVIRONMENT				
Affordable/ Safe Housing (Acevedo-Garcia et al., 2004; Bambra et al., 2010; Ludwig et al., 2011)	Affordable dwelling is one that a household can obtain for 30% or less of its income. A dwelling is considered "affordable" for low-income families if it costs less than 24% of the area median income	Strong association between better housing conditions and better over-all health, less substance abuse, less neighborhood disorder, less violence exposure, higher rates of employ-ment, and lower rates of public assistance.	Housing mobility. Zoning ordinances. Empowerment zones. Housing Choice Voucher Program. Tenant-based rental assis-tance programs	Support the Fair Housing Act and policies to eliminate redlining. Support increased funding for tenant-based rental assistance programs

Food Security (Gundersen & Ziliak, 2015; Kirkpatrick et al., 2010; Webb, 2012)	The availability and adequate access at all times to sufficient, safe, nutritious food to maintain a healthy and active life. When all people, at all times, have physical, social, and economic access to sufficient, safe, and nutritious food that meets their dietary needs and food preferences for an active and healthy life.	Food insecurity in children can lead to developmental impairments and long-term consequences such as weakened physical, intellectual, and emotional development. Food insecurity also related to obesity for people living in neighborhoods where nutritious food are unavailable or unaffordable	School Nutrition Programs (e.g., National School Breakfast/Lunch Programs) Federal nutrition programs (e.g., Supplemental Nutrition Assistance Program; Women, Infant and Child Program; Child and Adult Care Food Program) Public–private partnerships with local farmer's markets Community garden initiatives	Advocate for school subsidies to support free/reduced-price breakfast and lunches for school-age children Start/support a local community garden

ECE, early childhood education; FLSA, Fair Labor Standards Act; FMLA, Family and Medical Leave Act; OSHA, Occupational Safety and Health Act; SES, socioeconomic status.

Source: Reprinted with permission from Williams, S. D., Phillips, J. M., & Koyama, K. (2018, September 30). Nurse advocacy: Adopting a Health in All Policies approach. *OJIN: The Online Journal of Issues in Nursing, 23*(3), 1. https://doi.org/10.3912/OJIN.Vol23No03Man01

Quality, the CDC, the Centers for Medicare and Medicaid Services, the FDA, HRSA, and the Substance Abuse and Mental Health Services Administration.

The National Prevention Council, which consists of 17 federal agencies, including housing, transportation, and labor, launched a national healthcare strategy that is well aligned with the HiAP collaborative approach. (National Prevention Council, 2011). The national strategy involves a multisector structure across the federal government to address the social determinants (e.g., housing, transportation, labor, education) known to impact health inequities. The activities associated with the national prevention strategy are designed to reduce the leading causes of preventable death and major illness through tobacco-free living, the prevention of drug abuse and excessive alcohol use, healthy eating, active living, injury- and violence-free living, reproductive and sexual health, and mental and emotional well-being.

The Coronavirus Aid, Relief, and Economic Security Act of 2020 also known as the CARES Act is the most comprehensive piece of legislation signed into law since the 2010 ACA. The U.S. Congress appropriated more than $4 trillion in response to the COVID-19 pandemic that infected more than 18 million people and caused more than 325,000 deaths as of December 2020. The CARES Act began as a $2.2 trillion economic stimulus bill signed into law on March 27, 2020, in response to the economic fallout of the COVID-19 pandemic in the United States. To date, the *CARES Act* legislation is the largest economic stimulus package in U.S. history, amounting to 10% of total U.S. gross domestic product. The legislation attempted to mitigate the ballooning unemployment and housing crisis early in the pandemic. Later in December 2020, the U.S. Congress passed $900 billion in subsequent legislation, COVID-19 Emergency Relief, to provide additional financial support for a faltering economy and collapsing safety net. Hundreds of billions of dollars were allocated for critical social determinants, including unemployment, direct rental assistance, housing, nutrition assistance, and transportation. The massive cross-sectoral legislative investments made clear that social and economic policies, population health, and health inequities were inextricably linked.

Nurses should engage and support federal legislation such as the ACA and the CARES Act, which increase access to healthcare and reduce health inequities. However, opportunities to reduce health inequities also exist on the local level (see Policy on the Scene 13.1). The first step for nurses is to be aware of policies and resources within their own local communities. Nurses can share with their local legislators, the media, and policy decision-makers their firsthand knowledge of how social and economic determinants, such as low income, lower educational attainment, and limited access to healthcare and services negatively impact health outcomes. Nurses should advocate for the provision of resources to address social determinants that are negatively impacting disadvantaged populations in their communities. Cross-sectoral initiatives to reduce health inequities can only be strengthened with nurse involvement and nurse advocacy.

IMPLICATIONS FOR THE FUTURE

We have presented considerable evidence of the nature and impact of health inequities in our society. The following are trends that can have a powerful impact on health inequities: (a) increased demands for cross-sectoral partnerships to effect social and economic policies that increase equity, (b) a greater recognition of the role of community in reducing health inequities, (c) expanded and sustained implementation of healthcare reform, and (d) a greater recognition of environmental

POLICY ON THE SCENE 13.1: THE RACIAL EQUITY RAPID RESPONSE TEAM: INTERSECTION OF BIG-P AND LITTLE-P

The Racial Equity Rapid Response Team (RERRT) is a community-partnered approach to stopping the spread of the coronavirus (American Medical Association, 2021). No doubt, the COVID-19 pandemic has had a disproportionate impact on African Americans communities across the nation. Chicago's Department of Health data revealed that approximately 68% of the city's death from COVID-19 were among African Americans. While African American Chicagoans make up 30% of the city's population, they are more than six times likely to die from the virus when compared to White Chicagoans. The sobering statistics on COVID-19 in Chicago prompted a swift and targeted response from government and community leaders across the city, particularly in neighborhoods where large proportions of Blacks and other minorities reside (City of Chicago–Office of the Mayor, 2020).

The City of Chicago's Office of the Mayor collaborated with community organizations and leaders to deliver a robust public health response to eradicate the spread of the deadly virus by targeting three high-risk predominately African American communities. Community-engagement strategies focus on education, prevention, testing, treatment, and supportive services. The response team is responsible for creating culturally tailored messages, strengthening prevention, and tracing outreach initiatives, as well as coordinating the distribution of protective equipment and supplies to those in need. Since its creation in April 2019, the RERRT has secured $3.1 million in grant funding, hosted seven virtual town hall meetings in neighborhoods heavily impacted by the virus, and opened eight city testing sites in communities of color. U.S. cities have responded to the COVID-19 disparity in various ways, and Chicago's RERRT was a cross-sectoral initiative created to address the devastating impact of the virus in African American communities. Although the RERRT initiative has shown promise in mitigating the negative impacts of COVID-19, long-term and sustained public health policies and programs that offer redress to societal inequities way beyond the COVID pandemic are needed. Without resources and dedication, the goal of achieving health equity will remain far from becoming a reality for those most in need.

POLICY SOLUTION | The Case of Marquis: An Illustration of How Childhood Exposures to Toxic Environments Equals a Lifetime of Health Disadvantage

The Policy Challenge illustrated how legislation, especially when enacted without applying a consideration of equity, can perpetuate the ongoing inequities in health and healthcare experienced by communities of color. Marquis' story of addiction to menthol cigarettes began years ago while growing up in a poor, midwestern city neighborhood that was the subject of targeted and intense tobacco marketing campaigns. Members of his inner-city community had limited to no access to smoking cessation resources. The oversaturation of tobacco messages coupled with few antismoking resources has created the conditions for the disproportionate tobacco-related health risks for Marquis and members of his community.

Despite the grim tobacco-related equity data for African Americans and other disadvantaged populations, there has been limited progress relative to banning menthol-flavored tobacco products. In 2009, the Family Smoking Prevention and Tobacco Control Act (TCA) gave the U.S. FDA authority over tobacco products (U.S. FDA, 2020). This tobacco legislation called for a ban on flavored cigarettes but failed to direct a ban on menthol-flavored tobacco products. Some experts posit that as many as 237,000 African American tobacco-related deaths could have been prevented if provisions to ban menthol products were included in the 2009 legislation (Levy, et al., 2011). Ten years after the enactment of the 2009 TCA legislation, Massachusetts, in 2019, became the first state to restrict the sale of all flavored tobacco products, including menthol cigarettes. Yet, in 2020, in Marquis's Chicago hometown, the city council voted to prohibit the sale of all flavored e-cigarettes but failed to legislate a ban on menthol-flavored tobacco products. The continued failure to ban menthol-flavored cigarettes contributes to the excess mortality and morbidity already experienced among disadvantage and resource-poor African Americans.

The right policies and interventions are critical to interrupting the cycle of tobacco use among children and youth and thereby reducing the long-term sequela of chronic illness and premature death, regardless of racial ethnicity or community. Evidence-based, equitable policies can ensure healthier environments and communities and address the harmful effects of targeting and saturating a community with harmful products and devices. Beginning in January 2021, California will implement State Bill (SB) 793, legislation prohibiting the sale of flavored tobacco products, including vapes and menthol cigarettes (*Los Angeles Times*, 2020).

Marquis' story is emblematic of social disadvantage and targeted policies that are known to contribute harm to specific populations in society. Poor policies lie at the very root of most chronic diseases and other health inequities. The tobacco industry's tactics are not focused solely on the United States. Marquis' story is repeated in resource-poor and disadvantaged cultures and communities throughout the world. The key question for nurses then becomes, what implications does Marquis' story have for U.S. and global policies on health and healthcare inequities? What can nurses do as a profession and in collaboration with other stakeholders to address tobacco and other healthcare inequities? Nurses must be actively engaged in advocating for equitable policies that enable health and well-being for all populations in society. The right policies can change the trajectory of Marquis' health and others like him.

impacts on health. These trends will impact how nurses can and should work in the future.

Our society is increasingly interconnected. Although overall population health indices have improved, we have not made progress in all segments of societies with regard to increasing quality of life and overall life expectancy (USDHHS HRSA, Office of Health Equity, 2020). With an ever-growing and irrefutable body of research demonstrating that where one lives matters in terms of health, a greater focus will be on ensuring that our communities are healthy places to live and work. Success in improving health and reducing inequities will require engagement and commitment at a local level. Healthy communities will become increasingly critical when addressing the underlying causes of health inequities such as access to quality education, safe places for children to play, and work environments free of health hazards. Recognizing that health inequities harm everyone will result in an increase in collaborative partnerships of all types: government–private, local–state, education–health, and business–government, to name a few. These partnerships will bring together key stakeholders who recognize that each sector of the community has resources and expertise that can be used together to improve health.

The incidence of natural disasters, such as the COVID-19 worldwide pandemic, will continue to exert a disproportionately devastating impact on the physical, mental, and emotional health of the world's most vulnerable populations. Natural disasters such as the 2020 pandemic and unfolding disasters such as climate change will continue to burden, strain, and break down our community's safety net and healthcare infrastructure. Thus, any efforts to address health inequities must be coupled with efforts to address the effects of environmental impacts on health including climate change. Access to basic human needs, clean air, safe drinking water, sufficient food, and safe shelter are impacted by climate change, and these are most pronounced for those living in the margins of our society.

It is important for nurses to be aware of these trends and capitalize on the potential for promoting positive health outcomes for all people. As widely respected and trusted members of healthcare teams, their workplace, and their communities, nurses are in key positions to take a leadership role in working to reduce health inequities and their root causes. Nurses can change the trajectory of health and healthcare for future generations in the United States and the world. Embracing and engaging in policy actions are more than just a consideration, it is nurses' responsibility. Implementing *The Future of Nursing* (IOM, 2011) recommendations with its call to action for nurses to further their education and to step up to the plate in assuming leadership roles can serve as a vehicle for accelerating the necessary work to reduce health inequities.

KEY CONCEPTS

1. Health is a human right.
2. Health and social inequities are a matter of economics and social justice.
3. Health inequities are unfair differences in the health status of different populations closely linked with historical social and economic disadvantage.
4. SDOHs are the conditions in which people are born, grow, live, work, and age—including the health system—and are shaped by the distribution of money, power, and resources at global, national, and local levels, which are themselves influenced by policy choices.
5. Social and economic determinants drive population health inequities.
6. SDOHs have important implications for U.S. and global health policy.
7. Nurses need to be knowledgeable about healthcare and social policies that create inequities to be effective advocates for the populations and communities that they serve.
8. There are no biological or genetic reasons to explain why socially disadvantaged groups experience significantly poorer health outcomes compared with the socially advantaged.
9. The type of health insurance is a key indicator of SES and class status in the United States. The type of health insurance status is also strongly correlated with race, ethnicity, and SES.
10. SES has a direct influence on the type of health insurance one can obtain, and health insurance has a direct impact on health outcomes.
11. Effective health policy strategies should include education, housing, labor, commerce, urban development, and environmental initiatives.
12. Partnerships that extend beyond the boundaries of nursing and healthcare to include education, housing, and economic sectors must be engaged to effectively address population health inequities.

SUMMARY

Political advocacy and policy engagement on behalf of people, families, and communities are essential role functions for professional nurses. In the United States, social and economic health inequities are indeed real and present threats to the nation's health. Given the urgency of such inequities, it is important that today's nurses be prepared to actively engage in all aspects of the policymaking process where discussions and decisions take place regarding the social determinants of healthcare. Undoubtedly, the health inequity problem cannot be solved by nursing alone; despite being the largest workforce in the United States, nurses will not be able to eliminate health inequities by working in isolation. Rather, nurses have to work to create partnerships with other professions that not only span the healthcare landscape but also extend beyond the borders of healthcare. Diverse cross-sectoral partnerships will enable nursing to acquire the necessary knowledge, skills, language, and expertise to address the social and economic determinants of health inequities.

Once those partnerships are formed, we then must work to better understand the complexity of the deep-rooted drivers of inequities in health among social groups. We must actively engage beyond the boundaries of nursing to be effective and influential in seeking solutions to the persistent inequities in health. Partnerships with government, academia, business, industry, public and private partners, community, and faith-based organizations, to name a few, are needed to address the complexity of SDOHs. In recent years, the call for a partnership approach to advance health by the nursing community has gained momentum (Institute of Medicine (IOM [now the National Academies of Medicine]), 2011; Shalala & Vladeck, 2011; Williams et al., 2018). The value of diverse perspectives in addressing health- and nursing-related issues is reflected in the committee membership for the landmark report *Future of Nursing* report (IOM, 2011). The report committee was composed of a cadre of professionals from areas such as business, academia, healthcare delivery, and health policy. Each member of this diverse coalition collectively provided unique perspectives and experiences when shaping the robust action-oriented report. Shalala and Vladeck (2011) echoed a similar call to action when they emphasized the need for nursing to develop allies from a wide variety of fields to effectively garner the political support and capital needed to implement the recommendations outlined in *The Future of Nursing* report.

We must maintain our commitment to developing effective policies and interventions to address and redress societal health inequities. Developing effective policy and following up with policy implementation actions through policy-directed initiatives and strategies is how we achieve the goal of health equity for all.

END-OF-CHAPTER RESOURCES

LEARNING ACTIVITIES

1. Read the article on social justice and healthcare. Identify ways in which you can incorporate some of the principles into nursing practice. file:///C:/Users/jphilli3/Downloads/The_promotion_of_social_justice_in_healthcare.6.pdf

2. Identify the annual income and the life expectancy for men and women for the county/parish where you live. Then identify the counties/parishes in your state that have the highest and lowest annual income and the life expectancy for men and women in those counties/parishes. Compare these life expectancies in your state with two affluent countries such as Japan and Switzerland and then compare these results with two less affluent countries such as Algeria and Bangladesh.

3. Prepare a list of partnerships in your area that have developed programs for health inequities. Discuss nursing's roles and visibility or lack of roles and visibility in these partnerships.

4. Contact a local community-based organization to see how they are working to close the gap in one or more health inequities. Examples might include starting a food pantry, instituting an advocacy agenda, supporting an after-school tutoring program, or hiring locally.

5. Find one article that highlights a nurse-led initiative to help a vulnerable population with health inequities and identify the lessons learned for your specialty area.

6. Visit the websites of newly elected officials (state- and federal-levels) and identify their agenda for addressing social and economic health inequities.

7. Describe one type of project related to the reduction of health inequities that you could develop if you served as an intern in a U.S. Congressional Office or the WHO.

8. Determine if your employer has created a health equity agenda as part of their overall strategic plan. Identify the components of this plan. If your employer has not created a health equity agenda, explore the feasibility and opportunities to strengthen existing or future strategic plans to include a focus on health equity.

E-RESOURCES

- Alliance for Health Equity https://allhealthequity.org/leadership-workgroups/

- American Hospital Association https://www.aha.org/social-determinants-health/populationcommunity-health/community-partnerships

- American Public Health Association https://www.apha.org/topics-and-issues/health-equity

- Centers for Disease Control and Prevention—Health Equity https://www.cdc.gov/chronicdisease/healthequity/index.htm

- Ethnic Minority Fellowship Program http://www.emfp.org

- GovTrack.us: Tracking the Activities of the U.S. Congress https://www.govtrack.us

- Healthy People 2030 https://health.gov/healthypeople

- Medicaid http://www.medicaid.gov

- The Minority Health and Health Equity Archive http://health-equity.lib. umd.edu

- National Association of County and City Health Officials: Roots of Health Inequity http://www.rootsofhealthinequity.org/about-course.php

- National Conference of State Legislatures https://www.ncsl.org/research/ health/health-disparities-overview.aspx

- National Minority Quality Forum https://www.nmqf.org/

- National Stakeholder Strategy for Achieving Health Equity https:// minorityhealth.hhs.gov/npa/files/Plans/NSS/completenss.pdf

- United States Department of Health and Human Services Action Plan to Reduce Racial and Ethnic Health Disparities, 2011 https://minorityhealth. hhs.gov/npa/files/Plans/HHS/HHS_Plan_complete.pdf

- United States Department of Health and Human Services Health Resources and Services Administration, Health Equity Report 2019-2020. Special Feature on Housing and Health Inequalities https://www.hrsa.gov/sites/default/ files/hrsa/health-equity/HRSA-health-equity-report.pdf

ACKNOWLEDGMENTS

The views expressed are the authors' and not necessarily those of the Health Resources and Services Administration or the U.S. Department of Health and Human Services.

REFERENCES

Acevedo-Garcia, D., Osypuk, T. L., Werbel, R. E., Meara, E. R., Cutler, D. M., & Berkman, L. F. (2004). Does housing mobility policy improve health? *Housing Policy Debate*, *15*(1), 49–98. https://www.tandfonline.com/doi/abs/10.1080/10511482.2004.9521495

American Cancer Society. (2020). *Cancer facts and figures 2020*. American Cancer Society.

American Medical Association. (2021). COVID-19 health equity initiatives: Chicago Racial Equity Rapid Response Team. https://www.ama-assn.org/delivering-care/health-equity/ covid-19-health-equity-initiatives-chicago-racial-equity-rapid

Annas, G. J. (2013). Health and human rights in the continuing global economic crisis. *American Journal of Public Health*, *103*(6), 967. https://doi.org/10.2105/AJPH.2013.301332

Aron, L., Dubay, L., Zimmerman, E., Simon, S. M., Chapman, D., & Woolf, S. H. (2015). *Can income-related policies improve population health? Income and Health Initiative: Brief Two*. https:// societyhealth.vcu.edu/media/society-health/pdf/IHIBrief2.pdf

Avram, A. (2020, May 31). No, you're not "lucky" to dodge the coronavirus. Our rigged society shields you, *The Washington Post*, p. B5. https://www.washingtonpost.com/outlook/coronavi-rus-luck-inequality-privilege/2020/05/26/2dc48700-9b86-11ea-ac72-3841fcc9b35f_story.html

Babb, S., Malarcher, A., Schauer, G., Asman, K., & Jamal, A. (2017). Quitting smoking among adults—United States, 2000–2015. *Morbidity and Mortality Weekly Report*, *65*(52), 1457–1464. https://doi.org/10.15585/mmwr.mm6552a1

Bambra, C., Gibson, M., Sowden, A., Wright, K., Whitehead, M., & Petticrew, M. (2010). Tackling the wider social determinants of health and health inequalities: Evidence from systematic reviews. *Journal of Epidemiology and Community Health*, *64*(4), 284–291. https://doi.org/10.1136/ jech.2008.082743.

Bhala, N., Curry, G., Martineau, A. R., Agyemang, C., & Bhopal, R. (2020). Sharpening the global focus on ethnicity and race in the time of COVID-19. *The Lancet, 395*(10238), 1673–1676. https://doi.org/10.1016/S0140-6736(20)31102-8.

Bill and Melinda Gates Foundation. (n.d.). *What we do.* http://www.gatesfoundation.org/what-we-do

Braveman, P. (2014). What are health disparities and health equity? We need to be clear. *Public Health Reports, 129*(1 Suppl. 2), 5–8. https://doi.org/10.1177/00333549141291S203

Burgard, S. A., & Lin, K. Y. (2013). Bad jobs, bad health? How work and working conditions contribute to health disparities. *American Behavioral Scientist, 57*(8), 1105–1127. https://doi.org/10.1177/0002764213487347

Cai, Y., & Fremstad, S. (2020). *Pandemic leads to more precarious housing situation.* Center for Economic and Policy Research. https://cepr.net/pandemic-leads-to-more-precarious-housing-situation

Carroll-Scott, A., Henson, R. M., Kolker, J., & Purtle, J. (2017). The role of nonprofit hospitals in identifying and addressing health inequities in cities. *Health Affairs, 36*, 1102–1109. https://doi.org/10.1377/hlthaff.2017.0033

Case, B. G., Himmelstein, D. U., & Woolhandler, S. (2002). No care for the caregivers: Declining health insurance coverage for health care personnel and their children, 1988–1998. *American Journal of Public Health, 92*(3), 404–408. https://doi.org/10.2105/AJPH.92.3.404

Center for Public Health Systems Science. (2014). *Point-of-sale strategies: A tobacco control guide.* Center for Public Health Systems Science, George Warren Brown School of Social Work at Washington University in St. Louis and the Tobacco Control Legal Consortium. https://cpb-us-w2.wpmucdn.com/sites.wustl.edu/dist/e/1037/files/2004/11/CPHSS_TCLC_2014_PointofSaleStrategies1-2jps9wj.pdf

Centers for Disease Control and Prevention. (2017). *Childhood obesity facts.* https://www.cdc.gov/healthyschools/obesity/facts.htm

Centers for Disease Control and Prevention. (2020a). *Provisional death counts for coronavirus disease (COVID-19): Health disparities: Race and Hispanic origin – provisional death counts for coronavirus disease (COVID-19).* National Center for Health Statistics. https://www.cdc.gov/nchs/nvss/vsrr/covid19/health_disparities.htm

Centers for Disease Control and Prevention. (2020b). *African Americans and tobacco use.* https://www.cdc.gov/tobacco/disparities/african-americans/index.htm

Cha, A. E., & Cohen, R. A. (2020). Reasons for being uninsured among adults aged 18–64 in the United States, 2019 (NCHS Data Brief, No. 382). National Center for Health Statistics.

Chetty, R., Hendren, N., Kline, P., & Saez, E. (2013). *The economic impacts of tax expenditures: Evidence from spatial variation across the US.* http://citeseerx.ist.psu.edu/viewdoc/summary?doi=10.1.1.364.2184

Chou, C. F., Johnson, P. J., Ward, A., & Blewett, L. A. (2009). Health care coverage and the health care industry. *American Journal of Public Health, 99*(12), 2282–2288. https://doi.org/10.2105/AJPH.2008.152413

Chun, Y., Roll, S., Miller, S, Lee, H., Larimore, S, & Grinstein-Weiss, M. (2020). *Racial and ethnic disparities in housing instability during the COVID-19 pandemic* (Social Policy Institute Working Paper). https://openscholarship.wustl.edu/spi_research/38

City of Chicago-Office of the Mayor. (2020, April 20). *Mayor Lightfoot and the Racial Equity Rapid Response Team announce latest efforts to address racial and health disparities among minority communities* [Press release]. https://www.chicago.gov/city/en/depts/mayor/press_room/press_releases/2020/april/RERRTUpdate.html

Clinton Foundation. (n.d.). *Clinton health access initiative.* http://www.clintonfoundation.org/main/our-work/by-initiative/clinton-health-access-initiative/about.html

The Coronavirus Aid, Relief, and Economic Security Act. Pub. L. No. 116-136. 134 § 281-615. https://www.congress.gov/116/plaws/publ136/PLAW-116publ136.pdf

Couch, K. A., Fairlie, R. W., & Xu, H. (2020). Early evidence of the impacts of COVID-19 on minority unemployment. *Journal of Public Economics*, *192*, 104287. https://doi.org/10.1016/j.jpubeco.2020.104287

Council on Foreign Relations. (2013). *The global health regime*. http://www.cfr.org/world/global-health-regime/p22763

Crossley, T. F., Fisher, P., & Low, H. (2021). The heterogeneous and regressive consequences of COVID-19: Evidence from high quality panel data. *Journal of Public Economics*, *193*, 104334. https://doi.org/10.1016/j.jpubeco.2020.104334

de Brey, C., Musu, L., McFarland, J., Wilkinson-Flicker, S., Diliberti, M., Zhang, A., Branstetter, C., & Wang, X. (2019). Status and trends in the education of racial and ethnic groups 2018 (NCES 2019-038). U.S. Department of Education. National Center for Education Statistics. https://nces.ed.gov/pubs2019/2019038.pdf

Figueroa, J. F., Wadhera, R. K., Mehtsun, W. T., Riley, K., Phelan, J., & Jha, A. K. (2021). Association of race, ethnicity, and community-level factors with COVID-19 cases and deaths across U.S. counties. *Healthcare*, *9*(1), 100495. https://doi.org/10.1016/j.hjdsi.2020.100495

Food and Drug Administration. (2013). *Preliminary scientific evaluation of the possible public health effects of menthol versus nonmenthol cigarettes*. https://www.fda.gov/media/86497/download

Gallo, W. T., Teng, H. M., Falba, T. A., Kasl, S. V., Krumholz, H. M., & Bradley, E. H. (2006). The impact of late career job loss on myocardial infarction and stroke: A 10-year follow up using the health and retirement survey. *Occupational Environmental Medicine*, *10*, 683–687. https://doi.org/10.1136/oem.2006.026823

Gennetian, L. A., Sciandra, M., Sanbonmatsu, L., Ludwig, J., Katz, L. F., Duncan, G. J., Kling, J. R., & Kessler, R. C. (2012). The long-term effects of moving to opportunity on youth outcomes. *Cityscape: A Journal of Policy Development and Research*, *14*(2), 137–168. https://www.huduser.gov/portal/periodicals/cityscpe/vol14num2/Cityscape_July2012_long_term_effects_youth.pdf

Goodman, N., Morris, M., Boston, K. (2019). Financial inequality: Disability, race, and poverty in America. *The National Disability Institute*. https://www.nationaldisabilityinstitute.org/wp-content/uploads/2019/02/disability-race-poverty-in-america.pdf

Gouveia, N. (2016). Addressing environmental health inequalities. *International Journal of Environmental Research and Public Health*, *13*(9), 858. https://doi.org/10.3390/ijerph13090858

Greene, S., & McCargo, A. (2020). *New data suggest COVID-19 is widening housing disparities by race and income*. Urban Institute; Urban Wire: Housing and Housing Finance. https://www.urban.org/urban-wire/new-data-suggest-covid-19-widening-housing-disparities-race-and-income

Groeger, L. (2020). *What coronavirus job losses reveal about racism in America*. https://projects.propublica.org/coronavirus-unemployment/10.7936/v0xn-yr31

Gundersen, C., & Ziliak, J. P. (2015). Food insecurity and health outcomes. *Health Affairs*, *34*(11), 1830–1839. https://www.healthaffairs.org/doi/10.1377/hlthaff.2015.0645

Halfon, N., Aguilar, E., Stanley, L., Hotez, E., Block, E., & Janus, M. (2020). Measuring equity from the start: Disparities in the health development of US kindergartners. *Health Affairs*, *39*(10), 1702–1709. https://doi.org/10.1377/hlthaff.2020.00920

Harris, R., Cormack, D., Stanley, J., & Rameka, R. (2015). Investigating the relationship between ethnic consciousness, racial discrimination and self-rated health in New Zealand. *PLoS ONE*, *10*(2), e0117343. https://doi.org/10.1371/journal.pone.0117343

Health Resources and Services Administration, Office of Health Equity. (2018). *Health Equity Report 2017*. U.S. Department of Health and Human Services.

Healthy People 2030. (2020). *Social determinants of health*. U.S. Department of Health and Human Services, Office of Disease Prevention and Health Promotion. https://health.gov/healthypeople/objectives-and-data/social-determinants-health

Heroes Act. (2020). *H.R. 6800—116th Congress: The Heroes Act*. GovTrack.us. https://www.govtrack.us/congress/bills/116/hr6800

Heron, M. (2019). Deaths: Leading causes for 2017. *National Vital Statistics Reports*, *68*(6), 1–77. https://www.cdc.gov/nchs/data/nvsr/nvsr68/nvsr68_06-508.pdf

Hubert H. Humphrey quotes. (n.d.). *BrainyQuote.com*. https://www.brainyquote.com/quotes/hubert_h_humphrey_163688

Huizar, M. I., Arena, R., & Laddu, D. R. (2020, July 20). The global food syndemic: The impact of food insecurity, malnutrition, and obesity on the healthspan amid the COVID-19 pandemic. Progress in Cardiovascular Disease. Advanced online publication. https://www.ncbi.nlm.nih.gov/pmc/articles/PMC7347484/

Institute of Medicine. (2011). *The future of nursing: Leading change advancing health*. The National Academies Press. https://doi.org/10.17226/12958

Jones, C. P., Truman, B. I., Elam-Evans, L. D., Jones, C. A., Jones, C. Y., Jiles, R., Rumisha, S. F., & Perry, G. S. (2008). Using socially assigned race to probe white advantages in health status. *Ethnicity and Disease*, *18*(4), 496–504. https://www.ethndis.org/priorarchives/ethn-18-04-496.pdf

Kary, T. (2020, October 13). Lawsuit aims to ban menthols, big tobacco's bait for black smokers. *Bloomberg Businessweek*. https://www.bloomberg.com/news/features/2020-10-13/lawsuit-aims-to-ban-menthols-big-tobacco-bait-for-black-smokers

Kirkpatrick, S. I., McIntyre, L., & Potestio, M. L. (2010). Child hunger and long-term adverse consequences for health. *Archives Pediatric Adolescent Medicine*, *164*(8), 754–762. https://doi.org/10.1001/archpediatrics.2010.117.

Landrigan, P. J., Sly, J. L., Ruchirawat, M., Silva, E. R., Huo, X., Diaz-Barriga, F., Zar, H. J., King, M., Ha, E. H., Asante, K. A., Ahanchian, H., & Sly, P. D. (2016). Health consequences of environmental exposures: Changing global patterns of exposure and disease. *Annals of Global Health*, *82*(1), 10–19. https://doi.org/10.1016/j.aogh.2016.01.005

LaPar, D. J., Damien, J., Bhamidipati, C. M., Mery, C. M., Stukenborg, G. J., Jones, D. R., Schirmer, B. D., Kron, I. L., & Ailawadi, G. (2010). Primary payer status affects mortality for major surgical operations. *Annals of Surgery*, *252*(3), 544–551. https://doi.org/10.1097/SLA.0b013e3181e8fd75

LEAD Center. (2015). *Policy brief. The impact of employment on the health status and health care costs of working-age people with disabilities*. http://www.leadcenter.org/system/files/resource/downloadable_version/impact_of_employment_health_status_health_care_costs_0.pdf

Levy, D. T., Pearson, J. L., Villanti, A. C., Blackman, K., Vallone, D. M., Niaura, R. S., & Abrams, D. B. (2011). Modeling the future effects of a menthol ban on smoking prevalence and smoking-attributable deaths in the United States. *American Journal of Public Health*, *101*(7), 1236–1240. https://doi.org/10.2105/AJPH.2011.300179

Li, Q., & Keith, L. G. (2011). The differential association between education and infant mortality by nativity status of Chinese American mothers: A life-course perspective. *American Journal of Public Health*, *101*(5), 899–908. https://doi.org/10.2105/AJPH.2009.186916

Lorem, G., Cook, S., Leon, D. A., Emaus, N., & Schirmer, H. (2020). Self-reported health as a predictor of mortality: A cohort study of its relation to other health measurements and observation time. *Scientific Reports*, *10*, 4886. https://doi.org/10.1038/s41598-020-61603-0

Los Angeles Times. (2020, August 28). *California bans flavored tobacco sales in response to a surge in teen use*. https://www.latimes.com/california/story/2020-08-28/california-bans-flavored-tobacco-products-sales-newsom-signs-bill

Ludwig, J., Sanbonmatsu, L., Gennetian, L., Adam, E., Duncan, G. J., Katz, L. F., Kessler, R. C., Kling, J. R., Lindau, S. T., Whitaker, R. C., & McDade, T. W. (2011). Neighborhoods, obesity, and diabetes—A randomized social experiment. *New England Journal of Medicine*, *365*(16), 1509–1519. https://doi.org/10.1056/NEJMsa1103216

Maani, N., & Galea, S. (2020a). COVID-19 and underinvestment in the health of the US population. *Milbank Q*, *98*, 239–249. https://doi.org/10.1111/1468-0009.12462

Maani, N., & Galea, S. (2020b). COVID-19 and underinvestment in the public health infrastructure of the United States. *Milbank Q*, *98*, 250–259. https://doi.org/10.1111/1468-0009.12463

MacDorman, M. F., Hoyert, D. L., & Mathews, T. J. (2013). Recent declines in infant mortality in the United States, 2005–2011. *NCHS Data Brief, 2013*(120), 1–8. https://www.ncbi.nlm.nih.gov/pubmed/23759138

MacDorman, M. F., Mathews, T. J., Mohangoo, A. D., & Zeitlin, J. (2014). International comparisons of infant mortality and related factors: United States and Europe, 2010. *National Vital Statistics Reports, 63*(5), 1–6. https://www.ncbi.nlm.nih.gov/pubmed/25252091

Mackintosh, M. (2001). Do health care systems contribute to inequalities? In D. Leon & G. Walt (Eds.), *Poverty, inequality and health* (pp. 175–193). Oxford University Press.

Maness, S. B., Merrell, L., Thompson, E. L., Griner, S. B., Kline, N., & Wheldon, C. (2021). Social determinants of health and health disparities: COVID-19 exposures and mortality among African American people in the United States. *Public Health Reports, 136*(1), 18–22. https://doi.org/10.1177/0033354920969169

Marmot, M., & Allen, J. J. (2014). Social determinants of health equity. *American Journal of Public Health, 104*(Suppl. 4), S517–S519. https://doi.org/10.2105/AJPH.2014.302200

Marr, C., Huang, C. C., Sherman, A., & DeBot, B. (2015). *EITC and child tax credit promote work, reduce poverty, and support children's development, research finds.* Center on Budget and Policy Priorities. Center on Budget and Policy Priorities. http://www.cbpp.org/cms/?-fa=view&id=3793

Mathews, T. J., & Driscoll, A. K. (2017, March). Trends in infant mortality in the United States, 2005–2014 (NCHS Data Brief No. 279). National Center for Health Statistics. https://www.cdc.gov/nchs/data/databriefs/db279.pdf

Mathews, T. J., MacDorman, M. F., & Thoma, M. E. (2015). Infant mortality statistics from the 2013 period linked birth/infant death data set. *National Vital Statistics Reports, 64*(9), 1–30. https://www.cdc.gov/nchs/data/nvsr/nvsr64/nvsr64_09.pdf

Matijasevich, A., Victora, C. G., Lawlor, D. A., Golding, J., Menezes, A. M., Araújo, C. L., Barros, A. J. D., Santos, I. S., Barros, F. C, & Smith, G. D. (2012). Association of socioeconomic position with maternal pregnancy and infant health outcomes in birth cohort studies from Brazil and the UK. *Journal of Epidemiology and Community Health, 66*(2), 127–135. https://doi.org/10.1136/jech.2010.108605

Medicaid and Children's Health Insurance Program Payment and Access Commission. (2020). *Medicaid enrollment changes following the ACA.* https://www.macpac.gov/subtopic/medicaid-enrollment-changes-following-the-aca/

Moffitt, R. A., & Ziliak, J. P. (2020, October). *COVID-19 and the U.S. safety net.* National Bureau of Economic Research. NBER Working Paper No. w27911. https://www.nber.org/system/files/working_papers/w27911/w27911.pdf

Morales, D. X., Morales, S. A., & Beltran, T. F. (2020). Racial/ethnic disparities in household food insecurity during the COVID-19 pandemic: A nationally representative study. *Journal of Racial and Ethnic Health Disparities*, 1–15. https://doi.org/10.1007/s40615-020-00892-7

Musu-Gillette, L., de Brey, C., McFarland, J., Hussar, W., Sonnenberg, W., & Wilkinson-Flicker, S. (2017). Status and trends in the education of racial and ethnic groups 2017 (NCES 2017-051). U.S. Department of Education, National Center for Education Statistics. http://nces.ed.gov/pubsearch

National Prevention Council. (2011). *National prevention strategy.* U.S. Department of Health and Human Services, Office of the Surgeon General. http://www.surgeongeneral.gov/initiatives/prevention/strategy/report.html

National Research Council Panel on DHHS Collection of Race and Ethnic Data, Ver Ploeg, M., & Perrin, E. (Eds.) (2004). *Eliminating health disparities: Measurement and data needs.* National Academies Press.

Niu, X., Roche, L. M., Pawlish, K. S., & Henry, K. A. (2013). Cancer survival disparities by health insurance status. *Cancer Medicine, 2*(3), 403–411. https://doi.org/10.1002/cam4.84

Osypuk, T. L., Joshi, P., Geronimo, K., & Acevedo-Garcia, D. (2014). Do social and economic policies influence health? A review. *Current Epidemiological Reports, 1*(3), 149–164. https://doi.org/10.1007/s40471-014-0013-5

The Patient Protection and Affordable Care Act of 2010. Pub. Law No. 111–148. 124 § 119-1025. https://www.congress.gov/111/plaws/publ148/PLAW-111publ148.pdf

Quarells, R. C., Liu, J., & Davis, S. K. (2012). Social determinants of cardiovascular disease risk factor presence among rural and urban Black and White men. *Journal of Men's Health*, *9*(2), 120–126. https://doi.org/10.1016/j.jomh.2012.03.004

Robbins, A. S., Chen, A. Y., Stewart, A. K., Staley, C. A., Virgo, K. S., & Ward, E. M. (2010). Insurance status and survival disparities among nonelderly rectal cancer patients in the National Cancer Data Base. *Cancer*, *116*(17), 4178–4186. https://doi.org/10.1002/cncr.25317

Robert Wood Johnson Foundation. (2013). *Health policy snapshot—Issue brief. How does employment—or unemployment—affect health?* http://www.rwjf.org/content/dam/farm/reports/issue_briefs/2013/rwjf403360

Rudolph, L., Caplan, J., Ben-Moshe, K., & Dillon, L. (2013). *Health in all policies: A guide for state and local governments*. American Public Health Association and Public Health Institute.

Sanchez, R. (2020). *Coronavirus in Black America: Living in the eye of a "perfect storm."* CNN. https://www.cnn.com/2020/04/11/us/coronavirus-black-americans-deaths/index.html

Schnittker, J., & Bacak, V. (2014). The increasing predictive validity of self-rated health. *PLoS ONE*, *9*(1), e84933. https://doi.org/10.1371/journal.pone.0084933

Selden, T. M., & Berdahl, T. A. (2020). COVID-19 and Racial/Ethnic Disparities in Health Risk, Employment, and Household Composition. *Health affairs (Project Hope)*, *39*(9), 1624–1632. https://doi.org/10.1377/hlthaff.2020.00897

Shalala, D., & Vladeck, B. (2011). Leading change: How nurses can attract political support for the IOM Report on the future of nursing. *Nurse Leader*, *9*(6), 38–39, 45. https://doi.org/10.1016/j.mnl.2011.09.007

Singh, G. K., & Jemal, A. (2017). Socioeconomic and racial/ethnic disparities in cancer mortality, incidence, and survival in the United States, 1950–2014: Over six decades of changing patterns and widening Inequalities. *Journal of Environmental and Public Health*, *2017*, 2819372. https://doi.org/10.1155/2017/2819372

Singh, G. K., Daus, G. P., Allender, M., Ramey, C. T., Martin, E. K., Perry, C., & Vedamuthu, I. P. (2017). Social determinants of health in the United States: Addressing major health inequality trends for the nation, 1935–2016. *International Journal of MCH and AIDS*, *6*(2), 139–164. https://doi.org/10.21106/ijma.236

Singh, G. K., & Kogan, M. D. (2007). Persistent socioeconomic disparities in infant, neonatal, and postneonatal mortality rates in the United States, 1969–2001. *Pediatrics*, *119*(4), e929–e939. https://doi.org/10.21106/ijma.236

Sloan, C., Duddy-Tensbrunsel, R., Ferguson, S., & Valladares, A. (2020, September 16). *COVID-19 projected to worsen racial disparities in health*. Avalere. https://avalere.com/press-releases/covid-19-projected-to-worsen-racial-disparities-in-health-coverage

Sly, P. D., Carpenter, D. O., Van den Berg, M., Stein, R. T., Landrigan, P. J., Brune-Drisse, M.-N., & Suk, W. (2016). Health consequences of environmental exposures: Causal thinking in global epidemiology. *Annals of Global Health*, *82*(1), 3–9. https://doi.org/10.1016/j.aogh.2016.01.004

Smokefree.gov. (2015). *Menthol Cigarettes*. U.S. Department of Health and Human Services, National Institutes of Health, National Cancer Institute.

Subramanian, S. V., & Kawachi, I. (2004). Income inequality and health: what have we learned so far? *Epidemiologic Reviews*, *26*, 78–91. https://doi.org/10.1093/epirev/mxh003

U.S. Census Bureau, Current Population Survey. (2020). *Annual social and economic supplement (CPS ASEC)*. https://www.census.gov/library/visualizations/2020/demo/p60-271.html

U.S. Department of Health and Human Services. (2014). Healthy People 2020. *Disparities*. http://www.healthypeople.gov/2020/about/disparitiesAbout.aspx

U.S. Department of Health and Human Services, Health Resources and Services Administration, Office of Health Equity. (2020). *Health Equity Report 2019–2020: Special feature on housing and health inequalities*.

U.S. Department of Labor, Bureau of Labor Statistics. (2020). *Occupational outlook handbook, registered nurses*. https://www.bls.gov/ooh/healthcare/registered-nurses.htm

U.S. Department of Treasury. (2020). *The CARES Act works for all Americans*. https://home.treasury.gov/policy-issues/cares

U.S. Food and Drug Administration. (2020). *Family smoking prevention and tobacco control act*. https://www.fda.gov/tobacco-products/rules-regulations-and-guidance/family-smoking-prevention-and-tobacco-control-act-overview

U.S. Global Leadership Coalition. (2020). *COVID-19 Brief: Impact on the economies of developing countries*. https://www.usglc.org/coronavirus/economies-of-developing-countries/

Waddill, K. (2020, September 17). COVID-19 Amplifies racial disparities for coverage. Health Payer Intelligence. *Value-Based Care News*. https://healthpayerintelligence.com/news/covid-19-amplifies-racial-health-disparities-for-coverage

Webb, B. C. (2012). Moving upstream: Policy strategies to address social, economic, and environmental conditions that shape health inequities. *Joint Center for Political and Economic Studies*. https://jointcenter.org/moving-upstream-policy-strategies-to-address-social-economic-and-environmental-conditions-that-shape-health-inequities/

Wicks-Lim, J., & Arno, S. (2017). Improving population health by reducing poverty: New York's earned income tax credit. *Social Science and Medicine—Population Health, 3*, 373–381. https://doi.org/10.1016/j.ssmph.2017.03.006

Williams, S. D., Phillips, J. M., & Koyama, K. (2018, September 30). Nurse advocacy: Adopting a Health in All Policies approach. *OJIN: The Online Journal of Issues in Nursing, 23*(3), 1. https://doi.org/10.3912/OJIN.Vol23No03Man01

Wodon, Q., Montenegro, C., Nguyen, H., & Onagoruwa, A. (2018). *Missed opportunities: The high cost of not educating girls* (The Cost of Not Educating Girls Notes Series). World Bank. https://openknowledge.worldbank.org/handle/10986/29956; http://hdl.handle.net/10986/29956

Wolfson, J. A., & Leung, C. W. (2020). Food insecurity and COVID-19: Disparities in early effects for US adults. *Nutrients, 12*(6), 1648. https://doi.org/10.3390/nu12061648

World Bank. (2020). *COVID-19 to add as many as 150 million extreme poor by 2021*. https://www.worldbank.org/en/news/press-release/2020/10/07/covid-19-to-add-as-many-as-150-million-extreme-poor-by-2021

World Health Organization. (2013). *Health in All Policies: Framework for country action*. https://apps.who.int/iris/bitstream/handle/10665/112636/9789241506908_eng.pdf;jsessionid=B9E38E2EE5161A5C00A0B411E8E81C9E?sequence=1

World Health Organization. (2017). *10 facts on health inequities and their causes*. http://www.who.int/features/factfiles/health_inequities/en

World Health Organization, Commission on Social Determinants of Health. (2008). *Closing the gap in a generation: Health equity through action on the social determinants of health*. Final Report of the Commision on the Social Determinants of Health. https://www.who.int/publications/i/item/WHO-IER-CSDH-08.1

Yancy, C. W. (2020). COVID-19 and African Americans. *JAMA, 323*(19), 1891–1892. https://doi.org/10.1001/jama.2020.6548

CHAPTER 14

Valuing Global Realities for Health Policy

JUDITH SHAMIAN AND MORIAH ELLEN

I am no longer accepting the things I cannot change. It is now time to change the things I cannot accept.
—Angela Davis

OBJECTIVES

1. Examine the social responsibility of nursing in the context of global health policy.
2. Identify common issues that unite nurses globally.
3. Compare and contrast key international organizations relevant to health and nursing policy.
4. Describe collaborative strategies designed to advance the nursing profession internationally.
5. Appreciate and explore the role of the nurse as a global citizen.

Nurses are the largest sector of health professionals and the most trusted around the world. The nursing workforce is composed of more than 28 million people, including 19.3 million professional nurses caring for nearly 8 billion people across the globe (World Health Organization [WHO], 2020b). Despite these millions of nurses, many people do not have the care they need. Nurses, however, hold the keys to be a true force for healthcare transformation in their own communities and worldwide. Due to their numbers, earned public trust, unique skills, and nursing lens, nurses are uniquely positioned to influence healthcare and change the face of the medical establishment. More than policymakers, politicians, or even other healthcare workers, it is nurses who know best how to care for patients.

Now more than ever, nurses need to be "together" globally as we face natural disasters, cross-border violence, infectious diseases, travel, technology, and increasing migration. As emphasized in landmark reports by the WHO, in *The State of the World's Nursing 2020* (WHO, 2020b), and the National Academy of Sciences, Engineering and Medicine, in the *Future of Nursing 2020–2030: Charting a Path to Achieve Health Equity* (2021), the social determinants of health (SDOHs) are at the crux of health in all aspects of one's life no matter what country they live in. All nurses are facing challenges with one or more sectors of the populations they serve (e.g., maternal–child, aging, mental health) because of the large impact of SDOHs on healthcare beyond simple access to clinical care and services.

Nurses are prepared to act individually, through teams, and across sectors to meet challenges associated with an aging population, access to primary care, mental and behavioral health problems, structural racism, high maternal mortality and morbidity, and the elimination of the disproportionate disease burden carried by specific segments of the U.S. population. Nurses hold a unique role to improve health and contribute to the current and future development goals outlined by the United Nations. Despite the sheer number of nurses and the underlying potential power of nurses to advocate, individual nurses may not recognize, think or act as "global citizens" or value our global interconnectedness. Thus, nurses not be able to readily appreciate nursing's potential power to impact healthcare and nursing practice globally.

Nurses frequently express concern about healthcare issues as it relates to their personal practice, their communities, and their environment. Far too often, these concerns are discussed within local communities of practice and do not develop into measurable progress toward a common health goal. Nursing practice occurs within a complex environment of multicultural and multiethnic populations. Nursing has a social responsibility and professional practice obligation to impact health at a global level. Nurses are leaders and advocates in their communities who can shape health policy across the globe in order to ensure the achievement of the UN's Sustainable Development Goals (SDGs; Rosa et al., 2019).

Global citizenship unites people; it is not country- or continent-bound. It is defined as "awareness, caring, and embracing cultural diversity while promoting social justice and sustainability, coupled with a sense of responsibility to act" (Reysen & Katzarska-Miller, 2013, p. 858). The challenge that nurses face is understanding the world stage and the global actors participating in the production of healthcare. As we gain an appreciation of the plot and subplots behind health inequities, the nursing community needs to increase its focus on engaging key stakeholders in strategic partnerships to shape the global health agenda. See the section on Advocating as a Global Citizen.

OVERVIEW OF GLOBAL HEALTH ISSUES

On this planet, more than 7.8 billion people live in more than 194 countries with both unique and disparate profiles. These countries or nations have often been labeled using political, economic, or ethnic terms. There is no common definition of criteria for each category of a country's development; however, prominence is often determined relative to other countries using the gross domestic product (GDP) per capita and the Human Development Index (HDI) measure. The latter is a multifactorial statistic using a combination of life expectancy, education, and income factors.

Global health issues include a multitude of concerns that directly impact population health. Worldwide, healthcare systems are burdened by chronic underfunding and underdeveloped community and public healthcare, which leads to ever-escalating disease and associated costs (Langlois et al., 2020). Adding to this problem are complex stressors to the already burdened system (Langlois et al., 2020). Examples of these stressors are illustrated in Figure 14.1.

Socioeconomic, cultural, environmental, and equality factors all contribute to health whether positive or negative. Global health is concerned with SDOHs that are transnational in nature. Examples of global health issues include urbanization, climate change, gender equality, tobacco control, injury prevention, violence, human trafficking, migrant workers, obesity, infectious disease, chronic disease,

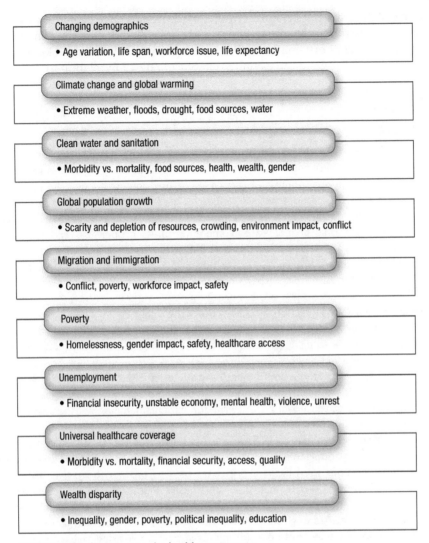

Changing demographics
- Age variation, life span, workforce issue, life expectancy

Climate change and global warming
- Extreme weather, floods, drought, food sources, water

Clean water and sanitation
- Morbidity vs. mortality, food sources, health, wealth, gender

Global population growth
- Scarity and depletion of resources, crowding, environment impact, conflict

Migration and immigration
- Conflict, poverty, workforce impact, safety

Poverty
- Homelessness, gender impact, safety, healthcare access

Unemployment
- Financial insecurity, unstable economy, mental health, violence, unrest

Universal healthcare coverage
- Morbidity vs. mortality, financial security, access, quality

Wealth disparity
- Inequality, gender, poverty, political inequality, education

FIGURE 14.1 Stressors to the healthcare system.

malnutrition, poverty, mental health, and motor vehicle accidents, to name a few. Global health issues are all-encompassing concerns that affect the healthcare of a population. This means that global health issues are also concerned with the infrastructure of healthcare systems and the global healthcare workforce. The maldistribution of healthcare workers worldwide directly affects the ability of a nation to handle the burden of disease. Migration and economics contribute to potential problems with inequality and the distributive justice of scarce workforce resources.

Globalization has led to extensive international travel and trade. Historically, epidemics may have taken weeks to months to a year to traverse a continent. However, as seen with COVID-19, a global pandemic can occur just in a span of few months. Although the initial cases were identified in November 2019, by January 2020, every country registered COVID-19 cases, with nearly 4 million deaths and 190 million people infected by July 2021 (Worldometer, 2021). National economies were brought to their knees and the impact will be felt for decades. This pandemic further tested the under-resourced healthcare system and once again demonstrated the tension and the gap between the healthcare community and policymakers. The COVID-19 pandemic exacerbated the need for nurses making it more visible to the public. Furthermore, while nurses have been the absolute front line and more than 2,200 nurses worldwide have died during the pandemic (ICN, 2021a), the role of nursing was still not recognized at decision-making tables. See the Policy Challenge for an examination of COVID-19 in relation to policy.

POLICY CHALLENGE	Pandemic Highlights Nurses as Global Citizens and Policymakers

What nurse will forget 2020 and the daily reality faced with COVID-19? With each global infectious disease, there has been uncertainty about the disease's progression and treatment. As the cases unfold, there is mounting concern about not only protecting the public but also protecting direct care and support staff.

Although rare and deadly, Ebola prior to COVID-19, created a heightened awareness of the importance of personal protective equipment (PPE), its proper use, and the dangers of inadequate protection. The image of improvised PPE provided a glimpse of some of the stark realities faced by healthcare workers in Africa during the Ebola crisis. See www.youtube.com/ watch?v=Nmja-QbMA4EA. Often, garbage bags and other everyday items were turned into makeshift PPE. Many individuals and professional groups across the globe were raising questions about the ability to prevent infections and to protect the public.

Fast-forward to 2020. Little did nurses imagine that the shortage of PPE would so soon be a global reality; countries with distinct economic advantage would lack crucial supplies—goggles, gowns, face shields, antiseptic wipes, specialized N95 masks, and equipment. Some of the most renowned health systems in the world did not have adequate PPE. This lack of supply and quality of equipment for frontline healthcare workers fighting COVID-19 was daily news across the world. Protection against the novel coronavirus for patients, families, and healthcare workers was a serious and ongoing concern.

Images associated with inadequate PPE are a constant reminder of these struggles. Vivid photos, stories, videos, and blogs detailed how individuals desperately tried to protect themselves from COVID-19 exposure. They used hacks like garbage bags to protect themselves from COVID-19 and improvised protections from bruises and ulcers from wearing masks hours on end. These images were shared globally across social and news media, creating much controversy, conversation, and outrage. Although some posts were forced to be removed, many of these images persist across the internet. See examples (a) nurses in London wearing garbage bags at nypost. com/2020/04/09/3-uk-nurses-forced-to-wear-trash-bags-get-coronavirus/?utm_source=dlvr. it&utm_medium=twitter and (b) nurses across the world at www.cbsnews.com/news/ coronavirus-health-care-bruised-faces-masks-ppe-hospitals-doctors-nurses-italy-new-york/.

Failure to provide healthcare workers with appropriate PPE and requiring its reuse was dangerous, increased employee risks, and threatened patient safety. Nurses and healthcare workers were angry, disillusioned, and distressed when policies, which were designed to protect them, abandoned them. Employee workload increased and stress levels were heightened. Caring for COVID-19 patients contributed to hospitals and healthcare workers feeling overwhelmed and unsafe and contracting and dying from COVID-19. No clinical setting in any country was spared from shortages and failed policies. According to Cockburn at Amnesty International (2021), "for one health worker to die from COVID-19 every 30 minutes is both a tragedy and an injustice.... far too many have been left unprotected and paid the ultimate price" (para. 3).

See Policy Solution

Nations no longer exist in complete isolation. Globalization requires rapid identification and control of potential public health threats to prevent the international spread of emerging infectious diseases. Although globalization has included extensive international travel and trade, and an increase in epidemics, global health reaches far beyond communicable diseases such as COVID-19, Ebola, or Zika. Selected global health issues briefly described here include poverty, universal health coverage (UHC), and noncommunicable diseases (NCDs), in the context of the SDGs 2030 (UN, 2015a, 2015b).

The Millennial Development Goals (MDGs) 2020 (UN, 2021a) and newer SDGs 2030 (UN, 2021b) describe the responsibilities of each country for the eradication of health inequality. Some of the noted accomplishments related to the MDGs were major declines in child and maternal mortality rates (WHO, 2021b), and progress in the prevention and treatment of HIV, tuberculosis (TB), and malaria (WHO, 2021c). While the MDGs accomplished some of the targets, they fell short in numerous areas. It was realized that a different approach was required to tackle global challenges. The MDGs were superseded by the SDGs 2030 as it was recognized that there was a need for a more comprehensive and integrated approach to advance the wellbeing of the global population.

The 17 SDG 2030 goals (see Figure 14.2) are far-reaching and include education, gender issues, environment, and more to be achieved by 2030 (UN, 2015a). These SDGs and targets aim for a much stronger synergistic integration. They focus on ending poverty, fighting inequality, and tackling climate change (UN, 2021b). The SDGs address the delicate balance between human prosperity and environmental protection in a sustainable plan of action. Notable is that the goals recognize the interrelated nature of factors that contribute to global poverty and the need for all countries at all levels of economic development to address poverty within an integrated agenda (Osborn et al., 2015).

In 2017, the WHO Department of Health Systems Governance and Financing projected outcomes based on the resource needs for 67 low- and middle-income countries, representing 95% of the total population of interest (Stenberg et al., 2017). Based on the model, approximately $371 billion per year every year through 2030 would be needed to be spent on healthcare to reach SDG targets. In 2019, the model projections estimated that an additional $200 to $328 billion would be needed to expand the service delivery and meet SDG targets (Stenberg et al., 2019). Model projections show that 75% of the costs are related to the healthcare

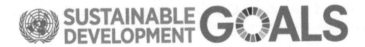

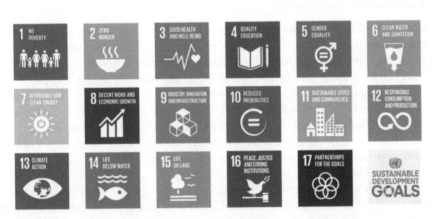

FIGURE 14.2 The United Nations Sustainable Development Goals.

Source: From United Nations. (2017). *Sustainable Development Goals: 17 goals to transform our world*. https://www.un.org/en/exhibits/page/sdgs-17-goals-transform-world

workforce and infrastructure, 97 million potential lives could be saved, and life expectancy could increase 3 to 8 years based on country (Stenberg et al., 2017). Achieving the SDGs will lead to a healthier and more productive population with a longer life expectancy and an ability to be more productive members of society (Griggs et al., 2017; Singh et al., 2018; WHO, 2018).

POVERTY

Poverty is the first of the 17 SDG 2030 Goals and exemplifies a health and socio-economic problem that all countries face, even those with relatively high GDPs. Beyond a lack of income and resources, poverty is manifested in hunger, malnutrition, limited access to education, social discrimination, exclusion, and limited decision-making (UN, 2021b). Highly developed countries in the world contain impoverished populations. For example, 10.5% (34 million) of the U.S. population lives in poverty; the poverty rate is the highest among women aged 18 to 24 (21.35%), Blacks (18.8%), and Native Americans 23% (Semega et al., 2020; U.S. Census Bureau, 2019). Worldwide, the poverty statistic is 10.7%; one in 10 people lives in poverty, which is defined as less than $1.90 per day per person (World Bank, 2017). The highest global poverty rates are seen in rural areas with poor educational systems and agricultural economies. The worst example of poverty can be seen in sub-Saharan Africa, where half (389 million) of the extreme poor reside (World Bank, 2017). As world and country leaders focus on international issues, they identify universal issues that drive global health, well-being, and equity.

It is well established that the poor across the world usually bear the brunt of global crises and stresses. Communicable diseases are often most prevalent in areas with high rates of poverty. Some communicable diseases do not have high per capita costs associated with their eradication, but these measures are not universally available to the most vulnerable. Likewise, there is a greater risk that emerging infectious disease threats will take hold in communities with limited resources devoted to health. Climate change, global economic changes, corruption, the privatization of public services, and austerity disproportionately impact the poor (UN Human Rights Council, 2017). Very often, children and older people are disproportionately represented among the poor.

Universal Health Coverage

More than half the world's population does not have access to essential health services; with more than 100 million people forced into extreme poverty due to healthcare expenses (WHO, people have no access to healthcare services; World Health Organization and International Bank for Reconstruction and Development, The World Bank, 2017). A lack of access is usually found among the poorest of the world's population regardless of their country of residence, even in high-income countries. The WHO constitution of 1948 declared "the highest attainable standard of health as a fundamental right of every human being," the first international instrument to take this stance (WHO, 2017a). Seventy years later, the world still struggles with this issue.

Care coverage is a central component of the global healthcare agenda. The WHO (2021e) defines *UHC* as "all people have access to the health services they need, when and where they need them, without financial hardship. It includes the full range of essential health services, from health promotion to prevention, to treatment, rehabilitation and palliative care" (para. 1). This definition of *UHC* embodies three related objectives: (a) equity in access to health services, which means that all who need, not just those who can pay for, services should get them; (b) the quality of health services should be good enough to improve the health of those receiving services; and (c) people should be protected against financial risk, ensuring that the cost of using services does not place people at risk of financial harm (WHO, 2021e). At the heart of the issue is access for all people on the planet to basic healthcare without suffering financial burden. The World Bank (2017, para 1) views UHC as "the foundation for individuals to lead productive and fulfilling lives and for countries to have strong economies." UHC has significant potential to impact multiple SDGs as noted in the next section. Specifically, the target is getting UN member states to commit to trying to achieve the provision of UHC by 2030. Since UHC has been identified as a global challenge, millions of people have been lifted out of absolute poverty (Ataguba & Ingabire, 2016; Wagstaff & Neelsen, 2020). It is difficult to predict the long-term impact of COVID-19 on UHC and poverty.

Noncommunicable Disease (NCDs)

NCDs, also known as chronic illnesses, are an important global agenda item to recognize in the context of world health. They have taken a more prominent role in the global health agenda as a result of the interaction of the many stressors as noted in Figure 14.1. Although the problem of NCDs in highly industrialized countries is well recognized, nurses need to also be aware of the impact of NCDs as a leading cause of premature death globally. In 2019, 41 million global deaths were due to an NCD, with 47% of NCD deaths occurring before the age of 70 in low- and middle-income countries (WHO, 2021c).

The NCD Alliance is an example of a mega-association of more than 2,000 non-governmental organizations (NGOs) brought together as a civil movement to create solutions for the NCD global agenda (NCD Alliance, 2021). Each of the 2,000 NGOs focuses on a specific and/or unique NCD factor. Based on its membership, the NCD Alliance is uniquely structured to leverage its expertise. The strategic pillars of the NCD Alliance (2021) include advocacy, accountability, capacity development, and knowledge exchange. Through strategic partnership, this advocacy network has developed policy and practice recommendations specific to the NCD agenda for global health.

The United Nations endorsed the WHO Global Action Plan for the Prevention and Control of NCDs from 2013 to 2020. This has a goal to reduce preventable and avoidable morbidity, mortality, and disability from NCDs by 25% by 2025 (WHO, 2013). The action plan depends on the following primary philosophies: human rights, equity, and national action with international cooperation, multisectoral action, life-course approach, empowerment of people and communities, evidence-based strategies, UHC, and managing of conflicts of interest. It is recognized that meeting the NCD targets will be challenging.

The UN's commitment to reducing NCDs was reflected in the establishment of a high-level global commission on NCDs in 2017 with a comprehensive review by the General Assembly of global and national progress regarding early mortality from heart and lung diseases, cancer, and diabetes in 2018 (WHO, 2017b, 2019a). The commission's aim was to identify innovative ways to curb the world's biggest causes of death and extend life expectancy for millions of people (WHO, 2019a). It is important to note that mental health was also recognized as an important element of NCDs. See Exhibit 14.1 for the key features of the commission's recommendations.

EXHIBIT 14.1   INDEPENDENT HIGH-LEVEL COMMISSION RECOMMENDATIONS FOR WHO ACTION TO ADDRESS NCDS AND MENTAL HEALTH

AREA	RECOMMENDATION
Whole-of-Society Focus	Encourage strategic NCD responses with a whole-of-government, health-in-all-policies for engaging stakeholders in whole-of-society action aligned with national NCD and SDG targets.
Empower Healthy Choices	Support country efforts to empower individuals to make healthy choices that are easy to make with enabling environments and promoting health literacy through policy, legislation, and regulation to mitigate NCD and mental health risks.
Country Investment	Encourage country investment in the prevention and control of NCDs and mental health conditions to enhance human capital and accelerate economic growth.
Health Coverage and Affordability	Advise countries on making NCDs and mental health conditions essential in universal health coverage and affordable health services with investments in social protection, primary healthcare, essential public health services, investment in the health workforce with increased accountability.
Social Protection	Promote social protection for all to ensure equity and economic security in preventing and controlling NCDs including protection from catastrophic health costs.
Engaging Private Sector	Engage the private sector to promote contribution to efforts to address NCDs across the globe and to contribute technical support for capacity-building.
Engage Civil Society	Encourage governmental engagement with civil society for prevention and control of NCDs and promotion of mental health.
Multi-Donor Trust Fund	Advocate for the establishment of a multi-donor trust fund for NCDs and mental health conditions.

NCD, noncommunicable diseases; SDG, Sustainable Development Goal.

Source: World Health Organization. (2019a). *WHO Independent high-level commission on noncommunicable diseases:* Final report: It's time to walk the talk. https://apps.who.int/iris/handle/10665/330023

GLOBAL HEALTH STAKEHOLDERS

Attainment of global health requires an interdisciplinary and interagency approach with collaboration from many organizations. *Global health* refers to "those health issues which transcend national boundaries and governments and call for actions on the global forces and global flows that determine the health of people" (Kickbusch, 2006, p. 561). *Global health stakeholders* include individuals or organizations with a vested interest in programs and plans affecting healthcare inequality and global health issues. Global health stakeholders may include governments, not-for-profit agencies, community groups, businesses, political parties, health insurance funders, donors, UN agencies, health workers, patients, and health service end users. Global health stakeholders can be categorized as intergovernmental organizations (IGOs) and international NGOs. All organizations in these categories maintain a global presence and agenda specific to their mission, vision, and organizational values. Global health issues require an interdisciplinary and interagency approach with collaboration from non-governmental organizations (NGOs) and IGOs for solutions to emerging health problems.

IGOs are often termed *international governmental organizations.* These organizations are composed of sovereign states (member states) representing a specific geographical area with a centralized government. Sovereign states simply stated are a country, nation, or nation-state. IGOs are established most often by treaty or an agreement defining the role and function of the group (Union of International Associations, 2017). Notable examples of IGOs include the United Nations, the World Bank, the International Labor Organization, the European Union, and the WHO.

International NGOs often exist by private philanthropy or as a support to an international organization's agenda. NGOs can be categorized by their primary function: advocacy, policymaking, community activism, issue awareness, or program delivery organization. They are often task-oriented by common interest groups to provide a range of services specific to their mission. Examples include international nonprofit organizations and worldwide companies such as Médecins Sans Frontières, the International Rescue Committee, and the Clinton Health Access Initiative. International nursing NGOs are discussed in the Global

EXHIBIT 14.2 SELECTED GLOBAL STAKEHOLDER ORGANIZATIONS IN HEALTHCARE

ORGANIZATION AND WEBSITE	MISSION
Intergovernmental Organizations	
International Labor Organization www.ilo.org	Promotes social justice and internationally recognized in human and labor rights. Enhances social protection and strengthens dialogue on work-related issues.
United Nations www.un.org	Takes actions on issues confronting humanity such as peace, security, climate change, sustainable development, human rights, terrorism, emergencies, gender equality, and food production.
World Bank www.worldbank .org	Works to end extreme poverty by reducing the share of the global population that lives in extreme poverty. Promotes shared prosperity by increasing the incomes of the poorest 40% of people in every country.
World Health Organization www.who.int	Works to build better health for people worldwide. Works to combat diseases and ensure the safety of food, air, and water.
Nongovernmental Organizations	
Bill & Melinda Gates Foundation www.gatesfoundation.org	Works to help all people lead healthy, productive lives. Improves health, hunger, and extreme poverty in developing countries. Provides access to opportunities to enhance education and improve life in the United States.
Clinton Foundation www .ilo.org	Works to improve global health, women's equality, preventable diseases, economic opportunity, and climate change through philanthropic initiatives.
Florence Nightingale International Foundation www.icn.ch/who-we-are/florence-nightingale-international-foundation-fnif	Supports ICN's work and objectives to advance nursing education, research, and services for the public good. Its GCEF focuses on primary and secondary education for girls in developing countries whose parent or parents have died.

(continued)

EXHIBIT 14.2 SELECTED GLOBAL STAKEHOLDER ORGANIZATIONS IN HEALTHCARE (CONTINUED)

Girl Child Education Fund™ www.icn.ch/what-we-do/ projects/girl-child-education-fundtm-gcef	Supports primary and secondary education for orphaned daughters of nurses in four sub-Saharan African nations: Eswatini, Kenya, Uganda, and Zambia.
Gretta Foundation www. grettafoundation.org	Supports nursing education for impoverished persons living in countries with a heavy disease burden to improve the healthcare workforce and improve patient care and outcomes.
International Committee of the Red Cross www.icrc.org	Provides humanitarian protection and assistance for victims of armed conflict and violence. Responds to emergencies and promotes respect for international humanitarian law.
Nippon Foundation www. nippon-foundation.or.jp/en	Provides funding for maritime sustainability, community development, social welfare, cultural preservation, public health, and education, in Japan and abroad.
Nurses Global Outreach, Inc. nursesglobaloutreach.org/ about-ngo/	Dedicated to engaging nurses in the care of the most vulnerable in the United States and abroad. Began with outreach to the homeless.
Tkiyet Um Ali www.tua.jo	Combats hunger and malnutrition in poor citizens through sustainable, healthy food programs, the first such initiative in the Arab world.
Tzu Chi Foundation tw.tzu-chi.org/en	Provides funding to better social and community services, medical care, education, and humanism in Taiwan and globally.

GCEF, Girl Child Education Fund; ICN, International Council of Nurses.

Nursing Leadership section. See Exhibit 14.2 for examples of IGOs and NGOs. Some of these are readily recognized, and others reflect the diversity of stakeholders across the world.

A basic understanding of the interconnectedness and relationships between NGOs and IGOs is required in order to understand how they may contribute to the advancement of the 2030 SDGs, UHC, fighting pandemics, and global health-related agendas. Often, agendas of these groups overlap and provide an opportunity for collaboration across networks and systems. Nurses have the opportunity to volunteer and work for these NGOs. Additionally, nurses associations with an international focus can and should be a part of these collaborations. Pooled resources through supportive partnerships create and synergize momentum toward shared goal attainment.

Although global decisions are made after complex multilevel and often years-long negotiation, they can directly affect daily lives. The trickle-down effect from global decisions regarding healthcare issues is usually the result of situations and problems identified in many countries. These situations become a global concern, leading to the creation of global policies and recommendations. As the trickle-down effect continues, these global policies eventually end up affecting countries, communities, societies, families, and, finally, individual patients. Understanding the connections and systems at play is part of determining where best the voice of nurses is to be heard to impact the issues at hand.

GLOBAL NURSING LEADERSHIP

Nursing leadership on the global stage includes international professional associations, nurses working in key positions in the WHO and other organizations, as well as nurses with significant roles in various international NGOs. International professional associations are those with an international membership, scope, or presence. Normally nonprofit, these groups represent a specific profession and their respective interests. For example, the ICN is a partnership of national nursing associations (NNAs) representing the interests and speaking on behalf of more than 19.3 professional nurses in the global health arena (WHO, 2020b). International professional nurses associations are also united by common goals of selected specialty nurse groups. Examples include Sigma Theta Tau International Honor Society of Nursing now known as Sigma, the International Federation of Nurse Anesthetists (IFNA), the International Nurses Society on Addictions, and the International Academy of Nursing Editors. Similarly, the World Medical Association is an international group that represents the interests of physicians. The common thread of international professional associations is the shared professional membership of the group. Some, such as the ICN, have special standing with IGOs and can make statements at their formal meetings.

Globalization involves the interaction and integration of persons or organizations from different nation-states pushed by international trade and investment largely driven by information technology and economic policy (Peterson Institute for International Economics, 2021). Globalization directly affects culture, environments, economic systems, healthcare, and society. One could argue the effects of globalization may have a negative or positive impact on the community, based on the transformation of local cultures from the global marketplace. Effective global nursing leadership requires an understanding of this globalization and its impact on healthcare systems, communities, and people. Global nurse leaders share the following qualities: system thinker, critical thinker, problem-solver, integrity, active listener, skillful communicator, courage, initiative, energy, optimism, perseverance, coping skills, and self-knowledge (Oulton, 2014). These leadership qualities enhance the global nurse leader's ability to influence and change the cultural and political landscape. Furthermore, there is a growing level of awareness of the importance of nursing's voice among various stakeholder groups including governments, NGOs, UN agencies, and beyond.

Global health issues discussed by IGOs, such as the UN or/and the WHO, and by international professional association groups, such as the ICN, are many of the same issues discussed by nurses providing direct patient care to affected populations. These global communities are linked directly to the nursing community, with each benefiting from the other's knowledge and experience. See Exhibit 14.3 for examples of key reports related to nursing. In spite of the obvious benefits of joint efforts, these groups work in parallel, with the nursing community on one side and the global community on the other, not crossing paths often enough. Everyone loses when no one collaborates. Most of all, the world population does not benefit from the collective experience, knowledge, and wisdom that nursing can provide to the conversation. This presents a challenge for the nursing community. Global nurse leaders, whether individually or at the organizational level, need to comprehend the larger systems at play and have a worldview philosophy that engages a broader constituency and partners with major stakeholders in shaping the global health agenda.

EXHIBIT 14.3   **SELECTED GLOBAL REPORTS ON NURSING**

REPORT	DESCRIPTION
International Council of Nurses. (2021). Nurses: A voice to lead a vision for future healthcare.	2021.icnvoicetolead.com/wp-content/uploads/2021/05/ICN-Toolkit_2021_ENG_Final.pdf
World Health Organization. (2021). Global strategic directions for strengthening nursing and midwifery 2021–2025. Draft.	cdn.who.int/media/docs/default-source/health-workforce/who_strategic-direc-tions-for-nursing-and-midwifery-2021-2025.pdf?sfvrsn=a5ffe81f_5
World Health Organization. (2021). Strengthening nursing and midwifery: Investments in education, jobs, leadership, and service delivery.	apps.who.int/gb/ebwha/pdf_files/WHA74/A74_ACONF3-en.pdf
World Health Organization. (2020). State of the world's nursing 2020: Investing in educa-tion, jobs and leadership.	www.who.int/publications/i/item/9789240003279
World Health Organization. (2019). It's time to walk the talk: WHO independent high-level commission on noncommunicable diseases final report.	apps.who.int/iris/bitstream/handle/10665/330023/9789241517003-eng.pdf?sequence=11&isAllowed=y
Kennedy, A. (2018). Nurses play a central role in arresting and controlling NCDs. Statement of the Commissioner, noncommunicable diseases and their risk factors. World Health Organization.	www.who.int/ncds/governance/high-lev-el-commission/statement-of-annette-ken-nedy.pdf?ua=1

International organizations, associations, and collaborations are often formed to fill the gaps when healthcare systems reach their stretching points and can no longer meet demands for services. Whether governmental or nongovernmental, international organizations often lack the knowledge and professional expertise of nursing. Organizations like the ICN, for example, are the global voice of nurses. On the other hand, collaborative working groups provide opportunities to share resources, such as access, knowledge, expertise, and funding. To address this issue, nursing collaborations have been formed with key worldwide networks and programs. These mutually beneficial partnerships and initiatives operate to com-plement the strategic plans and actions of the other. Examples include the nursing specialty networks within the ICN, NNAs, Sigma, the Commission on Graduates of Foreign Nursing Schools (CGFNS), international specialty nurses' associations, and the WHO Nursing Leadership.

INTERNATIONAL COUNCIL OF NURSES

The ICN, founded in 1899, is a federation of more than 130 NNAs, the voice of the more than 28-million-member nursing workforce worldwide (ICN, 2021e; WHO, 2020b). The ICN is operated by nurses to represent the nursing profession and influ-ence health policy. The ICN is committed to visionary leadership, innovativeness, solidarity, accountability, and social justice as core organizational values. The ICN has three core areas of active engagement: professional nursing practice, nursing regulation, and socioeconomic welfare for nurses. The vision of the ICN is to be the voice of international nursing by influencing health, social, and economic policy at all levels (global, regional, country) by communicating evidence and best practices (ICN, 2021d). The ICN conducts one of its NNA meetings in advance of the World Health Assembly to strategize its positions and approaches to ensure that the voice of nursing is heard (ICN, 2021c) (www.icn.ch/news/icn-world-health-assembly-74). See section on Nursing's Role in the Global Health Infrastructure.

The ICN has been active in social projects that addressed the MDGs and continuing to do so as it relates to SDG 2030. The ICN is also a forceful voice at times of local and global crisis, as during the global COVID-19 pandemic (Anders, 2020; Catton, 2020; Gagnon & Perron, 2020). Under the ICN's auspices is the Girl Child Education Fund (GCEF), which provides education to orphaned girls of nurses in four developing countries in Africa (ICN, 2021b). The GCEF works in partnership with a country's NNA to manage the allocation of funds. This illustrates how partnering can make a difference on the world stage. The ICN also addresses healthcare workforce issues as noted later. ICN also provides leadership programming through its Global Nursing Leadership Institute™. This is specifically designed to strengthen nurses' political and policy understanding and influence, with a particular emphasis on the SDGs and, more recently, the COVID-19 pandemic. The ICN is also becoming more active at the United Nations at its headquarters in New York not only with nurses in leadership roles but with nurses' regular attendance at many of its forums.

Housed within the ICN is the Nurse Practitioner/Advanced Practice Nursing Network focused on providing international resources for nurse practitioners. The key goal of this network is to advocate for advanced practice nursing in both academia and practice. It provides a forum for knowledge, experience, and expertise in advanced practice nursing to be shared with other practitioners, educators, policymakers, regulators, and health planners.

NATIONAL NURSES' ASSOCIATIONS

NNAs form the ICN membership base. An NNA is an association representing nursing in a specific country, state, or republic. NNAs are formal, nurse-led entities representing the interests of their constituents. The importance of NNAs is immeasurable to nursing practice worldwide because there is no individual membership in the ICN. Nurses with membership within an NNA that is a member of the ICN are automatically part of the ICN. NNA leaders have the opportunity to assume leadership roles in ICN. For example, the first author of this chapter (J. S.) served as the president of the Canadian Nurses Association before assuming the role of ICN president. Pamela Cipriano, a past president of ANA, co-author of the foreword, is now the president of the ICN. The core business of the ICN is to strengthen and support NNAs in professional nursing practice, nursing regulation, and the socioeconomic welfare of nurses. NNAs work through the ICN to collaborate for strategic alliances with governmental and nongovernmental agencies, foundations, regional groups, and other NNAs to advocate for nursing globally. The following are some of the current member NNAs: the American Nurses Association (ANA), the Canadian Nurses Association, the Ethiopian Nurses Association, the Finnish Federation of Nurses, the Australian College of Nursing, and the Singapore Nurses Association. The complete list is available at www.icn.ch/who-we-are/membership.

SIGMA

Sigma is a global health leader for nursing. Sigma (2021) has more than 135,000 members in over 100 countries, with 540 chapters in 700 institutions of higher education. Membership is by invitation to community leaders and students in baccalaureate and graduate nursing programs who have demonstrated scholarship excellence and high achievement. Sigma offers nursing research grants, supports education and research conferences, provides online nursing continuing education, houses the Virginia Henderson Global Nursing e-Repository, mentors with leadership programs, publishes peer-reviewed journals, and provides resources for career development. Sigma influences the global agenda in healthcare through partnerships with IGOs (e.g., UN Economic and Social Council, WHO), NGOs (e.g., JBI [Joanna Briggs Institute], American International Health Alliance), and international professional organizations. Sigma also functions as an international connection hub for nurses so that it can network globally in multiple areas of nursing practice.

COMMISSION ON GRADUATES OF FOREIGN NURSING SCHOOLS

The CGFNS is an NGO that provides verification and knowledge-based practice competency assessment of the healthcare workforce. In the late 1960s, the United States experienced an influx of nurses migrating from other countries. To address the competency assessment of foreign-educated nurses, the W. K. Kellogg Foundation provided funding to the ANA and the National League for Nursing to create the CGFNS in 1977. The main objectives of CGFNS (2018) include (a) predictive testing and evaluation for foreign-educated nurses (outside the United States), (b) credential evaluation for foreign healthcare workers, (c) data collection and distribution service for international nursing education and licensure, and (d) research studies pertinent to internationally educated nurses.

INTERNATIONAL SPECIALTY NURSES' ASSOCIATIONS

Intentionally, some nursing specialty organizations are established as international organizations to represent nurses globally (e.g., Wound, Ostomy, and Continence Nurses Society, IFNA). The missions of these organizations recognize the responsibilities and commitment to advancing educational standards and practices to the nurses and public they serve. Furthermore, they are the nursing voice with the larger international clinical and healthcare community within their specialty. Several of the U.S.-based national specialty nurses' associations, such as the Oncology Nursing Society and Association of periOperative Registered Nurses, recognize the global nature and impact of their associations' work. Their programs extend beyond the U.S. boundaries to support nurses globally with evidence-based knowledge and standards of care. In addition, some specialties have global associations, such as the IFNA for nurse anesthetists. The IFNA has developed practice standards and has created a voluntary anesthesia program approval process.

WHO COLLABORATING CENTRES

WHO Collaborating Centres are institutions within an international collaborative network established to support the WHO's programs within countries, between countries, and globally. Each institution is designated by the WHO director-general with the agreement of the director of the independent institutions and after consultation with the national government (WHO, 2021a). Designation as a WHO Collaborating Centre initially lasts 4 years, with possible redesignation for the same or a shorter period. Each WHO Collaborating Centre strives to strengthen countries' resources and provide strategic support to the WHO's (2017a) programming and ongoing work. Designated centers may apply for grants for specific programs linked to WHO objectives. WHO Collaborating Centres provide two primary functions: (a) implementation of WHO's mandated program objectives and (b) development of institutional capacity in countries/regions (WHO, 2021a). Networks of WHO Collaborating Centres have also been created around specific professional fields, with more than 800 in 80 countries. Examples of these networks include food safety, nursing and midwifery, traditional medicine, international classification, radiation, occupational health, and communicable diseases (WHO, 2021a). The Collaborating Centres have expanded their work from bilateral relations to encompass a broader interrelated focus with multilateral networks.

NURSING'S ROLE IN THE GLOBAL HEALTH INFRASTRUCTURE

The central component of the global health infrastructure is the United Nations and its agency, the WHO. Since its inception in 1948, the WHO, a UN agency, has been considered the global voice and authority on health issues. The WHO is governed by member states, which are the countries and their official governments. Nurses leaders hold positions within the WHO that includes a chief nurse, among others. Policy setting for the WHO is done once a year at the World Health Assembly that takes place annually in Geneva. The World Health Assembly is the decision-making body that provides directions for the WHO's policies. It can last up to 2 weeks, during which reports are tabled and debated, resolutions are submitted, revised, voted on, and adopted, and each country's health minister or selected representatives (e.g., Department of Health and Human Service in the United States) make statements about the health status of their nation. Member countries are not obligated to comply with any of the resolutions passed. Although it is expected that if a country supports a resolution, it would also integrate it into its national strategies, the evidence shows that too often, countries do not give a high priority to WHO resolutions. However, in many countries, the influence of health ministries on the national agenda is variable.

On the other hand, there are WHO agendas that are embraced and often supported by major donors and other UN agencies. One of the significant events for nursing took place in 2019 when the World Health Assembly designated 2020 the International Year of the Nurse and the Midwife, and then extended it through 2021.

Passing this designation was extremely significant as it was supported by each member country. This declaration gives the respective nursing communities in each country the opportunity to further advance the nursing agenda and public profile in both the policy and the practice arenas.

Although the WHO had many reports and resolutions about nursing since its establishment. The *State of the World's Nursing 2020* (WHO, 2020b) report was the World Health Day publication in 2020. This is very important because each year on World Health Day, the WHO publishes its leading publication of the year, which garners world attention, from policymakers, other global organizations, the healthcare community, media, and beyond. These publications are considered to be seminal, nonpartisan, reliable evidence-based documents used by other global agencies, organizations, foundations, and others to build their individual agendas. It is also important to note that the report was published by WHO in collaboration with the ICN and "Nursing Now." This three-way collaboration further strengthened the impact that such a report could have on the state of nursing in the world.

The *State of the World's Nursing 2020* (WHO, 2020b) report provides the latest, most up-to-date evidence on the global nursing workforce and related policy options. It presents a compelling case for considerable—yet feasible—investments in nursing education, jobs, and leadership (WHO, 2020b). The report includes data from 191 member countries and progress in relation to the projected shortfall of nurses by 2030 and policy options to strengthen the nursing workforce to achieve the SDGs by 2030 and the primary healthcare workforce in order to attain UHC and global health. See Exhibit 14.4.

EXHIBIT 14.4 MAJOR RECOMMENDATIONS OF THE STATE OF THE WORLD'S NURSING 2020 REPORT.

1. Countries affected by shortages will need to increase funding to educate and employ at least 5.9 million additional nurses.
2. Countries should strengthen the capacity for health workforce data collection, analysis, and use.
3. Nurse mobility and migration must be effectively monitored and responsibly and ethically managed.
4. Nurse education and training programs must graduate nurses who drive progress in primary healthcare and universal health coverage.
5. Nursing leadership and governance are critical to nursing workforce strengthening.
6. Planners and regulators should optimize the contributions of nursing practice.
7. Policymakers, employers, and regulators should coordinate actions in support of decent work.
8. Countries should deliberately plan for gender-sensitive nursing workforce policies.
9. Professional nursing regulations must be modernized.
10. Collaboration is key.

NURSING WORKFORCE

The issue of the nursing workforce has been on the national and international agenda for decades. Many reports address the challenges associated with the nursing workforce; they continuously project significant shortages. As noted above, the State of the World's Nursing 2020 report is the most significant.

The common denominator that ties the numerous health workforce reports together is the projected shortages and the healthcare workforce requirements needed. To address the SDG 2030s, 40 million new healthcare workers, in addition to replacements for those who leave the workforce, will be needed. Significant differences in the availability of healthcare workers and resources are seen globally.

Human resources for health is a concept that is concerned with having the right number of healthcare workers to give the right care to the right people at the right time. Heads of state and global organizations recognize the enormous urgency for focusing on the human resources for health as a cross-cutting solution to all other global agendas.

The issue of human resources for health is multifaceted because the global healthcare workforce is a complex system. This means that components of the healthcare system may or may not interact because the system's supply and demand varies over time depending on factors such as relationships, pressures, adaptation, and feedback loops. The problem with this complexity is that the outcomes and behavior of that system are highly unpredictable because the workforce components of the system are interdependent and the components often self-organize and change based on the environment. Factors that directly affect the healthcare workforce in the global healthcare system will push the system to behave in a particular way, resulting in negative or positive outcomes.

One component of the human resources for health concept is workforce migration. A maldistribution of qualified healthcare workers results from nurse migration internationally and abroad. Multiple factors influence the decision to practice out of country. Organizational infrastructure, job security, manageable workloads, workplace safety, compensation, gender inequality, harassment, violence, and discrimination have all contributed to the migration of the workforce for better working conditions and a better way of life. In addition, high-income countries faced with nursing shortage concerns have aggressively recruited foreign nurses, often from low- to middle-income countries (Thompson & Walton-Roberts, 2019). The Philippines has led the nurse export globally since the 1950s. Historically, the preparation and export of Filipino nurses have been driven by market demand. Between 1992 and 2003, close to 88,000 Filipino nurses went overseas to work in 31 different countries (Brush & Sochalski, 2007). For vulnerable countries, migration of the nurse workforce has a detrimental effect on the community. Countries in sub-Saharan Africa have experienced the void created by migration to the point that urban hospital units are understaffed and unable to meet the current health demands of already impoverished communities. The end result of nurse migration is inequitable access to care and maldistribution of resources. To address issues surrounding nurse migration, the WHO *Global Code of Practice on the International Recruitment of Health Personnel* enacted in May 2010 promotes ethical practices in international recruitment based on social justice and equitable distribution of health workers (WHO, 2014).

The WHO (2016a) developed a global strategy for guiding policymakers in meeting the healthcare workforce needs for 2030. Challenges identified include (a) equitable distribution of healthcare workers, including numbers and skill mix; (b) competency in practice, including training issues; (c) quality of care; and (d) healthcare system support in the work environments, including socioeconomics and demographics (Kabene et al., 2006; WHO, 2016a).

EQUITABLE DISTRIBUTION

The distribution of the nursing workforce presents its own challenges. First and foremost is the shortage of nursing professionals worldwide when the demographics of the population are drastically changing. Furthermore, the ratio of nurses per population is drastically different in different parts of the world. The aging workforce, especially of nurses, is a mismatch to the booming population of elderly. Socioeconomic barriers also exist where the workforce is unequally distributed, leaving some of the most impoverished and highly populated areas without adequate care (WHO, 2016b). This problem is further compounded by the migration of healthcare workers to countries with better working conditions. There is an ever-increasing gap between the supply and the demand of healthcare workers. This problem is not solved by just increasing the number of workers (Edmonson et al., 2017). As discussed in Policy on Scene 14.1, the nursing workforce issue demands an innovative approach.

COMPETENCY AND QUALITY OF CARE

The quality of the healthcare services provided is directly related to the competence of nurses professionals and the healthcare workforce. This, in turn, is influenced by the socioeconomic environment and access to education. The problem with measuring nurse competency indicators is multidimensional. Worldwide, nursing education is not standardized. There is no global accreditation standard

POLICY ON THE SCENE 14.1: EAST, CENTRAL, AND SOUTHERN AFRICA EDUCATION AND LABOR MARKETS FOR NURSES

Erica Burton, RN, MPH, BScN, GCNC
Senior Analyst, Nursing and Health Policy
International Council of Nurses
Geneva, Switzerland

Being under-resourced is a reality faced by nurses every day. This is not unique to any single country; it is a global issue. Being under-resourced is often seen as only a nursing problem to be handled by nurses. However, problems in nursing have broad societal impacts requiring a broader approach that includes nurses and a variety of other stakeholders.

However, the most severe challenges for healthcare workforce needs are in Africa (WHO, 2016b). Nurses and midwives provide over 80% of health services that are deemed to be essential to health in the East, Central, and Southern Africa (ECSA) region. It is expected that the shortage of nurses and midwives in Africa will worsen by 2030 (Drennan & Ross, 2019). Investment in nursing education and labor markets in the region is essential. Much like other countries, the region needs to increase the production and quality of preservice nursing education and, like many countries, still ensure the entering workforce is employed, retained, and allowed to work to their full scope of practice. This requires complementary investments in nursing governance, regulation and the production of data, and analytical capability to empower countries to plan and manage their nursing labor markets and then guide ongoing investments accordingly.

A unique partnership was created to tackle this persistent regional problem. Under the presidency of Dr. Judith Shamian, the International Council of Nurses (ICN) engaged with the World Bank (WB) because it has a very strong influence on many countries through its lending power. Because healthcare and socioeconomic issues are some of the main issues in many developing countries, the WB is a major funder and adviser in these areas. It was deemed essential that the ICN and the WB develop a partnership. Then two additional organizations were recruited, Jhpiego, a nonprofit organization for international health affiliated with Johns Hopkins University, and ECSA-ECSACON, an intergovernmental health organization that fosters and promotes regional cooperation in health among member states. These states include Eswatini, Kenya, Lesotho, Malawi, Mauritius, United Republic of Tanzania, Uganda, Zambia, and Zimbabwe. It is noteworthy that Jhpiego has a presence in most of the ECSA countries and that its president, Dr. Leslie Mancuso, is a nurse and a strong supporter of both the ICN and the International Council of Midwives.

This distinctive partnership focused on the nursing workforce was distinctive. It brought together four groups: a strong African nursing voice through ECSACON, strong global nursing input through ICN, a strong nongovernmental organization (NGO) contribution through Jhpiego, and the World Bank for its ability to provide loans and grants to low-income countries. The report provides several recommendations related to nursing governance, education, and the labor market which are summarized here.

- Health workforce information systems for comprehensive and systematic data should be strengthened to support evidence-based policy decision-making. Data will also inform human resource planning to effectively monitor and manage migration in the region, in particular out-migration.

- Nurses each representing the government, educator, the regulator, and the professional association (called the Quad) should be strengthened at the country level, and each representative must be involved in all policy discussions and decision-making. The region will benefit from building on existing regional models for planning and cooperation.

- Countries in the region must ensure decent working conditions and occupational health and safety for nurses. Nurses cannot be expected to deliver, improve, and sustain quality healthcare when working without basic infrastructure and feeling safe; both are also necessary to attracting and retaining nurses. Improved accountability mechanisms for quality improvement are necessary and should be informed by both patient and provider experience and outcomes.

- As an important resource to address health system challenges, the advanced practice nurse (APN) role should be developed, strengthened, and expanded, including recommendations about creating regional curriculum frameworks for APN education. Encourage policy that fosters nurse entrepreneurship in order facilitate developing nurse-owned private clinics, thus providing income-generating opportunities, expanding access to services, and supporting the economic empowerment of women.

- Investments expanding nursing education should be targeted toward institutions producing nurses who are most critical for attaining universal health coverage (UHC) and the Sustainable Development Goals (SDGs) in each country, including opening new schools in underserved areas.

- Countries must start to innovate academically and invest in high-quality, transformative educational models (e.g., competency-based, incorporation of technology) supported by meaningful student loan programs. There must be stronger regulatory mechanisms for curriculum and accreditation. The need to retain and grow the nursing faculty workforce must be addressed.

to assess nursing educational programs. Licensure is not consistent across and within nations, leading to a variety of skill levels, clinical experiences, and scope of practice expectations. This has the potential to be problematic in disaster situations. For example, nurses in a high-income country working in primary care clinics caring for patients with heart failure might have to deal with a mass influx of refugees due to armed conflict and war. These nurses would have to quickly adapt their skills sets to care for victims of disaster. Would they be familiar with the culture-specific care required by the refugee population? Would nurses be trained to handle mental health issues resulting from violence and trauma? Would the communities impacted have the resources to provide education and emergent training?

Differences in socioeconomic environments and educational backgrounds create inconsistency and potential gaps in quality healthcare. Socioeconomics has a profound effect on the education of a healthcare workforce. Nations lacking the necessary infrastructure for training and development risk having a workforce that does not provide evidence-based best practices in the care delivered. Quality care mandates workforce infrastructure that includes creating healthy, safe work environments, such as safe staffing and adequate resources. Healthy work environments incorporate occupational health and physical safety with discrimination-free, culturally integrated practices. Nurses should be provided opportunities to collaborate interprofessionally without fear of retaliation or violence as protocols across disciplines vary from country to country. Each country must examine and address this global issue.

The structures in place to support a healthy workforce within healthcare systems are crucial for recruitment and retention. Healthy work environments support optimal health and safety in both the patient and healthcare worker through respect, empowerment, and a safe environment (ANA, 2017). During the COVID-19 pandemic, we witnessed having insufficient protective gear for nurses and other healthcare personnel, which does not create a trusting and positive healthy work environment. Workplace policies in a safe environment are designed to protect the healthcare worker. Examples of policy topics for creating a healthy environment include staffing plans, workload, caregiver skill mix, nurse fatigue, worker safety, diversity, bullying, harassment, and workplace violence.

Globally, healthcare systems have not invested in the workforce, leading to a reduction in sustainability (WHO, 2016a). This chronic lack of training and education in some countries contributes to the continuous shortage of workers. Undeveloped or inadequate protocols for rural and remote care add to the imbalance of resources available and population needs. In some countries, nurses are not paid for months, and violence is a daily reality. Economic hardship, policy change, political systems, and civil unrest often contribute to the instability of the workforce in low- and middle-income countries. Given these impacts, it is perhaps not surprising that leading organizations that cut across healthcare are promoting healthy work environments. The WHO, for example, clearly articulates that a healthy workplace framework "is the right . . . smart . . . and . . . legal thing to do" (Burton, 2010) and that practice guidelines need to be developed. The Institute for Healthcare Improvement has a white paper discussing the importance of a healthy work environment and looking for "joy" in our work, not merely working to eliminate problems such as burnout (Perlo et al., 2017). Nurses must advocate for healthy work environments in their settings and across the world.

ADVOCATING AS A GLOBAL CITIZEN

Global citizenship requires an awareness of the world, a respect for diversity, and a desire for social justice from the local level to the worldwide stage (Oulton, 2014). Global health goes beyond geographic boundaries and is concerned with the health of populations. The nursing profession has a social responsibility and commitment to care for society. This social responsibility extends to global health issues and the SDOHs for the world population. Collaboration, cooperation, negotiation, and leadership are necessary skills for global nurse advocates. Tact and diplomacy, along with the ability to articulate ideas, meaning, and intention, are required for enhancing productive communication to influence a global agenda. The most important attributes for a global leader to cultivate are vision, passion, and emotional intelligence. Vision provides clarity about where you are going. People invest in a process when confident about the direction and path to a successful conclusion. Passion inspires a person to commit to the journey. Your passion around a vision engages others to the cause. Emotional intelligence gives a leader the ability to leverage their strengths while investing wisely in relationships.

An interprofessional approach to a global health issue increases the chance of success. Interprofessional teams provide an opportunity to view the same issue from multiple perspectives to create a "whole" picture. They provide a means of engaging multiple system stakeholders in the process for maximum impact and help communicate the vision so that the team can act on it. Plan for the team or teams to grow as people unite to the cause. Often, coalitions can help grow and sustain momentum and add personnel to achieve your goal.

Every person is a global citizen, and as such, we all have a stake in the outcome. As a starting point, decide which global issue most closely aligns with your personal interests, competencies, and professional goals. Whether it is cancer, traffic accidents, children's health, or any other topic, you need to ask yourself which global organizations are positioned for engagement with these problems. Initially, consider focusing on organizations within your country or region. Examine what you know about the organizations, reflect on their stakeholders and interactions, determine who influences whom, and analyze their business, public, and professional interests. Then determine your involvement and leverage relationships. You can have a voice and an impact on an issue once you have committed to engagement. See Exhibit 14.5 for action steps to start or increase your global citizenship.

EXHIBIT 14.5 STRATEGIES FOR ENHANCING GLOBAL CITIZENSHIP

STRATEGY	ACTION EXEMPLARS
Educate	■ Plan a course of action to increase knowledge on global issues. ■ Invite a global expert to speak at a program or class. ■ Intentionally review global news, podcasts, and books that highlight other cultures. ■ Seek out balanced reporting about global healthcare systems.
Support	■ Create mentor programs for global visitors/workers. ■ Participate in a health fair or clinic for migrant workers and immigrants. ■ Support and volunteer for disaster relief. ■ Donate resources for global initiatives (i.e., book drives for a specific setting).
Travel	■ Investigate opportunities to travel abroad with specialty organizations or churches. ■ Participate in a short-term mission trip. ■ Escort global visitors to local healthcare and culture sites in the community. ■ Volunteer as a chaperone for a group traveling abroad.

POLICY SOLUTION | Pandemic Highlights Nurses as Global Citizens and Policy Makers

The shortage of personal protective equipment (PPE) and exposure to COVID-19 were at the tip of the policy iceberg. With a woefully underestimated death toll of healthcare workers due to COVID-19 at 17,000 and rising, healthcare workers were "silenced, exposed and attacked" (Amnesty International, 2020). However, that did not stop nurses from speaking out and taking action individually and collectively in response to the collapse of health policies during the pandemic. Individually, nurses were some of the first on the scene taking great risks in using social media calling attention to the crises within their midst. Nurses associations across the world, including the International Council of Nurses (ICN) magnified this outcry and then took action by issuing reports, recommendations, and providing resources for nurses.

The World Health Organization (WHO), the ICN, and the National Academy of Medicine all issued major reports in 2020–2021 with policy recommendations clearly based on the experiences of the last year in response to the COVID-19 pandemic. These reports are not issued in isolation but reflect the input of stakeholders across broad sectors of their constituencies. A WHO report on strategic directions for nursing and midwifery acknowledges the impact of the COVID-19 pandemic and its strain on nurses and the healthcare infrastructure. This culminated in policy recommendations to increase job creation, strengthen leadership capacity and education, and encourage nursing service delivery based on country-wide collaboration (WHO, 2021d). This report complements a 2020 WHO report, dedicated to the health workers fighting for and dying from COVID-19, that prioritized healthcare worker safety as a prerequisite to patient safety (WHO, 2020a). Its five broad recommendations include establishing synergies between health worker safety and patient safety policies and strategies, occupational safety for health workers, violence protection, mental health support, and hazard protection (WHO, 2020b).

The ICN (2020a) report, developed from a survey of member national nursing associations (NNAs), identified seven recommendations focused on protecting nurses on the frontlines caring for patients with COVID-19. These include (a) standardized data collection on healthcare worker infections and deaths; (b) recognizing COVID-19 exposure as an occupational illness; (c) adequate PPE and infection control training; (d) zero-tolerance approach to violence, discrimination against healthcare workers (HCWs) and nurses; (e) prioritize nurses and HCWs for vaccinations; (f) prioritize nurses and HCWs for testing; and (g) provide mental health support services and counseling for HCWs and nurses.

The *Future of Nursing 2020–2030* report (National Academies, 2021) whose release was delayed because of the desire to capture the impact of COVID-19 on nurses and nursing. This report, also dedicated to the nurses who died caring for patients with COVID-19, highlights not only the impact on nurses but also the disparity of impact on nurses of color, indicating that the solutions that the U.S. health system needs to focus on are addressing equity and "doing better for nurses" (National Academies, 2021). Within the broad goal of nurses becoming involved in efforts to achieve health equity, three of the nine recommendations have specific details in response to the COVID-19 pandemic. These include (a) a recommended action permanently changing institutional, state, and federal policies adapted in response to the COVID-19 pandemic by 2022 (e.g., telehealth, scope of practice, insurance, payment parity); (b) a recommendation focused on the protection of the nursing workforce in response to public emergencies such as the COVID-19 pandemic, disasters, and climate change; and (c) identifying the impact of COVID-19 on healthcare organizations as an area needing further research (National Academies, 2021).

Nurses associations, collectively responded with voice and outrage, marshaling their forces in response to the urgent needs of nurses. In the United States, the American Nurses Association, working in conjunction with its charitable arm, the American Nurses Foundation, provided extensive educational resources that were free to the public. Its leaders were included in policy discussions at key government agencies. The ANA, state nurses' associations, specialty nurses' associations, and nurses' unions helped nurses expand their voices at all levels by encouraging and supporting their engagement in policy roles, providing accurate and timely information to the public, and sharing their insights and recommendations with the media.

These organizations, the WHO, the ICN, and NNAs, represent the tip of the profession's iceberg. While these reports reflect a distillation of policy, it is the nurses represented by these organizations who need to individually and collectively stand together in order to make progress in dealing with the expected and the unexpected in global health. This includes keeping alert, finding and providing accurate information, monitoring policy erosion in the face of political pressure, building and expanding one's capital, and taking action by joining forces with and supporting associations and other groups.

IMPLICATIONS FOR THE FUTURE

The future of nursing in policy and practice extends beyond the domestic agenda and involves full engagement in global health and its implications. The first Institute of Medicine (2011) *Future of Nursing: Leading Change, Advancing Health* report recommended that nurses lead the change in healthcare reform, engage in lifelong learning, and practice to the full extent of licensure and education. Viewing these recommendations from a national perspective is too narrow a view. As seen with recent world epidemics and pandemic, the downstream effects of a catalyst are felt by everyone. Based on these assumptions, the nursing profession is at a tipping point. The *Future of Nursing 2020–2030* report (National Academies, 2021) indicates that it is more important than ever for nurses to advocate for the profession as a cohesive, global voice. Worldwide, nurses must lead the effort to transform healthcare through UHC, which has the potential to achieve multiple SDGs.

Multifaceted approaches are needed to meet the world population's goals for health. Two of nursing's contributions lie in ensuring the appropriate preparation of the nurse workforce and an adequate number of nurses. As a profession, we must ensure that the training and competence of every nurse meet current standards of practice. Work toward building a global framework for nursing education content, standards, competencies, and accreditation. Internationally, nurses must practice to the full extent of their licensure and education. In each country and region, nursing needs to identify the minimum standards for education and practice. Too few healthcare workers are available for the world population, especially in rural and remote regions. Nurses have the potential to meet this growing demand for services if the proper policies and legislation are enacted and if the economic impact of nursing to a nation's health is recognized by policymakers. Therefore, it is incumbent on nurses to ensure that the proper policies are put into place to make these a reality. There are new emerging agendas over the last couple of years that require further attention from the global nursing community and some consensus regarding the impact of those new global agendas on nursing education, practice, leadership, policy, and the profession overall. A few of these agendas include gender equality, equity, ethnicity, race equality, and violence against women. Leaders of diverse ethnic and racial backgrounds are not sufficiently represented in powerful policymaking positions. Women and nurses are not represented in a balanced form in healthcare leadership (WHO, 2019b).

Although it is essential to have policies and a vision for the future, it is important to recognize that reality may modify plans. Globally, there are many unexpected events such as natural or man-made disasters, famine, and other tragedies that can slow, modify, or completely change national priorities and agendas. The WHO designated 2020 as the Year of the Nurse, and Midwife to commemorate the 200th anniversary of Florence Nightingale's birth, but instead of celebrations, 2020 was a year that will be marked by history as the "pandemic of the century." While natural and man-made disasters are often localized to specific regions, the COVID-19 pandemic engulfed the globe with heartbreaking carnage and devastating health, social and economic impacts that will be felt for the coming decade. The celebrations for the Year of the Nurse and Midwife 2020 were altered and then the year was extended into 2021.

KEY CONCEPTS

1. The SDGs 2030 recognize the responsibilities that each country must assume to eradicate health inequality and the unique role that nurses hold in improving health.

2. Nurses are uniquely positioned in roles to assess, advocate, evaluate, and partner with individuals, populations, legislators, and organizations to address global health issues.

3. Nurses have a social responsibility and professional practice obligation to participate in global healthcare.

4. Global health stakeholders are individuals or organizations that have a vested interest in programs and plans that affect healthcare inequality and global health issues.

5. Globalization involves the contact and integration of individuals and organizations from different countries, and it has far-reaching impacts on culture, healthcare, environments, economic systems, and society.

6. Global nurse leaders must comprehend the larger systems at play and have a worldview philosophy to engage and partner in shaping the global health agenda.

7. Global health goes beyond geographic boundaries and is concerned with the health of populations and equity in the distribution of health resources.

8. Global health issues require an interdisciplinary approach with collaboration from NGOs and IGOs for solutions to emerging health problems.

9. UHC is a central component of the global healthcare agenda.

10. Human resources for health is concerned with having the right number of healthcare workers to give the right care to the right people at the right time.

11. Collaboration, cooperation, negotiation, and leadership are necessary skills for global nurse advocates.

12. Every person is a global citizen and as such has a stake in global health outcomes.

SUMMARY

The world is increasingly shrinking. The expansion of borders, globalization, migration, demographic shifts, and technology have had impacts on the healthcare environment. Global health issues are no longer isolated within single nations or patient populations. The health of low-income nations can directly impact large, economically advantaged countries. Awareness is the first step in addressing a global health agenda. The challenge lies in how best to maximize nursing expertise to impact global health.

Nurses are fundamental and recognized as essential in strategies to improve health. Whether acting as an individual or working within an organization, nurses all over the world demonstrate the power of and contribute to the global health policy. Organizations such as the United Nations and the WHO have publicly highlighted nursing contributions and have invested in the nursing profession to advance global health. Examining the economic value of nurses' contributions to the well-being of a country's citizens and investing in the nurse workforce are key to improving health and prosperity. Nurses can work to ensure the appropriate investment in the nursing workforce. Likewise, by valuing global realities, you can today join the efforts to advance global health through health policy.

Despite the visibility afforded nursing by the Year of the Nurse and Midwife designation, an ongoing barrier is that nurses are often regarded as "just a nurse" by themselves and others, and thus, not use their voice or are not given a voice to advance policy and decisions. During the COVID-19 pandemic, it was clear that nursing did not have seats at decision-making tables in most countries. This is a universal phenomenon that must be reversed as global health continues to suffer due to the lack of nursing perspectives and knowledge in contributing to health policy. Nurse all have a professional responsibility to make every effort to contribute, participate, and expect to have a voice in making policy and practice decisions that will contribute to the well-being of close to eight billion people on this planet.

END-OF-CHAPTER RESOURCES

LEARNING ACTIVITIES

1. Review the World State of Nursing Report (https://www.who.int/publications/i/item/9789240003279) and identify how many of the recommendations are applicable to your setting.

2. Consider the multiple issues contributing to the global workforce shortage (e.g., migration, education, economics, working conditions, workplace violence, gender inequality, restrictions in scope of practice). Research one contributing factor. Create an action plan to address the factor identified. How can you create awareness? Is there legislation already in place to address the issue? If not, what legislation could be enacted?

3. Review the WHO website for Global Health Observatory data. Select a global health priority and review the global trends associated with it.

4. Research the SDGs for 2030. Select one SDG. Create an educational infographic around a specific target or goal for the population directly affected.

5. Review the ICN networks on the ICN website. Find the mission statement and strategic goals for a network related to your area of clinical practice. Is there an opportunity to collaborate? How might you participate in the network?

6. The UN is involved in more than 20 campaigns. Visit the UN website and select a campaign of interest to you. Perform a stakeholder analysis (https://www.un.org/sustainabledevelopment/campaigns/). If you were a change agent, what objectives would you need to be aware of for a successful outcome?

7. The World Bank is a global partnership for sustainable solutions to global health concerns. Select a region. What are the priorities the World Bank is focused on in that region? Who has the World Bank partnered with to address these priorities?

8. How do emergency temporary standards issued by OSHA impact practice? See www.osha.gov/coronavirus/ets. Using this example, what are your recommendations for transition to a permanent standard?

E-RESOURCES

- Centers for Disease Control and Prevention https://www.cdc.gov
- Civicus: World Alliance for Civil Participation https://civicus.org
- Commission on Graduates of Foreign Nursing Schools http://www.cgfns.org
- Forum of University Deans of South Africa (FUNDISA) http://fundisa.ac.za
- Global Health Workforce Alliance http://www.who.int/workforcealliance/en
- High-Level Commission on Health Employment and Economic Growth (HEEG) http://www.who.int/hrh/com-heeg/en
- International Council of Nurses http://www.icn.ch
- International Council of Nurses at the World Health Assembly https://www.icn.ch/news/icn-world-health-assembly-74
- International Council of Nurses Membership https://www.icn.ch/who-we-are/membership
- International Labour Organization http://www.ilo.org

- Jhpiego https://jhpiego.org
- NCD Alliance https://ncdalliance.org
- Our World in Data https://ourworldindata.org
- Our World in Data Global Extreme Poverty https://ourworldindata.org/extreme-poverty
- Sigma http://www.sigmanursing.org
- Union of International Associations http://www.uia.org
- United Nations http://www.un.org
- World Health Anchoring Universal Health Coverage in the Right to Health. What difference would it make? Policy Brief https://www.who.int/gender-equity-rights/knowledge/anchoring-uhc.pdf?ua=1
- World Health Organization Stakeholder Analysis Guidelines http://www.who.int/workforcealliance/knowledge/toolkit/33.pdf

REFERENCES

American Nurses Association. (2017). *Healthy work environment*. https://www.nursingworld.org/practice-policy/work-environment

Anders, R. L. (2020). Engaging nurses in health policy in the era of COVID-19. *Nursing Forum*, 56(1), 89–94. https://doi.org/10.1111/nuf.12514

Amnesty International. (2020). *Exposed, silenced, attacked: Failures to protect health and essential workers during the COVID-19 pandemic*. https://www.amnesty.org/download/Documents/POL4025722020ENGLISH.PDF

Amnesty International. (2021, March 5). *COVID-19 healthworker death toll rises to at least 17000 as organizations call for rapid vaccine rollout*. https://www.amnesty.org/en/latest/news/2021/03/covid19-health-worker-death-toll-rises-to-at-least-17000-as-organizations-call-for-rapid-vaccine-rollout/

Ataguba. J. E., & Ingabire, M. G. (2016). Universal health coverage: Assessing service coverage and financial protection for all. *American Journal of Public Health*, 106(10), 1780–1781. https://doi.org/10.2105/AJPH.2016.303375

Brush, B., & Sochalski, J. (2007). International nurse migration: Lessons from the Philippines. *Policy, Politics, and Nursing Practice*, 8(1), 37–46. https/doi.org/10.1177/1527154407301393

Burton, J. (2010). *WHO healthy workplace framework: Background and supporting literature and practices*. World Health Organization. http://www.who.int/occupational_health/healthy_workplace_framework.pdf

Catton, H. (2020). Nursing in the COVID-19 pandemic and beyond: Protecting, saving, supporting and honouring nurses. *International Nursing Review*, 67(2), 157–159. https://doi.org/10.1111.inr.12673

Commission on Graduates of Foreign Nursing Schools. (2018). *About us. Who we are*. http://www.cgfns.org/about

Drennan, V. M., & Ross, F. (2019). Global nurse shortages-the facts, the impact and action for change. *British Medical Bulletin*, 130(1), 25–37. https://doi.org/10.1093/bmb/ldz014

Edmonson, C., McCarthy, C., Trent-Adams, S., McCain, C., & Marshall, J. (2017). Emerging global issues: A nurse's role. *OJIN: The Online Journal of Issues in Nursing*, 22(1), 2. https://doi.org/10.3912/OJIN.Vol22No01Man02

Gagnon, M., & Perron, A. (2020). Nursing voices during COVID-19: An analysis of Canadian media coverage. *Aporia*, 12(1), 109–113. https://doi.org/10.18192/aporia.v12i1.4842

Griggs, D. J., Nilsson, M., Stevance, A., & McCollum, D. (2017). *A guide to SDG interactions: From science to implementation.* International Science Council. https://council.science/publications/a-guide-to-sdg-interactions-from-science-to-implementation/

Institute of Medicine. (2011). *The future of nursing: Leading change, advancing health.* National Academies Press. https://doi.org/10.17226/12956

International Council of Nurses. (2020a). *Protecting nurses from COVID-19 a top priority: A survey of ICN's member national nursing associations.* https://archive.nursingnow.org/wp-content/uploads/2018/01/Analysis_COVID-19-survey-feedback_ICN.pdf

International Council of Nurses. (2021a). *COVID-19 effect: World's nurses facing mass trauma, an immediate danger to the profession and future of our health systems.* https://www.icn.ch/publications?year=2021&category=68

International Council of Nurses. (2021b). *Girl Child Education Fund.* http://www.icn.ch/what-we-do/girl-child-education-fund

International Council of Nurses. (2021c). *ICN at World Health Assembly 74.* https://www.icn.ch/news/icn-world-health-assembly-74

International Council of Nurses. (2021d). *Strategic plan 2019-2023.* https://www.icn.ch/sites/default/files/inline-files/Strategic%20plan.pdf

International Council of Nurses. (2021e). *Who we are.* http://www.icn.ch/who-we-are

Kabene, S., Orchard, C., Howard, J., Soriano, M., & Leduc, R. (2006). The importance of human resources management in healthcare: A global context. *Human Resources for Health, 4*(20). https://doi.org/10.1186/1478-4491-4-20

Kennedy, A. (2018). Nurses play a central role in arresting and controlling NCDs. WHO Independent High-level Commission on NCDs. World Health Organization. https://www.who.int/ncds/governance/high-level-commission/statement-of-annette-kennedy.pdf?ua=1. World Health Organization.

Kickbusch, I. (2006). The need for a European strategy on global health. *Scandinavian Journal of Public Health, 34*(6), 561–565. https://doi.org/10.1080/14034940600973059

Langlois, E. V., McKenzie, A., Schneider, H., & Mecaskey, J. W. (2020). Measures to strengthen primary health-care systems in low-and middle-income countries. *Bulletin of the World Health Organization, 98*(11), 781–791. https://doi.org/10.2471/BLT.20.252742

National Academies of Sciences, Engineering, and Medicine. 2021. *The Future of Nursing 2020–2030: Charting a Path to Achieve Health Equity.* The National Academies Press. https://doi.org/10.17226/25982

NCD Alliance. (2021). *Making NCD prevention and control a priority everywhere.* https://ncdalliance.org

Osborn, D., Cutter, A. & Ullah. F. (2015). *Universal Sustainable Development Goals: Report of a study by stakeholder forum.* https://sustainabledevelopment.un.org/content/documents/1684SF_-_SDG_Universality_Report_-_May_2015.pdf

Oulton, J. (2014). Leading nursing globally. *Health Emergency and Disaster Nursing, 1,* 29–33. https://doi.org/10.24298/hedn.2014-1.29

Perlo, J., Balik, B., Swensen, S., Kabcenell, A., Landsman, J., & Feeley, D. (2017). *IHI framework for improving joy in work* (IHI White Paper). Institute for Healthcare Improvement. http://www.ihi.org

Peterson Institute for International Economics. (2021, August 24). What is Globalization? https://www.piie.com/microsites/globalization/what-is-globalization

Reysen, S., & Katzarska-Miller, I. (2013). A model of global citizenship: Antecedents and outcomes. *International Journal of Psychology, 48*(5), 858–870. https://doi.org/10.1080/00207594.2012.701749

Rosa, W. E., Upvall, M. J., Beck, D. M., & Dossey, B. M., (2019). Nursing and sustainable development: Furthering the global agenda in uncertain times. *OJIN: The Online Journal of Issues in Nursing, 24*(2), 1. https://doi.org/10.3912/OJIN.Vol24No02Man01

Semega, J., Kollar, M., Shrider, E. A., & Creamer, J. F. (2020). *Income and poverty in the United States: 2019* (Report No. P60-270). U. S. Census Bureau, Current Population Reports. https://www.census.gov/library/publications/2020/demo/p60-270.htm

Sigma. (2021). *Sigma organizational fact sheet*. https://www.sigmanursing.org/why-sigma/about-sigma/sigma-organizational-fact-sheet

Singh, G. G., Cisneros-Montemayor, A. M., Swartz, W., Cheung, W., Guy, J. A., Kenny, T. A., McOwen, C. J., Asch, R., Geffert, L. J., Wabnitz, C. C. C., Sumaila, R., Hanich, Q., & Ota, Y. (2018). A rapid assessment of co-benefits and trade-offs among Sustainable Development Goals. *Marine Policy, 93*, 223–231. https://doi.org/10.1016/j.marpol.2017.05.030

Stenberg, K., Hanssen, O., Bertram, M., Brindley, C., Meshreky, A., Barkley, S., & Tan-Torres Edejer, T. (2019). Guideposts for investment in primary health care and projected resource needs in 67 low-income and middle-income countries: A modelling study. *The Lancet Global Health, 7*(11), e1500–e1510. https://doi.org/10.1016/S2214-109X(19)30416-4

Stenberg, K., Hanssen, O., Edejer, T., Bertram, M., Brindley, C., Meshreky, A., Rosen, J. E., Stover, J., Verboom, P., Sanders, R., & Soucat, A. (2017). Financing transformative health systems towards achievement of the health Sustainable Development Goals: A model for projected resource needs in 67 low-income and middle-income countries. *Lancet Global Health, 5*, e875–e887. https://doi.org/10.1016/s2214-109x(17)30263-2

Thompson, M., & Walton-Roberts, M. (2019). International nurse migration from India and the Philippines: The challenge of meeting the Sustainable Development Goals in training, orderly migration and healthcare worker retention. *Journal of Ethnic and Migration Studies, 45*(14), 2583–2599. https://doi.org/10.1080/1369183X.2018.1456748

Union of International Associations. (2017). *What is an intergovernmental organization?* https://uia.org/faq/yb3

United Nations. (2015a). *Transforming our world: The 2030 agenda for sustainable development*. https://sdgs.un.org/2030agenda

United Nations. (2015b). *Resolution adopted by the General Assembly on 25 September 2015*. https://sdgs.un.org/2030agenda

United Nations. (2017). *Sustainable development goals: 17 goals to transform our world*. https://www.un.org/en/exhibits/page/sdgs-17-goals-transform-world

United Nations. (2021a). *Millennium development goals and beyond 2015*. http://www.un.org/millenniumgoals

United Nations. (2021b). *Sustainable development goals: 17 goals to transform our world*. http://www.un.org/sustainabledevelopment

United Nations Human Rights Council. (2017). *Report of the special rapporteur on the right to human development*. http://www.ohchr.org/Documents/Issues/Development/SR/SRRightDevelpment_IntroductiontoMandate.pdf

U.S. Census Bureau. (2019). *American Community Survey. ACS 1-Year selected population profiles*. Table S0201. https://data.census.gov/cedsci/table?q=american%20community%20survey&tid=ACSST1Y2019.S0101

Wagstaff, A., & Neelsen, S. (2020). A comprehensive assessment of universal health coverage in 111 countries: A retrospective observational study. *The Lancet Global Health, 8*(1), e39–e49. https://doi.org/10.1016/S2214-109X(19)30463-2

World Bank. (2017). *Poverty*. http://www.worldbank.org/en/topic/poverty/overview

World Health Organization. (2013). *Global action plan for the prevention and control of non-communicable diseases 2013–2020*. https://www.who.int/publications/i/item/9789241506236

World Health Organization. (2014). *Migration of health workers: WHO code of practice and the global economic crisis*. http://www.who.int/hrh/migration/14075_MigrationofHealth_Workers.pdf

World Health Organization. (2016a). *Global strategy on human resources for health: Workforce 2030*. https://apps.who.int/iris/bitstream/handle/10665/250368/9789241511131-eng.pdf;jsession-id=E8F3F4371366CD6ADCF0192C77C0B7FA?sequence=1

World Health Organization. (2016b). *Health workforce requirements for universal health coverage and the Sustainable Development Goals*. https://apps.who.int/iris/bitstream/handle/10665/250330/9 789241511407-eng.pdf

World Health Organization. (2017a). *Human rights and health. Fact sheet*. https://www.who.int/news-room/fact-sheets/detail/human-rights-and-health

World Health Organization. (2017b). *WHO to establish high-level commission on non-communicable diseases*. http://www.who.int/mediacentre/news/statements/2017/ncd-commission/en

World Health Organization. (2018). *Towards a global action plan for healthy lives and well-being for all: Uniting to accelerate progress towards the health-related SDGs*. https://apps.who.int/iris/handle/10665/311667

World Health Organization. (2019a). *WHO Independent High-level Commission on Noncommunicable Diseases: Final report: It's time to walk the talk*. https://apps.who.int/iris/handle/10665/330023

World Health Organization. (2019b). *Delivered by women, led by men: A gender and equity analysis of the global health and social workforce* (CC BY-NC-SA 3.0 IGO). https://apps.who.int/iris/handle/10665/311322

World Health Organization. (2020a). *Charter: Healthcare worker safety a priority for patient safety*. https://www.who.int/docs/default-source/world-patient-safety-day/health-worker-safety-charter-wpsd-17-september-2020-3-1.pdf?sfvrsn=2cb6752d_2

World Health Organization. (2020b). *State of the world's nursing 2020: Investing in education, jobs and leadership*. https://www.who.int/publications/i/item/9789240003279

World Health Organization. (2021a). *Collaborating centers*. https://www.who.int/about/partnerships/collaborating-centres

World Health Organization. (2021b). *Global health observatory data: Health workforce*. http://www.who.int/gho/health_workforce/en

World Health Organization. (2021c). *Noncommunicable diseases*. The Global Health Observatory. https://www.who.int/data/gho/data/themes/topics/topic-details/GHO/ncd-mortality

World Health Organization. (2021d). *Health workforce: Global strategic directions for nursing and midwifery*. Report by the Director-General. Seventy-Fourth World Assembly Provisional Agenda Item 15. https://apps.who.int/gb/ebwha/pdf_files/WHA74/A74_13-en.pdf

World Health Organization. (2021e). *Universal health coverage*. https://www.who.int/health-topics/universal-health-coverage#tab=tab_1

World Health Organization and International Bank for Reconstruction and Development, The World Bank. (2017). *Tracking universal health coverage. 2017 global monitoring report* (CC BY-NC-SA 3.0). IGO. https://documents1.worldbank.org/curated/en/640121513095868125/pdf/122029-WP-REVISED-PUBLIC.pdf

Worldometer. (2021, July 3). *COVID-19 coronavirus pandemic*. https://www.worldometers.info/coronavirus/

Taking Action, Shaping the Future

REBECCA M. PATTON, MARGARETE L. ZALON, AND RUTH LUDWICK

The future isn't what it used to be.
—Yogi Berra

OBJECTIVES

1. Examine the critical role and responsibility of all nurses to advance policy to address patient, professional, and societal needs.
2. Investigate strategies that enhance nursing's leadership to influence policy.
3. Compare and contrast the development of nurses' policy roles in different settings and at different points in their careers in relation to their personal goals.
4. Evaluate the roles in nursing and healthcare organizations for political activism.

When each nurse takes one step and joins with other nurses, then more than 4.3 million nurses will be taking steps together to strengthen nursing, improve health. To fulfill nursing's contract with society the standards nursing practice assert that nursing includes "advocacy in advocate for the care of individuals, families, groups, communities, and populations" (American Nurses Association [ANA], 2021, p. 1). The involvement of all nurses in policy provides the best strategy for creating the preferred future for nursing practice and the advancement of health for all. Numerous strides have been made in policy when nurses are involved, but the reality is that to keep pace with the numerous changes in healthcare, it is imperative that all nurses across all settings be involved in policy.

Nurses in all settings, including those in leadership roles, advanced practice registered nurses (APRNs), nurse managers, administrators, educators, and researchers have tremendous opportunities and responsibilities to influence future generations of nurses. Each nurse must not only be involved individually but also bear the broader obligation as leaders to help put in place the structural and process components that encourage and support nurses in a variety of direct care roles to become involved in policymaking. Thought leaders in nursing in the United States and beyond have called for more active nurse involvement in policy (Benton, 2012; Institute of Medicine [IOM], 2011; Kunavikitul, 2014). This is critical not only for policy at the little-p level but also for the future strength of nursing influence at the big-P level.

Widespread involvement requires a paradigm shift to nurses' active widespread involvement in policy. In the new norm, large numbers of nurses are active in policy, tackling the issues and solving problems at work, in the community, nationally, and globally. Becoming a policy advocate, to rephrase the words of Dwight Eisenhower, 34th president of the United States, ought to be the part-time profession of every citizen or as we believe, every nurse. The purpose of this chapter is to more closely examine the creation of a paradigm shift to nurses' greater involvement in policy, creating the structures and processes to facilitate such involvement. We hope to engender a commitment from you, our readers, about the active roles that should be taken in policy now and in the future as your careers evolve. The Policy Challenge illustrates how the commitment to policy can

---

POLICY CHALLENGE | **Transitioning to a Lifelong Policy Activist**

Karen Daley, PhD, RN, FAAN
Past President, American Nurses Association

I grew up in the Boston area, where I often took on the role of caretaker in my family. I chose nursing after seeing my mother's numerous hospitalizations and witnessing firsthand the impact of nurses. After 25 years in direct care as an RN in the one Boston teaching hospital, in 1998 I experienced a work-related sharps injury that resulted in my infection with HIV and hepatitis C.

That life-changing moment transported me into an unfamiliar world—one in which I was no longer the caregiver but rather an individual in need of care and advocacy. To describe that sudden transition from caregiver to patient as difficult is an understatement, especially given how much loss I experienced as a direct result in my health and life. Circumstances forced my transition from a healthy, successful, productive existence and career to a relative world of uncertainty. Suddenly, my days and weeks largely consisted of a life consumed by medical appointments, painstaking waits for lab results, and the constant fatigue and unpredictable toxicity of potent drug regimens. My ability to cope felt tenuous at times. More than anything, I worried I might not survive. After being immersed in this world for several months, my condition stabilized. As less of my energy was expended dealing with adverse effects of powerful multidrug therapies, for the first time I found myself thinking beyond my immediate health to the circumstances that led to my injury along with the nature of sharps injuries in healthcare. I also realized that, in order to make some sense of it and to prevent other nurses from having the same experience I had, I needed to educate myself about these injuries. Shifting my focus to injury prevention would also help me find greater meaning and purpose in what was happening to me—especially given how common and avoidable my injury was.

In 1998, sharps injuries were everyday occurrences (about 385,000 every year) for healthcare workers. Research also revealed something startling to me—that safety-engineered sharps devices were available and many had demonstrated effectiveness in preventing injuries. However, those devices were only available for at-risk workers in approximately 15% of U.S. hospitals. Most important, I learned that injuries like mine could be prevented if employers would be required to make sharps safety devices available. Thus, my advocacy journey began.

Armed with data, personal experience, and resolve, I began a policy reform journey in partnership with the American Nurses Association (ANA) and its leaders. I was already active in the Massachusetts Nurses Association—the state affiliate of the ANA—and had held numerous leadership positions, including the presidency at the time of my injury. My advocacy with the Massachusetts legislature, other state nurses associations, and at the federal level led to my participation in congressional hearings as well as face-to-face meetings with state legislative, congressional, and hospital leaders, and stakeholders.

I witnessed firsthand the power of the ANA—a respected voice and expert in health policy—as it launched a national campaign to update the Bloodborne Pathogens Standard in an effort to reduce healthcare worker sharps injuries. Within one year, as the result of concerted efforts by the ANA, state nurse leaders, industry stakeholders, and federal policy and congressional leaders, I was among those privileged to attend the White House Oval Office ceremony along with then ANA president Mary Foley to witness President Bill Clinton sign the Needlestick Prevention and Safety Act (Pub. L. 106-430) into law on November 6, 2000.

unfold and grow. Increasing nurses' engagement in policy is vital to advancing policy for the profession and the health of the public.

NURSES' CRITICAL ROLE IN ADVANCING POLICY

Some 30 years ago, Dr. Margretta Madden Styles, EdD, RN, FAAN, who served as president of the ANA and then as president of the International Council of Nurses challenged us to think about nursing's essential role in society by stating "Imagine a world without nurses." After the COVID-19 pandemic of 2020–2021, there was no doubt that the world could not survive without nurses. United by the images seen during the pandemic, the public sees nurses as credible sources of information and believes that nurses should have a great influence on policies as it relates to the pandemic. This downstream visibility and credibility need to be extended to policy tables for real meaningful change.

There are far too many examples at the little-p and big-P levels in which nurses have been intimidated, or have been held back with the words, "you're only a nurse" that prevent the implementation of policies with negative or unintended consequences. Some policies have long-standing implications for how nursing is practiced. Nurses have a critical role in advancing policy that directly impacts the profession and addresses the Quadruple Aims of quality and safety, improved health, reduced cost, and improved work life of healthcare providers (Bodenheimer & Sinsky, 2014).

ADVANCING POLICY FOR THE PROFESSION AND PATIENTS

To advance nursing, promote health, and protect patients, nurses need to be proactive with clinical issues, like quality and safety, and monitor and address issues related to the state of the profession of nursing. Ignoring or not addressing issues can have significant policy implications. Protecting patients and the profession are intimately intertwined. The examples of title protection, and quality and safety are examined in relationship to advancing policy.

Protecting Titles

Advocacy for the profession should be the priority so nurses can be the strong advocates needed for the patient. One example that impacts both the patient and profession is title protection, a global problem. Not all who use the title nurse are indeed nurses. It is not unusual to have an encounter at a healthcare provider's office with someone who identifies themselves as the "nurse" but does not have a nursing license.

It is easy to take the title *nurse* for granted. This title is still not protected in 11 states, meaning that anyone can call oneself a nurse (ANA, 2013). See states with "nurse" title protection in Figure 15.1. This practice is a common occurrence in healthcare providers' offices, where medical assistants might be called *nurses* or refer to themselves as a *doctor's nurse*. When people who are not nurses call themselves by this title, it, at minimum, creates confusion in the eyes of the public. It is very often illegal but clearly unethical, deceitful, and potentially harmful. A number of state nurses associations have marshaled considerable efforts to block

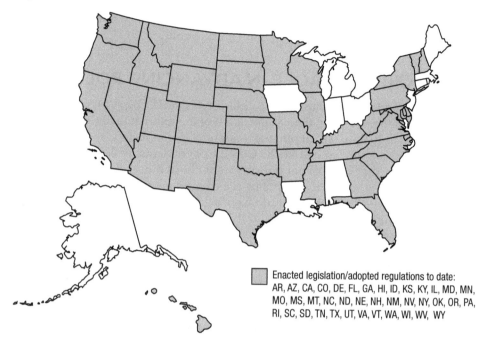

FIGURE 15.1 States with nurse title protection.

legislation that would allow laypersons to use the title *Christian Science nurse*. Each of us has a duty to not only identify ourselves as an RN or as an APRN in all our interactions with the public and other healthcare providers but to also address the improper use of the title *nurse* in our daily encounters with the healthcare system.

Language issues also directly impact APRNs. The term *midlevel provider* is used quite often when referring to APRNs in discussions regarding their titling and practice. However, using *midlevel provider* does not reflect the roles and responsibilities of APRNs and perpetuates a focus on hierarchy instead of interprofessional collaboration. Is anyone called a *high-level* or *low-level providers*? Using this term, and allowing the continued use of this term, creates confusion for the public, insurers, and other key stakeholders.

Ensuring Quality and Safety

Nurses, as the largest group of healthcare professionals, have a reach that is pervasive and has a significant influence on quality and safety; however, this reach is not necessarily matched by their influence on policy. No matter the setting, nurses are at the sharp end of healthcare because of their direct impact on patients when they provide care. However, the blunt end of care is where policy decisions are most often debated and made. Any discussion of quality and safety and any implementation of strategies to improve healthcare must include nurses as the gatekeepers at the sharp end.

The IOM's (2000) classic report *To Err Is Human: Building a Safer Health System* dramatically publicized the statistic that 98,000 deaths occur annually from medical errors. This number equates to a jumbo jet crash every day. Prior to the COVID-19 pandemic, medical error was deemed to be the third-leading cause of death in the United States (Makary & Daniel, 2016). The IOM report indicated that safety was an integral component of quality and that quality could not be improved without addressing safety. Although the IOM report did not begin the patient-safety movement, its release put the spotlight on safety organizations such as the Institute for

Healthcare Improvement and the National Patient Safety Foundation (now merged) and the Institute for Safe Medication Practices. The report spawned the release of subsequent reports such as *Keeping Patients Safe: Transforming the Work Environment of Nurses* (IOM, 2004). Patient-safety advocates have long recommended a systems approach to patient safety, recognizing that major errors were most likely due to a series of faults within a system and that blaming individuals for major errors did not prevent them from happening again.

The IOM's (2000) classic report *To Err Is Human: Building a Safer Health System* dramatically publicized the statistic that 98,000 deaths occur annually from medical errors. This number equates to a jumbo jet crash every day. Prior to the COVID-19 pandemic, medical error was deemed to be the third-leading cause of death in the United States (Makary & Daniel, 2016).

These quality and safety initiatives have certainly saved lives. However, we know that the adoption of a safety culture and achievement of successful outcomes are quite complex and frustratingly slow, as often, a disconnect exists among education, point of care, and policy decisions. The healthcare system is full of intricacies and hazards involving not only the unpredictability of people but also a myriad of interacting and competing parts not limited to equipment, organizations, policies, and financial issues. If one component breaks down in this dynamic arena of healthcare, expectedly or unexpectedly, the potential for downstream failure of more components may result. Failures can and do harm patients and caregivers, resulting in lost credibility and trust in the healthcare system.

Two approaches often used in working toward the goals of improved safety and quality in such a complex environment are the Quality and Safety Education for Nurses (QSEN) initiative and the high-reliability organization (HRO) approach to care. The QSEN initiative established quality and safety competencies for education and subsequently for practice at the system level. The six competencies, modeled after the IOM's (2003) health professionals' competencies, include (a) patient-centered care, (b) teamwork and collaboration, (c) evidence-based practice, (d) quality improvement, (e) informatics, and (f) safety (Dolansky & Moore, 2013).

HROs consistently and over time work at and achieve reductions in the number accidents that cause harm so that having a serious or catastrophic accident is very rare. They are embodied in the culture of the organization and are part of its matrix. Maintaining safety is of the utmost importance, and underpinning this goal are five pervasive ways of thinking: (a) preoccupation with failure; (b) reluctance to simplify explanations for operations, successes, and failures; (c) sensitivity to operations (situation awareness); (d) deference to frontline expertise; and (e) commitment to resilience (Agency for Healthcare Research and Quality [AHRQ], 2019).

The watchword for both approaches (QSEN and HROs) is vigilance, which includes systems thinking. In using these systems, nurses and other providers are expected to view how the components of an organization relate and fit together as part of a bigger whole or process. We have often heard that the whole is greater than the parts, and this requires constant vigilance and many eyes to help anticipate, monitor, evaluate, and improve it.

Despite views on systems thinking, a lack of input at various levels within and beyond the organization continues to be a challenge for nurses. For example, nurses serving as the early-warning system for infectious disease provides an example of how important it is for organizations to have nurses' input. Although the impact of nursing on patient health outcomes is well documented through research and program evaluation, having one's voice heard can still be a challenge.

Improving quality and safety requires much more than providing excellent performance in one's respective work arena; it requires being a thought leader and driver of change and policy. The link of nurse-sensitive quality indicators to the work of nurses and the importance of economic evaluations were discussed in Chapter 12. These same measures and economic evaluations can help make the case much stronger when nurses seek policy changes and want to enforce policy. Hospital-acquired infections are one nurse-sensitive indicator that can be used to illustrate this interplay among cost, quality, and the need for policy. Another area is the increasing call for nurses to be actively engaged in antibiotic stewardship in both frontline work and patient education (ANA & Centers for Disease Control and Prevention [CDC], 2017).

Safety is another area in which nurses' policy input is critical. Nurses are at the sharp edge of safety, frequently the first to make note of safety issues as discussed in Karen Daley's Policy Challenge, and often the first to act on preventing harm to a patient. To achieve a safety culture, nurses need to not only advocate on behalf of their individual patients but also speak up within their organizations and beyond. Being silent in an organization has been recognized as a serious threat to patient safety; communication errors and adverse events may be related to hesitancy in speaking up (Bell et al., 2018).

Being a leader requires being an advocate. Nurses can be the leaders and drivers of change in advancing policy related to safety initiatives. Although there is much value in implementing safety programs, nurses need to be at policy tables, setting the agenda for efforts to improve safety. An example of a safety practice being adopted in some hospitals where nurse advocacy is needed is the adoption of red rules (i.e., rules that cannot be broken). If these rules are broken, the outcome may be serious patient harm. The practice of red rules was adopted from highly reliable industries (e.g., airlines), but they should not be confused with organizational policies such as infection control. A common red rule across a hospital might be patient verification technique or time-out before an invasive procedure. An important role for nurses in the development of red rules is the guidance they can provide in (a) working to ensure that the approach to evaluating a red rule is applied uniformly across departments and (b) conducting studies of the impact of red rules on safety and on nurses beliefs about blame in a safety culture (Jones & O'Connor, 2016).

LEADERSHIP STRATEGIES TO ADVANCE NURSING'S POLICY INFLUENCE

Now is the time to bank on nurses' respected credibility and trustworthiness to lead the way. Leadership strategies to advance nurses' policy influence include understanding the policy competencies of new nurse graduates and new hires of an organization; increasing participation in health policy through professional development; and fostering membership and active involvement in associations, organizations, or specialty interest groups in nursing, across disciplines and with the public.

Previous chapters detailed how nurses can become involved in policy and strategies that can be taken at each step of the policy-making process. Nurses' collective impact is much greater when the potential in nursing's power of numbers is maximized. Thus, one step at the time taken by an individual nurse can become 4.3 million steps taken together. Getting to these steps together requires nurse leaders, at every level and in every setting, creating the expectation that nurses will be policy activists. All nurses, from bedside to boardroom and across settings must be prepared and committed to innovate for nursing policy.

POLICY ON THE SCENE 15.1: Taking the Perspective of Others

Deborah Gross, DNSc, RN, FAAN, Leonard and Helen Stulman Endowed Professor in Psychiatric and Mental Health Nursing, School of Nursing, School of Medicine, Bloomberg School of Public Health, Johns Hopkins University, Baltimore, Maryland

Being a leader in policy requires understanding the perspectives of others and realizing that policy work is never done. When I started my career, I did not think of policy. My goal was to make a difference for families with young children through research. I was looking to expand the Chicago Parent Program (CPP), which was initially created as a research intervention. The research team presented its findings and economic data at a congressional hearing in 2009 in an effort to get Medicaid reimbursement. As compelling as the data was, what stole the show was the presentation by a mother with her 2-year-old and a nurse about their experiences with the program. Not a single research or economic question was asked of the researchers, all the questions were directed to the mother and the nurse. It drove home for me that while research data and the economic evaluation are essential for opening the door, the personal context made the difference in convincing the legislators about the program's value. Now, I use personal stories when possible. What nurses bring to policy is that their research is linked to practical problems that are often couched in the stories of real people and their perceptions.

When I moved to Baltimore, these lessons about the personal connection through stories came with me. They change to address the concerns of different stakeholders. This is what nurses do; they listen and know what people care about. When I talked with school principals about implementing the CPP, I first asked them about their worries and what keeps them up at night. Then, you can frame the discussions to address those concerns. I am careful to keep my approach positive, recognizing that parenting is hard for everyone and that the program will make things easier for them as parents or will save time or money.

Just as with research, every time you do policy work, there is a next step. We compared the group-based format of the CPP to another program considered to be "the gold standard," which uses an individual parent–child coaching model. We had equally effective outcomes but with a 50% cost reduction, and it was reimbursed through Medicaid because the children had a diagnosed behavior problem. Our struggle has been getting it reimbursed for prevention when the child does not have a psychiatric/mental health diagnosis. In Baltimore schools, Department of Education Title 1 funding is used to cover the costs of CPP because that funding targets parent engagement in schools with a large percentage of low-income students. We continue to search for other sources of funding for prevention, but because payment systems in our country are very siloed, each funding stream (education, primary care, Head Start, etc.) requires a different set of rules/requirements.

My efforts to improve health now begin with deliberate thoughtfulness at the front end of policy, and I often work incrementally to change regulations. The lessons learned are listening to the voices of those impacted, telling stories about the personal impact, and leveraging influence through networking to determine the best policy solution. It is important to think about policy at the front end, the front end of your projects, and early in your career. Resources are available to help you. Informal and formal networking, mentoring, and education are keys to policy work. Even though I backed into my policy journey, I am now driving policy, looking forward to the next problem, connection, and policy solution.

Policy Competencies of New Graduates and New Hires

A first step in expanding the number of nurses involved in policy is for nurse leaders to understand the beginning health policy competencies of nurses.

One avenue for understanding these beginning competencies is to examine *The Essentials: Core Competencies for Professional Nursing Education* by the American Association of Colleges of Nursing (AACN, 2021). What is notable about this revision is that in the transition from essentials to domains, policy is not a distinct domain, but health policy is a concept for practice integrated into the document. Health policy is specifically identified as a competency within the population health domain with subcompetencies found in other selected domains. These competencies are articulated at both Level 1 (entry-level professional nursing education subcompetencies) and Level 2 (advanced-level nursing education subcompetencies and specialty/role requirements/competencies). Therefore, it is especially incumbent on educators to ensure that robust attention is given to policy so that the profession continues to march forward on the policy front.

As noted throughout the book, nurses' health policy roles and obligations are grounded in the ANA *Code of Ethics for Nurses* (2015). Ethically, nurses are expected to participate in improving healthcare environments, collaborating with others in meeting healthcare needs, and shaping social policy (see Chapter 2). These expectations require nurses to take an active role in policy, as an individual, as a member of a team, and in designated leadership roles. This may mean redesigning not just clinical policies but also processes such as orientation for new nurse hires, yearly and/or merit performance reviews, or clinical ladders.

Understanding the health policy competencies of nurses is a necessary step in marshaling the strength of numbers. The profession can ill afford the hard-earned health policy competencies being left at the door as nurses graduate from educational programs and move into their new roles. These competencies can be marshaled by taking a lesson from our colleagues in the military, where the expectation is not only that nurses develop and refine their skills for a specific clinical role but also that they assume leadership roles to take policy action. The growth of nurse residency programs provides a ready-made mechanism for incorporating the expectation of leadership and policy engagement. The IOM's (2011) *Future of Nursing* report recommends the establishment of residencies for new nurses, new APRNs, and nurses who are switching to a new specialization. Developers of these programs should consider including content and experiential learning activities supporting the policy role of nurses at the little-p level within an organization and beyond. This can be accomplished by transitioning some of the structured activities of nurse residency programs to add a focus on policy involvement.

Likewise, expectations for professional growth, which have been increasingly incorporated into job descriptions, can include involvement in professional activities. Policy work can be enhanced by harnessing the competencies of new graduates of prelicensure and advance nursing education programs to support organizational initiatives. An example is illustrated with the Legislative Action Interest Group (LAIG) developed at Boston Children's Hospital, which partners the hospital's nursing department with its governmental relations office (Waddell et al., 2016). This partnership involves nurses learning about health policy, engaging in policy activities with policymakers, and collaborating with the hospital's lobbyists. This involvement creates more informed nurses who bring their knowledge to the practice arena, which, in turn, strengthens nursing within their own healthcare organizations. Replicating the LAIG model can lead to more nurses becoming engaged in policy work. Other opportunities for policy involvement should be considered by nurses taking on new roles (e.g., employment at pharmaceutical companies, retail pharmacies, insurance companies). Thus, when nurses advance their education through formal program enrollment or advance in organizational leadership, their involvement in policy will not be a brand-new competency needing development; instead, policy advocacy can be built on a solid foundation.

Health Policy Professional Development

Numerous programs exist to enhance the professional development of nurses in health policy. Some programs are of a general nature and are open to nurses with a requirement to develop a specific area of expertise. The American Academy of Nursing (AAN)/American Nurses Foundation/ANA/ National Academy of Medicine (NAM) Scholar-in-Residence is specifically available to nurses. In Chapter 1, Joan O'Hanlon Curry describes her experience in the Nurse in Washington Internship.

However, there are many more opportunities for gaining policy expertise. Each has a defined focus that can be used as a stepping-stone to wider policy involvement. It is important that nurses be well represented in these programs and take advantage of the available opportunities. Policy fellowships are also available in public health through the CDC, as well as in health services research. Some states also have policy fellowships. One aspect of health policy development is learning to take the perspective of others through programs such as those mentioned in Exhibit 15.1.

EXHIBIT 15.1 **SELECTED HEALTH POLICY FELLOWSHIP PROGRAMS**

American Academy of Nursing—Jonas Policy Scholars *	https://www.aannet.org/resources/scholars/academy-jonas-policy-scholars
Centers for Disease Control and Prevention Fellowships and Training Opportunities	https://www.cdc.gov/Fellowships
David A. Winston Health Policy Fellowship	https://www.winstonfellowship.org/about-us/
GW Nursing Fellowship in Health Policy and Media*	https://nursing.gwu.edu/fellowship-health-policy-and-media
Harvard Medical School Fellowship in Health Policy and Insurance Research	https://www.populationmedicine.org/teaching/fellowships/fellowship-health-policy-and-insurance-research
Health and Aging Policy Fellows	https://www.healthandagingpolicy.org/fellowship-application/fellowship-overview/
National Academy of Medicine Nurse Scholar-in-Residence*	https://www.healthandagingpolicy.org/fellowship-application/fellowship-overview/
National Center for Health Statistics (NCHS)/ Academy Health Health Policy Fellowship Program	https://academyhealth.org/NCHS/Scholar
National Clinician Scholars Program (NCSP)	https://nationalcsp.org
New York Academy of Medicine Margaret E. Mahoney Fellowship	https://www.nyam.org/fellows-grants/grants-awards/student-grants/margaret-e-mahoney-fellowships/
Partners for Better Health Randall Lewis Health & Policy Fellowship	https://p4bhealth.org/randall-lewis-health-policy-fellowship/

(continued)

EXHIBIT 15.1   **SELECTED HEALTH POLICY FELLOWSHIP PROGRAMS** (*CONTINUED*)

Pozen-Commonwealth Fund Fellowship in Health Equity Leadership at Yale University	https://som.yale.edu/programs/emba/curriculum/areas-of-focus/healthcare/pozen-commonwealth-fund-fellowship
Robert Wood Johnson Foundation Health Policy Research Scholars	https://healthpolicyresearch-scholars.org/about-the-program/

*Nursing-specific.

Other avenues for professional development are conferences, continuing education offerings, and individual college-level courses. These types of opportunities are too numerous to list. However, resources to find these types of educational opportunities abound through ANA and specialty nurses associations. Various organizations also offer conferences and/or breakout sessions that provide policy content and subsequent contact hour credits. There are stand-alone continuing education policy offerings available for all practice roles.

Fostering Membership in Associations and Active Involvement in Policy

Increasing the numbers of nurses involved in policy is vital to leveraging our full advocacy policy potential as nurses. Much of our policy work is accomplished through numbers achieved by membership in associations, specialty organizations, or grassroots groups. Whether a nurse is an educator who requires student nurses to attend professional meetings or encourages them to join nursing (e.g., National Student Nurses Association [NSNA]) or other student groups, an agency manager or administrator who fosters staff nurses' involvement in shared governance (as described in Chapter 9), or a staff nurse who covers for other nurses so that they can attend a meeting or who invites a colleague to attend a shared governance or professional meeting, all nurses have a role in fostering engagement and involvement in policy.

Policy involvement provides nurses with the opportunity to learn about practice standards and to engage with other nurses to obtain guidance and information about addressing policy issues of serious concern. Nurses can work together to create a paradigm shift so that practice problems are acknowledged, discussed, and addressed. Nurses who participate in professional associations build on the policy advocacy foundation begun in educational programs and bring their expertise to enhancing the environments in which they live and work. Many times, nurses become inspired about an issue but are not familiar with the processes for advancing the policy process. Although this book outlines many of the steps in policymaking, the ANA, state nurses associations, specialty associations, and their affiliates have their own spheres of influence and provide critical expertise on the nuances of policy processes within that sphere.

Nursing has the numbers to be a powerful influence. The profession has a well-established, respected national association (ANA) with state and local affiliates. In addition to the ANA, many associations at the national, state, and local levels address the special interests of nurses. Working together, these groups can be leveraged to strengthen nursing's influence across healthcare at the organizational, local, state, national, and international levels. Considerable effort has been made through the Nursing Community, a coalition of more than 60 associations representing over than 1 million nurses; the Campaign for Action at the Center to Champion Nursing in America; and the Nurses on Boards Coalition to expand nursing's influence through the placement of nurses in key positions. Nurses associations are working on key appointments at the state level. Often, these positions are perceived to be only hospital- or health-focused boards. However, relevant experience and/or influence can be garnered by serving on boards of community-based affiliates of nonprofit organizations, schools, libraries, food banks, and agencies related to environmental hazards, to name a few. These efforts can expand influence into all the communities where nurses live and work.

An important strategy for helping foster involvement is acknowledging the policy work and outcome that resulted from nurses' activism. The purpose is not only to provide recognition for an individual's contributions to policy efforts but also to enhance visibility in a selected community. Recognition within organizations or associations creates excitement and fosters member engagement. It also provides additional opportunities to bring the policy to the attention of key stakeholders. Most important, recognizing the work of policy activists creates a culture in which policy advocacy becomes the norm rather than the exception.

When key issues emerge, stakeholders such as state associations, specialty associations, educational institutions, healthcare systems, and other groups have convened summits and other high-level, high-visibility activities, along with the attendant media activities, to heighten the publicity around a specific issue. These activities often lead to the production of a white paper, position statement, or policy brief that has an enduring influence on the profession and beyond. An example of such a well-known document is the 1965 ANA position paper on entry to practice. Fast-forward to 2017 to the signing into law of the requirement for RNs in New York to obtain a BSN within 10 years of initial licensure. Although this is a landmark achievement, it also illustrates the long path to achieving policy goals that combine the use of evidence, perseverance, and political skill.

The work of nursing cuts across disciplines. There are numerous opportunities for interdisciplinary policy work. Examples include the Gerontological Society of America and Academy Health, which recognize the integral role of policy in their conferences and other activities. Opportunities for interprofessional collaboration in policy are available in nearly every specialization (e.g., critical care, cardiovascular care, pain management, patient safety, long-term care).

CONFRONTING FAILED POLICY AND REENERGIZING ENGAGEMENT

Policies do fail. It is often nurses at the sharp end who see the consequences of policy failures. Nurses at all levels, those in direct care and nurse administrators, have a role in addressing policy failure. It starts with reporting the failure, but depending upon the policy and the nature of nursing's role in the failed policy, taking additional steps is often necessary. These advocacy actions can be hard and may necessitate moral courage (Davidson et al., 2020).

Given the complexity of healthcare, it is perhaps no surprise that policy failures cannot be avoided. The extent of failure is such that "even policies that have become known as classic policy failures also produced small and modest successes" (McConnell, 2015, p. 231) One set of helpful parameters to examine the good, the bad, and the ugly of failed policies includes "overly optimistic expectations; implementation in dispersed governance; inadequate collaborative policy-making; and the vagaries of the political cycle" (Hudson et al., 2019, p. 2).

Another detailed approach to examining policy failure by Porter-O'Grady et al. (2019, pp. 251–253) is presented in the following paragraphs. Some of the factors they recommend in order to examine policy failure include inappropriate objectives, asymmetrical information, moral hazard, adverse reactions, and clear communication.

Often a policy is doomed for failure at the outset, driven by the primary process failure in establishing *objectives that are inappropriate* (Richtermeyer, 2010). Focusing a policy on service provision directed to specific populations rather than to clearly defined and well-articulated health outcomes, expectations, or impact is a mistake often replicated in healthcare. Establishing strong helmet laws to reduce accidental head injury is not nearly as specific a policy objective as is the establishment of such laws to reduce crippling and costly brain damage. Additionally, health laws that focus on cause or prevention are more effectively defined than those emphasizing treatment.

Asymmetrical information, with some individuals having different or varying amounts of information, also contributes to policy failure. COVID-19 vaccination information and disinformation are an example that will be studied for years. However, the classic example in the United States is the duplicity shown by drug companies when recommending the use of their drugs to the general population. While this information may be objectively correct, its accuracy and veracity are particularly limited when viewed through the lens of individual patient conditions, circumstances, and drug interactions. One of the most prescribed powerful psychotropics is prescribed by primary care providers because of patient demand rather than carefully delineated clinical need. One notable erectile dysfunction drug is generally prescribed for those who want it but who present little evidence of actual erectile dysfunction; advertising a side effect of prolonged action led to a boon in demand. Both are examples of this information asymmetry resulting in behaviors that have little relationship to purpose or intent.

An important threat to the integrity of policy formation is the issue of *moral hazard*. There are many cases in the United States in which the Food and Drug Administration (FDA)–approved drugs have been used for off-label purposes or in which the data supporting the use of drugs for specific purposes have been inadequate or inaccurate. Often, the interest in generating a large volume of sales or the exciting potential effects of one of these drugs overwhelms careful judgment regarding appropriateness, safety, and efficacy. Problems lie both in policy, which governs the approval process, and in issues with the effectiveness related to countering opportunity enthusiasm, elements of groupthink, or inadequacies in review or process leading to a negative impact or outcome.

Often driving policy failure are issues of *adverse selection* regarding who, how, and where policy is managed and executed. Forming policy often portends a legitimate response to a public need. That good intention is sometimes lost in the dynamics of politics, competition, lowest bidder vendor selection, hidden agendas, and so on. Implementation and application of policy can be disciplined through clear management, budgetary parameters, and precise metrics, which validate the relationship among intent, impact, and outcome expectations. A classic example of the conflict between policy and resources is that which relates to the wide variety of nursing staffing mechanisms and approaches. Frequently, policies related to staff-to-patient ratios do not include valid measures of preparation, competence, intensity, and demand, resulting in generalized staff-to-patient ratios that may not best fit the clinical conditions or requirements of patients or populations. As a result, wide variation exists in the appropriate use of resources and a good fit with patient needs.

Failing to effectively *communicate* is one of the challenges to successful policy implementation. Communication throughout the process from design to implementation and evaluation is critical. A thorough and complete generation of relevant information related to the character, content, and intent of the policy gets lost or altered in the transition and communication process. Ineffective communication, in all its forms, can result in unintentional modification of the policy. In effect, the policy being implemented is frequently not the policy designed, and either the structure of implementation leads to a perversion of the policy or the processes of application implement a policy format that looks little like its origination. Clear communication processes are necessary to ensure that policies are efficient, appropriately applied, impactful, and therefore less likely to fail.

Ongoing *monitoring* is essential as policies move into the rituals and routines of organizational systems and human practices. They can often devolve into patterns of behavior and action that little resemble the purpose, intent, or origination that drove policy formation. A structured, regular, consistent review of an individual policy is a corollary for the effective management of policy. This review can serve to determine the policy's ongoing value and relevance. Some institutions may bar nurses from using cell phones while at work. Yet, nurses are now using their personal smartphones to access online information about medications, diseases, and laboratory tests, as well as applications to help patients manage their illnesses. An unintended consequence of limiting access to such resources is that it could have a negative impact on the quality of care received by patients. Policy is as dynamic as the circumstances it addresses; when circumstances change and policy fails to change along with them, people become cynical, lax, and noncompliant, and their action becomes increasingly situational (Scott, 2004). (See Exhibit 15.2.)

EXHIBIT 15.2 SUGGESTIONS FOR AVOIDING POLICY FAILURE

- Make sure the use of policy to address the behavior is necessary.
- Define objectives in a way that clearly relates to policy outcomes.
- Make sure there is a tightly related interaction between cause and effect in policy formation.
- Define a clear relationship among cost–benefit, outcome efficacy, and effectiveness.
- Invest and engage stakeholders in policy design and construction.
- Ensure that there is an effective communication model that affirms a strong relationship between intent and implementation.
- Establish a continuous and ongoing mechanism for monitoring policy effectiveness and relevance.

Source: Porter-O'Grady, T., Malloch, K., & Johnson, I. (2019). Changing organizations, institutions, and government. In R. Patton, M. Zalon, & R. Ludwick (Eds.), *Nurses making policy from bedside to boardroom* (2nd ed., pp. 251–253). Springer, American Nurses Association.

POLICY ROLES

Nurses historically have played a suboptimal role in influencing policymaking (Rasheed et al., 2020). To change this trajectory, policy activities and expectations must be at the least incorporated into existing educational institutions and organizational structures. Voting is a civic responsibility in which it is known that some subgroups in nursing take very seriously. Of nurse practitioners, for example, 94% reported voting in the 2012, and 95% planned to vote in the 2016 presidential election (O'Rourke et al., 2017). Other easily achievable individual or group activities include active engagement in meetings and discussions, outreach to educate and influence stakeholders, activism in professional and consumer groups, and advocating for patients and nurses at the policy forums and with policymakers at all levels. All nurses can help foster policy activities and expectations. In this section, the roles of direct care, nurse, educators, and nurses with graduate education that hold managerial and advanced practice roles are highlighted because the work of these groups is necessary to avoid a continuing gap between education and practice related to policy.

Direct Care Nurse

All nurses in direct care roles have responsibilities to foster policy advocacy in their environments. Resources and structure vary across settings and locations. For example, ambulatory surgery and endoscopy centers typically have less support and individual nurses must take on a greater role with vigilance and oversight. One of the worst infection-control lapses occurred at the Nevada endoscopy clinics owned by a single gastroenterologist. This lapse created a public health crisis of enormous proportions, in which up to 63,000 patients might have been exposed to hepatitis C. Only one nurse, who was employed at the clinic for less than 1 week, reported her concerns about improper charting practices (Leary & Diers, 2013). In this environment, rife with breakdowns in practice standards, nurses were too intimidated regarding their advocacy responsibilities to address these concerns. Lest we think that this was an isolated incident, the CDC (2019) reports that more than 200,000 patients have been advised of their potential exposure to blood-borne pathogens since 2001. In response, the CDC leads the Safe Injection Practices Coalition, which created the *One & Only Campaign* to raise public and professional awareness. Given the sheer number of notifications, it is likely that many nurses were involved with or observed breakdowns in practice.

A positive work environment is necessary to foster policy advocacy. A poor work environment results in nurse burnout, high turnover, job dissatisfaction, and negatively affects patient outcomes (Lake et al., 2019; Shin et al., 2018). Nurses and others in healthcare organization leadership roles have a responsibility to create healthy environments (ANA, n.d.) to foster advocacy, which is critical to patient safety, quality outcomes, and a safe work environment for nurses. One type of leader indispensable to improving the work environment is the clinical nurse specialists (CNSs), who have been called "liquid gold" for their multiple roles, such as the ability to foster healthy work environment standards (Ulit et al., 2020).

With the expansion of primary care, attention is now being drawn to factors critical to establishing a positive work environment in these settings. Not surprisingly, better nurse practitioner (NP)–physician relations, independent practice and support, professional visibility, and NP–administrative relations scores are associated with a lower risk of burnout (Abraham et al., 2021). The practice environments have also been examined for certified registered nurse anesthetists (Boyd & Poghosyan, 2017), nurse midwives (Thumm et al., 2020), and CNSs (Thurby-Hay et al., 2020). Creating a work environment that ensures opportunities for nurses to take an active role in controlling their practice and to positively influence the critical factors in that work environment will entail policy knowledge and work.

The challenge as a profession is to help nurses understand the policy implications of day-to-day practice and the way that organizational, legislative, and regulatory initiatives can, in turn, impact policy in everyday practice. The issues need continued activism and monitoring for new developments that are on the horizon as the nature of healthcare and the myriad of providers evolve.

Nurse Educator

To increase the number of nurses well versed in policy, a two-pronged approach is needed: faculty preparation for teaching policy and meaningful engagement of students at all levels in policy. Over and over in this book, the authors and editors make the case for increasing policy content, both didactic and experiential, in nursing education. Strategies to increase policy knowledge and competencies are included in text's content, learning activities, and e-resources. One area that has not been addressed is the policy education of nursing faculty. A lack of preparation of students in nursing programs is an often-cited barrier to policy, but less talked about is the lack of faculty preparation to teach policy.

Recognizing the need to address policy in nursing education, the AACN (2017) convened a think tank of policy curriculum nurse experts to advise its board. The think tank created a set of recommendations for the board's consideration that included strategies to increase both nurse faculty and students' expertise in health policy so that future nurses will understand the drivers of health policy and be able to set forth nursing expertise at all levels of policy. Then in 2018, the Nursing Now campaign launched a 3-year program (see Chapter 14) to raise the visibility of nursing and give it a stronger voice in policy discussions globally. Despite the report by the think tank and the work of the Nursing Now campaign, policy involvement on a large scale remains elusive for faculty and students alike.

A hallmark of quality nursing education is that faculty possess the necessary qualifications to teach their assigned courses in the curriculum. Accreditation criteria and regulatory standards provide guidance for faculty qualifications by education and experience for their teaching responsibilities. Someone who has never been involved in policy or is not a member of a professional association is not qualified. The assumption is that if there is a student expectation for certain competencies, then the faculty would have at least those competencies and expertise beyond the minimum. Just as nurse educators teaching maternal–child health nursing are expected to have the appropriate educational preparation and experience to support that teaching assignment, one would expect that faculty would have commiserate preparation for teaching health policy. Evidence indicates that a strong foundation in policy led by educators who are well grounded in policy has the potential to increase the policy competencies of nurses (Byrd et al., 2012; Perry & Emory, 2017; Primomo, 2007).

Evidence about faculty preparation in health policy is sparse. Staebler et al. (2017) found that faculty may not be fully prepared to teach policy but that nursing education administration does not value policy expertise; 46% of the respondents indicated lack of expertise was a barrier to teaching policy. The lack of expertise is exemplified by this comment, "Much of the time, the faculty have little 'real' policy experience" (Staebler et al., 2017).

A lack of educational preparation, coupled with a lack of administrative support and the dialectic of new faculty pursuing traditional research scholarship to the exclusion of all other work may systematically erode nurse faculty contributions to health policy advocacy and the development of policy competencies. Other factors contributing to this problem include faculty shortages and abundant use of part-time and adjunct faculty. Furthermore, it is also not known to what extent programs are held accountable for ensuring that faculty assigned to teach policy have sufficient expertise or preparation to do so. Nor is there consensus on the nature of such faculty qualifications and the best strategies for preparing faculty for teaching responsibilities related to health policy.

To address long-standing issues of adequate faculty preparation, we propose that it includes the theoretical underpinnings of policy (e.g., policy analysis, policy decision-making, policy evaluation): an understanding of civics and global citizenship; historical and current events influencing the trajectory of healthcare and nursing; competencies in the policy and political arenas; and active engagement in the ANA, state and specialty associations, and other stakeholder groups. School and program leadership have a critical role to play in ensuring that not only are faculty prepared but that the school environment also promotes a culture of active engagement in policy. In order to achieve the goals set forth in the *Future of Nursing 2020–2030: Charting a Path to Achieve Health Equity* report (National Academies, 2021), it is critical that academic nurse leaders and accrediting bodies advocate that faculty be prepared in all phases of the policy process. Faculty have a pivotal role in teaching, modeling, and mentoring students in advocacy and policy, but they must also have basic policy competencies themselves if they and the nursing profession are to be successful in the policy arena.

Likewise, a concerted effort is needed to ensure that educational strategies are substantive and meaningful and engage students to use advocacy skills in multiple policy arenas. It is not surprising that new graduates, who often are focused on honing clinical skills and who may not have had a strong acclimatization to policy, will have limited policy involvement. These complementary findings indicate that significant investment in the value of policy education for nurses, with the implementation of policy content in nursing curricula, has the potential to reap rewards for the profession.

Strengthening policy-related activities in nursing educational programs requires a staged approach that is matched to the educational level of the student as recommended by Ellenbecker et al. (2017). Faculty and students can use the Patton–Zalon–Ludwick (PZL) Policy Assessment Framework (see Chapter 1) as a guide for assessing and tailoring policy-related learning activities.

Some strategies for developing policy expertise includes establishing and strengthening health policy courses, integrating policy learning activities across courses, creating expectations for professional association involvement, and expanding the emphasis on civic or service-learning that focuses on upstream activities to advance health advocacy. The use of a variety of strategies creates more dynamic engagement in policy discussions at the big-P and little-p levels, upstream/downstream, and Health in All Policies (HiAP) that contribute to an overall culture that values policy.

Education for policy can take place in dedicated coursework in both nursing and with other disciplines, as well as through experiential learning accomplished with professional activities and involvement in specific policy issues germane to clinical content. Incorporating policy activities always begs the question: If we add to the curricula, what might be deleted or changed? Although adding to health policy curricula might be a long-term solution, there are opportunities to incorporate a policy focus within the existing curricula. These include service-learning activities, as well as strengthening support for leadership activities through the student nurses association, state nurses associations, and specialty associations.

Courses with heavy clinical content can include the policy implications drawn from healthcare disparities, genetics, and access to care, as well as quality and safety initiatives. The latter almost always includes implications for policy. Other healthcare professional groups have the same issues in preparing their workforce for policy activism amid calls to action by their leaders. A policy course can include formal lectures and classroom exercises, integrating real-world experiences, guest lecturers with direct policy experience, and a culminating experiential learning activity.

Infusing policy-related content into nursing curricula can be accomplished by incorporating a policy focus into clinically-oriented discussions. This can be accomplished on a regular basis in clinical settings as students learn about the processes of care. When issues related to common clinical problems, such as safety, documentation, and pain relief, are discussed, policy can and should be addressed. Reviewing the policies associated with these topics can help students see how policy can guide the resolution of care problems, how policy can be developed, or where there are gaps between practice and policy.

Likewise, students' policy awareness can be enhanced by the consistent inclusion of health policy implications in classroom discussions. Other avenues for emphasizing the importance of policy are including upstream approaches to policy (e.g., food insecurity policy vs. the provision of meals for an individual) and identifying strategies for a HiAP approach (e.g., repairing sidewalks across a community vs. encouraging exercise). Incorporating policy discussions into clinical conferences also means that adjunct faculty, who often provide clinical teaching, need to be well versed in policy. Policy content and expectations should be included in preceptor orientations.

Service-learning activities, which have been widely incorporated into nursing curricula, can increase students' sensitivity and awareness of social justice issues. Very often, these activities focus on providing individual service to members of disadvantaged communities. Systematically expanding this focus to include upstream activities and a HiAP approach within volunteer experiences is synergistic with efforts to improve understanding of the social determinants of health. This larger, more proactive approach can help students learn about the vital role of policymaking in advancing health. Education is needed to facilitate the use of this broader approach. A community and/or health promotion focus can be used as a service-learning structure for the development of health policy competencies at the undergraduate level (Broussard, 2011; O'Brien-Larivée, 2011). Similarly, the NSNA's (n.d.) Leadership University provides a structured mechanism for providing course credit for leadership-related learning activities that include, among others, shared governance, legislation, and community health and disaster projects. Creating an expectation of policy advocacy and involvement needs to happen across a curriculum so that the value of advocacy in health policy can be internalized. When health policy is only a strategy mentioned or addressed in a final capstone course, students have difficulty understanding the connections to their daily practice and may see participation in health policy advocacy as an unnecessary and boring impediment to the development of the competencies required to transition to a new practice role.

Embedding policy-related content at the master's level should also occur in clinical and classroom settings. Interest and involvement in policy by nurse faculty serve as important modeling of policy activist behaviors. APRN education requires the three "Ps," physical assessment, pathophysiology, and pharmacology as a common foundation. It strongly encouraged here that a fourth "P" of policy be added to demonstrate the value of policy in every APRN's education.

An exemplar of effective role modeling for professional development in relation to policy is the American Association of Nurse Anesthesiology (American Association of Nurse Anesthesiology). The AANA maintains a membership penetration well over 90%, enabling it to have a large presence in Washington with one of the largest healthcare Political Action Committee (PAC) funds. Much of this is accomplished with a strong educational foundation in health policy in their educational programs. This advocacy and policy work is replicated in their state affiliates across the nation. As has been demonstrated, important policy advances for the profession occur at the state level. Many opportunities for policy work present themselves at the doctoral level. In DNP programs, the final scholarly project or capstone might focus on a policy issue. Policy implications, as noted by Gross earlier in the Policy on the Scene 15.1, should be identified at the front end of a project.

The growth of programs offering nursing doctorates with an emphasis on the health policy and leadership roles of nurses provides unique opportunities for strengthening policy advocacy. Policy courses and capstone courses in policy provide the opportunities for immersion experiences in policy, allowing students to explore issues in depth and engage in multiple steps of the policymaking process. The growth of these programs also creates the need to develop the policy competencies of faculty across the curriculum.

Nurses in Advanced Organizational Roles

Equally important to the full realization of nurse policy engagement is the role of nurses in organizations through which care is delivered (e.g., hospitals, community). Nurse managers and nurses with advanced degrees have critical roles for active policy engagement not only individually but also in mentoring, coaching, role modeling, and creating structures and processes that facilitate direct nurse care involvement in policy. As the group of nurses most often responsible for developing, monitoring, evaluating, and changing policy, nurses in advanced organizational roles are in a unique position to help other nurses understand policy not only within the work setting but also outside the organization in associations and community work. Their advanced role and often advanced education provide opportunities for engagement that direct care nurses frequently or readily do not see.

A strong commitment from organizational nurse leaders is needed to incorporate policy expectations into orientation, residency programs, and performance reviews. The shared governance model provides a structure for nurses to have input into their practice and work environment, and input related to policy is one of the vital elements to success. Through shared governance, nurse leaders can empower nurses to use and develop their intellectual and social capital, which are necessary skills to move policy advocacy from the little-p to the big-P.

It is, therefore, necessary to make sure that nurses understand the shared governance structure of the nursing organization and can not only tell you where to locate the documents that describe this structure but also identify all the parts and the interconnections. Nurses need to know how to get involved and to have the support they need (e.g., time back, coverage, paid time) to attend and carry out the work of the council or committee of shared governance to which they belong. These activities require organizational leaders to demonstrate that they believe in the value of shared governance and that they are willing to expend resources and energy to implement and provide ongoing support for shared governance. This support starts with the chief nurse officer and extends across all leadership. These resources include professional development for direct care nurses so that they can better understand shared governance and the necessary space, time, and financial resources to do so. With the increasing emphasis on interprofessional practice and shared governance for patient care across disciplines, it is important that nursing's voice and perspective are not lost (see Chapter 11).

A clear example of when the organization has failed in shared governance is when whistle-blowing occurs. This issue can be seen in the hepatitis C story shared earlier in the Work Environment section. This story is a clear example of why internal policies to address nurse concerns are vital for protecting patients and nurses. Shared governance makes it hard for nurses to work in silos, and working in silos makes it easier for bad behavior to go undetected and violations to be unreported. As Fletcher et al. (1998) succinctly state, "our underlying premise is that when whistleblowing occurs there is an institutional failure" (para. 11).

Organizational nurse leaders can also help build a culture that values policy advocacy by using several strategies: role modeling, coaching, and mentoring. First, as a leader, take inventory of your policy activities and memberships for self-evaluation and for the potential that they may have for being shared. If, for example, you are an APRN, consider inviting a nursing student who works at your agency or a student you precept in your advanced practice area to attend a local membership meeting. For new members of shared governance committees, remember to have an established orientation process (see Chapter 11).

Finally, providing recognition for nurses involved in policy, while noted earlier, bears repeating, specifically as it relates to the organization. Through organizational and unit newsletters, the accomplishments in policy, appointments to boards, memberships, and offices held should be noted. Imagine working in perioperative nursing and not knowing a colleague was on a national subcommittee of the Association of periOperative Registered Nurses (AORN). The names of nurses sitting on shared governance councils or committees should be highlighted in the areas where they work and posted on easily accessible resources such as an organization's intranet and/or internet site.

All nurses have roles in policy, and nurses with advanced education have not only individual roles but also roles in assisting direct care nurses in policy advancement. The important contributions of nurses to the development of policy occur at the local, state, and national levels. In an increasingly global, changing, and often uncertain world, nurses around the world face similar challenges in advancing health policy, within the context of their unique environments. Leadership development provides a foundation for the development of competencies in policy.

POLICY ROLES IN TIMES OF CHANGE AND UNCERTAINTY

Many people, including nurses, avoid talking about politics and complain that they "hate" politics. "Yet politics can no more be avoided than traffic on a freeway. It always exists" (Condon, 2015, p. 115). Although politics may create instability in a number of arenas, the reality is that change and uncertainty are omnipresent both in our professional practice and in health policy. Regardless of the setting, when nurses assume responsibility for the care of patients, there is uncertainty, whether it is related to trying to figure out what is happening with a patient, to predicting what strategy might work best for patient teaching, to determining best method for delivering anesthesia, or to reducing the incidence of opioid addiction in our communities. We address uncertainty in practice by developing and practicing our competencies so that we are prepared to handle new and unexpected situations. Similarly, we can address uncertainties in the policy arena by developing and performing policy competencies. As citizens and professionals, we must know the policy process and, most important, participate in advocacy efforts throughout our careers. Being informed and engaged prepares us for new challenges in the ever-changing healthcare landscape, as well as obstacles created under the guise of normal political differences that are cleverly designed to deliberately derail the goal of healthcare for all. See the Policy on Scene 15.2 by Pearce, Gordon, and Summers, cofounders of Healing Politics, an organization designed to educate nurses to run for public office.

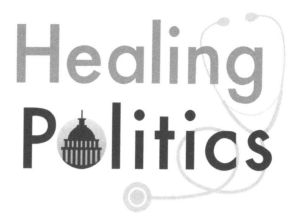

FIGURE 15.2 Healing politics

POLICY ON THE SCENE 15.2: Healing Politics: An Initiative to Increase the Number of Nurses Elected to Political Office

Sharon Pearce, DNP, CRNA
Kimberly Gordon, DNP, CRNA
Lisa Summers, DrPH, FACNM

Most nurses are aware that nursing is consistently rated as the most ethical profession in the United States. Did you know, however, that nurses are the only group the public trusts to reform the healthcare system? Despite that trust, the 4.3 million RNs in the United States are vastly underrepresented in elected office, comprising less than 3% of state legislators and less than 1% of federal legislators. Since the 1970s, the American Medical Association has trained more than 1,500 physicians and their spouses to run for elected office. There has never been a candidate training program for nurses—until now.

In 2016, Sharon Pearce, CRNA ran for the North Carolina state house of representatives; her colleague Kimberly Gordon, CRNA managed her campaign. Although Sharon's bid was unsuccessful, their experience piqued the interest of their advisor, Lisa Summers, when they entered the DNP program at Yale University's School of Nursing in 2018. Their DNP project focused on the problem of underrepresentation of nurses in elected office and how they could equip nurses with the skills and resources to become successful political candidates.

The project was developed with expert advice from political scientists; nurse legislators serving at the local, state, and federal levels; and campaign operatives who have practical experience in fields ranging from fundraising to digital strategy. The first-ever Candidate School for Nurses and Midwives was to be piloted in May 2020. The COVID-19 pandemic postponed its plans but did not dampen its enthusiasm.

We have created an initiative to help nurses understand and use their power to create change at the local, state, and national levels while creating a pipeline of nurses to run for elected office. See Figure 15.2 Healing Politics will

- raise awareness of the degree to which nurses are underrepresented in elected office, from school boards to Congress,

- highlight the characteristics of nurses that make them eminently qualified for elected office,
- inspire nurses to run for office up and down the ballot,
- identify nurses who will run and build a community of nurses to help them,
- provide nonpartisan training and support to help nurses who run *win*,
- promote a culture within the profession where we support our nurse colleagues who enter politics, and
- partner with researchers to add to what we know about nurses in elected office, including initiating and maintaining a database of nurses in elected office.

Reflecting the importance of interdisciplinary work, Healing Politics will be housed at Duke University's Polis: Center for Politics (polis.duke.edu).

Whether it's the need for bike paths, additional bus, and train routes (how many times does noncompliant really mean socially disadvantaged?) or affordable housing options, nurses see their communities through the eyes of their patients. Nurses already have the skills and expertise to develop better public policy. Your community and school board/city council/county commission/library board/state legislature need you!

Increasingly, nurses face real-world events either in person or through the news. Mass shootings, terrorism, disasters, military conflict, partisan divisions, economic issues, and changing technology require change and may result in personal insecurity. A lack of supplies ranging from basic medicine shortages to electricity add to uncertainty. The news itself is overwhelming, with technology immediately alerting us when a story breaks. Aside from dealing with these extreme conditions, it is also necessary to develop skills in sifting through and making sense of what you are experiencing and what you are hearing in the news.

Being able to discern legitimate sources of information and make informed opinions about the best policies is an important skill. The spread of "fake news" with inaccurate information has contributed to the uncertainty and impactful world consequences. The spread of "fake news" is believed to be exacerbated by individuals' overconfidence in the ability to recognize misleading information, with three out of four people overestimating their ability to distinguish between legitimate and false news headings; if people do not realize that news is misleading or incorrect, they may then be more likely to share it (Lyons et al., 2021). News challenged as fake, whether true or not , impacts how people interpret and respond to policy topics and elected representatives. Fake news is dangerous and can lead to conflicting information, which creates bias and a citizenship prone to political apathy and uncertainty. It can have unintended consequences (e.g., if citizens in the path of a hurricane were advised to ignore evacuation orders). Developing policy competencies enables nurses to become more discerning in evaluating legitimate sources of information.

It is not only leadership development that is important for health policy advocacy. Also important are paradigm shifts and a culture that creates expectations and rewards nurses for their active engagement in policy. The challenge for the future is for all nurses to recognize and embrace their roles and to support each other individually and in groups to move the policy agenda for the profession

Karen Daley, PhD, RN, FAAN

Wish I could say that was the end of my sharps injury prevention journey, as there was still much to be done. Despite enactment of the 2000 law, my advocacy has continued as have preventable injuries. As a result, I continue to engage around opportunities to improve sharps injury safety for healthcare workers.

In the years following Congressional passage of the federal legislation, I earned my PhD from Boston College Wm. F. Connell School of Nursing and was elected the 35th president of the ANA. My election as ANA president occurred shortly after the Affordable Care Act (ACA) was enacted and a few months prior to the release of the *Future of Nursing* report in the fall of 2010. Both safe patient care and safe work environments were ideals I was and to which I remain committed. Both are consistent with policy reforms and recommendations within the ACA and the *Future of Nursing* report. As ANA president, one of my roles was to educate the public and nurses about the benefits of such reforms, including improving access to safe, quality healthcare by assuring advanced practice RNs practice to the full scope of their license, enabling nurse-led innovative patient care models, and measuring outcomes to advance patient quality and safety.

In my role as ANA president, I was also able to expand my efforts to many other workplace issues. Some of these issues we were able to focus on programmatically through ANA included safe patient handling and mobility and safe staffing initiatives, as well as workplace bullying and preventing exposure to toxic chemotherapeutic agents.

As ANA president for 4 years, I was privileged to engage with nurses around the world on issues of concern to all of us as we care for patients. I learned more than I can share here. As was the case with every ANA president before and after me, I had hopes of "changing the world." On my journey, I did learn some valuable advice: *It's not always possible to get to the goal line—because the goal can be hard to reach—but it is always important to keep moving forward.* As a profession, it is critical that we work together to continue to move our goals and vision for better, more accessible healthcare forward.

Like with my advocacy around sharps safety, it is essential to progress forward. For those who seek legislative and regulatory solutions to issues, we know effective policy advocacy requires vigilance in surveillance and enforcement. It is every nurse's opportunity and ethical obligation to know their workplace rights under the law and to advocate for changes that will improve health and safety, not only for patients but also for those who provide the care.

and healthcare for all forward. Nurses occupy a place of trust. To build on that trust, we must advance our health policy and advocacy skills. It requires that we improve our ability to negotiate and compromise. Often, this can be accomplished by choosing words and planning action thoughtfully and with a purpose. As stated in Policy Challenge in Chapter 4, words matter. The sensitivity of language can make the difference in not only understanding the issue but also building relationships rather than creating divisions.

IMPLICATIONS FOR THE FUTURE

Continuing the march of nurses in policymaking will depend on the extent to which nurses are actively involved in policy. All nurses together need to vigorously monitor, refine, and develop healthcare policy at all levels. Nurses must capitalize on their long-standing status as the most trusted healthcare professionals and become the most trusted source for health policy and advocacy. Pioneering efforts will be needed to develop new competencies and skills for future health policy work given the increasing complexity of the world, the need for upstream approaches, and the importance of addressing the social determinants of health. With all the challenges and changes in healthcare now and into the future, nurses and nurses associations are called on to step up their policy engagement. It requires an openness to innovation, new ways of working, delivering care, and embracing technology to support that care including the policies that enhance progress. The public demands a response beyond passivity: "healthcare professionals need to get into the trenches of civic life for the long run, participating in community organizations and professional organizations to move public policy forward" (Hersh & Horn, 2020).

Nursing is at a moment of reckoning in taking on a leadership role in policy. The next frontiers for nurses to conquer include enhancing nurse well-being, expanding regulatory statutes affecting nurses (e.g., full practice authority, payment models, telehealth, environment); focusing on diversity, equity, and inclusion, (e.g., elimination of structural racism, increasing nursing workforce diversity); addressing the political determinants of health to improve the social determinants of health; using data to drive decision-making, and leveraging nurse participation at more policy tables. *Political determinants of health* refers to the upstream examination of the political dynamics (e.g., voting, laws, regulations, legal decisions, etc.) that then, in turn, influence social determinants of health (Dawes, 2020). For nurses to be in prominent policy frontiers, it requires hard work, commitment, collective action, education, and an understanding of the political determinants of health.

Consider the policy accomplishments of the nurses highlighted throughout the book. See Figures 15.3 and 15.4 and reflect on how the influence and status of nurses in healthcare policy have changed more than 50 years. While these accomplishments are laudable, they do not reflect the collective involvement of all nurses. The pace of progress for nurse involvement in policy needs to be accelerated. Imagine the progress that could be made in just the next 5 years if all 4.3 million nurses were mobilized at a higher level than they are now.

Leading the way in policy is an immersion experience in life that it is not easy; it is often messy and evolving. It requires vigilance in monitoring policies, not being silent and speaking up, and opening the windows of opportunity without

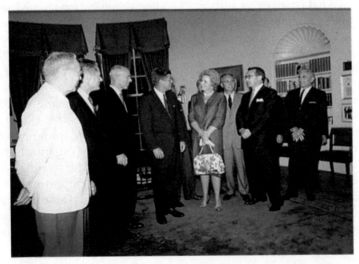

FIGURE 15.3 Early healthcare reform discussion in the Oval Office with President Kennedy and one nurse, ANA president Margaret Dolan.

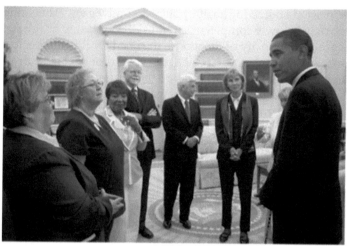

Photo Credit: ANA.

FIGURE 15.4 Fifty years later, President Obama in the Oval Office discussing healthcare reform with members of Congress, including nurse representatives Lois Capps, RN; Eddie Bernice Johnson, RN; and Carolyn McCarthy, RN; along with ANA president, Rebecca M. Patton and other ANA members.

waiting for an invitation. *Vigilance* means that at every juncture across sectors, nurses must be prepared to formulate, implement, monitor, and evaluate policies to advance global health and strengthen nurses' ability to provide safe, quality care. We know that being silent within an organization has repercussions for the safety and well-being of our patients (Henriksen & Dayton, 2006). Likewise, being silent within our society, our organizations, our associations, our community, and our government has repercussions for the advancement of our profession and the well-being of the patients entrusted to our care. Taking an active role in policy is every nurse's responsibility as a member of our profession. Opening the windows of opportunity means recognizing problems, taking advantage of the political landscape, and demonstrating political courage to achieve policy goals.

The Year of the Nurse and Midwife in 2020, and its extension through 2021, along with the critical role of nurses in the COVID-19 pandemic, brought attention to needed changes for nursing. Leading organizations issued seminal reports highlighting nursing as an integral player in health policy on the world stage. These include the Tri-Council for Nursing[1] report (Tri-Council for Nursing, 2021), *Transforming Together: Implications and Opportunities from the COVID-19 Pandemic for Nursing Education, Practice, and Regulation,* on opportunities for nursing education, practice, and regulation; the World Health Organization's (2021) *Health Workforce: Global Strategic Directions for Strengthening Nursing and Midwifery*; and the *Future of Nursing 2020–2030: Charting a Path to Achieve Health Equity* report (National Academy, 2021; see Chapter 14 for additional examples of reports). All these reports emphasize the critical role of healthcare organizations and professional associations in achieving the desired outcomes for healthcare. These initiatives require the commitment of individual nurses in supporting the work of these organizations. This support includes joining professional associations and actively engaging in its work, by providing time, talent, and treasure (human and financial capital) to leverage strength in numbers. The challenge in moving forward

---

[1] Alliance between the AACN, the ANA, the American Organization for Nursing Leadership (AONL), the National Council of State Boards of Nursing, and the National League for Nursing.

with the far-reaching recommendations in these reports is mobilizing the nation's 4.3 million nurses, nurses associations, and other key stakeholders in a collective effort to transform healthcare through policy.

KEY CONCEPTS

1. All nurses in all settings need to be actively engaged in policy to achieve important health goals.

2. Active involvement in professional associations is necessary to capitalize on the potential of more than 4 million nurses taking steps together to advance policy.

3. Nurses need to be the thought leaders in policy, speaking up and participating in the formulation of policy at policy tables.

4. Nurses' involvement in policy must include participation in professional associations, community, and consumer groups to leverage the power of collective action.

5. All nurse leaders have a dual role in being policy activists and creating the expectation and support for nurses to become policy activists.

6. Nurse educators, who must be prepared in policy, have a foundational role in the preparation of students by facilitating the examination of policy issues across the curriculum and courses in policy.

7. Expectations for policy involvement should be incorporated into job descriptions and annual and promotion reviews as all nurses need to be involved in policy issues at work to enhance safety, quality, and work environments.

8. Ongoing vigilance in developing, monitoring, and evaluating policies is an important step in detecting policy failure.

9. The PZL Policy Assessment Framework can be used for assessing and tailoring one's activities to address policy goals.

10. Policy engagement requires efforts at the little-p and big-P levels and upstream and downstream strategies, as well as an HiAP approach, to address not only the social determinants of health but also the political determinants of health.

11. Change and uncertainty are omnipresent in professional practice, policy, and healthcare as vividly demonstrated during the COVID-19 pandemic.

12. Policy competencies include the ability to discern legitimate sources of information and effectively communicate credible and accurate information to stakeholders.

13. Policy work requires a spirit of innovation and the demonstration of political courage to achieve policy goals.

SUMMARY

The roles of nurses individually and collectively are basic to healthcare transformation and the necessary policy needed to achieve the Quadruple Aim of healthcare: enhancing patient experience, improving population health, reducing cost, and improving the work life of healthcare providers. It is indefensible for nurses to be told or to believe their only duty for care is direct service. Ethically, we are bound to be at the policy table. If not invited, we must knock loud and hard on the door and, when necessary, just walk in. The policy journey is never over. New structures and processes in education and work settings are needed to facilitate the development of policy competencies for all nurses. The gap between education and practice needs to be bridged for nurses to fully take action and expand policy horizons.

END-OF-CHAPTER RESOURCES

LEARNING ACTIVITIES

1. Develop a one-page resume that highlights your policy activities that can be used to accompany an application to serve on a state or national health policy committee.

2. Compare and contrast and undergraduate and graduate roles related to policy as outlined in the AACN essentials.

3. Develop a plan for two policy activities at any level that you can achieve within 6 months and then within 1 year. Identify the amount of effort it will take and your strategies for accomplishing the activities, as well as your rationale for selecting the activities.

4. Compare your progress in policy using the PZL Policy Assessment Framework since the beginning of the class. Critically analyze your participation in terms of personal growth and your contribution to an association, cause, or organization.

5. Explore a policy fellowship experience that matches your interests, background, and future goals.

6. Analyze a failed workplace policy with rationale for subsequent recommendations for action.

7. Formulate talking points for use with nurse colleagues who, when learning that you are enrolled in a health policy class, complain that they hate politics.

8. Identify two areas of uncertainty in healthcare that can serve as springboards for policy-change opportunities. Provide rationales for your selections.

9. Examine how a clinical problem in your setting is influenced by the social determinants of health and the political determinants of health.

E-RESOURCES

- American Association of Colleges of Nursing https://www.aacnnursing.org
- American Association of Nurse Anesthesiology https://www.aana.com
- American Association of Nurse Practitioners https://www.aanp.org
- American Nurses Association https://www.nursingworld.org
- American Nurses Association, Healthy Work Environment https://www.nursingworld.org/practice-policy/work-environment
- American Organization for Nursing Leadership https://www.aonl.org
- Barton Associates: Scope of Practice Laws: Interactive Nurse Practitioner (NP) Scope of Practice Law Guide http://www.bartonassociates.com/nurse-practitioners/nurse-practitioner-scope-of-practice-laws
- Duke University's Polis: Center for Politics https://polis.duke.edu
- Future of Nursing Campaign for Action at the Center to Champion Nursing in America https://campaignforaction.org
- National Association of Community Health Centers: Jessica's Story: Illustrating the Political Determinants of Health https://www.nachc.org/jessicas-story-illustrating-the-political-determinants-of-health/

- National Association of Clinical Nurse Specialists https://www.nacns.org
- National Council of State Boards of Nursing https://www.ncsbn.org
- National League for Nursing https://www.nln.org
- National Student Nurses Association https://www.nsna.org
- Nurses on Boards Coalition https://www.nursesonboardscoalition.org
- The Nursing Community https://www.thenursingcommunity.org
- Tri-Council for Nursing https://tricouncilfornursing.org

REFERENCES

Abraham, C. M., Zheng, K., Norful, A. A., Ghaffari, A., Liu, J., & Poghosyan, L. (2021). Primary care practice environment and burnout among nurse practitioners. *JNP: The Journal for Nurse Practitioners, 17*(2), 157–162. https://doi.org/10.1016/j.nurpra.2020.11.009

Agency for Healthcare Research and Quality. (2019, September 7). *High reliability*. PSNet Patient Safety Network. https://psnet.ahrq.gov/primer/high-reliability

American Association of Colleges of Nursing. (2021). *The essentials: Core competencies for professional nursing education*. https://www.aacnnursing.org/Portals/42/AcademicNursing/pdf/Essentials-2021.pdf

American Nurses Association. (n.d.). *Healthy work environment*. https://www.nursingworld.org/practice-policy/work-environment.

American Nurses Association. (1965). *A position paper*. Author.

American Nurses Association. (2021). *Nursing: Scope and standards of practice* (4th edition). Author.

American Nurses Association. (2013, December 12). *Title "nurse" protection*. https://www.nursingworld.org/practice-policy/advocacy/state/title-nurse-protection/

American Nurses Association. (2015). *Code of ethics for nurses with interpretive statements*.

American Nurses Association & Centers for Disease Control and Prevention. (2017). *Redefining the antibiotic stewardship team: Recommendations from the American Nurses Association/Centers for Disease Control and Prevention Workgroup on the role of registered nurses in hospital antibiotic stewardship practices*. https://www.cdc.gov/antibiotic-use/healthcare/pdfs/ANA-CDC-whitepaper.pdf

Bell, S. K., Roche, S. D., Mueller, A, Dent, E., O'Reilly, K. Sarnoff Lee, B., Sands, K., Talmor, D., & Brown, S. M. (2018). Speaking up about care concerns in the ICU: Patient and family experiences, attitudes and perceived barriers. *BMJ Quality and Safety, 27*(11), 928–936. https://doi.org/10.1136/bmjqs-2017-007525

Benton, D. (2012). Advocating globally to shape policy and strengthen nursing's influence. *OJIN: Online Journal of Issues in Nursing, 17*(1), 5. https://doi.org/10.3912/OJIN.Vol17No01Man05

Bodenheimer, T., & Sinsky, C. (2014). From Triple to Quadruple Aim: Care of the patient requires care of the provider. *Annals of Family Medicine, 12*(6), 573–576. https://doi.org/10.1370/afm.1713

Boyd, D., & Poghosyan, L. (2017). Measuring registered nurse anesthetist organizational climate: Instrument adaptation. *Journal of Nursing Measurement, 25*(2), 224–237. https://doi.org/10.1891/1061-3749.25.2.224

Broussard, B. B. (2011). The bucket list: A service-learning approach to community engagement to enhance community health nursing clinical learning. *Journal of Nursing Education, 50*(1), 40–43. https://doi.org/10.3928/01484834-20100930-07

Byrd, M. E., Costello, J., Gremel, K., Schwager, J., Blanchette, L., & Malloy T. E. (2012). Political astuteness of baccalaureate nursing students following an active learning experience in health policy. *Public Health Nursing, 29*(5), 433–443. https://doi.org/10.1111/j.1525-1446.2012.01032.x

Centers for Disease Control and Prevention. (2019). *The one and only campaign*. https://www.cdc.gov/injectionsafety/1anonly.html

Condon, B. (2015). Politically charged issues in nursing's teaching-learning environments. *Nursing Science Quarterly, 28*(2), 115–120. https://doi.org/10.1177/08943184155716

Davidson, J. E., Marshall, M. F., & Watanabe, J. H. (2020). Policy impact: When policy fails. *Nursing Forum, 55*(1), 37–44. https://doi.org/10.1111/nuf.12380

Dawes, D. E. (2020). *The political determinants of health*. Johns Hopkins University Press.

Dolansky, M. A., & Moore, S. M. (2013). Quality and Safety Education for Nurses (QSEN): The key is systems thinking. *OJIN: The Online Journal of Issues in Nursing, 18*(3), 1. https://doi.org/10.3912/OJIN.Vol18No03Man01

Ellenbecker, C. H., Fawcett, J., Jones, E. J., Mahoney, D., Rowlands, B., & Waddell, A. (2017). A staged approach to educating nurses in health policy. *Policy, Politics and Nursing Practice, 18*(1), 44–56. https://doi.org/10.1177/1527154417709254

Fletcher, J., Sorrell, J., & Silva, M. (1998). Whistleblowing as a failure of organizational ethics. *OJIN: Online Journal of Issues in Nursing, 3*(3), 3. https://ojin.nursingworld.org/MainMenuCategories/ANAMarketplace/ANAPeriodicals/OJIN/

Henriksen, K., & Dayton, E. (2006). Organizational silence and hidden threats to patient safety. *Health Services Research, 41*(4 Pt. 2), 1539–1554. https://doi.org/10.1111/j.1475-6773.2006.00564.x

Hersh, E., & Horn, D. (2020, September 11). Health care workers need to engage on politics. It's the only way to fix mounting problems. *USA Today*. https://www.usatoday.com/story/opinion/2020/09/11/covid-politics-health-care-workers-must-vote-to-get-change-column/5758672002/

Hudson, B., Hunter, D., & Peckham, S. (2019). Policy failure and the policy-implementation gap: Can policy support programs help? *Policy Design and Practice, 2*(1), 1–14. https://doi.org/10.1080/25741292.2018.1540378

Institute of Medicine. (2011). *The future of nursing: Leading change, advancing health*. National Academies Press.

Institute of Medicine. (2003). *Health professions education: A bridge to quality*. The National Academies Press. https://doi.org/10.17226/10681

Institute of Medicine. (2004). *Keeping patients safe: Transforming the work environment of nurses*. The National Academies Press. https://doi.org/10.17226/10851

Jones, L. K., & O'Connor, S. J. (2016). The use of red rules in patient safety culture. *Universal Journal of Management, 4*(3), 130–139. https://doi.org/10.13189/ujm.2016.040306

Kunavikitul, W. (2014). Moving towards the greater involvement of nurses in policy development. *International Nursing Review, 61*(1), 1–2. https://doi.org/10.1111/inr.12092

Lake, E. T., Sanders, J., Duan, R., Riman, K. A., Schoenauer, K. M., & Chen, Y. (2019). A meta-analysis of the associations between the nurse work environment in hospitals and 4 sets of outcomes. *Medical Care, 57*(5), 353–361. https://doi.org/10.1097/MLR.0000000000001109

Leary, E., & Diers, D. (2013). The silence of the unblown whistle: The Nevada hepatitis C public health crisis. *Yale Journal of Biology and Medicine, 86*(1), 79–87. https://www.ncbi.nlm.nih.gov/pubmed/23483090

Lyons, B. A., Montgomery, J. M., Guess, A. M., Nyhan, B., & Reifler, J. (2021). Overconfidence in news judgments is associated with false news susceptibility. *Proceedings of the National Academy of Sciences, 118*(23), e2019527118; https://doi.org/10.1073/pnas.2019527118

Makary, M. A., & Daniel, M. (2016). Medical error—the third leading cause of death in the US. *BMJ, 353*, i2139. https://doi.org/101136/bmj.i2139

McConnell, A. (2015). What is policy failure? A primer to help navigate the maze. *Public Policy and Administration, 30*(3-4), https://doi.org/10.1177/0952076714565416

National Academy of Sciences, Engineering, and Medicine. (2021). *The future of nursing 2020–2030: Charting a path to achieve health equity.* National Academies Press. https://doi.org/10.17226.25982.

National Student Nurses Association. (n.d.). *Leadership.* https://www.nsna.org/leadership-university.html

O'Brien-Larivée, C. (2011). A service-learning experience to teach baccalaureate nursing students about health policy. *Journal of Nursing Education, 50*(6), 332–336. https://doi.org/10.3928/01484834-20110317-02

O'Rourke, N. C., Crawford, S. L., Morris, N. S., & Pulcini, J. (2017). Political efficacy and participation of nurse practitioners. *Policy, Politics, and Nursing Practice, 18*(3), 135–148. https://doi.org/10.1177/1527154417728514

Perry, C., & Emory, J. (2017). Advocacy through education. *Policy, Politics and Nursing Practice, 18*(3), 158–165. https://doi.org/10.1177/1527154417734382

Porter-O'Grady, T., Malloch, K., & Johnson, I. (2019). Changing organizations, institutions, and government. In R. Patton, M. Zalon, & R. Ludwick (Eds.), *Nurses making policy from bedside to boardroom* (2nd ed., pp. 225–260). Springer, American Nurses Association.

Primomo, J. (2007). Changes in political astuteness after a health systems and policy course. *Nurse Educator, 32*(6), 260–264. https://doi.org/10.1097/01.NNE.0000299480.54506.44

Rasheed, S. P., Younas, A., & Mehdi, F. (2020). Challenges, extent of involvement, and the impact of nurses' involvement in politics and policy making in in last two decades: An integrative review. *Journal of Nursing Scholarship 52*(4), 446–455. https://doi.org/10.1111/jnu.12567

Richtermeyer, S. B. (2010, February 8). Top 5 reasons why strategic initiatives fail. *Industry Week, 1,* 1. https://www.industryweek.com/leadership/change-management/article/21959964/top-five-reasons-why-strategic-initiatives-fail

Scott, W. G. (2004). Public policy failure in health care. *The American Academy of Business Journal, 5*(1/2), 88–94. http://www.journalbrc.com/journal.htm

Shin, S., Park, J. H., & Bae, S. H. (2018). Nurse staffing and nurse outcomes: A systematic review and meta-analysis. *Nursing Outlook, 66*(3), 273–282. https://doi.org/10.1016/j.outlook.2017.12.002

Staebler, S., Campbell, J., Cornelius, P., Fallin-Bennett, A., Fry-Bowers, E., Kung, Y. M., LeFevers, D., & Miller, J. (2017). Policy and political advocacy: Comparison study of nursing faculty to determine current practices, perceptions and barriers to teaching health policy. *Journal of Professional Nursing, 33*(5), 350–355. https://doi.org/10.1016/j.profnurs.2017.04.001

Thumm, E. B., Shaffer, J., & Meek, P. (2020). Development and initial psychometric testing of the Midwifery Practice Climate Scale - Part 2. *Journal of Midwifery and Women's Health, 65*(5), 651–659. https://doi.org/10.1111/jmwh.13160

Thurby-Hay, L., Whitehead, P., & Nelson, K. (2020). A statewide survey of clinical nurse specialist practice: Opportunities and challenges. *Clinical Nurse Specialist, 34*(6), 290–294. https://doi.org/10.1097/NUR.0000000000000559

Tri-Council for Nursing. (2021, May 6). *Transforming together: Implications and opportunities from the COVID-19 pandemic for nursing education, practice, and regulation.* https://tricouncilfornursing.org/publications

Ulit, M. J., Eriksen, M., Warrier, S., Cardenas-Lopez, K., Cenzon, D., Leon, E., & Miller, J. A. (2020). Role of the clinical nurse specialist in supporting a healthy work environment. *AACN Advanced Critical Care, 31*(1), 80–85. https://doi.org/10.4037/aacnacc2020968

Waddell, A., Audette, K., DeLong, A., & Brostoff, M. (2016). A hospital-based interdisciplinary model for increasing nurses' engagement in legislative advocacy. *Policy, Politics, and Nursing Practice, 17*(1), 15–23. https://doi.org/10.1177/1527154416630638

World Health Organization. (2021). *Health workforce: Global strategic directions for nursing and midwifery* (Report by the Director-General. Seventy-Fourth World Assembly Provisional Agenda Item 15). https://apps.who.int/gb/ebwha/pdf_files/WHA74/A74_13-en.pdf

Index